critical care nursing

CONTRIBUTING AUTHORS

Allen C. Alfrey, M.D.
Associate Professor
University of Colorado School of Medicine

John H. Altshuler, M.D.
Assistant Clinical Professor of Medicine
(Hematology and Pathology) University of
Colorado School of Medicine

Margaret Ann Berry, R.N., M.A., M.S.
Physiologist
Heritage High School
Littleton, Colorado
Formerly with University of Colorado School
of Nursing

Anne T. Bobal, R.N., B.S.
Clinical Specialist
Hemodialysis Unit
Veterans Administration Hospital
Denver, Colorado

H. L. Brammell, M.D.
Project Director, RT-10
Associate Professor of Medicine and Physical
Medicine and Rehabilitation
University of Colorado Medical Center

**Patricia K. Brannin, R.N., M.S.N.,
A.A.R.T.**
Pulmonary Nurse Clinician
Adult Nurse Practitioner
Clinical Instructor
University of Colorado School of Nursing
Denver, Colorado

Joseph O. Broughton, M.D.
Clinical Instructor in Medicine
University of Colorado School of Medicine
Medical Director, Inhalation Therapy
Department
Mercy Hospital
Denver, Colorado

Helen C. Busby, R.N.
Critical Care Practitioner
Head Nurse, ICU
West Nebraska General Hospital
Scotts Bluff, Nebraska

Donald E. Butkus, M.D.
Chief of Nephrology Service
Walter Reed Army Medical Center
Washington, D.C.

Corinne A. Cloughen, R.N.
Neuro Trauma ICU/CCU
Swedish Medical Center
Englewood, Colorado

Lane D. Craddock, M.D.
Associate Clinical Professor of Medicine
University of Colorado School of Medicine
Director, Cardiopulmonary Department
General Rose Memorial Hospital
Denver, Colorado

Alva R. Degner, R.N.
Assistant Director of Nursing
Former Head Nurse, CCU/ICU
Aurora Community Hospital
Aurora, Colorado

Karen Busch Driver, R.N., M.S.
Associate Professor
Louisiana State University
New Orleans, Louisiana

Velarie Richard Frusha, R.N., B.S.
Graduate Student
Louisiana State University School of Nursing
New Orleans, Louisiana

Robert W. Hendee, Jr., M.D.
Assistant Clinical Professor of Neurosurgery
University of Colorado School of Medicine

Shirley J. Hoffman, R.N., B.S.
Cardiac Clinical Specialist
Denver, Colorado

Carole K. Johnson, M.A.T., C.C.C. – Sp.
Speech Pathologist
Craig Hospital
Englewood, Colorado

Cynthia Johnson, M.A., C.C.C. – Sp.
Speech Pathologist
Craig Hospital
Englewood, Colorado

Janet Kerkman, R.N., A.R.I.T., E.M.T.
Critical Care Practitioner
Consultant and Educator
Professional Medical Consultants
Denver, Colorado

Margaret Kersenbrock, R.N., B.S.N.
Director of Nursing Service
Rocky Mountain Regional Spinal Injury
Treatment Center
Craig Hospital
Englewood, Colorado

Mary Susan Kudla, R.N., M.S.
Clinical Specialist
Emergency Department
Denver General Hospital
Denver, Colorado

Barbara Lockwood, R.N., M.S.
Manager, Critical Care Services
Formerly, Supervisor of Flights
Flight Nurse and Critical Care Practitioner
St. Anthony Hospital System
Denver, Colorado

Cary Lou Martinson, R.N., B.S.N.
Assistant Head Nurse
Neuro Trauma Unit
Swedish Medical Center
Englewood, Colorado

M. Lynn McCracken, R.N., M.S.
Director of Patient Care
Swedish Medical Center
Englewood, Colorado

Naomi D. Medearis, B.S., M.A., M.B.A.
Educational Consultant and Vice President
Associates for Continuing Education, Inc.
Denver, Colorado

Joan Mersch, R.N., M.S.
Clinical Nursing Coordinator, CCU
Stanford Medical Center
Palo Alto, California

Marilynn Mitchell, R.N., B.S.N.
Head Nurse, Neuro ICU
Denver General Hospital
Denver, Colorado

Virginia S. Paulson
Executive Director
Colorado Nurses' Association

Ann Marie Powers, R.N., B.S.N.
Graduate Student
University of Connecticut School of Nursing
Storrs, Connecticut

Karen Choate Robbins, R.N., B.S.N.
Clinical Specialist
Renal Transplantation
Hartford Hospital
Hartford, Connecticut

Janice S. Smith, R.N., M.S.
Instructor in Nursing
Community College of Denver, North
Denver, Colorado

Rae Nadine Smith, R.N., M.S.
Clinical Nursing Specialist
Gould Inc., Statham Instruments Division
Oxnard, California

Marilynn J. Washburn, R.N., B.S.N.
Neuro Trauma Unit
Swedish Medical Center
Englewood, Colorado

Phillip S. Wolf, M.D.
Associate Clinical Professor of Medicine
University of Colorado
Director, Coronary Care Unit
General Rose Memorial Hospital
Denver, Colorado

critical care nursing

SECOND EDITION

Carolyn M. Hudak, R.N., M.S.
Associate Professor of Nursing
Assistant Professor of Medicine
Adult Nurse Practitioner
University of Colorado Medical Center
Denver, Colorado

Thelma "Skip" Lohr, R.N., M.S.
Manager, Patient Care Services, Education
St. Anthony Hospital Systems
Nursing Consultant, Educator
Associate Director, Psychodrama, Sociometry, Sociatry
Denver, Colorado

Barbara M. Gallo, R.N., M.S.
Project Director, COPD Program
Visiting Nurse Association of Hartford, Inc.
St. Francis Hospital
Hartford County Lung Association
Hartford, Connecticut

J. B. Lippincott Company
Philadelphia
New York   San Jose   Toronto

Distributed in Great Britain by
Blackwell Scientific Publications
London   Oxford   Edinburgh

ISBN 0-397-54207-0

Library of Congress Catalog Card Number 77-23009

Printed in the United States of America

  2 3 4 5 6 7 8 9

Library of Congress Cataloging in Publication Data
Main entry under title:

Critical care nursing.

  Includes bibliographies and index.
  1. Intensive care nursing.   I. Hudak, Carolyn M.
II. Lohr, Thelma.   III. Gallo, Barbara M.
RT120.I5C74   610.73'6   77-23009
ISBN 0-397-54207-0

To those nurses who feel and
respond to the challenge of
caring for the critically ill

and

To Mom who has her own very special talents,
Carolyn

To my family of friends,
Skip

To my son, Brian,
Bobbie

contents

preface to the second edition

During the past few years, our lives have taken each of us into new areas of nursing. Working more directly with the nurse who is experiencing an expansion of her role, we found that new technologies have produced new knowledge. This new knowledge has necessitated new practices of care which demand increased problem solving of the nurse for now there is an even wider range of information from which to make decisions.

The response to the first edition of this book confirmed our belief that nurses are indeed eager for sophisticated material which helps prepare them for their very important role in health care delivery. Our initial prediction that certain expanded role functions would soon become the expected level of practice for all nurses is materializing. Our current premise holds that this role evolution will continue, particularly for the critical care nurse practitioner, and will involve the incorporation of more highly technical and intellectual skills to match the increasing responsibilities in the patient care arena. This second edition is based on that premise.

To this end, major portions of the book have been revised and updated. The core body systems have not only been revised and updated but extensively expanded. The respiratory section now contains broader coverage of pathologies commonly encountered in the critical care setting, along with appropriate assessment and aggressive management modalities for the nurse. In the cardiovascular section, the material on arrhythmias has been updated, expanded and new rhythm strips incorporated. A section on hemodynamic pressure monitoring techniques has been added which will assist the nurse in increasing the ability to utilize this parameter in patient care. The chapter on transplantation included in the renal section should provide extremely useful information on a procedure which is now becoming fairly commonplace. The neurological section has been extensively revised. We have added a section on spinal cord injuries which includes some revolutionary ideas on rehabilitative care that should begin while the patient is in the critical care unit. Additionally, information on invasive intercranial monitoring techniques has been added.

The section on specific crisis situations now includes material on a number of common problems and management techniques including GI bleeding, hyperalimentation, hepatic failure, burns, and disseminated intravascular coagulation.

It is well known that when individuals are in crisis, other key persons, such as family and staff, become involved in the dynamics of that crisis through a series of successive relationships. Recognizing this process, we have included a chapter dealing with families in crisis and with the occupational stresses on the critical care nurse.

As educators, we like to see content flow in a rational sequence. Being practitioners and learners as well, we are aware that real world situations often do not present in this fashion. Thus, the book is built on realities, and its approach moves from crisis to the understanding that underlies the critical care process. As in the first book, this edition maintains a holistic approach through the interrelatedness of the body systems. Its purpose remains to assist the critical care nurse practitioner to acquire the knowledge base necessary to carry out the responsible role of patient guardian and advocate.

Our sincere appreciation is expressed to the contributing authors who have shared their expertise with you. It is especially gratifying to pull together a book which represents the efforts of many who are not only colleagues, but also special friends.

We wish to thank Dana Morse, Suzanne Flake, Sharon Swanson and Beverly Johnson who typed major portions of the manuscript for us.

As in the first edition, David T. Miller of J.B. Lippincott has continued to give us valued counsel and support, and we continue to appreciate his special talents.

Carolyn M. Hudak
Thelma L. Lohr
Barbara M. Gallo

preface to the first edition

The idea and materials for this book have evolved from four years experience with intensive care nursing content for the practicing nurse. Through the Continuing Education Department of the University of Colorado School of Nursing, we have conducted a five-week, ongoing course, "Intensive Care Nursing—A Core Program" for registered nurses. Our approach has been a holistic one based on the interrelatedness of the four major body systems—respiratory, cardiovascular, renal, and nervous—with man's hierarchy of needs as a framework. Continuous use of evaluation tools has helped to identify the strong points of the content and that which needed revision. This has led to the design and content appearing in this book.

The intent in the preparation of this work was to focus on the rational bases underlying medical and nursing intervention. We support the premise that in the illness state, when the patient can no longer effectively control his own environment and requires assistance from an outside source, the nurse is the appropriate health team member to assume the role of patient negotiator. This role will be especially challenging in the critical care setting where the patient's internal and external environment is in a constant state of change. In order to accept this challenge, the nurse's practice must be geared to predicting and anticipating possible events in a patient's clinical course based on understanding of the patient's underlying pathology. To this end we have moved from a review of normal system functioning to a more detailed coverage of pathophysiological, psychological, and social aspects of various illness states. The major emphasis is on the change from normal body functioning as a basis for therapeutic intervention. Laboratory data and its significance for the nurse as well as pharmacologic information are integrated throughout the text.

Some material in the book, such as the chapter on arrhythmias, is presented in work manual form to allow the reader to "digest" it at an individual pace and to provide an exercise for periodic review.

This book should be a major resource for the practicing nurse dealing with any patient in crisis, whether inside or outside the critical care unit. It will also be helpful to students who need a resource for increasing their understanding of a specific patient-care aspect, as well as to educators and those persons involved in inservice and continuing education programs related to crisis nursing.

We wish to express our appreciation for the assistance and involvement of the contributing authors and to those colleagues and past course participants who were a vital part of the Intensive Care Program and whose contributions are reflected throughout this work. We wish to acknowledge the expert assistance of Janet Kerkman, R.N., and Fern DeLouche, R.P.T., in preparing the material on the respiratory system. We are particularly grateful to our secretary, Mrs. Maxine Evertz, for her perseverance in typing the manuscript and keeping us "consistent," and to Miss Cindy DeCounter for her secretarial aid. To David Miller, Managing Editor, Nursing Department, J. B. Lippincott Company, a special thanks for his unique ability to provide encouragement and support.

Carolyn M. Hudak
Barbara M. Gallo
Thelma L. Lohr

introduction

(Thelma "Skip" Lohr)

Not so many years ago, there was one term to describe the care offered to seriously ill patients. The word was INTENSIVE. As units and services have become more sophisticated and specialized, many nursing groups have selected different words to convey what they mean and to differentiate themselves from other similar groups. Are you aware of how many descriptive terms we have in use? For example, "critical," "crisis," and "coronary" are descriptive of the person's condition; "emergency" and "intensive" are descriptive of the situation; while "dialysis" and "pulmonary" are more descriptive of some aspect within the environment. Then there are true mixtures of terms, like "neuro-intensive," "medical intensive," "surgical intensive," and "pediatric intensive."

The question "What is intensive care?" seemed to mean a variety of things to hospital personnel, depending upon the criteria they used to define it. Anticipating that at least one aspect of *care*, common to all, would surface, we were surprised to find that the common denominator everyone agreed upon was the *person* as a patient who is in crisis or who is critical and has the potential to be in crisis. Webster defines *intensive* as "highly concentrated . . . involving the use of large doses or substances having great therapeutic values." Perhaps the term *intensive* best describes the environment hospitals and units provide.

Crisis is defined as "an emotionally significant event or radical change of status in a person's life . . . an unstable state of affairs in which a decisive change is impending." And *critical* is defined as "exercising or involving careful judgment or judicious evaluation; discriminating, careful, exact . . . indispensable for the weathering, the solution, or the overcoming of a crisis . . . of doubtful issue: attended by risk or uncertainty." The terms *crisis* and *critical care* commonly have a close association. They are so frequently interchanged in nursing discussions that many do not recognize the differences, only the similarities. Although both of those terms broaden the activities of nursing to include more of the nurse's intellect and decision-making processes, the essence of the differences begins with the purpose.

	CRISIS CARE	CRITICAL CARE
PURPOSE	Life-saving.	Life-maintaining.
ORIENTATION	Treat the presenting crisis symptoms and stabilize.	Treat the first presenting symptoms and prevent a crisis.
FOCUS	On body systems in failure— to reverse the failure and/ or maintain the system.	On all body systems—to support those in trouble and to maintain those in health.
ASSESSMENT	Discriminating for presenting signs and symptoms.	Discriminating, exact, careful for subtle signs and symptoms before they become grossly presenting.
INTERVENTIONS	Continuous until life is stabilized for transportation to a unit, or until death occurs (hours).	Continuous with a wider range, until adaptation to a higher level of wellness is attained, or death occurs (days/weeks).

Even though our efforts are directed toward using terms which accurately portray the specific nursing care that we offer, the words in our language are *static* and thus cannot convey the *processes* that make up the care. The following chapters will verify this. So our words are limiting; the word CRITICAL still seems the most appropriate term for the ROLE nurses take and for the CARE nurses offer to patients who are critically ill (and who have the potential to be in crisis) in INTENSIVE care units.

new horizons in critical care nursing

MARGARET ANN BERRY, R.N., M.A., M.S.

1

fantasy?

The sun shone on the gleaming white edifice called *The Hospital.* The tele-recorder rang sharply in the receiving heliport and the teletype began its nervous chatter. The receiving room nurse walked over to read the message: "Caucasian, male; fifty-five years of age; shortness of breath; crushing chest pain; collapsed over desk; history of two previous similar attacks." She punched out the message on the electronic call board, indicating the estimated time of arrival.

When the sound of the helicopter blades increased to a deafening level, the nurse moved out to the landing pad. As the copter touched down, the doors in the fuselage opened and the life-support capsule was lowered into the waiting cradle car on the track. As soon as the nurse removed the sky hooks from the ends of the capsule, the helicopter lifted off with a pulsing roar. The nurse activated the electronic conveyor track and the capsule moved into the receiving room.

Once inside, the nurse quickly opened the capsule and took from the pocket the field-punched computer cards. As she passed the call board, she activated the call switches from The Learned Ones who would be concerned with #125-A-70-90056, the newly arrived case. While she awaited their arrival, she fed the cards into a computer and the information was instantaneously displayed on the video screen in all four corners of the receiving room and at the diagnosis console. Suddenly the doors marked "Biological, Psychological, and Sociological" burst open and The Learned Ones and their assistants quickly entered the room. Glancing furtively at the video printouts, each addressed his attention to the problems of #125-A-70-90056 which were in the area of his specialty. One by one they took their respective problem area in its minicapsule and left by way of the doors "Biological, Psychological, and Sociological." When all had left and only the capsule and clothing of #125-A-70-90056 remained at the diagnostic console, the nurse signaled for the sanitation specialist to prepare the room for the next arrival.

In white coveralls and armed with a collection of aerosols filled with various sanitizers, the specialist began to clean the life-support capsule, assisted by the receiving room attendant. The two chatted cheerfully as they did their work. After they had folded the clothing left inside the capsule they noticed an ethereal cloud inside the capsule. Selecting a stronger sanitizer, the specialist sprayed the cloud more thoroughly. Much to his dismay the cloud did not disappear. A second glance showed that the clothing was no longer neatly folded.

The specialist summoned the nurse from the receiving room office. She too tried without success to disperse the cloud and fold the clothes. Then she notified the offices of the director of nurses and the supervisors of biological, psychological, and sociological nursing problems. They arrived from the various areas, but they too were unsuccessful. The Learned Ones were recalled, but again all efforts met with failure. As the crowd of professionals stood pondering over the puzzling conditions inside the capsule, a small voice was heard:

"But what about me? I am MORE than the sum total of my parts!"

BARBARA LOCKWOOD, R.N., M.S.

2 2

new horizons: flight nursing

Persons experiencing a medical emergency have in the past had to await treatment until they arrived at a hospital or clinic. Now, what once was dreamed of in fantasy is a reality at St. Anthony Hospital Systems, Denver, Colorado.

Prior to October, 1972, the only "flight nurses" most people had heard of were Air Force officers. However, during the past several years, a number of people in Colorado and across the nation have come in contact with a hospital flight nurse from St. Anthony's "Flight For Life" program. This program came about because a small group of people were dedicated to the idea of delivering quality emergency care to the victim at the scene, no matter where the situation occurred.* Typically, nurses had very little to do with the planning of the program, even though the registered nurse was to play the vital role. As the primary care deliverer, the nurse developed into the focal point of the endeavor—the ultimate factor which determined its success or failure.

The most significant aspect of the "Flight For Life" program is that it is not primarily a transportation system. It is a system that responds to victims wherever they are and continues to care for them until they are placed in the care of a physician in a medical facility. This system delivers sophisticated

*The "Flight For Life" program would not have been possible without the continuous encouragement and support of the medical staff, the Administration, and the Board of Directors of St. Anthony Hospital Systems, and the Sisters of Saint Francis. Their innovative ideas and input were vital to the development of the nurse's role as it is today. Their willingness to support such a program and the participating nurses is truly unique.

medical equipment and a highly trained, well-educated nursing team. Symptomatic reversal of the crisis begins as soon as the team arrives at the scene. Once the victim is stabilized, (s)he is transported by helicopter or fixed-wing aircraft under the close supervision and care of the nursing team.

The need for rapid transportation and easy access to the scene, as well as the rugged terrain of the Rocky Mountains, made the helicopter the perfect vehicle for this service. As the service expanded, regulation fixed-wing aircraft were added to accommodate longer flights. The concept underlying the flight nurse program has been realized. Today the program transports 200 patients per month and continues to grow. The majority are local helicopter transports. Longer regulation aircraft flights have taken the nurses into 20 states, to both coasts of the country and to Costa Rica.

The purpose of this chapter is to explore the role of the flight nurse and to outline the qualifications that nurses assuming this role must possess. Background training and education, special knowledge and skill, personality characteristics and the personal commitment necessary to fill the role will be discussed. This exploration would be incomplete without a discussion of the mechanisms incorporated into the program for maintaining reliability and ensuring accountability of the nurse.

The flight nurse is a critical care nurse practitioner, skilled in intervening in emergency situations of all kinds. The ultimate aim, of course, is to get the patient to a hospital alive. She is well versed in all aspects of critical care and crisis intervention. Therefore, a generalist approach to nursing is an absolute necessity. The flight nurse is able to care for the cardiopulmonary arrest victim as well as for the patient with crushing trauma or the child with epiglottitis. The care she delivers is directed at the immediate crisis. *Longer term care* will be undertaken by others upon arrival at the hospital.

In order to meet the above expectations, a broad experience base is helpful. This gives the nurse basic knowledge that she can build upon so that she can develop, over several months, into an excellent flight nurse. Nurses of various professional backgrounds have become flight nurses. They have all worked several years in emergency rooms, intensive care units, and/or coronary care units. One requirement is experience with critically ill patients with both medical and surgical problems. Expertise in trauma makes it easier to assimilate all the new material the nurse is required to learn. Another desired experiential element is having worked with patients of all ages—newborn to aged.

Assimilating past clinical experiences and education into the skills and theoretical knowledge required for flight nursing is accomplished by several processes. The desired end result is to develop a critical care nurse practitioner, capable of assessing all emergencies, choosing the appropriate method of intervention, and reversing the crisis in unpredictable, unstable surroundings. In order to develop this expertise, the flight nurse undergoes an intensive, rigorous orientation period. Much of this orientation involves an "unlearning" process. She must learn to work outside of the more comfortable hospital surroundings, where equipment is stable and where there are many experienced people on whom to rely. The typical working environment of the flight nurse is ever changing. It may be a vibrating helicopter, a small fixed-wing airplane in turbulent weather, a bathroom floor, a garage, an interstate highway, the interior of an overturned vehicle, or a small rural hospital with very limited facilities. Her supplies and equipment must be portable and are packed away into a multitude of small cases. The people the flight nurse must rely on will probably have less expertise than she does. These people also change with the location of the crisis. Most likely those who are at the scene will be emergency medical technicians, firemen, paramedics, law enforcement agents, onlookers, and the family of the victim.

During the early phase an enormous amount of learning is still going on, both on and off the job. For example, each flight nurse must complete a nine-month critical care practitioner course offered at the hospital. The course is directed at preparing the nurse who will work in areas where sophisticated facilities are nonexistent and where physicians are not immediately available. It stresses a systems approach to illness and injury and a review of physiology, common and not-so-common emergencies and the appropriate interventions that a nurse may initiate in these situations. After the orientation process is completed, the nurse begins to fly on her own.

None of her education and training lies fallow. The flight nurse must have her entire knowledge base at her disposal at all times. There is no way to second guess what types of patients will be seen in an eight-hour shift. One rule everyone learns early is "always expect the worst." The chances of being unprepared are minimized by this philosophy.

While the knowledge base of the flight nurse has been described in general, a review of her specific areas of expertise gives a more complete picture of what makes her as effective as she is. A solid understanding of anatomy and physiology, as well as of anatomical abnormalities and pathophysiology, of all body systems is essential. In order to determine where a victim is bleeding internally one must know what organs lie under the injured exterior. For example, several crushed lower left ribs should alert the nurse to a possible splenic injury. Anticipation of this potential problem may save the victim's life. It is also extremely difficult to assess a distressed newborn if one has had no experience in caring for a normal infant.

The flight nurse must have a firm command of the care of the patient with respiratory embarrassment, whatever the cause. She must be able to recognize and clear an obstructed airway. The obstruction may be caused by emesis or blood, a foreign body, or trauma, and it may be of the upper or the lower airways. Once the nurse has cleared the airway, she must be sure that it remains open. This may simply involve positioning the victim on his or her side and applying frequent suctioning, or it may require intubating the patient and assisting ventilation with a hand ventilator (Ambu bag). The intubation procedure is taught by anesthesiologists in the calm controlled environment of the hospital. It is up to the flight nurse to become proficient enough to intubate in any circumstance. Most people do not collapse in "convenient" places. They are usually on the floor, requiring the nurse to intubate on her knees or stomach, or outside in the bright sunlight, where it is difficult to visualize with a laryngoscope's small bulb. (The latter problem can be solved by having a large person block the sunlight during the procedure.)

Regardless of where or under what circumstances intubation is done, the same principles apply. All the necessary equipment must be available. The procedure must be done quickly to reduce the risk of hypoxia. The intubator must be accurate, and must recognize immediately if the endotracheal tube is correctly positioned. Trauma must be kept to a minimum. These principles require the nurse intubating in untoward circumstances to possess the greatest expertise possible.

The most important aspect of intubation, however, is not performing the skill well, but knowing when and when not to intubate. It is difficult to maintain a tight seal on a face mask when bagging a patient and moving him or her from the scene to the helicopter, flying in high winds, and moving him or her from the helicopter to the hospital. When the patient requires constant ventilation and transport is difficult, intubation may be indicated prior to transport. The unconscious patient with emesis or bleeding into the oral cavity obviously needs intubation to maintain a patent airway. Swelling of the neck from burns or hematomas may warrant intubation as a prophylaxis against an occluded airway, particularly if the trip to the hospital is long. Regardless of the problems inherent to transporting the critical patient, some patients are better off if intubation is not attempted in the field. The child with epiglottitis may experience complete upper respiratory occlusion once the laryngoscope blade is placed in the mouth. Unless the nurse is prepared to do a tracheostomy, and she is not, the better plan is to support respiratory status as well as she can with a partially open airway and avoid intubation. To prevent the risk of injury to the spinal cord, patients who may have cervical spine fractures are not always intubated. A tracheostomy done at the hospital will be safer for such patients. Each patient is different, and whether or not the nurse intubates is dependent upon her judgment of the patient's condition, the time transport will take, and other factors such as weather conditions and mode of transportation. Flight nurses try to avoid intubating the patient in flight. Hitting an air pocket during the procedure may rid the patient of his front teeth, or worse. The nurse's skill, judgment and anticipation of problems which may occur in flight can save the patient from unnecessary complications or further injury.

In order to interpret placement of the endotracheal tube without the benefit of x-ray, the nurse has expertise in using auscultation to evaluate breath sounds. This skill is also useful for determining the extent of pulmonary congestion from chronic lung disease, pulmonary edema or fluid overload, and for recognizing pneumothorax and ruptured diaphragm. One obstacle frequently prevents the use of auscultation: noise. The helicopter and fixed-wing aircraft are very noisy. Even the atmosphere outside the aircraft may be so permeated with the sounds of traffic, extrication equipment, and the aircraft itself that the ears are rendered useless. The flight nurse learns to adapt other senses to make up for this loss. The senses of sight and touch become primary assessment tools. If the sides of the chest are not rising equally, there is probably a pneumothorax, or the endotracheal tube is in the right mainstem bronchus. A deviated trachea can alert the nurse immediately to a pneumothorax or hemopneumothorax. The nurse develops the ability to *feel* rales and rhonchi. The color of the patient's skin is observed closely for the slightest change which may indicate improvement or deterioration of respiratory status. Should the nurse discover a pneumothorax, she can needle the affected side of the chest with an angiocath to evacuate the trapped air.

Reversing acute problems of the respiratory system requires an in-depth understanding of oxygen transport problems. The nurse must know when to apply oxygen and how much is appropriate. Since Denver, Colorado, sits one mile above sea level, the amount of oxygen is less than that of sea level communities, and the residents' blood gas levels are different. Many people served by the "Flight For Life" program live in mountain communities at higher elevations. Colorado also has a large tourist trade, bringing people from all over the country. The flight nurse must be familiar with oxygen transport variances caused by altitude changes. The history taken from the patient or family should include place of residence. Many oxygen transport problems occur in people from sea level communities when they come to Colorado. Some chronic illnesses, like emphysema, are aggravated. The most common problem occurs on the ski slopes. The cold, in combination with relative hypoxia in individuals accustomed to a more heavily oxygen-laden atmosphere, frequently produces high altitude pulmonary edema. Hypoxia also causes high altitude psychosis. Each flight nurse cares for several of these victims each ski season. Problems peculiar to transporting the critically ill at high altitudes in unpressurized aircraft will be dealt with later in this chapter.

As would be expected, the flight nurse is also proficient in intervening in cardiac emergencies. Many patients with acute myocardial infarctions are treated every year. This requires that the nurse interpret electrocardiograms and treat life-threatening arrhythmias. The appropriate drugs (lidocaine, atropine, isoproterenol [Isuprel], sodium bicarbonate, adrenalin and morphine sulfate) are carried for these emergencies. A portable monitor-defibrillator is always on board the aircraft for the observation and treatment of these patients.

While the electrocardiogram is an important aspect of monitoring the acute infarct patient, the flight nurse cannot always rely on her equipment. Altitude plays tricks with portable medical equipment. Very few such machines work reliably above 10,000 feet. The rotor blade action of the helicopter and radio communications can also cause inaccurate readings. Because of these variables, the flight nurse learns to watch the patient. She rarely takes her eyes off the patient, or her fingers off the femoral pulse. Talking to the patient constantly, she explains the flight, outlines what will happen at the hospital, and monitors patient perceptions of what is happening minute by minute. Many people have expressed concern that transporting the victim of acute myocardial infarction by air is dangerous and anxiety-producing for the patient. Surprisingly, most of the awake patients do very well in flight. The close monitoring and one-to-one relationship with the nurse seem to comfort the patient and ease anxiety.

The flight nurse must also participate in many cardiopulmonary resuscitations. These may occur in small rural hospitals, in the aircraft, on the golf course, and in every other conceivable location. The cause may be ventricular fibrillation due to acute myocardial infarction, cerebral vascular accident, and poisoning, drowning, electrocution, or trauma. The victim may be an infant, a child, a teenager or an adult of any age. Most of the arrests are not witnessed by the flight nurse, for they have occurred before she arrives on the scene. When the flight nurse arrives, she follows the protocol outlined by the hospital for cardiopulmonary resuscitation. She becomes the team leader and assigns duties to paraprofessional personnel and/or persons on the scene; one fireman to do closed chest massage, one to bag the victim after she has intubated, and so on. She carries out the protocol where appropriate, starts intravenous fluids, and gives the appropriate drugs. When all that is feasible is done at the scene, she prepares for transport.

CPR is continued enroute to the hospital while the nurse receives and carries out instructions from the Emergency Room physician. Upon arrival at the hospital, she and the patient are met by the "Cor Zero" team who continue resuscitation efforts if indicated.

At the scene, the leadership abilities of the flight nurse can determine the outcome for the victim. If she can direct the people at the scene effectively, the chances of saving the victim increase. This requires all her knowledge and expertise, a calm approach and continual observation of the procedure. She must correct ineffective closed chest massage, teach at the spur of the moment, and coordinate every person's activity for the benefit of the patient. In a highly charged emotional atmosphere, this takes a great deal of patience and is not easily done. Experience helps the nurse turn an excited crowd of paraprofessionals and laypeople into a very effective life-support team.

Accidents are one of the foremost causes of death for all ages. The intervention of the flight nurse can significantly decrease morbidity and mortality caused by accidents. All aspects of traumatic injury are in the nurse's repertoire. Of primary importance to the well-being of the victim is an initial, thorough assessment from head to toe. All injuries are noted and treated when appropriate. In order to properly evaluate the patient's condition, the nurse must elicit as complete a history as possible. She must know how long ago the accident occurred, if there were witnesses, if the victim was moved, how much blood there was, whether or not seat belts were worn, and specific body areas which were bluntly injured. Many times, the victim is still trapped in the vehicle upon arrival of the nurse. This necessitates initiation of appropriate therapy prior to extrication. After climbing into the vehicle, she makes her assessment and establishes the airway, stops any visible bleeding, and begins replacing fluid for hypovolemic shock, if indicated. Earlier it was mentioned that the flight nurse's ears often become useless in the field. For this reason, blood pressures are difficult to obtain. One can still palpate to assess blood pressure, but this is extremely time consuming if the victim is bleeding to death. Most flight nurses rely more upon the rate and quality of peripheral and central pulses. Young adults can maintain their blood pressures until exsanguination occurs. A rapid thready pulse will indicate impending death much earlier than a change in blood pressure.

Only absolutely necessary procedures are done at the scene. Many victims of trauma will die if surgery is delayed. In such cases, the airway is opened, IVs are started, and large fractures are immobilized. This type of emergency requires the nurse to call on all her experience and best judgment. If a hospital can be reached within 10 minutes, fluid resuscitation can wait until nurse and patient are airborne. Longer flights require the nurse to do more for the victim at the scene, but she must work quickly and deftly while the patient is still bleeding. Air transportation of these victims expedites the trip; often the helicopter is used for this type of injured patient. Upon arrival at the hospital, the surgeon and surgical team take over.

Flight nurses also see a large number of victims with head and/or spinal cord injuries. Besides immobilization and transportation, a thorough assessment is extremely important. The condition of the patient—level of consciousness, degree of sensation, motor abilities, vital signs, and pupillary reaction—must continually be monitored. Any changes must be noted. When the patient arrives at the hospital, the physician will be better able to assess his or her neurological status if an accurate record has been kept. In order to care for the victim of neurotrauma more effectively, each flight nurse has received additional instruction at the regional center for neurotrauma in Denver. Nurses have learned to insert Gardner-Wells tongs to immobilize cervical fractures, apply traction, pad and utilize a portable Stryker frame. Instructions for this sophisticated therapy are received from a physician in Denver via telephone or radio.

Many medical emergencies in and around Denver require more than the expertise of the flight nurse. The most common of these are poison ingestions and poisonous bites. When these occur close to the hospital, the nurse treats the symptoms as indicated. Those emergencies occurring outside the Denver area require consultation with the Rocky Mountain Poison Control Center. A physician or a nurse from this team accompanies the flight nurse to the rural hospital requesting assistance. The flight nurse administers life support while the poison control personnel initiate therapy directed at reversing the effects of the particular poison. Utilization of the expertise of both teams simultaneously has proved extremely effective in decreasing morbidity and mortality in poison cases.

Two other types of emergencies call into play the participation of other experts available in the city. Care of the critical neonate requires constant input from neonatologists and personnel in neonatal intensive care nurseries in Denver. The flight nurse is taught to assess the neonate and to correct the common problems of these tiny patients: ventilation, circulation, temperature control and maintenance of adequate glucose levels. During transport, she receives specific instructions from a neonatologist in Denver, as she relays her assessment of the infant's condition and describes the infant's symptoms. The neonatal nurseries provide the clinical experience for the flight nurses; their personnel are the instructors.

Recently, the program has also begun to participate in the transportation of high-risk mothers to Denver hospitals specializing in their care. Medical personnel from these hospitals accompany the flight nurse on these flights. The team is always prepared not only to treat the mother, but to deliver a distressed infant. Adding this service has required further education of flight nurses so they can appropriately evaluate the high-risk mother, anticipate problems she may have, and intervene in any potential or realized emergency during transport. Many hospital critical care nurses are required to have a good deal of the above described knowledge base and expertise.

One area of expertise unique to the flight nurse is the ability to understand and apply the principles of aerospace medicine to the care of her patients. She also must be acutely aware of the effects altitude has on her performance. Most of the regulation aircraft used are pressurized; however, the helicopter, which is used in the majority of flights, is not. In order to gain access into many of the mountain communities serviced, altitudes of 15,000 feet are reached. Anytime the helicopter flies above 10,000 feet, oxygen masks must be worn by the pilot and the nurse. Without oxygen, hypoxia would adversely affect the nurse's judgment, impede her ability to care for the patient, and even cause unconsciousness. The nurse frequently works outside the helicopter at high elevations, such as on mountain rescues, or in Leadville, Colorado, which has an elevation of 10,000 feet. It is not practical to wear an oxygen mask under these circumstances, and, because she is not acclimatized to these elevations, she must conserve her strength and continually be aware of how the altitude is affecting her performance. Other factors affect the nurse's performance at high altitudes, such as whether or not she has eaten and the amount of sleep she has had. Flight nurses frequently work in excess of their eight-hour shifts and miss meals because of flights. If the nurse is tired and has a low blood sugar level, the effects of altitude-induced hypoxia will hinder performance more rapidly. All of these factors influence whether or not the nurse makes the right decision at the appropriate time.

Altitude affects the patient as well as the nurse. All patients are given oxygen if flying above 8,000 feet. The patient with an oxygen transport problem such as pulmonary edema, chronic lung disease, or flail chest has higher oxygen requirements. Hypovolemic patients also have higher oxygen requirements, because they have fewer red blood cells and less hemoglobin to carry oxygen to the tissues. Patients who have received medications which depress the respiratory system such as morphine and diazepam (Valium) require greater amounts of oxygen. The flight nurse closely observes each patient for any signs of hypoxia during these high-altitude flights and adjusts the level of inspired oxygen accordingly. Many patients become anxious when the nurse tries to apply oxygen, for they fear their condition has suddenly worsened. A brief explanation of the effects of altitude and the nurse's simultaneous use of oxygen usually allay the patient's fears.

Besides decreased oxygen supply, high altitudes are accompanied by an overall decrease in atmospheric pressure. This causes a number of problems for patients with specific injuries. Complications increase as altitude increases and decrease as altitude decreases. For example, increased intracranial pressure from a closed head injury rises higher as altitude increases. The patient may become stuporous and later obtunded. As altitude decreases, the level of consciousness improves. This phenomenon makes it very difficult to evaluate a closed head injury. Altitude may not be the only factor influencing the level of consciousness. The patient may truly be deteriorating independently of the effect of altitude.

Decreased atmospheric pressure also has adverse effects on open injuries. An enucleated eye may lose more vitreous humor as altitude increases. These patients should never be transported in unpressurized aircraft unless another injury will cause death before safer transportation can be arranged. Bleeding will also increase as altitude does. This may require more rapid fluid replacement at high altitudes. The nurse must take extra precautions not to overload the patient. Fluid replacement itself becomes a problem at altitudes in excess of 10,000 feet. Intravenous fluids do not run correctly. For this reason plastic IV bags are used. Blood pumps must be applied to the bags and the pressure adjusted to obtain the correct rate of flow. Edema also increases with decreased atmospheric pressure. Casts may have to be bivalved before transportation to prevent cutting off circulation to the limb.

Closed drainage systems cannot be used at high altitudes, because the fluid or air will not move from the body to the receptacle. Adequate drainage is obtained by venting all drainage systems to the air—Foley bags, nasogastric tubes, and so on. Decompression of the stomach may have to be assisted manually by the nurse. Normal chest tube drainage systems are replaced with a one-way valve apparatus to release air trapped in the pleural cavity. This is extremely important because pneumothoraxes extend as altitude increases.

The complications caused by decreased atmospheric pressure and decreased oxygen supply play a continual role in the flight nurse's decision-making processes. Both she and the patient are affected. Continual observation of the patient for any adverse signs and symptoms, plus awareness of her own response to the environment, is essential. Anticipating potential problems prepares the nurse to take corrective action when necessary. All knowledge of various illnesses and injuries is collated with an in-depth understanding of aerospace medicine.

Along with the foregoing, the nurse has a healthy respect for the potential hazards the aircraft she works on and around holds for her and her patients. She works within stated safety regulations enforced by the pilots and the Federal Aviation Association (FAA). Because she works outdoors much of the time, she must understand the influence of environment on the human body. Excessive temperatures, either hot or cold, will affect her performance as well as her patient's condition. She must be prepared to survive in the wilderness if something should go wrong with the aircraft. Survival training is part of flight nurse orientation, and a special survival kit is taken on every flight into the mountains.

It takes most nurses several months to learn the required material and skills and assimilate them into a framework within which they can perform. All the material must be readily available to the nurse, in order for her to assess the patient, arrive at a conclusion, appropriately intervene in the emergency, continue to monitor the patient, and respond to any changes. The ultimate goal is to deliver the patient to the hospital in better condition than (s)he was at the time of the crisis.

To realize this goal, the flight nurse must be able to concentrate on several areas at once. Knowledge and skill combined with the data obtained from various sources provide the basis for the split-second decisions the nurse needs to make. The importance of excellent observation skills cannot be over-emphasized. Any overlooked symptom, no matter how minor it appears, may change the outcome for the patient. Observation of the patient has always been one of nursing's primary responsibilities. Accurate observation, however, is much more difficult for the flight nurse, because of the working environment.

The flight nurse makes her assessment without the luxuries many nurses take for granted. There are no x-rays to confirm a fracture or check for endotracheal tube placement, no blood gas studies to confirm respiratory acidosis, no blood work to confirm electrolyte imbalance, hematocrit and hemoglobin levels, or serum glucose. It has been noted how useless the ears become when confronted with the high noise level at the scene and on board the aircraft. Performance of common procedures such as listening for breath sounds and measuring blood pressures is impossible. Monitoring equipment is also less reliable in the field than in the hospital. It is subject to interference, not only from the patient's movements, but also from the aircraft's vibration and radio communications. As stated earlier, equipment does not function properly above certain altitudes.

Few nurses consider working in well-lighted facilities a luxury. The flight nurse, however, will see at least half of her patients after dark. A flashlight may be the only source of light available. Once aboard the helicopter, the nurse cannot use bright lights, because the pilot would be blinded and unable to navigate. After several months, the flight nurse is able to note even skin color changes in the dark almost as well as she does in light.

Observing the patient is hindered not only by the absence of light, but also by the inability to examine the injured portions of the body. During the winter months, many patients' injuries are hidden under layers of bulky clothing. It is unwise to undress the patient in freezing temperatures. The nurse learns to feel for fractures and other injuries through the clothing. If she is in doubt, it is safer to immobilize a suspected fracture than to assume the limb is uninjured.

The flight nurse works around these obstacles to accurate observation of the patient. She assumes nothing and suspects the worst. To appropriately evaluate the patient requires the nurse's constant vigilance and the ability to substitute other senses when one is rendered inefficient. Most patients can save the nurse frustrating minutes by relating what is wrong. The patient's subjective appraisal of his or her body is extremely accurate. Nurses frequently forget this, but many times the patient can save his or her own life if someone is willing to listen. Flight nurses have learned patients who say they are going to die will do so with extreme rapidity if the crisis is not reversed.

Whether or not the crisis is reversed is the ultimate responsibility of the flight nurse. The survival of the patient is dependent on how well the nurse interprets her observations and on what measures she takes to stabilize the victim prior to transportation. No one wants to lose a patient in the air because something was left undone at the scene. Long-term survival also depends on what is done during transport. A misplaced endotracheal tube will doom the patient to certain anoxic brain death. A fracture which is not immobilized may cause the loss of a limb.

Physicians at Saint Anthony Hospital Systems have established protocols for the treatment of every imaginable emergency. These are not standing orders. Standing orders limit the nurse's judgment. Protocols allow the nurse room to incorporate knowledge, observation and assessment of the patient, and nursing judgment into treatment. Flight nurses do not make differential diagnoses. Rather they evaluate the symptoms presented and treat them accordingly. If the patient is bleeding, they try to stop the bleeding and replace fluid loss, and so on.

No two emergencies or patients are alike. In order to make the best decision and to reverse the crisis effectively, the nurse must call on prior knowledge, past experience, all observable data, including patient history, and all the common sense available to her, and then "tailor-make" a given protocol to meet the needs of the patient. An example of this decision-making process is the treatment of the patient with a flail chest. The protocol states that the method of stabilizing a flail chest is intubation with assisted mechanical ventilation. If the patient is comatose and has severe paradoxical respiration, the flight nurse would intubate and ventilate with a hand ventilator (bag resuscitator) until the patient could be placed on a mechanical ventilator at the hospital. However, this patient is wide awake, frightened and having moderate paradoxical respiration. Assume that the hospital is three minutes away by air. The nurse cannot intubate because the patient would resist frantically. The nurse has two choices: (1) wait until the patient becomes comatose or (2) administer large amounts of oxygen by nasal cannula and mask, splint the patient, if possible, and get to the hospital as fast as possible. The second choice is clearly the best for the patient. Once at the hospital, the physician can administer a paralytic respiratory drug, intubate, and place the patient on a mechanical ventilator. Should the patient lose consciousness in flight, the trip is very short, so (s)he can be ventilated with a bag and mask until landing at the hospital where (s)he can be intubated and supported properly.

Decisions made by the flight nurse are always countered by an element of risk. Each action taken may cause yet another complication. In the example above, the nurse is counting on the patient's remaining awake and cooperative during the flight. The nurse must have alternative actions prepared if her expectations are incorrect. She must also balance one alternative against another, sometimes choosing the one least likely to harm the patient. There are no easy formulas to follow. The nurse does whatever is necessary to intercede in the crisis within the scope of her abilities. Accountability is a word each flight nurse understands intimately. The patient's welfare is the nurse's responsibility. Each decision made must be justified and evaluated. The final analysis lies with the patient. The most difficult decision for the flight nurse to make is to decide to do nothing. Action may harm a patient more than watching and waiting. To accompany a patient screaming in pain is terrifying. It would be easier on the nurse to medicate the patient for pain. However, that very pain will help the physician to recognize and correct the problem. In mass casualty accidents or disasters, it is extremely difficult for the nurse to leave the dying victims in order to save others.

Decision making is vital to the flight nurse's role. If the nurse cannot mobilize others at the scene of the crisis to help carry out the decisions made, the effort is futile. The helicopter draws hundreds of onlookers everywhere it lands. The people who called for the flight nurse are anxious to help but generally are less skilled and less knowledgeable. Leadership by a calm, experienced, critical care practitioner will turn chaos into an environment conducive to the survival of the patient. Mastery of this kind of situation takes a very long time. It is the most difficult thing a flight nurse has to do and the hardest thing to learn.

A strong leader has to have excellent communication skills. The nurse must translate medical terminology into words the laypeople helping can understand. In order to direct patient care, the nurse must give orders that are clear and to the point. A good communicator also listens to witnesses to learn the history of the situation and the minute-by-minute changes they observed. Communication with the receiving hospital is vital to continuity of care. The nurse radios the condition of the patient to the hospital and receives orders from physicians, while the hospital prepares whatever is necessary for the patient. If the nurse communicates incorrectly, the hospital may not be prepared. For example, the patient has a thoracic-aortic aneurysm diagnosed by a physician in a small rural hospital. The nurse phones the receiving hospital and states the patient has an aortic aneurysm. Upon the patient's arrival, a general surgeon is ready to revise an abdominal-aortic aneurysm, but a chest surgeon must be called in, delaying the operation another 30 minutes. The only thing that will save this patient is surgery, which was delayed by the nurse's faulty communication.

Much has been written about the impact a crisis has on family members and loved ones. The flight nurse must deal with this daily, for many crises occur with loved ones present. When the helicopter and flight nurse arrive, families must stand by helplessly watching the painful, sometimes almost barbaric, process of saving their loved one's life. There is no place like a hospital waiting room for the family. There are no curtains to draw around the victim. Many people cannot bear to watch and leave voluntarily. Others stand fixed, unable to move from the spot. Some are victims with their own injuries asking what happened to their son or wife. Whatever the situation, the flight nurse tries to help the family cope with the crisis. Families who lose loved ones after heroic efforts have been made by the flight team are sometimes angry. Flight nurses frequently feel guilty when the family of a deceased victim receives a bill for services rendered. Many times, however, the family thanks the team. Their loved one died, but they know that had there been any chance of survival (s)he would have lived. They do not have to wonder, "Could something more have been done?"

Flight nursing is an expanded role for the registered nurse. She has skills and makes decisions that may never be required of other nurses. All nursing roles must build in a system of checks and balances to ensure optimum care and safety for the patient; this expanded role requires an even more elaborate system. For the nurse who works under little direct supervision, the process must provide for quality control, ensure that expertise of the nurse is maintained, evaluate success and/or failure, and provide a continuous learning situation for all.

An elaborate audit system provides those checks and balances necessary for the flight nurse role. This consists of peer review, supervisor review, and review by the medical director and any other physician he consults. Each flight record is audited daily by the nursing supervisor and medical director. The flight nurse may be called on at any time to justify what she did for any given patient. Statistics are also kept on each patient transport, breaking down what was done for the patient, diagnosis made by the receiving physician, and outcome for the patient. It would be impossible to evaluate the actions taken by the nurses without a thorough follow-up of the patients.

Perhaps the most important part of the audit system is the bimonthly flight nurse meeting. During these meetings, the nurses review flights together. They discuss the patient's history, the crisis which required the team, the assessment the nurse made, the problem-solving process used to decide on treatment, and patient outcome. These dialogues allow the nurses to explore and rehearse alternatives with their peers. The nurses learn from each other how they might approach a problem the next time they encounter it. More experienced nurses give helpful hints to those new to the program. The atmosphere is safe for openness, allowing the nurses to question and explore without ridicule. It takes a strong nursing leader to ensure that this atmosphere is maintained, and that each nurse is given the opportunity to learn and develop professionally.

The medical director also attends these meetings. Serving as a resource person, he answers questions, adds medical input to case reviews and provides the medical support necessary for the success of the flight nurse. The flight nurse meeting is also utilized to provide in-service education. The statistics, the patients, the medical director and the nurses themselves determine what subjects are to be reviewed and what new areas of knowledge need to be taught.

implications

The "Flight For Life" program is successful. It has provided a system which begins to reverse the crisis before the patient arrives at a hospital, and it continues to expand its service area. Expanding the role of the nurse to the role of the flight nurse has been instrumental in developing the program into what it is today. Without the expertise of the nurse, her commitment to her beliefs, her involvement with the community, and her willingness to work long hours in extreme environmental conditions, the program could not have been as successful.

The existence of "Flight For Life" has stimulated the community's ambulance companies, fire departments and even the state patrol to become aware that moving a patient to a hospital rapidly without treatment is not always compatible with life. People are now concentrating on stabilizing the patient prior to transportation. Many private ambulances, fire departments, and rescue squads call the helicopter when they realize that the patient is too critical for them to handle. With increasing community awareness, the "Flight For Life" program is utilized for the right patient at the right time. Emergency care at the scene has improved immensely in the Denver metropolitan area since the program has been in existence. Those patients who do not require the flight nurse's skills are getting better, more comprehensive care by paraprofessionals prior to hospital arrival than ever before.

Flight nursing is a NEW ROLE on the horizon. Only a few women and men have had the opportunity to experience it. Flight nurses have proved that a nurse can perform in areas only physicians worked in before. They have not become, as many feared, little doctors. Instead they have brought into the role all their past education and experience as nurses, and have become well-educated, highly skilled crisis/critical care practitioners. Each nurse is acutely aware of her limitations and her responsibilities. Within the framework of the role, the nurses are contributing to the well-being of the community. They are helping save lives by being the second link in the life support chain: (1) basic life support given by those first on the scene, (2) advanced life support given by the flight nurse, (3) definitive therapy administered by the physician and (4) maintenance of life support provided by intensive care nurses and other hospital personnel.

Many people have said, "Why use a registered nurse? An emergency medical technician or a paramedic could do the same thing." With this the author strongly disagrees. While skills can be taught to anyone, the commitment to use them judiciously and to maintain accountability to the patient cannot. The entire nursing educational process is directed at developing people who will be committed to the patient's welfare before anything else. It has been a relatively successful socialization process. The basic nursing material presented gives each nurse enough theoretical and experiential background to build on, to develop into any nursing role. No paraprofessional is as ready to take on the extra knowledge, new skills and formidable responsibility as is the professional nurse. The role, if held by anyone else, would cease to be a nursing role. Nurses DO make the DIFFERENCE.

holistic approach to critical care nursing

CAROLYN M. HUDAK, R.N., M.S.
THELMA L. LOHR, R.N., M.S.
BARBARA M. GALLO, R.N., M.S.

3

critical care nursing: what makes it special?

It is our contention that the essence of the concept of critical care nursing lies not in special environments or amid special equipment but rather in the decision-making process of the nurse and her willingness to act upon her decisions.

Critical care nurses have been pioneers in what professional circles are now calling the "expanded role." From the days of the 24-hour recovery room which substituted for the absence of an intensive care unit, nurses in these areas have had to look beyond just "taking vital signs." Before the term "critical care nursing" evolved, the critical care nurse was the one who could see beyond the patient's blood pressure, pulse, and respiration. She felt a pulse and noted its quality; she made a mental note of the temperature of the skin and its state of hydration; she compared the pulse rate with the temperature and blood pressure and asked "why?" if the anticipated correlation was not there. In short, she functioned according to her intellect. She anticipated events based on what she knew about normal physiology and her patient's condition, and if findings other than those she anticipated materialized, she asked herself "why?" and proceeded to gather additional clinical data to answer that question. If she did not answer the question, her response was based on intuition, "That patient just doesn't look good to me!" We believe that predictability based on intuition actually involved a response to clinical cues which nurses had not attempted to identify concretely. For example, the patient doesn't "look good" because:

  his respirations are more shallow;
  his color is duskier than previously;
  his eyes have an anxious stare;

he is more restless now;

he is perspiring.

The critical care nurse of today seeks the *rational base* for all her interpretations and actions.

What are the processes a nurse goes through to arrive at a decision which guides her intervention? A postoperative patient presents with a blood pressure of 88/60, pulse 100, respirations 28, and diaphoresis. How does the nurse arrive at a decision to medicate the patient for pain as opposed to alerting the physician that the patient may be hemorrhaging? What findings are there to support either premise? Does he complain of pain? Does he "splint" the area when he moves? Is his dressing wet? Is urine output diminished? Is there any evidence of bleeding into the incisional area? What is the pulse quality? Does the CVP lend any clues? Depending on her findings, the nurse may decide to medicate the patient for pain.

In turn, critical care nursing also involves evaluating the outcome of a given intervention and proceeding appropriately. For example, after medicating the postop patient described above the nurse will *anticipate* a given outcome. If the vital sign parameters noted above are due to pain, the nurse will anticipate a return to that patient's previous "normal" values if pain relief is achieved. If this anticipated outcome is not realized, she then asks "why?" and proceeds to gather additional data to answer that question. We believe that the essence of critical care nursing is to be found in that decision-making process, which is based on a sound understanding of physiological and psychological entities.

The expression of the decision is the art of nursing intervention which will produce a given clinical picture. This art of intervention requires the ability to deal with critical situations with a rapidity and precision not usually necessary in other health care settings. It requires adeptness at integrating information and establishing priorities, for when illness strikes one body system, other systems become involved in the effort of coping with the disequilibrium. The person admitted to an acute care unit usually receives excellent care for the affected body system, but problems in other systems are not recognized early, if at all. Critical illnesses will always endanger and involve the respiratory, cardiovascular, renal, and central nervous systems as well as the self-esteem of each person.

We believe the nurse needs to actively engage her mental image of the person and his body processes to gather all the data possible for the decision-making process. Therefore, the framework outlined in Fig. 3-1 is proposed as a basis for the study of persons with critical illnesses and of *critical care nursing.*

Individuals seek to preserve their lives by directing all their energies toward the most basic unmet needs. For example, all the compensatory mechanisms of a person with inadequate cardiac output will work to maintain the circulation of oxygen, thus meeting the most basic requirement for life. In this situation, energy is directed away from subsystems such as the gastrointestinal, skin, and kidney functions, creating a degree of physiological amputa-

Self-Preservation

The Nurse as the Negotiator

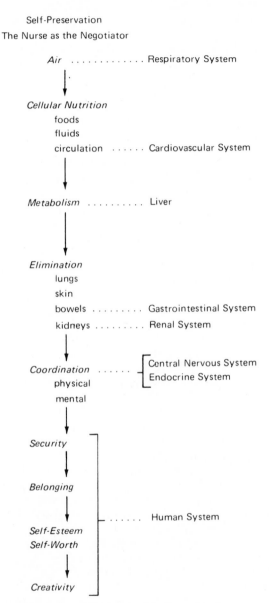

Air . . . . Respiratory System

Cellular Nutrition
    foods
    fluids
    circulation . . . . . . Cardiovascular System

Metabolism . . . . Liver

Elimination
    lungs
    skin
    bowels . . . . Gastrointestinal System
    kidneys . . . . Renal System

Coordination . . . . . . ⌈ Central Nervous System
    physical   ⌊ Endocrine System
    mental

Security

Belonging

    . . . . . . Human System

Self-Esteem
Self-Worth

Creativity

Fig. 3-1. Hierarchy of human needs for critical care nursing.

tion. The need for a sense of security to allay anxiety is always present, but it is not the most basic need at this time. Later, when needs for air, cellular nutrition, and elimination are met, the efforts of the individual are directed toward seeking security, a sense of belonging, and self-esteem. Although each of us has physiological and psychological mechanisms which compensate for disequilibrium, there are situations in which we cannot adapt without outside intervention. It is in these situations that the critical care nurse becomes the patient's advocate and fosters adaptation.

The individual's attempts to cope with the environment include avoidance, in which one flees from the situation; counteraction, in which body defenses try to destroy the stressor, often at the expense of other systems; and adaptation, in which one seeks to establish a compatible response to the stress and still retain a steady state. Although all mechanisms foster self-preservation, nursing intervention is aimed at adaptation. By fostering responses that encourage useful functioning both physiologically and emotionally, nurses enhance adaptation and aid the patient in conserving energy. On the other hand, when nursing intervention or lack of it does not foster adaptation, the patient's energy is wasted and a state of entropy exists; that is, the patient will have a diminished capacity to deal with a changing situation. Thus, entropy is increased when a patient's energy is devoted to maladaptive functioning which perpetuates the disequilibrium, and entropy is minimized when the patient expends energy which fosters adaptation to the disequilibrium. An example of maladaptation versus adaptation is seen in the patient with restrictive lung disease who develops a lung infection resulting in $\uparrow CO_2$ and $\downarrow O_2$. This patient cannot compensate because of his restrictive lung disease; thus his established pattern of breathing is maladaptive, perpetuating the problem of gas exchange. On the other hand, adaptive nursing intervention involves helping the patient to breathe more deeply and to foster the drainage of secretion either by having him do breathing exercises or by use of mechanical aids. Although the energy is still expended, it is expended usefully. This concept of minimizing entropy is consistent with the ultimate goal of health care—to restore the person to a steady state with minimal stress to the rest of the body.

Because of the degree of patient contact, critical care nurses have more influence than other health care personnel in either fostering adaptation or encouraging entropy. That influence may be a burden as well as a challenge. It does not however negate the responsibility of other health care personnel to act on behalf of patient adaptation.

Fostering adaptive functioning means that the nurse negotiates for the patient. She becomes his advocate. Because the critically ill patient often cannot effectively cope with both the physiological problem *and* the rest of his environment, it becomes necessary for the nurse to do for the patient what he is unable to do for himself so that his energy is conserved. As negotiator, the nurse must refrain from adding burdens which increase the patient's need to interact when such interaction will not foster adaptation. For example, patient energy spent in fearful suspense about the equipment nearby is not as helpful as energy spent in asking about it and then listening to a reply. Or, energy spent in persistently requesting a loved one to be present may not be as helpful as energy spent interacting with that person.

Fostering safety for the critically ill patient involves decreasing his vulnerability both physiologically and emotionally. The feeling of security is lost or at least significantly decreased whenever there is a decrease in one's control of body functions. Loss of control may vary from fatigue and weakness to paralysis. It may result from pathology, from the environment (such as restraint by IV tubing or machinery), or both; from fatigue and sleeplessness caused by physical discomfort; or from physiological fatigue, e.g., dyspnea and sensory overload. Regardless of the decrease or loss of control, the nurse intervenes in order to increase the patient's feeling of safety. She may accomplish this by using technical skill, tools, medication, interaction; by providing assisted breathing with a respirator; by encouraging breathing exercises; or by staying with the patient during a time of anxiety or loneliness. Recognizing a patient's safety needs is an important element in the holistic approach to patient care. In addition, it is this very consideration of the "whole" patient which allows us to establish priorities as patient negotiators.

Negotiating for the patient is not without its hazards. This kind of caring and giving requires our energies in place of those which the patient is temporarily lacking. Therefore, to maintain our own emotional reserves, we also need to support one another as colleagues in the critical care unit and to enhance one another's feelings of belonging and self-esteem. Other hazards involve speaking on behalf of the patient often as a minority voice and in the face of administrative, physician, or peer pressure. It means experiencing the joy of patients who recover or the sadness and anger of those who do not.

It is apparent to us that this philosophy of nursing need not and should not be confined to acute care areas. It is every patient's right to expect this type of intelligent care; it is the nurse's responsibility and challenge to provide it.

In the first edition of *Critical Care Nursing* we predicted that the responsibilities then defined as the expanded role would soon be the standard level of practice for the professional nurse. This has indeed happened. Meanwhile, we continue to develop the *thinking* part of nursing while also blending it with the *doing* part of patient care.

We continue to see a reversal of the trend of centralizing patients receiving critical care nursing. The rationale for this reversal lies in the desire to maintain consistency in providing care. This purpose is lost if the patient is moved from one area to another with different staff along the course of his hospitalization. The critical care nurse may eventually find herself delivering care both in the hospital and in the community. This is already happening because of earlier hospital discharge, often directly from critical care units. Critical care and community health nurses work side by side in order to provide a continuous high level of care. Regardless of the setting, with her background of technical, intellectual and psychosocial skills the critical care nurse is invaluable.

KAREN BUSCH DRIVER, R.N., M.S.
BARBARA M. GALLO, R.N., M.S.

4

emotional response to illness

When an individual's dynamic stability is threatened or impinged upon and his usual coping mechanisms begin to fail him, he enters a state of illness. Much of this book is focused on supporting and implementing the patient's response to the threat of illness through physiological maintenance and adjustments. It is the purpose of this chapter to consider the intimate relationship between one's emotional response to illness and its effect upon one's adaptation to temporary or permanent limitations. Concepts of anxiety, grief, and adaptation to illness will be presented for the purpose of developing related nursing interventions based on principles of sound theory.

Illness, or the threat of it, acts as a stressor which leads to an ambient state of tension. The existence of tension produces a response toward adaptation, and this tension state is known as *entropy*. For example, if a man is dehydrated, he drinks when he becomes aware of his thirst. The tension state of thirst activates his response of drinking. If he drinks salt water, neither the stressor nor the tension state of thirst will be relieved and his state of entropy will increase. If he drinks fresh water, his dehydration will be relieved and therefore his thirst, and he will place himself in a state of negative entropy, thus freeing his energies to cope with other stressors of life (Fig. 4–1).

Just as thirst is the motivating tension state to relieve dehydration, the phenomenon of anxiety is the tension state which activates one's response to the threat of illness. When energy is channeled toward *reducing the stressor*, it minimizes entropy. But energy is often directed toward merely relieving the tension state and may only perpetuate entropy, as with the thirsty, dehydrated man who drinks salt water.

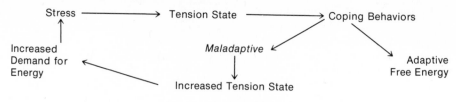

Fig. 4-1. Negative entropy.

anxiety

Any stressor which threatens one's sense of wholeness, containment, security, and control will bring anxiety into play. Illness is such a stressor. The physiological responses of rapid pulse rate, increased blood pressure, increased respirations, dilated pupils, dry mouth, and peripheral vasoconstriction may go undetected in the seemingly cool, calm, self-controlled patient. These autonomic responses to anxiety are always a reliable index when behavioral responses do not conform to the professional's expectations. Behavioral responses indicative of anxiety are often familial and culturally learned. They vary from quiet composure in the face of disaster to panic in the presence of a honeybee.

Nevertheless, such extremes of control or panic utilize valuable energy; and when this energy is not directed toward eliminating the stressor it serves only to perpetuate the state of entropy. Thus the goal of nursing care is always to promote physiological and emotional equilibrium, thereby minimizing entropy and freeing the patient's energy resources for healing and recuperation.

Whenever possible the threatening stressor is reduced or eliminated. When this is done the problem is quickly resolved and the patient is returned to equilibrium. Usually, however, the stressor is not so easily eliminated; instead many other stressors are introduced for the purpose of remedying the original state of entropy. For most people hospitalization is that kind of secondary stressor. Their presence in the critical care unit is to them the tangible proof that their fears are justified, that their life may be in jeopardy, and that they are wholly at the mercy of strangers who, they feel, must regard them as inferior for not understanding what is happening or how those awesome gadgets work their reputed cures.

When it is impossible to remove the provocative stimuli, it is the nurse's function to make an assessment of the coping mechanism that the patient might utilize in his current precarious state. Those coping behaviors may be directed toward eliminating either the stressor of illness or the stressor of the anxiety state itself. Thus the nurse must evaluate each behavior in the light of whether or not it functions to restore a steady state. She can support or encourage those behaviors which are consistent with movement toward a steady state; or she may need to modify or find substitutes for those behaviors which are disruptive to or threaten a steady state. And at times it is necessary to teach or introduce new coping mechanisms to enhance movement to the overall goal of homeostatic equilibrium.

For example, in an acute period a patient may be more capable of experiencing concern and worry over the variety of equipment which surrounds him rather than of focusing on the threat to his life. This activity may allow him some necessary denial of the reality of the crisis, but the worry itself may drain him of needed energy. Information and explanation of the machinery may serve to reduce his secondary anxiety, while expert nursing care may serve to reassure him nonverbally of his security without stripping him of his defense of denial.

Anxiety is commonly experienced when there is a threat of helplessness or lack of control. Thus nursing measures which reinforce every possible control the patient may have help to increase his sense of autonomy and reduce the overpowering sense of loss of control. Providing order and predictability allows the patient to anticipate and prepare for what is to follow. Perhaps it creates only a mirage of control, but anticipatory guidance keeps the patient from being caught off guard and allows him to muster those coping mechanisms which he can bring to bear.

Allowing small choices when the patient is willing and ready decreases the patient's feeling that he is totally at the mercy of others. Is he ready for pain medication? Would he prefer to lie on his right or left side? In which arm would he like his IV? How high does he want the head of his bed? Does he want to cough now or in 20 minutes following pain medication? All serve to let the patient participate in ways which allow him to exert a certain amount of control and predictability. It may also help him accept his lack of control of procedures for which he has little choice. Minute decisions like these allow him to exercise some controls in a way designed to help reduce the anxiety-provoking sense of helplessness.

A second overriding cause of anxiety is a sense of isolation. Rarely is one more lonely than in the midst of a socializing crowd of strangers. In such a situation individuals either attempt to include themselves, remove themselves, or distance themselves with feigned interest in a magazine, scenery or anything else that offers them relief from the sense of not belonging. The sick person surrounded by active and busy persons is in a similar situation but with fewer available resources to reduce his sense of isolation. Serious illness and the fear of dying separate the patient from his family. The reassuring cliche "You'll be all right" serves to enhance the sense of distance the patient is experiencing. It shuts off his expression of fears and his questions of what is to come next. The efficiency and activity engulfing him reinforce his sense of separateness as he lies isolated in his bed.

A third category of anxiety-provoking stimuli includes those which threaten the individual's security. Needless to say, entrance into the critical care unit serves as dramatic confirmation to the family and patient that their security on all levels is being severely threatened. Most individuals associate the critical care unit with a life-and-death crisis; many associate it with the deaths of relatives and friends.

But to the nurse the unit may represent a closer and safer vigilance of life. Her attention is directed more to the preservation of life than to the fears of and preparations for dying that may be occupying the minds of the patient and his family. Upon the patient's admission to the unit, insecurity is undoubtedly about life itself. Later, questions of length of hospitalization, return to work, well-being of the family, permanent limitations and the like arise, so that the state of insecurity is ever present.

response to loss

The threat of illness precipitates the coping behaviors associated with loss. For some patients it is an adaptation to dying; for others it is the loss of health or loss of a limb, a blow to one's self-concept, or the necessity to change one's life style. All of these require a change in one's self-image — a loss of the familiar image and its replacement with an altered self-image. Nevertheless, the dynamics of grief present themselves in one form or another. Engel has conveniently categorized the response to loss in four phases: shock and disbelief, development of awareness, restitution, and resolution.[1] Each phase has characteristic and predictable behaviors which dynamically take the patient step-by-step through the healing process. Through the recognition and assessment of the various behaviors and an understanding of their underlying dynamics the nurse can plan her intervention to support the healing process.

shock and disbelief

In this stage the patient demonstrates the behaviors characteristic of denial. He fails to comprehend and experience the emotional impact and rational meaning of his diagnosis. Because the diagnosis has no emotional meaning the patient often fails to cooperate with precautionary measures. For example, he may attempt to get out of bed against the doctor's orders, may deviate from his diet, may fail to inform the nurse of minor pain, and may assert that he is there for a *rest!* Denial may go so far as to allow the patient to project his difficulties onto what he perceives as ill-functioning equipment, mistaken lab reports, and — more likely — on the sheer incompetence of physicians and nurses.

When such blatant denial occurs it is apparent that the problem is so anxiety-provoking to the patient that it cannot be handled by the more sophisticated defense mechanism of rational problem solving. Thus the stressor is obliterated. This phase of denial may also serve as the period when the patient's resources, temporarily blocked by the shock, can now be regrouped for the battle ahead. The principle of intervention consists not in stripping away the defense of denial but in supporting the patient and acknowledging his situation through nursing care.

The nurse accepts and recognizes his illness by watching the monitor or changing the dressings. She communicates her acceptance of the patient through her tone of voice, her facial expression, and her use of touch. She can reflect back to the patient his statements of denial in a way that allows him to hear them—and eventually to examine their incongruity and apply reality—as by saying, "In some ways you believe that having a heart attack will be helpful to you?" She can also acknowledge the patient's difficulty in accepting his restrictions by such comments as, "It seems hard for you to stay in bed." By verbalizing what the patient is expressing she gently confronts his behavior but does not cause anxiety and anger by reprimanding and judging him. Thus in this phase the nurse supports denial by allowing for it, but she does not perpetuate it. Rather she uses herself to acknowledge, accept, and reflect the patient's new circumstance. It is interesting to note that although denying illness can prevent adaptation at a new level, denial also has its advantages. High deniers with myocardial infarctions have a higher survival rate than moderate or low deniers.[2] They also often return to work sooner and reach higher levels of rehabilitation. This points out the effectiveness of denial as a coping mechanism as well as the hazards of stripping it away before the patient is ready.

development of awareness

In this stage of grief, the patient's behavior is characteristically associated with anger and guilt. He may present himself as overtly angry. His anger is most likely to be directed at the staff for oversights, tardiness, and minor insensitivities. Demanding and whining in this state often serve to alienate the nurse. The patient who does not demand or whine has probably retreated into the withdrawal of depression. He will demonstrate verbal and motor retardation, will have difficulty sleeping, and may prefer to be left alone.

At this time the ugliness of reality has made its impact. Displacement of the anger on others helps to slow the impact. The expression of anger itself helps give the patient a sense of power in a seemingly helpless state. The depression is characteristic of other depressions, such as anger turned inward. The demanding and whining are attempts to regain the control the patient senses he has lost.

During this phase the nurse is likely to hear irrational expressions of guilt. The patient seeks to answer, "Why me?" He will attempt to isolate his human imperfections and attribute the cause of his malady to them. He and his family may participate in looking for a person or object to blame.

Guilt feelings around one's own illness are difficult to understand unless one examines the basic dynamic of guilt. Guilt arises when there is a decrease in the feeling of self-worth or when the self-concept has been violated. In this light, the nurse can understand that what is behind an expression of guilt is a negatively altered self-concept. Blame thus becomes nothing more than projection of the unbearable feeling of guilt.

Nursing intervention in this phase must be directed toward supporting the patient's basic sense of self-worth and allowing and encouraging the expression of direct anger. Nursing measures which support a patient's sense of self-worth are numerous: calling the patient by name, introducing him to strangers (particularly when they are to examine him), talking *to* rather than *about* him, and most of all providing and respecting his need for privacy and modesty. The nurse needs to guard against verbal and nonverbal expressions of pity. She will do better to empathize with the patient's specific feelings of anger, sadness, and guilt rather than with his condition.

The nurse can create outlets for anger by listening and by refraining from defending either herself, the doctor, or the hospital. A nondefensive, accepting attitude will decrease the patient's sense of guilt, and the expression of anger will avert some of the depression. Later when the patient is apologetic for his irrational outburst the nurse can interpret the necessity of this kind of verbalization as a step toward rehabilitation.

restitution

Engel called this phase the "work of mourning." In this stage the griever puts aside his anger and resistance and begins to cope constructively with his loss. He tries new behaviors consistent with his limitations. His emotional level is one of sadness, and much of his time may be spent crying. As he adapts himself to his new image he spends considerable time going over and over significant memories relevant to his loss. Behaviors in this stage should include the verbalization of fears regarding his future. Often these go undetected because they are unbearable for the family to hear. After severe trauma which includes scarring or removal of a body part or loss of sensation, the patient may question his sexual adequacy and the future response of his mate to his changed body. He probably also questions his new role in his family and job and has a variety of concerns that are specific to his own life style.

Thus in the mourning process such manifestations as reminiscing, crying, questioning, expressing fears, and trying out new behaviors serve to help the patient modify his old self-concept and begin working with and experiencing his revised concept.

Nursing intervention in this stage should again be supportive to allow this adaptation to occur. Listening to the patient for lengthy periods of time will be necessary. If the patient is able to verbalize his fears and questions about the future, he will be better able to define his anxiety and to solve his problems. Furthermore it will help him put his fears into a more rational perspective as he hears himself talk about them. He may require privacy, acceptance, and encouragement to cry so that he can find respite from his sadness.

During this stage the nurse might have the patient consider meeting someone who has successfully adapted to similar trauma. This measure would provide the patient with a role model as he begins to take on a new identity, which often occurs after the crisis period.

Additionally, the patient with appropriate support from the nurse will begin to identify and acknowledge changes that are arising out of his adaptation to illness. Relationships can and do change. Because friends respond to an invalid differently, the patient will not feel or believe that he is being treated like his old self. During this time the family has also been going through a similar process. They too have experienced shock, disbelief, anger, and sadness. When they are ready to try to solve their problems, their energies will be directed toward wondering how the changes in the patient will affect their mutual relationship and their life style. They too will experience the pain of turmoil and uncertainty. Nurses must help the family also. By providing ventilation and acceptance of their feelings of repulsion and fear, the nurse can help the family to be more useful to and accepting of the patient. Through intensive listening the nurse provides a sounding board and then redirects the members of the family back to each other so that they can give and receive support.

resolution

Resolution is the stage of identity change. At first the patient can be observed to be overidentifying himself as an invalid. He may discriminate against himself and make derogatory remarks about his body. Another method is to detach the traumatized part such as a stoma, prosthesis, scar, or paralyzed limb by naming it and referring to it in a simultaneously alienated and affectionate way. The patient is alert to the ways in which health care workers respond to his body and to his comments about himself, and may be testing out their acceptance before he ventures into the outside world. Chiding him or telling him that many others share his problem will be less helpful than acknowledging his feelings and indicating acceptance by continuing to care for and talk with him.

As the patient adapts with the passage of time, the sting of the endured hurt leaves and the patient moves toward identifying himself as an individual who has certain limitations due to his illness, rather than as a "cripple" or "invalid." He no longer uses his defect as the basis of his identity. As the resolution is reached, the patient is able to depend on others when necessary, and he should not need to push himself beyond his endurance or to overcompensate for his inadequacy. Often the individual will look back upon the crisis as a growing period. He will have hopefully achieved a sense of pride at accomplishing the difficult adaptation. He is able to reflect back realistically upon his successes and disappointments without discomfort. At this time he may find it useful and gratifying to help others in the stage of restitution during their identity crisis by sharing himself as a role model.

Unfortunately the hospital nurse is rarely in a position to observe the successful outcome. It is useful for her to know the process in order that she may work with and communicate an attitude of hope, especially when her patient is most self-disparaging.

The goal of nursing care in this stage is to help the patient attach a sense of self-esteem to his rectified identity. Nursing intervention revolves around helping the patient find the degree of dependence that he needs and can accept. She must accept and recognize with the patient his vacillation between independence and dependence, and must encourage a positive emotional response to his new state of modified dependence. Certainly she can support and reinforce his growing sense of pride in his rehabilitation. For those nurses who have had the experience of working through the process with one individual, the problem will be to stand back and allow the patient to move away from them.

adaptation to illness

Another method of assisting and evaluating a patient's response to his illness is described by Martin and Prange.[3] By comparing emotional adaptation to physical state of illness or well-being, it is easy to identify problem areas.

Martin and Prange theorize that there is an emotional lag, by which a person becomes physically ill before he adapts emotionally; it follows that in the process of recuperation the person becomes well before he adapts emotionally. Thus in the shaded area of Fig. 4-2 the patient is likely to be denying his illness. Again, he is likely to be uncooperative in his treatments and resist restrictions placed upon him. As he adjusts to his sick role things should go fairly smoothly. As the patient improves physically, the nurse and others begin to raise their expectations for his activity and independence. However, since his emotional adaptation has not caught up with his physical state the patient will move forward only with trepidation. He will demonstrate greater concern over his physical state and increase his demands for help. Preparation for his return to health, acknowledgment of his concerns about increased activity, and the reassurance of watchful eyes will help alleviate his anxiety as he progresses.

One principle that greatly affects understanding of the patient's response is the fact that during stress the patient will regress as an attempt to conserve

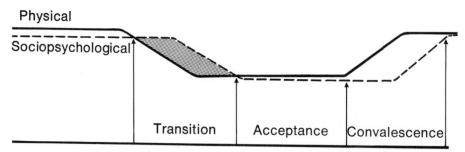

Fig. 4-2. The solid line represents a normal level of physical well-being, the broken line a corresponding degree of sociopsychological integration.

his energies. Thus during times of acute exacerbation or the raising of expectations, or during any significant change, the initial response will be to regress to an earlier emotional position of safety. Weaning from a respirator, removal of monitor leads, or increased activity and reduction in medication often trigger anxiety and regression. This regression may even include a retreat into increased dependency, depression, and anger. At that time comfort may be found in regressing into a state the patient has already discovered he can live through and/or master. The regression is usually temporary and brief and serves to pinpoint the cause of anxiety. At this time health personnel may become disappointed, anxious, or angry with the patient's backsliding and may wish to retreat from him. It is more helpful, however, to acknowledge that regression is inevitable and to support the patient with intervention appropriate in earlier stages.

Each person's electrocardiogram has common characteristics as well as individual differences. Similarly, each person's response to illness, if put into a graph, would have both common and unique points. There will be variations in time and in the congruence between physical and sociopsychological responses, but the stages will occur predictably. Like the electrical events of the heart, responses to illness, both adaptive and maladaptive, can be anticipated and hopefully minimized.

The prevalence of anxiety and depression as part of the response to illness is documented in a study by Cassem and Hackett.[4] During this research project, any patient whose outlook or behavior endangered his physical or emotional well-being was referred for psychiatric consultation. Of 441 patients who were admitted to the coronary care unit because of myocardial infarction, 145 (32.7 percent) were referred because of anxiety, depression or behavior problems. Referrals because of anxiety were highest on the patients' first and second days in the unit, with referrals for depression peaking on days three and four. Behavior problems were the third most common reason for consultation. The greatest number were referred on day two, with fewer on day four. The behaviors included: denying illness by threatening to leave the hospital, euphoria, sexually suggestive comments, and conflicts about hospital or treatment restrictions. This supports the premise that anxiety accompanies transition into illness and that depression emerges as people recognize the impact of the illness.

Although these responses occurred in patients who had myocardial infarctions, they may be generalized to include other persons who have a sudden onset of illness and who need intensive care. In addition, the authors noted that the interventions which helped patients deal with their situation did not have to be carried out by psychiatrists alone.

Both doctors and nurses were invited to make referrals. Not only did nurses make more referrals than doctors, but all those referred by doctors had already been referred earlier by nurses. This fact points out that nurses made early and astute observations about coping mechanisms. Because of their expertise and proximity to the patient, nurses should continue both to intervene and to make referrals.

teaching and learning

Recognizing the patient's response to illness helps predict the time at which information will be best absorbed and most helpful to him. Learning is most likely to occur during quiet stages when the patient's emotional outlook corresponds to his physical condition. This can be seen in Fig. 4-2 where the lines representing sociopsychological and physical functioning are in close proximity. This means that the patient feels just about as sick (or well) as he is. Providing information in this phase of illness will help him move on to the next phase of recovery. When there is less congruence between the patient's emotional outlook and his physical condition, the lines representing sociopsychological and physical functioning are farther apart. Providing information at this time may increase the patient's vulnerability and either reinforce his defenses, causing resistance, or diminish them enough to cause regression. Both responses result from anxiety and will further increase the gap between sociopsychological and physical functioning.

As the patient adjusts to the sick role he will be receptive to learning about his illness. Because progress heightens anxiety, teaching is usually more effective during the period of acceptance than during the times in which the patient is moving either into or out of the sick role. Whenever there is movement forward or backward on the health-illness continuum there is likely to be an emotional response of anxiety, worry or depression which will interfere with concentration and learning. Therefore, admission, transfer or readmission to the critical care unit, as well as hospital discharge, are poor times for learning to occur. During periods of anxiety, it is useful to ascertain the patient's perceptions of what is happening so that misunderstandings which may cause unnecessary worry can be corrected.

Informal teaching and the provision of information which serves to enhance equilibrium while promoting a minimum of entropy are best woven into the other nursing procedures occurring throughout the patient's stay in the critical care unit. For effective learning to take place, the high levels of anxiety commonly found in critical care units must be decreased to no more than mild anxiety states in which the patient demonstrates alertness without fear, motivation to learn, and interest. The more facts there are to absorb and the more behavior change is implied by the information, the more likely the patient is to respond with increased levels of anxiety; and therefore, the greater the need to teach during periods of only mild anxiety.

Anxiety levels, physiological function, and the patient's own priorities must be assessed when the readiness of the patient-learner is evaluated. Anxiety, worry, pain and some medications will interfere with the patient's ability to learn. Informal teaching and rehabilitation programs which may involve structure and extended periods of time should occur after the crisis, when the patient has reached a fairly stable period of adjustment. In order to provide this type of essential health teaching, hospital-based personnel can conduct programs for patients to return to after hospital discharge. In addition, community-based classes can be conducted, as well as individualized teaching in the home, where the patient's and family's learning and ability to apply the information can be evaluated. An effective approach includes a combination of informal teaching, group instruction, and individualized learning and evaluation at home. Teaching can be started during the hospital stay, but it can rarely be completed.

The hierarchy of needs described in Fig. 3-1 (p. 23) is another guide to keep in mind when predicting receptivity to teaching. During the stage of severe physiological limitations, when the patient's energies are directed at maintaining basic physiological functions, teaching which involves upper levels of functioning will probably be unsuccessful. Learning occurs more easily when security, a sense of belonging, and self-esteem are high. Often learning about illness means that the patient and family must not only learn facts and techniques but must also synthesize, apply and adapt what is said to their own lives. This will be difficult when there are high degrees of anxiety, depression or acute physical dysfunction. It will be impossible for patients to respond creatively while they are struggling to maintain basic physiological needs.

transference

There are some types of irrational behavior directed toward nurses which cannot be explained by adaptation or grieving. It appears that in times of stress, as well as at other times, some patients attribute to the nurses feelings, desires, characteristics, attitudes and fears which they have encountered in the past. This phenomenon is called *transference.*[5] Exhibitionism, extreme dependency, and irrational demands are some behaviors which can often be accounted for by transference. It may be that in times of crisis and regression, reality testing is impaired, and the patient is more likely to act and react to the irrational fears and feelings that originated when he was a helpless child. In such instances, the patient must be treated and addressed as an adult and helped to test reality in the current environment. For example, if the patient fears that the nurses do not care about him, he can be encouraged to ask specific nurses how they feel or he can be helped to identify what it is about the nurses that suggests to him that they do not care for him. At that time, specific explanations can be given about nurses' behavior. This type of intervention satisfies the patient's need to be cared about far better than global reassurance and generalizations that the nurses do care about him.

Just as patients may transfer feelings which originated from their earlier experiences, so too do nurses. This process is called *countertransference* and should be considered whenever a nurse's behavior toward a particular patient differs from her usual pattern. Inappropriate or intense feelings, including anger, the desire to argue and extreme protectiveness should signal the possibility that countertransference is occurring.

transfer from the critical care unit

Regression is often elicited when the patient is told that he is ready to be transferred to the general unit. The stage of illness greatly influences the patient's response to transfer. If the patient is transferred while he is denying his illness, the move will be done with ease since it further fortifies his feeling that he isn't very sick. On the other hand, if the patient is transferred when he is improving physically more than he acknowledges emotionally, then anxiety will be heightened. The patient is saying, "I'm sick, and being transferred means you think I'm getting better when I'm not." In trying to cope with the anxiety generated by the move, he will regress and become more dependent. Transferring a patient when he first acknowledges the severity of his illness may create discomfort for nurses, since the patient is likely to be frightened, angry, uncooperative, and demanding.

preparing the transfer

Regardless of the timing, in preparing for transfer both nurses and patients need to accept the fact that their relationship with each other will be ending. This may be done by reminiscing over an initial meeting or a special moment and by talking about the move.

If the patient is feeling dependent, then more time may be needed to talk about how it will be to leave. Often, because of discomfort at saying goodbye, nurses withdraw under the guise that it is easier for the patient to ignore the termination process. This unexplained withdrawal may be interpreted by the patient as a lack of interest or anger over earlier unresolved outbursts when he had been experiencing a change in body image and lowered esteem because of his illness.

The news of transfer often comes without warning or preparation. Even though the patient may be pleased with his progress, he is at the same time concerned about losing the reassurance of special equipment, close surveillance, and the presence of familiar faces. It has long been advocated that continuity of care be provided by thoughtful preparation. Introduction to the new nurses who will take over care of the patient, as well as follow-up visits by the critical care nurses, will increase familiarity, enhance security, and let the patient know that he is important. Removing equipment before the time of transfer will lessen the strain of having to give up his room, equipment, and nurse all at the same time.

Urine catecholamine studies on patients transferred to a general unit from a coronary care unit indicated that increased stress with transfer occurred in five out of seven patients.[6] All five of these patients had a cardiovascular complication such as arrhythmia. In a follow-up study however, seven patients were prepared for transfer from the beginning of their stay. They had follow-up visits by the nurse and care by the same physician. No cardiovascular complications occurred and only two had a rise in urine catechols at the time of transfer. Even with preparation for transfer, regression and anxiety may occur; however, by acknowledging his concerns and receiving support from the nurse, the patient will again mobilize his energy.

Because these processes have proven predictable, they give the nurse a basis for her care and provide rationale for appropriate intervention. In spite of the predictability of these responses in human behavior, they still have an impact upon the individual and are unique to him. By the time they are modified by his personality and by sociocultural and economic variables, they have become a significant part of his life, and are indeed made unique as they are made a historical and living part of his identity.

REFERENCES

1. George L. Engel, "Grief and Grieving," *American Journal of Nursing,* Vol. 64, No. 9 (September 1964), pp. 93–98.
2. Thomas Hackett, N. H. Cassem, and Howard Wishnie, "The Coronary Care Unit—An Appraisal of Its Psychological Hazards," *New England Journal of Medicine,* Vol. 279, No. 25 (December 19, 1968), pp. 1365–1370.
3. Harry W. Martin and Arthur J. Prange, "Adaptation to Illness," *Nursing Outlook,* Vol. 10 (March 1962), pp. 168–171.
4. N. H. Cassem and Thomas P. Hackett, "Psychiatric Consultation in a Coronary Care Unit," *Annals of Internal Medicine,* Vol. 75, No. 1 (July 1971), pp. 9–11.
5. Joan J. Kyes and Charles K. Hofling, *Basic Psychiatric Concepts in Nursing,* ed. 3 (Philadelphia: J. B. Lippincott Company, 1974), p. 426.
6. Robert F. Klein et al., "Transfer from a Coronary Care Unit—Some Adverse Responses," *Archives of Internal Medicine,* Vol. 122 (August 1968), pp. 104–108.

KAREN BUSCH DRIVER, R.N., M.S.

5

families in crisis

A holistic approach to critical care nursing must include the patient's family. For the purposes of this chapter, *family* means any persons who share intimate and routine day-to-day living with the critical care patient—in other words, those persons whose social homeostasis is altered by the patient's entrance into the arena of critical illness or injury, and who are a significant part of the patient's normal life style and therefore must be a part of holistic care.

The patient's entrance into a life-death sick role threatens and alters the family's homeostasis for many reasons. The patient's responsibilities will now have to be added to the responsibilities of others, and therefore will demand an alteration in their schedules and activities. When these responses are left undone, the members experience various degrees of discomfort and annoyance. Financial concerns are usually major; also, daily activities which previously were of little consequence to family members now become important and often difficult to manage. Such activities as packing school lunches for children, keeping the family car filled with gasoline, taking out the garbage, and balancing the checkbook can, when unfulfilled, all become critical incidents with the right timing.

In addition to the responsibilities the patient normally carries, the social role the patient plays in the family will also be missing. Disciplinarian, provider of affection, lover, humorist, time keeper, motivator, comforter, and so on are all important roles; when they are missing, considerable havoc and even grief in the family may ensue.

The family enters into a crisis situation under the following conditions:
1. A stressful event occurs, which threatens lasting changes for the family.[1]
2. Usual problem-solving activities are inadequate and therefore do not lead rapidly to the previous state of balance.[2]
3. The present state of family disequilibrium cannot be maintained and will lead either to improved family health and adaptation or to decreased family adaptability and increased proneness to crisis events.[3]

41

By using these conditions to identify and define families in crisis, the stress of normal maturational events of family life such as marriage, pregnancy, enrollment in school, and retirement can be appreciated in a different light. Holmes and Rahe have scored stressful life events which can be predictors of illness.[4] These life events all require readjustment and include such things as marital reconciliation, change in finances, and trouble with the in-laws or the boss. Thus, it is not only situations of disease and injury that propel families into crisis. A family who has been coping adequately with unemployment may not be able to deal with the added stress of a critically ill family member. What appears to be a family's overreaction to a small stress may be explained as having a "last straw" effect added onto a maturational crisis.

Some families experience many more crises than others. Often the challenges and demands that face these families are similar to the ones that present themselves to all families. There appears to be an additional factor of *cognitive appraisal* which must be considered. Some persons or families appear to assign catastrophic meaning to some events that others would not. If family members appraise a situation by giving it the proportions and labels of crisis events, then the emotions, stress, and anxiety associated with a crisis, as well as attempts to cope, will follow.[5] This phenomenon then implies that crises based on cognitive appraisal are individual and unique—i.e., a crisis for one family is not necessarily a crisis for another. The wide range of family behaviors and reactions observed by critical care nurses can in large part be explained by this concept. Cultural and age variables can also be accounted for in this way.

Brose makes four important generalizations about crises which can form a basis for nursing care of families dealing with them:

1. Whether a person emerges stronger or weaker as a result of a crisis is not based so much on his previous character as on the kind of help he receives during the actual crisis.
2. People become more amenable to suggestions and open to help during actual crises.
3. With the onset of a crisis situation, old memories of past crises may be evoked. If maladaptive behavior was used to deal with previous situations, the same type of behavior may be repeated in the face of a new crisis.
4. The only way to survive a crisis is to be aware of it.[6]

Roberts states, "Families of patients in a critical care unit attempt to continue in a steady state. They accomplish this goal either by minimizing the significance of the patient's illness, or by being overprotective of him. The critically ill patient enters the hospital in biological crisis. Unlike the patient, the family enters the same hospital, or critical care unit, in psychological crisis."[7] Roberts also makes the point that as stress increases, the family system at first improves; as stress continues, disintegration of the family system may occur.[8]

Reactions to crisis situations are difficult to categorize because they depend on individual responses to stress; and within a family, several mechanisms to handle stress and anxiety will be employed. In general, the nurse may observe behaviors which indicate emotions signifying helplessness and urgency. An inability to make decisions and mobilize resources can be noted. A sense of fear and panic pervades. Irrational acts, demanding behavior, withdrawal, perseveration, and fainting all have been observed by critical care nurses. Just as the patient is experiencing shock and disbelief about his illness, so too is the family. A nurse must herself perceive the feeling a crisis victim is experiencing, particularly when that person cannot identify the problem or feeling to himself or others.

nursing intervention

Nursing intervention must be designed to help families (1) reach a higher level of adaptation by learning from the crisis experience, (2) regain a state of equilibrium, and (3) experience the feelings involved in the crisis to avoid delayed depressions and allow for future emotional growth.

assessment

The critical care nurse can expect to deal with large numbers of persons who can be defined as being in a crisis. Almost all patients and families who populate the waiting room will fit the crisis conditions described above. The problem will be to assess the immediate events causing the disruption and then to help the families assign priorities to their needs, so that they can act accordingly.

The nurse will need to identify current methods of coping and evaluate them in terms of adaptation (see Chapter 4). The nurse will need to determine, and sometimes point out to the clients, chronic problems resulting from the threatening crisis. When the situational crisis seems inconsequential or obscure, the nurse must attempt to discern and understand the meaning the clients have attributed to the event. Furthermore, it will help to evaluate current maturational problems with which the family may be attempting to cope. Understanding the parameters of the crisis may give the direction for action.

the use of the relationship

Establishing an emotionally meaningful relationship with people in crisis tends to be easier than at any other time. Persons in crisis are highly receptive to an interested and empathic helper. In the first meeting with the patient's family, the nurse must demonstrate that she can help.

The family must be prepared for their experience in the critical care unit. The patient's condition, alertness and appearance should be described in terms suitable to the family's level of understanding. Any equipment should be explained before the family views the patient. At the bedside further explanation can be made.

Other specific help can be given at this time to demonstrate the nurse's interest. Looking up telephone numbers can be extremely difficult for the highly anxious family member. Even deciding who is to be notified of the patient's status can be an overwhelming decision at these times.

With this kind of timely intervention, the family will begin to trust and depend on the nurse's judgment. This process then allows family members to believe the nurse when she conveys a feeling of hope and confidence in their ability to deal with whatever is ahead of them in the days to come. It is important to avoid giving false reassurance; rather, the reality of the situation can be expressed in statements like, "This is a complicated problem; together we can work on it."

defining the problem

As the relationship develops from one interaction to another, the nurse can formulate for herself the dynamics of the problem. The formulations would include such items as (1) the meaning the family has attached to the event, (2) other crises with which the family may be already coping, (3) the coping mechanisms previously used in times of stress, with an idea of why these behaviors are or are not working at this time, and (4) the normal resources of the family which may include friends, neighbors, relations, colleagues, etc. The nurse, having identified these areas, will best use them with the family to help them deal with their predicament.

A vital part of the problem-solving process is to help the family clearly state what their immediate problem is. Often people feel overwhelmed and immobilized by the free-floating anxiety or panic caused by acute stress. Stating the problem in words helps the client achieve a degree of *cognitive mastery*. Regardless of the difficulty or threat the problem implies, being able to state it as such reduces anxiety by helping the family to feel that they have achieved some sort of understanding of what is happening.

Defining and redefining the problem or problems must occur many times before resolution of the crisis occurs. Stating the problem clearly automatically helps the family to assign priorities and direct the needed actions. For example, finding a baby-sitter may become the number one priority, superseding notification of close relatives of a tragic accident. Goal-directed activity will further help to decrease anxiety and the irrational acts that sometimes go with it.

In high levels of stress, some people expect themselves to react differently. Rather than turning to the resources they use daily, they become reluctant to involve them. Simply asking people who they usually turn to when they are upset, and finding out what has gotten in the way of turning to these people now, helps direct the client back to the normal mechanisms that he uses to maintain homeostasis. When the client is reluctant to call on a friend, the nurse can help with the indecision by asking, "Wouldn't you want to help her if she were in your place?" Most families are truly not without resources; they have only failed to recognize and call on them.

Defining and redefining the problem may also help to put the problem in a different light. It is possible in time to view a tragedy as a challenge, and the unknown as an adventure.

The nurse can also help the family call on their own strengths. How have they handled stress before? Have they used humor, escape, exercise, or friendship? Do they telephone close friends and relatives who are far away? Even though the family may be threatened financially at this time, some expenditures of this sort may be well worth the money.

problem solving

A problem-solving technique which emphasizes choices and alternatives will help the family achieve a sense of control over part of their lives. It will also serve to remind them, as well as clarify to them, that they are ultimately responsible for dealing with the event, and that it is they who must live with the consequences of their decisions.

Helping the family focus on feelings is extremely important in order to avoid delayed grief reactions and protracted depressions later on. The nurse can give direction to the family to help each other cry and to share their fear and sadness. Reflection of feelings or active listening will be necessary throughout the crisis. If the nurse can start a statement by saying, "You feel . . .," she will be reflecting a feeling. If she says, "You feel *that* . . .," she will be reflecting a judgment instead of a feeling. Describing and recognizing one's feelings will decrease the need to look for someone to blame. Valuing the expression of feelings may help the clients avoid the use of tranquilizers, sedatives, and excessive sleep to escape painful feelings. In sad and depressing times the nurse can authentically promise the family that they will feel better with time. Depression is self-limiting.

During the difficult days that a person is critically ill, the family may become very dependent on the judgment of professionals. It may be difficult for them to identify the appropriate areas in which to accept others' judgments. The nurse can best handle inappropriate expectations like, "Tell me what I should do?" by acknowledging the feelings involved in an accepting manner and stating the reality of the situation, e.g., "You wish I could make that difficult decision for you, but I can't, because you are the ones who will have to live with the consequences." This type of statement acknowledges the clients' feelings and recognizes the complexity of the problem, while emphasizing each individual's responsibility for his or her own feelings, actions and decisions.

Once the problem has been defined and the family begins goal-directed activity, the nurse may help further by asking them to identify the steps they must take. This anticipatory guidance will help reduce anxiety and make things go more smoothly.

Crisis victims must always be left with a specific plan of action. This plan may be as simple as, "Call me tomorrow at 2:00 P.M."; regardless of its simplicity, it implies hope, responsibility, and a reason to get through the night.

The critical care nurse's time with families is often limited due to the nature of her work, so it is important to make every interaction as useful to the family as possible. She will have to take responsibility for directing the conversation and focusing on the here and now. She will need to avoid the temptation of giving useless advice in favor of emphasizing a problem-solving approach. However, she must use her judgment and recognize those moments when direction is vital to health and safety. It is often necessary to direct families to return home to rest. This can be explained by saying that by maintaining their own health they will be more helpful to the patient at a later time. To make each interaction meaningful, she must focus on the crisis situation and avoid getting involved in long-term chronic problems and complaints. For example, she would help the family of the overdose patient deal with the events immediately preceding the suicide attempt rather than with long-standing family problems.

referral

Regardless of the nurse's ability in this area, there will be some families who will profit most by referral to a mental health nurse clinician, a social worker, a psychologist, or a psychiatrist. A nurse can best help the client accept help from others by acknowledging the difficulty of the problem emphatically and providing a choice of names and phone numbers. At times it even may be appropriate for the nurse to set up the first meeting; however, the chances of follow-through are greater when the client makes his own arrangements.

conclusion

Crisis intervention for families undergoing acute stress is an important preventive mental health function that nurses can provide. Their knowledge of and proximity to the problem allow them to be first-line resource professionals. As patient advocates, their role will be to realize and point out that dealing with a psychological crisis in the family greatly affects the recovery and well-being of the patient, as well as decreases the chances for further disequilibrium in the family unit.

REFERENCES

1. Lydia Rapoport, "The State of Crisis: Some Theoretical Considerations," *Crisis Intervention: Selected Readings,* Howard J. Parad, ed. (New York: Family Service Association of America, 1965), p. 24.
2. *Ibid.*
3. Carolyn Brose, "Theories of Family Crisis," *Family Health Care,* Debra P. Hymovich and Martha Underwood Barnard, eds. (New York: McGraw-Hill Book Company, 1973), p. 271.
4. Thomas H. Holmes and Richard H. Rahe, "Social Readjustment Rating Scale," *Journal of Psychosomatic Research,* Vol. II (1967), pp. 213–218.
5. Richard S. Lazarus, "Cognitive and Personality Factors Underlying Threat and Coping," *Social Stress,* Sol Levine and Norman A. Schotch, eds. (Chicago: Aldine Publishing Company, 1970), pp. 143–164.
6. Brose, *op. cit.,* pp. 279–282.
7. Sharon L. Roberts, *Behavioral Concepts and the Critically Ill Patient* (New Jersey: Prentice-Hall, Inc., 1976), p. 359.
8. *Ibid.,* p. 355.

JANICE S. SMITH, R.N., M.S.

6 | 9

adverse effects of critical care units

part I: the patient

The necessity of employing highly technical and precise measures to preserve life in a crisis situation commonly found in critical care units can create an environment totally alien and threatening to the patient. The complicated equipment necessary for maintaining life requires unquestionable expertise on the part of personnel involved in patient care. However, if life-preserving measures are to have any value for the patient, the nurse must be aware of aspects of care in addition to the patient's physical needs and the mechanical workings of the ever increasing array of machines which medical technology is producing.

The psychosocial support needed by the patient in the critical care unit demands more than assistance in dealing with a critical illness. The sounds and activities of the unit are bombarding the patient 24 hours a day; in addition, the patient must cope with the effects of fear concerning illness. Normal defense mechanisms which allow us to cope with threatening situations are diminished in all patients (and absent in the unconscious patient). The ability to run from a frightening or painful stimulus is gone, as is the ability to analyze a situation objectively and take action to control it.

To appreciate how devastating confinement to a critical care unit can be, the nurse needs only to think of her own feelings about reversing roles with a patient. When asked if they would volunteer to spend 24 hours in the patient role in the crisis care unit, nurses respond readily with a definite "No!" In view of their awareness of the environmental threats of such units, nurses must function as the negotiator for the patient. To be an effective negotiator the nurse must acquire knowledge about the effects of sensory input on the human organism.

sensory input

The broad concept of sensory input deals with stimulation of all of the five senses: visual, auditory, olfactory, tactile, and gustatory. Stimuli to all of the senses may be perceived in a qualitative manner as pleasant or unpleasant, acceptable or unacceptable, desirable or undesirable, soothing or painful. Individual perceptions of stimuli may vary drastically. Some individuals may consider the sounds and smells of a metropolitan business section to be pleasant, acceptable, desirable — or painful. Everyday activities including the choice of food or drink are based on the individual's perception of what is liked or disliked. Thus people tend to choose, whenever possible, the environment or stimuli from the environment most acceptable to them, but patients in the critical care unit have no control over the choice of their environment or many of its stimuli.

In addition to the quality of a stimulus, the nurse must also consider the quantity. Too much of a desirable stimulus can become as unacceptable as a little of an undesirable stimulus. An example of excessive quantity of a good thing is gorging oneself with a favorite food to the point of revulsion. In the critical care unit, excessive and constant noise, bright light and hyperactivity can be as distorting and bothersome as gloom, silence, and indolence.

In dealing with the control of environmental stimuli in a critical care unit, the nurse must then be aware of both the quality and the quantity of sensory input. If sensory stimuli are diminished too drastically, the patient is exposed to sensory deprivation, which can cause severe disorganization of normal psychological defenses.[1] When sensory stimuli occur in excessive quantity, the phenomenon of sensory overload will create an equally undesirable response to the environment including confusion and withdrawal.

sensory deprivation

Sensory deprivation is a general term used to identify a variety of symptoms which occur following a reduction in the quantity and/or the degree of structure or quality of sensory input.[2] Other terms used to denote sensory deprivation or some form of it include *isolation, confinement, informational underload, perceptual deprivation,* and *sensory restriction.* A variety of symptoms or changes in behavior has been noted in normal adults following exposure to sensory deprivation for varying lengths of time. These include loss of sense of time; presence of delusions, illusions, and hallucinations; restlessness; and any of the types of behavior or symptoms present in psychoses.

Sensory deprivation need not be present for a period of days or weeks for psychopathological reactions to occur. In one study conducted on a normal young male subject, an 8-hour period of sensory deprivation elicited an acute psychotic reaction followed by continuation of delusions for several days, and severe depression and anxiety for a period of several weeks.[3] The degree of sensory deprivation possible in a laboratory setting is greater than that likely in a critical care unit, but it must be remembered that the subject was aware of the time involved in the experiment and also possessed clinically normal defense mechanisms, whereas hospital patients do not have these advantages.

It is not presently known how the stress of illness will affect human subjects exposed to sensory deprivation, but there is no reason to assume that such stress will make patients any less susceptible to adverse reactions to such deprivation. On the contrary, it would appear more logical to assume that patients faced with coping with illness would have increased susceptibility to more severe responses to sensory deprivation. The main types of patients most susceptible to the adverse effects of sensory deprivation would appear to be the defenseless or unconscious patient, the very young patient, the very old patient, and the postoperative patient.

Although it has been known for more than 20 years that sensory deprivation can lead to psychotic behavior, the nursing profession has done very little to apply this knowledge to its planning for patients in critical care units. Hospital personnel have long demonstrated at least a passing concern over the control of excessive noise causing sensory overload by the use of the familiar "Quiet, Please" signs in hospitals and other health care facilities, but a survey of the literature and an examination of many critical care units fails to demonstrate a similar concern for creating an environment intended to diminish the effects of sensory deprivation.

If unstructured sound or noise was all that was necessary to prevent the phenomena caused by sensory deprivation, most crisis care units would never need to be concerned with the concept at all. It is not, however, *quantity* alone that must be considered; even more important is the inclusion of planning the *quality* of stimuli in the external environment. A British investigator supports such a conclusion by stating, "Reality testing can only occur when there is a continual input of meaningful information from the outside world. When this is markedly reduced, as under experimental conditions of sensory deprivation, reality testing is impaired and internal mental events are taken to be events in the external world."[4]

REALITY TESTING

For reality testing to occur there must be familiar environmental stimuli. However, the sounds of the critical care unit cannot be said to be meaningful to more than a few medical and nursing personnel who spend long periods of their working life in such an environment. Therefore the nurse in the critical care unit should be certain that the environment offers the patient adequate stimuli to provide for reality testing. As human beings we take our physical environment for granted, but if we suddenly awoke in a world without grass or sunlight or the sounds of traffic or human speech we would not have the necessary stimuli to keep our minds in contact with reality. We would try to interpret the unknown stimuli on the basis of what we have always been familiar with. In reality, however, our interpretations may be wrong. This is especially true of patients who suffer temporary loss of any of the senses, particularly vision or hearing, since we normally utilize a combination of senses to interpret our environment.

This lack of reality testing may offer at least partial explanation for the high incidence of psychosis in patients commonly assigned to critical care units for long-term care due to an "unconscious state." The fact that no physical reason has ever been identified to explain post-traumatic psychosis offers additional support to such an assumption. Nursing is limited in its consideration of the unconscious patient who is often found in critical care units because authorities in the field have perpetuated the concept that such patients are insensitive to their environment and have perceptual disturbances that affect their responses to the environment. In view of the necessity of reality testing and the lack of meaningful information to allow such testing in the critical care unit, it is reasonable to explain some of the reactions of patients, including even the unconscious patient, as being caused by the lack of meaningful input which can be referred to as sensory deprivation. There is more empirical data to support this assumption than there is evidence for believing that post-traumatic psychosis is due to physical phenomena.

One example of such a situation caused by sensory deprivation in the critical care unit occurred during an experiment conducted by the writer with an unresponsive patient assumed to be unconscious by both the medical and nursing team members. She was a 20-year-old college student with severe basal skull trauma and multiple injuries who was unresponsive throughout the 8-day period she spent in a critical care unit. When she began responding verbally, her first words to her mother were: "Am I free now? I was in the hands of the Soviet Union!" An immediate interpretation of such a statement could reasonably be that she was totally out of contact with reality due to the injury and had dreamed such an episode. It is just as reasonable to assume that she could have perceived that the actions in the unit and treatments she received due to her condition were related to torture and she was the victim for some unknown reason. She had no noticeable motor control of her facial muscles, so she was "blind." She had a tracheostomy that required frequent suctioning. She was almost immobile because of fractures and spasticity necessitating plaster casts or cloth restraints on all extremities. It is reasonable to assume that such a situation could cause her to believe she was being tortured, since she had no means of interpreting her experience realistically from meaningful cues in the environment.

Many other situations and case histories can be reported to stress the importance of planning for and providing meaningful sensory stimulation for the patient cared for in all hospital units but especially the ones in critical care units. Nurses can play a significant role in alleviating the unnecessary stress caused by sensory deprivation by recognizing the need for the structuring of sensory input. The use of auditory stimuli such as the explanation of any treatment or procedure to be performed on a patient is a basic requirement and must not be overlooked as insignificant; but explanation alone is not adequate to prevent adverse effects of sensory deprivation. This type of communication can be considered a minimal requirement in a broader area of communication which can be called security information.

SECURITY INFORMATION

Security information helps prevent unnecessary anxiety and disorientation regarding date, time, and place. It also includes explanation of treatment and procedures. This is particularly important for patients with deviations in levels of consciousness due to trauma, drugs, or toxicity. Orientation to date and time could be encouraged not only by including the information in conversation but by providing large-faced clocks that are readily visible to the patient, and similar placement of large calendars displaying the day, month, and year in large figures. The simplicity of such information sometimes causes it to be overlooked, but it can affect the patient's comfort by providing information we take for granted. In addition, it is essential to provide this information because an assessment of the patient's state of orientation is often based on his answers to those questions.

A nursing history included in the initial phase of planning can help make nursing intervention an effective part of the total care. Such a history requires that individualized questions be asked of both patient and family members. A brief outline of a normal 24-hour period of activity and sleep habits gives a good starting point in compiling a useful nursing history. A concerned and well-informed nurse can determine the times when the individual's physiological functions are at both maximal and minimal levels. For example, urine output is minimal during the night when sleep normally occurs. Treatment and procedures not predicated by moment-to-moment conditions and necessary activities such as bathing can then be performed when maximum energy is available—or avoided if possible when lower energy levels are present. Physiological functions reach their lowest levels in the middle of the night, whereas in the early morning hours functions are beginning to move up to a maximum level. Therefore normal fluctuations in vital signs should be expected and patients should not be subjected to activity or stressful procedures in the early morning hours. Such predictability of peaks and troughs of physiological functions is possible due to increasing knowledge of periodicity, a topic which is briefly discussed later in this chapter.

Additional information which may be included in the nursing history could be anything from food likes to dislikes to favorite type of music or TV programs. It would be desirable to provide exposure to familiar stimuli such as playing a favorite record from home or finding the right radio station to listen to if the patient is not able to do it, or requesting a taped message sent from a loved one who cannot visit. Such action will offer meaningful sensory stimulation to the patient in an otherwise unfamiliar environment. A simple rule to use in collecting a nursing history is to determine what is significant or familiar to the patient and expose him to it if possible.

The family and friends should be involved in planning and providing such sensory input, especially for unconscious patients. One of the most miserable feelings must be that of uselessness on the part of a family member or friend at the bedside of an unresponsive loved one. During a survey conducted in critical care units preceding a research project on unconscious patients, this writer was repeatedly impressed by the scene of a mother, father, husband, wife, or other close relative standing at the bedside and staring with a variety of emotions at the unconscious patient. A simple direction, or granting of permission in some cases, to touch the patient's hand and talk to him brought a look of relief and gratitude to their faces. With further assistance on what to say to the patient, the visitor became very effective in diminishing sensory deprivation by discussing people or subjects familiar and of interest to the patient.

The value of simple conversation about everyday activities is underestimated in the care of the unconscious patient in critical care units. This is pointed out vividly in the following incident recorded in "A Study of Sensory Response in the Unconscious Patient":*

Critical Incident

Interest in nursing implications inherent in care of the unconscious patient beyond the physical dimensions was initiated while caring for a patient in her late fifties, comatose as a result of metastatic carcinoma of the brain. The investigator carried on a one-sided conversation about many things, including a daily introduction of self, explanations of care to be given, and discussion of the day and the weather. There was no perceptible response from the patient. Her condition appeared to be slowly deteriorating. Contact with the patient was lost after four days due to an assignment change.

About two months later while boarding a train the investigator was approached by a woman on crutches who called the investigator's name and asked if she were a nurse. Following an affirmative response and recognition of the previous nurse-patient interaction the investigator and the patient conversed for several hours. The discussion revealed much about the initial relationship between them. The patient expressed how she had felt during the days she lay in the hospital bed totally defenseless and at the mercy of those on the nursing team and that the investigator had been the only person who had identified herself and talked to the patient.

Of particular interest to the patient was information as to the nurse's time of leaving and when she would return. When the investigator had informed her she would be leaving for another assignment she said she had felt like crying because she anticipated receiving no further information about the outside world. The patient recalled much more about the interaction than the investigator.

---

* Janice Shirley Smith, "A Study of Sensory Response in the Unconscious Patient," thesis submitted to the faculty of the Graduate School of the University of Colorado in partial fulfillment of the requirements for the degree of Master of Science, School of Nursing, 1970.

Such experiences indicate that even in today's modern nursing world the little things, such as consideration of the patient as an individual deserving common courtesies, are still important to patients. It cannot be taken for granted that such behavior should be automatic since nurses are conditioned to be comfortable around the hectic environment of a critical care unit, and rapidly forget the sense of awe or fear that was present the first time they saw the unit. It might be helpful for the nurses in the critical care unit to stop for a moment each day and project themselves mentally into the patient's role to determine what information or activity might be desirable. Such an act might be effective in salvaging whatever human dignity is left for the patient after being subjected to the regressive procedures of being bathed, fed, and forced to meet toileting needs in bed shielded from other patients only by a cloth curtain with wide openings at top and bottom.

sensory overload

The area of sensory overload has not received as much attention as that of sensory deprivation, but some of its effects on humans are known. One of the best documented adverse effects is that of decreased hearing following long-term exposure to high noise levels such as those found in factories or machine shops. It is also recognized that tension and anxiety increase when an individual is exposed to noise for continuous periods of time without quiet periods of rest. Edgar Allan Poe capitalized on such knowledge in horror stories dealing with the effect of continuous rhythmical sounds such as the dripping of water or the whirring of machinery, as in "The Pit and the Pendulum." In more recent periods we have heard of the use of continuous noise as a means of torturing prisoners of war. We too must capitalize on this information. When patients become increasingly anxious or restless, environmental causes such as noise as well as physiological reasons such as hypercarbia must be considered in trying to determine the cause of such behavior.

Many years ago Florence Nightingale expressed her awareness of the effects of noise on patients: "Unnecessary noise is the most cruel absence of care which can be inflicted on either sick or well."[5]

Clues about the significance of both the quantity and quality of noise are offered by a study conducted in a recovery room. It was found that high levels of noise increased the need for pain medication. It is interesting to note, however, that the most pronounced reaction on the part of the recovery-room patient was that of resentment of the sound of occasional laughter from the recovery-room personnel.[6]

The presence of continuous noise in crisis care units must be minimized at least for some time in every 24-hour period. The cardiac monitors with their beeping should not be kept in areas where patients must hear them continuously. The physical planning for units must include provision for facilities where patients on continuous respirators are not in the same open area as other patients. However, ways have not yet been devised for protecting patients who are on the respirator from the machine's incessant cycling noise. Nor is it presently known how or if the sound of the machine has any adverse psychological effect on the patient. In view of the recent and ongoing advancement in technical methods necessary for retention of life, problems such as this will continue. As technology becomes more advanced and heroic life-saving measures succeed in significant numbers of patients, we will then be able to focus attention on their less apparent psychological needs.

The effect of continuous sound on the intricate physiological functions of the human organism is not fully known, but assumptions can be made that a variety of adverse responses can be expected. Even without such empirical data to support the need to control unnecessary noise we can look at our own life style to see how we react to continuous or loud noise. It is normal to attempt to plug our ears in the presence of a loud noise such as a firecracker, and it is just as normal to choose to sleep in a quiet room with the sounds of the outside world shut out by well-constructed walls or special soundproofing. It is perhaps not feasible to control noise in the environment of critical care units to the same extent the patient is accustomed to, but it is both feasible and essential that nurses exert a conscious effort to avoid unnecessary noise in such an environment.

Another facet of controlling unnecessary noise involves preventing exhaustion. There is adequate knowledge available in the areas of sleep research to prove that sleep is essential for both physical and mental well-being. Therefore nurses need to plan for and provide an environment which will not only allow but also encourage sleep for patients in critical care units. This sounds deceptively simple until one realizes what is necessary in meeting such a need. A darkened room makes it impossible to have the security of visual observation of the critically ill patient, but few people can sleep in a lighted room even if the lighting level is low or soft. Normal practice is to sedate many patients in such a unit, but the nurse must realize that drug-induced or interrupted sleep is not adequate for any significant period of time. The human organism must have normal uninterrupted periods of sleep that are long enough to allow all stages of sleep to occur. This normally means a period of a minimum of three to four hours, but even that is probably not adequate for most people for a period of more than a day or two.

the hospital phenomenon

The hospital environment is one that should be conducive to rest and recuperation from illness, but it is no surprise to any nurse that such a myth has long been dispelled. A bitter joke frequently heard from patients is that a hotel room is cheaper, has better food and service, and provides a better chance to get a rest.

The fact is that the hospital environment is one that deprives the patient of normal sensory stimuli while it bombards him with continuous strange sensory stimuli not found in the average home environment. This situation is a combination of sensory deprivation and sensory overload which will be referred to as the *hospital phenomenon.*

Normal sounds at home include voices of loved ones and friends, barking of neighborhood dogs, automobile, bus and train traffic and horns, the television or radio on a familiar station, children at play, the washing machine or dishwasher, the daytime telephone calls, and many other sounds and sights which do not diminish until night comes. Sounds in critical care units include voices of strangers in large numbers, movement of bed rails, beeping of cardiac monitors, paging systems calling strange names, suctioning of tracheostomies, telephones ringing at all hours, whispering and muffled voices. These are accompanied by continuous lighting, strange views of other areas, and fear and pain.

The combination of the loss of familiar stimuli and continuous exposure to strange stimuli elicits varying types of defensive responses from the patient.

Additional research is needed in this area, but it is fairly safe to assume that some degree of withdrawal from the frightening reality of the situation is a common defense mechanism. On the assumption that many patients cope by withdrawing, nurses should anticipate a delayed response when calling the patient's name and should provide extra environmental objects to orient the patient to time, date, and place.

periodicity

Another area of knowledge necessary for the nurse in the critical care unit deals with the broad concept of periodicity. Other terms include: *circadian rhythm, biological clock, internal clock,* and *physiological clock.* It has been recognized for a number of years that all living creatures have not only an identifiable life cycle but also short-term cycles which are rhythmical in nature; disruption of that rhythm can cause deviations from the normal or cessation of life. The human organism possesses a 24-hour cycle that is resistant to change, and long-term disruption can be fatal. Each of the biochemical and biophysical processes of the human body possesses a rhythm with peaks of function or activity which occur in consistent patterns within the normal 24-hour day we are accustomed to. Knowledge of when physiological functions are at their lowest level would allow for more intelligent assessment of the significance of vital-sign fluctuation, and even the quantity of urine output, since the kidneys possess their own unique rhythm as demanded by sleep and activity patterns. Drug dosage, sleep periods, and stressful procedures such as surgery may also someday be based on knowledge of individual circadian rhythms, thus avoiding further stress in the most vulnerable part of the cycle and capitalizing on the strongest parts of the cycle.

Even though the critical care environment traditionally shows lack of regard for the 24-hour cycle of the human organism by ignoring the need for a period of undisturbed sleep, the fact remains that the human organism cannot adapt to any other cycle. There are both physiological and psychological necessities for sleep that affect humans' potential for maximal recovery from illness in minimal time. Adverse side effects are numerous in individuals who are deprived of the stages of deep sleep and rapid-eye-movement

(REM) sleep for even a few days. The adverse effects include irritability and anxiety, physical exhaustion and fatigue, and even disruption of metabolic functions, including adrenal hormone production.

Such adverse effects indicate the necessity for providing an environment conducive to all stages of sleep including the REM stage. Because a cycle of sleep measured from REM stage to REM stage requires from 90 to 100 minutes, it is important to provide periods of a minimum of 2 hours of uninterrupted sleep during the night.[7] More frequent arousal can cause enough disruption to deprive the patient of essential cyclic rest and activity periods and create a situation incompatible with life.

When assessing the patient's condition, consider whether or not there have been adequate uninterrupted time periods for all stages of sleep to occur. The plan must provide such periods as early as possible following admission to the unit. The necessity of taking vital signs every 1 or 2 hours during the night must be weighed against the damage caused to the human organism when it is deprived of sleep. Only the most critical condition could warrant ignoring the equally fatal outcome when exhaustion causes disequilibrium of physiological functions. Intelligent nursing care will provide rest periods for the patient with the same emphasis as providing assessment of cardiac status or other aggressive physical measures of care.

The usual critical care environment disregards the need to control the 24-hour sounds, light and activity by having open units for six to ten patients who require care at variable times. Commitment to controlling the activity of the environment can diminish the constant level of noise, but additional measures may be necessary. If the patient is receptive to wearing darkened eyeshades and earplugs to shut out light and sound, he may be able to tolerate the environment with less stress. This is the least we can offer a patient to minimize the adverse effects of the environment until units can be developed which consider rest and sleep for the critically ill patient. No patient needs such consideration more, but the irony of the situation is that this critically ill patient is placed in the least desirable environment for meeting such needs.

patients with special problems

Patients assigned to critical care units are acknowledged as having special problems which cannot be cared for in the usual hospital setting. They need almost constant observation and/or special life-saving equipment requiring specialized training and knowledge. Some patients have additional needs because they are especially susceptible to the environmental influences of the critical care unit. As noted above, the patients most likely to be adversely affected by the environment include: (1) the unconscious or defenseless, (2) the very young, (3) the elderly, and (4) the postoperative.

The areas of care discussed in this chapter are relevent to the child with some variation in degree of significance; however, further discussion is outside the scope of this book. The information also applies to patients coming out of anesthesia in the recovery room. The main difference is that the time in the recovery room does not usually exceed a few hours, while patients in intensive care units stay for days and in some instances for weeks. Special emphasis will be given to the elderly patient and to the defenseless or unresponsive patient.

the elderly patient in critical care

Because of the large number of elderly people who need intensive care, critical care nurses need knowledge about the special problems of the elderly. Since the elderly often have some deterioration of their senses, nurses who are not aware of and sensitive to these problems can contribute to the stresses they have already experienced.

In order to diminish the potentially adverse effects of the critical care environment for the elderly it is necessary for the nurse to (1) assess the senses, (2) recognize the symptoms of acute brain syndrome, (3) use reality orientation therapeutically, and (4) know the views on death and dying held by elderly people.

It is essential to fully assess the senses of each elderly person, particularly for a history of visual and auditory deficits.[8] If the elderly patient is unable to filter out environmental sounds in order to hear soft spoken sounds, talking louder or asking the patient to use a hearing aid may help. It will not help, however, to talk loudly (or yell) at the elderly person whose hearing is intact but whose motor responses are blocked by injury such as from a cerebral vascular accident.

If glasses are worn by the elderly patient, it is important to provide the glasses even if the patient is not able to request them. Clean eyeglasses placed on the patient will provide the opportunity of viewing the unknown and frightening environment rather than requiring imagination to interpret the area. Many elderly persons may be dependent on glasses to "hear" since it is not uncommon for them to rely on lipreading to communicate.

The response to vocal requests may be significantly delayed in the elderly. It is normal for motor responses to be slowed in these patients and this along with the tendency to withdraw from the hyperactivity of the critical care unit may further extend their response time. It is necessary to allow a longer period of time for any motor response, including a vocal response to a question. It is reasonable to wait a full minute before repeating a request.

Actions that appear to denote disorientation of a pathological nature may be prematurely labeled *chronic brain syndrome* when they may actually be *acute brain syndrome*. In view of the grave consequences of hopelessness projected on the patient with chronic brain syndrome, it is imperative that adequate historical data be collected to differentiate between the two conditions. The primary difference between them is that acute brain syndrome has a rapid onset but is considered reversible, while chronic brain syndrome is slow in onset and is irreversible. The significance of such differences has a great impact on nursing care.

Symptoms of acute brain syndrome include: (1) fluctuation in the level of awareness, (2) visual hallucinations (auditory hallucinations are not present), (3) misidentification of persons (usually in the form of thinking a nurse is some close relative such as a sister or daughter), and (4) severe restlessness.[9]

A sudden change in the elderly person's life, such as removal from familiar surroundings or administration of certain sedative and tranquilizing drugs, can precipitate these symptoms. The following situation reported by Dr. William Kiely illustrates these points.[10]

> A 78-year-old retired schoolteacher was knocked down by a purse snatcher while on her way to a neighborhood grocery store. There was no physical injury evident but the event triggered an episode of paroxysmal tachyarrythmia accompanied by vascular collapse with a blood pressure of 79/30 mm. Hg.
>
> At the emergency room she was able to coherently recount her experience and seemed more upset by the loss of her eyeglasses than her purse. She seemed mildly disoriented about time and place. A comprehensive physical and laboratory exam revealed only a low blood pressure and atrial flutter. With treatment, both of these returned to normal.
>
> The patient's mental status, however, continued to deteriorate. She became increasingly disoriented and demanded that nursing personnel explain their presence in her "apartment." She became restless, climbed over the bedrails and when soft restraints were applied, became even more restless. Then she heard voices and screamed that people were trying to kill her. Sodium Amytal, 500 mg. IM initially sedated her but later heightened her arousal.

The very close correlation of these symptoms with the symptoms of sensory deprivation discussed earlier creates a situation that makes it impossible to differentiate the cause initially. A concerted effort at reality orientation by the nursing staff must be started immediately as a primary treatment for either condition.

Reality orientation requires a rigid, repetitive regime of giving security information at predetermined times around the clock. The monotony of the procedure may make nurses want to give up the regime when there is no positive response after a few days. For the benefit of the patient, however, it must continue until she can repeat the information on request (or until death releases the nurse from the responsibility). After a few days, repetition is more comfortable if the information is prefaced by a statement to the patient that you know the information has been stated many times but that it is important to the patient so it will be repeated until she is able to say it to you.

The elderly patient must adapt to a major change in her spatial perception and territory when placed in the critical care unit. The frequently existing problems related to diminished vision and hearing combined with disruption of territory create greater vulnerability to adverse effects from sensory deprivation and sensory overload.

At a time in life when adapting to change becomes increasingly difficult and painful, the patient is confronted with a limitation of territory that exceeds any such limits in the past. Even the patient coming from a long-term care facility has had more space to call her own and greater freedom to organize it in the manner she desires than she will have in the critical care unit. The historically diminishing size of the territory possessed and controlled by the elderly creates psychological pain and a decrease in self-esteem. The nurse in a critical care unit can be sensitive to this by avoiding unnecessary intrusion into the patient's now further diminished territory.

Limitation of the space available to the patient in the critical care unit is severe enough, but further limits occur because extensions of territoriality are unavailable in this setting. Examples of extensions utilized frequently by the elderly patient include radio, television, and telephones. Both televisions and telephones are normally denied to the patients in these units. However, the availability of small television sets with earplugs for sound control and telephones with wall jacks makes the use of both easily feasible in the critical care unit. Nursing assessment can determine the patient's ability to benefit from their use without harmful effects.[11] The nurse who recognizes the potentially great therapeutic effect of such territorial extensions will incorporate them in the humanistic plan of care for all patients, with special awareness of the unique needs of the elderly.

Intrusions into the critically limited territory of the elderly patient also occur in the form of impersonal equipment kept at the bedside (suction machines, monitors, oxygen equipment, IV equipment, etc.) which the patient does not view as his possessions. This creates a situation in which his spatial orientation is limited to the confines of the bed and possibly a bedside stand. For this reason, the patient usually clusters all of his personal possessions in the bed or on the small stand. Nurses should tolerate such space-occupying items since their importance to the patient far exceeds their interference to the nurse.

A visit to the home or room of an elderly person characteristically reveals the presence of multiple treasures on walls, tables, and shelves, including pictures, books, glass items, etc. No matter how poverty-stricken the person is there will be some highly prized items. These objects develop increased value for the elderly as the years pass, and the nurse must protect such possessions brought to the unit and allow the patients to position them wherever they wish within the pathetically small territory they are able to cling to.

The informed and sensitive nurse will preface any intrusion into the personal territory of the patient with appropriate conversation, including an explanation of the reason for invading the space, and then await the cue that the patient is ready and receptive to the invasion. Such cues can be vocal or projected through body language, including facial expressions and body posturing. A receptive cue could be in the statement, "Well, if it has to be done then go ahead," or a beginning movement to turn over to expose the area for the shot. Cues that you are rushing too much may include the question, "Why do I have to have that?" or a movement to tighten the covers near the neck. Such cues demand more explanation and less haste.

Being aware that dying is looked upon as the final stage and natural outcome of life by many elderly persons may help the staff when it has been decided that death should occur without further intervention. While this problem of when to withhold further intervention is certainly not unique to the elderly, there are certain aspects of the problem generally more common in the elderly. Certainly the 80-year-old with a history of a CVA will have dealt more directly with his feelings of dying (and his family with their feelings of losing him to death) than will have the 18-year-old and his family. No implication is intended, however, that age alone is a criterion for determining the extent of the heroic effort to sustain life, but rather that age is a highly significant factor to be considered along with factors such as previous state of health and current cause of illness.

It is important that whenever possible the patient's feelings about dying must be listened to, and the family must be included in discussions and decisions. Enforcement of restrictive visiting rules should be ignored in such a situation to prevent further adverse effects of isolation on the patient and to assist the family in dealing with the common feelings of guilt at such a time. The family also suffers from adverse effects caused by the critical care environment. No hospital policy should be allowed to remove humanistic values from nursing care.

Roberts has expressed an opinion that perhaps we ignore the patient's wishes and prolong the process of dying rather than doing what we see as prolonging life.[12] She also reminds us that many aged patients have control over their lives until they lose control when admitted to the critical care unit. The role of the nurse becomes vital and she must resolve her own feelings about death as she works with the patient and family in an advocacy role. Perhaps the elderly see what we cannot when they plead with us to let them die. It is wrong to project our personal fear of death on the patient who repeatedly pleads with us to stop our heroic efforts to sustain a poor quality of life manifested many times by constant pain and exhaustion.

the unresponsive patient

The patient most likely to suffer greatest psychological trauma related to the adverse effects of the environment is the patient traditionally labeled "unconscious." While the disease processes causing unconsciousness are widely diversified, the more common causes are usually related to trauma of extracranial or intracranial origin. Such primary disease processes are frequently accompanied by multiple traumas such as fractures, lacerations, and unknown soft tissue damage. This patient requires care which considers both physical and psychological needs and which is given by a nurse who believes that human dignity is a basic right to be preserved.

Few patients place as many significant and continuous demands on the nurse as the unconscious patient, but too often the only emphasis of care is on the patient's physical needs. There is no desire to minimize the physical needs, since the patient depends totally on the nurse and other members of the health care team for life preservation. If we wish to give optimal care, however, more concern must be focused on the psychosocial needs of unconscious patients in critical care units.

The first precept that must be developed is that the most descriptive diagnostic label for such a patient is *unresponsive* since that is the only condition that can be demonstrated by assessment methods currently utilized in the health care fields. The term *unresponsive* means that motor and sensory coordinated responses are not currently identifiable in a particular patient. The term *unconscious* denotes a lack of sensory awareness that cannot currently be measured in the absence of concurrent motor response.

Replacing the label unconscious with the term unresponsive removes the connotation of lack of awareness which is automatically associated with the term unconscious. Taber's *Cyclopedic Medical Dictionary* gives a literal translation of unconscious as "not aware." It further defines the word as, "A state of being insensible or without conscious experiences." A survey of other such reference books by current health care authorities reveals similar definitions. This mental set is being perpetuated in spite of documented incidents that invalidate such a definition for many patients who are labeled unconscious. (See the Critical Incident described above.)

The probability that some unresponsive patients are also unconscious is very likely. However, in view of the current lack of ability to make such an assessment, the only logical approach for nurses to take is that *no patient is unconscious*. From that assumption the care required is the same as that needed by the patient with an intact communication process.

The assessment and control of pain is a major problem area in nursing. Pain is rarely acknowledged as existing in unresponsive patients who are totally defenseless due to the absence of meaningful motor activity. That such a patient is defenseless is clearly evidenced by the fact that he cannot demand something for pain or refuse any invasive procedure that is performed regardless of how severe the pain may be. The author has observed a physical debridement of tissue, through a window cut in the cast from the site of an open fracture of the proximal end of the radial bone, on an "unresponsive" patient. No anesthesia or pain medication was utilized. This would never be tolerated by any person with the ability to manifest a motor response by vocally rejecting it (loudly!) or by fleeing from the procedure.

In view of the knowledge that pain can be severe enough to be fatal in instances where the injury itself is not lethal, it appears that such procedures are contraindicated without appropriate pain control measures. Much more investigation of pain is needed for the development of a safe and humane plan of care for such a patient. If the current assumption that the patient who does not scream with pain is not capable of feeling pain is replaced by the more likely assumption that pain is felt but response to it is blocked, then survival rates of multiple trauma patients may improve.

Due to the inability to prove the *absence* of sensory functioning in the unresponsive patient, it is imperative that nursing care be planned in the context that sensory function exists in some form. All senses should be considered rather than just hearing. The traditional belief that hearing may be the last sense lost may have prevented some unnecessary conversations in the presence of the patient, but historically it has done very little to develop a theoretical framework of nursing care which acknowledges the existence of sensory functioning.

Use of the more logical term *unresponsive* for the patient who cannot respond to commands due to motor-sensory pathology could initiate a refreshingly new positive approach to care. It is certainly the word best suited to directing nursing care.

summary

The environment of a critical care unit possesses the unique ability to deprive a patient of meaningful sensory input while exposing him to a continual bombardment of unfamiliar stimuli causing potential sensory overload. A period of casual observation of sounds and activity in such a unit will identify a wide variety of sounds not present in the normal environment outside the hospital setting. The only readily identifiable familiar sound is that of the ringing of the telephone, and even that can create frustration. For example, think about your internal response to a ringing telephone. After years of conditioning, a ringing telephone elicits an automatic movement to answer it and a feeling of frustration when it is left unanswered. This can create additional stress for an immobile patient in a strange environment.

The unfamiliarity of the environment is a potential double threat to patients already faced with coping with a severe crisis that demands more energy than may be available. The challenge is in recognizing the potential for using the presently rampant environment of the crisis care unit as a controlled and therapeutic tool in the total care of the patient in the unit.

Effective planning can reverse the current traumatic situation present in most critical care units. Total control of the sounds and activities is not possible in the physical setting present in most units used in hospitals today, but the nurse can exert her influence in the knowledgeable planning of future units. It is not possible to give concrete directions that will fit all situations, but it is important to know that sensory input can be hazardous if it is excessive, meaningless, or too continuous. This knowledge, combined with the awareness that the patient is probably not familiar with the life-saving but noisy technical machinery, will make the nurse in the critical care unit a knowledgeable and effective practitioner and negotiator for the patient.

A great number of nursing measures are presently possible, and identification of them will result in a significant advance in the area of individualization of care. Nursing has used the phrase "individualization of care" for a long time, but now needs to apply it to the critical care units more extensively than ever before. The area of individualization of physical care has been more tangible, and was therefore the initial area of care focused on. However, the psychological care of the patient should now receive more emphasis. Some of our actions have been traditional rather than logical with empirical data supporting them. Knowledge available today indicates that actions must be justified in light of weighing their potential adverse effects against their validity and necessity. In other words, it is necessary to determine whether or not the omission of the act is more threatening than its commission, as in arousing a patient to take a BP at the expense of disrupting the REM (rapid eye movement) stage of sleep. The robot action of following a routine without theoretical knowledge involved in decision making is no longer a function of the nurse. Instead it is necessary to make decisions based on sound rationale, with knowledge of the consequences and evaluation of the effects.

future hope

The near future should see many important improvements in the care provided the patient in critical care units. Rapidly developing technology will undoubtedly reach levels that only a few of the most creative dreamers will foresee. Three areas needing major change and for which adequate knowledge and technology appear already available are:
1. Nursing utilization of a method of measuring physiological activity in order to assess the unresponsive patient's awareness of the environment. This is no more impossible than the use of the ECG appeared to the nurse 15 years ago. Such assessment will significantly enhance care of the patient who has loss of coordinated motor response necessary for communication in the current movement-bound manner.
2. Use of the term unresponsive rather than unconscious. As assessment techniques advance, so too will the description of our findings. Meanwhile, unresponsive is the term which better describes a total lack of motor response.
3. Provision of environmentally controlled units for all critically ill patients offering full control of sound, light, and temperature. With the sophistication of patient monitoring equipment rapidly advancing, it will be possible to assess and monitor life signs without the use of contact instrumentation such as blood pressure cuffs and thermometers. Such procedures now normally require disturbing the patient on a 24-hour basis or not collecting such data during the periods of sleep which are necessary for restoring energy.

When soundproof units with life-function monitoring devices of a noninvasive nature are a reality, nurses can focus on providing therapeutic structuring of the environment, since they will be free of the routine, repetitive functions now consuming a significant amount of time in each 24-hour period. Patients will not have to suffer the adverse effects of the hospital phenomenon to the same degree, and can receive the benefits of care planned to fit within their personal 24-hour cycle of biological rhythmicity.

REFERENCES

1. G. C. Curtis et al., "A Psychopathological Reaction Precipitated by Sensory Deprivation," *American Journal of Psychiatry*, Vol. 125 (August 1968), pp. 255–260.
2. H. B. Adams et al., "Sensory Deprivation and Personality Change," *Journal of Nervous and Mental Disease*, Vol. 143 (September 1966), p. 256.
3. G. C. Curtis, et al., *op. cit.*
4. J. P. Leff, "Perceptual Phenomena and Personality in Sensory Deprivation," *British Journal of Psychiatry*, Vol. 114 (December 1968), pp. 1499–1508.
5. T. W. Hurst, "Is Noise Important in Hospitals?" *International Journal of Nursing Studies,* Vol. 3 (September 1966), pp. 125–131.
6. Barbara Minckley, "A Study of Noise and Its Relationship to Patient Discomfort in the Recovery Room," *Nursing Research*, Vol. 17, No. 3 (May–June 1968), pp. 247–250.
7. Gay Gaer Luce, *Body Time: Physiological Rhythms and Social Stress* (New York: Pantheon Books, 1971), p. 86.
8. Irene Mortenson Burnside, "The Special Senses and Sensory Deprivation," *Psychosocial Nursing Care of the Aged*, Irene M. Burnside, ed. (New York: McGraw-Hill Book Company, 1976), pp. 387–394.
9. Robert N. Butler and Myrna L. Lewis, *Aging and Mental Health* (St. Louis: C. V. Mosby Company, 1973), pp. 71–72.
10. William F. Kiely, "Critical Care Psychiatric Syndrome," *Heart and Lung*, Vol. 2, No. 1 (January–February 1973), pp. 54–55.
11. Sharon L. Roberts, "Territoriality: Space and the Aged Patient in Intensive Care Units," *Psychosocial Nursing Care of the Aged*, Irene M. Burnside, ed. (New York: McGraw-Hill Book Company, 1973), pp. 72–83.
12. Sharon L. Roberts, "To Die or Not to Die: Plight of the Aged Patient in ICU," *Psychosocial Nursing Care of the Aged*, Irene M. Burnside, ed. (New York: McGraw-Hill Book Company, 1973), pp. 96–106.

BIBLIOGRAPHY

Adams, H. B., et al., "Sensory Deprivation and Personality Change," *Journal of Nervous and Mental Disease*, Vol. 143 (September 1966), pp. 256–265.
Benoliel, J. Q., et al., "As the Patient Views the ICU and CCU," *Heart and Lung*, Vol. 4, No. 2 (March–April 1975), pp. 260–264.
Blake, Florence G., "Immobilized Youth," *American Journal of Nursing*, Vol. 69, No. 11 (November 1969), pp. 2364–2369.
Catlin, Francis, "Noise and Emotional Stress," *Journal of Chronic Diseases*, Vol. 18 (June 1965), pp. 509–518.
Comer, Nathan L., Leo Madow, and James J. Dixon, "Observations of Sensory Deprivation in a Life-Threatening Situation," *American Journal of Psychiatry*, Vol. 125 (August 1967), pp. 164–169.
Curtis, G. C., et al., "A Psychopathological Reaction Precipitated by Sensory Deprivation," *American Journal of Psychiatry*, Vol. 125 (August 1968), pp. 255–260.

Gerdes, Lenore, "The Confused or Delirious Patient," *American Journal of Nursing,* Vol. 68 (June 1968) pp. 1228–1233.

Golub, Sharon, "Noise, the Underrated Health Hazard," *R.N.* (May 1969), pp. 40–45.

Hackett, Thomas P., "Pain and Prejudice: Why Do We Doubt that the Patient Is in Pain?" *Medical Times,* Vol. 99, No. 2 (February 1971), pp. 130–141.

Humphries, J., "Thoughts on Care of the Elderly: A Life Worth Living," *Nursing Times,* Vol. 71, No. 42 (October 16, 1975), pp. 1661–1662.

Hurst, T. W., "Is Noise Important in Hospitals?" *International Journal of Nursing Studies,* Vol. 3 (September 1966), pp. 125–131.

Jacox, Ada, and Mary Stewart, *Psychosocial Contingencies of the Pain Experience,* H.E.W., The University of Iowa, 1973.

Kiersnowski, Cynthia, Donna Martsolf, and Patricia O'Brien, "Miss Greene Thought We Were 'Torturing' Her," *Nursing '76* (September 1976), pp. 58–60.

Leff, J. P., "Perceptual Phenomena and Personality in Sensory Deprivation," *British Journal of Psychiatry,* Vol. 114 (December 1968), pp. 1499–1508.

Minckley, Barbara, "A Study of Noise and Its Relationship to Patient Discomfort in the Recovery Room," *Nursing Research,* Vol. 17, No. 3 (May–June, 1968), pp. 247–250.

part II: the nurse

VELARIE RICHARD FRUSHA, R.N., B.S.

Just as the effects of the critical care unit can create havoc with both the physical and the mental well-being of the critically ill patient, so too can the critical care unit become a stressful work environment which poses serious and damaging effects on the physical and mental health of critical care nurses.

Social critics blame stressful work situations on the frantic pace of contemporary American life style: the crowding, the hurried pace, the pressure to achieve. We, through lack of specific methods to minimize stress, become the victims of our reactions to it. Occupational stress increases the risk of illness, decreases work satisfaction, and results in the loss of many dollars and work hours each year. The results of occupational stress in nursing are also seen in high rates of attrition and absenteeism and in a decline in morale. In addition, nurses under stress are unable to give support to critically ill patients and their families. For these reasons, nurses must look for the causes of their occupational stress and find solutions to alleviate the problems.

Several factors affect occupational stress in nursing, particularly critical care nursing. One is the nurse's individual philosophy about nursing. Some nurses strive for the ultimate goal in nursing, quality care, regardless of the price they pay with their own physical and mental health. Nurses who continually support critically ill patients, physically and mentally, day-in and day-out, begin to deplete their own coping mechanisms. Few nurses who develop high standards for their care will give less care without some sense of guilt. Because of their commitment, many nurses continue to work in stressful situations in spite of the occupational hazards.

The influences of our technological society compound and abet the problem of occupational stress in critical care nursing. As part of society, nurses are affected by issues, trends, problems, and changes of society in general. Some of the changes, such as scientific and technological advances, have directly influenced the evolution of critical care units. The intricate machinery combined with an often too hectic environment adds to the occupational stress experienced by nurses.

Women's liberation along with the expanding role of the nurse has created new conflicts and enhanced the stress experienced by many women in critical care nursing. As a result of these changes, women have recently allowed themselves to accept newly created nursing roles—roles that require advanced nursing knowledge and decision making, and that entail added responsibilities and pressures. At the same time, preparation for these new roles often focused only on knowledge and skills and rarely on helping nurses, as women, deal internally and externally with increased levels of responsibility.

A lack of congruity between nursing education and nursing practice is another factor that has contributed to the stress of critical care nursing. For many nurses there continues to be a large gap between what they are taught in their educational institutions and the actual opportunities provided for practice in the hospital setting. The pressures and frustrations often arise from the conflict between the services which nurses wish to provide and those which are possible to provide in an understaffed, underfinanced, and under-equipped facility.

All of these forces have contributed to the stress which occurs in (a) the individual nurse, (b) the critical care environment, and (c) the interactions that occur between the two.

Several hospital situations produce anxiety in nurses and are potentially stressful. These include being in constant contact with the physically ill person, working with patients whose rehabilitation is uncertain, and dealing with psychological stress in patients, their families, and colleagues. However, the major influencing force behind the nurse's stress is the social organization of the hospital structure.[1]

Nursing Service often attempts to protect nurses from disturbing emotional experiences by fragmenting nursing care through patient care assignments, and by limiting the amount of interpersonal contact and communication between nurse and patient. Depersonalization of patients by identifying them by numbers or disease entities further removes nurses from developing a personal and emotional alliance with the patient. Furthermore, nurses themselves are often identified by their position or status in the organization rather than by name, e.g., the *Supervisor* says . . . . This type of overprotection only evokes stress by never allowing nurses to fully utilize their personal capacities and professional skills. The hospital social structure is nonsupportive of the nurse in stress, and it is the professional situation in which the nurse works rather than the nurse's personality which is often the source of emotional and psychological stress.[2]

In order to identify stresses in both intensive and nonintensive nursing care settings, Gentry and colleagues gave a battery of tests to a group of nurses from each setting.[3] No differences were found between nurses working in intensive and nonintensive care settings in general personality patterns, conditions of guilt, or self-esteem. However, intensive care nurses reported more anxiety, depression and hostility than nonintensive care nurses. This supports the premise that the work situation rather than the nurse's personality is the source of stress. The occupational stress was related to an overwhelming workload, increased responsibility, lack of continuing education, a limited work area, and poor communication between coprofessionals.

Other sources of tension were identified by a group of nurses working in a coronary care unit.[4] Heavy lifting was listed as the most frequent cause of stress. Bad schedules, required participation in research, too hectic a pace, families annoying the staff, the patient's prognosis, a patient's troublesome personality, conflicts with coprofessionals, the unavailability of physicians when needed, and a feeling of incompetence were other stresses identified by these nurses.

intervention

Different critical care units will have varying sources and levels of stress. Each unit will host its own unique conflicts and pressures depending on its structure, purpose, and staff. Some specialized units will be more stressful than others. Regardless of these differences, interventions must be developed for the support of personnel who work in these areas. Specific steps can be taken to reduce occupational stress in critical care personnel.

A good place to start is with the unit personnel and their immediate supervisors. Nurses who choose to work in a specialized setting must possess certain qualifications: they must be motivated, healthy, and competent in their field, able to rely on the skills and judgments of one another, and willing to give of themselves during patient-nurse interactions.

The unit supervisors, head nurses and coordinators should be trained in the area of humanistic supportive techniques. Developing such techniques involves advanced training in interpersonal relationships and in dealing with the emotions and conflicts of personnel. In addition, provisions should also be made for supplying the units with behavioral experts.[5] A psychiatric nurse clinician or psychiatric consultant can be of value in leading group discussions and teaching staff members methods of solving patient and staff conflicts. The following steps should be included in resolving group conflicts:

1. Identification and acknowledgment of feelings;
2. Sharing of these feelings;
3. Review of the experience with criticism, support and praise;
4. Integration of what is learned with application in future experiences.[6]

To further reduce stress for nurses in critical care units, auxiliary personnel should be hired to do nonnursing functions. This will allow nurses the freedom to interact with patients and their families in crisis. Once nurses achieve the freedom and time to give this type of care, work satisfaction will increase and fear of involvement will decrease.

In order to help units function better, one physician should be in authority as medical director.[7] This physician should fill the role of practitioner, teacher, gatekeeper, supporter, and adviser to the staff in the unit. This physician can play a key role in keeping conflicts between medical colleagues to a minimum by screening the patients that will be admitted into the unit. The physician's main function is to act in the best interest of the patient and the critical care staff.

Nursing Service can directly support the critical care staff in several different ways. It must recognize the fact that nurses in high-risk areas need regular rest and relaxation apart from the unit. For example, Nursing Service must insist on better staffing, better schedules, and opportunities for temporary rotation to other areas of the hospital.

Nursing Service can keep environmental stress to a minimum by adequately staffing the unit with competent nurses and supervisors. The nurse-patient ratio should remain small to prevent work overload so that nurses are able to maintain alertness to subtle patient changes. Lines of communication need to be kept open between critical care nurses and Nursing Service administration. This kind of communication can be accomplished by having a unit representative meet routinely with the medical staff and Nursing Service. Competent and informed nurses have fewer reasons for becoming frustrated and pressured in highly charged areas. In addition, Nursing Service must support continued education by providing regular staffing patterns.

Critical care units must take into consideration patients' and staff's privacy needs. Units should be constructed with spatial needs in mind. Specialty units are hectic enough without the compounding problem of limited work areas. Lounges must be provided as areas for withdrawal and rest periods, as well as places to hold staff conferences. These lounges should be designed into the unit so that nurses have both easy access to patients and privacy. This careful placement of rest and meeting rooms is essential because it is difficult to arrange for qualified coverage in the critical care unit.

Nurses must come to grips with the reality that nursing, like other professions, has stressful components attached to it. Nursing Service can provide leadership in identifying high-risk areas and in formulating, instituting and evaluating plans to reduce occupational stress.

evaluating occupational stress

A tool for nurses to evaluate their own unit stress must be developed. Measurements of attrition rates, absenteeism, requests for transfer and intrastaff conflicts are reliable indicators of occupational stress. Research which compares levels of patient care to levels of stress in critical care personnel is needed to document nurses' needs for nonhazardous working conditions. Finally, nurses must demonstrate that the quality of patient care improves as the working conditions become less stressful.

summary

Intensive care units have become a vital part of the hospital organization, even though they have added to the stress experienced by nurses. It is, therefore, most important that nurses make it their responsibility to see that these units are not the cause of their demoralization, but become the major impetus to the development of more competent, healthy, and autonomous nurses.

REFERENCES

1. I. Menzies, "Nurses Under Stress," *International Nursing Review,* Vol. 7, No. 6 (December 1960), pp. 9–16.
2. *Ibid.*
3. W. D. Gentry, S. B. Foster, and M. S. Froehling, "Psychologic Response to Situational Stress in Intensive and Nonintensive Nursing," *Heart and Lung,* Vol. 1 (November–December 1975), pp. 793–796.
4. N. H. Cassem and T. P. Hackett, "Sources of Tension for the CCU Nurse," *American Journal of Nursing,* Vol. 72 (August 1972), pp. 1426–1430.
5. P. Holsclaw, "Nursing in High Emotional Risk Areas," *Nursing Forum,* Vol. 4, No. 4 (1965), p. 44.
6. N. H. Cassem and T. P. Hackett, "Stress on the Nurse and Therapist in the Intensive Care Unit and the Coronary Care Unit," *Heart and Lung,* Vol. 4 (March–April 1975), p. 258.
7. D. Hay and D. Oken, "The Psychological Stresses of Intensive Care Nursing," *Psychosomatic Medicine,* Vol. 34 (March–April 1972), p. 117.

BIBLIOGRAPHY

Bilodeau, C., "The Nurse and Her Reactions to Critical Care Nursing," *Heart and Lung,* Vol. 3 (May–June 1973), pp. 358–363.
Colls, J., "Future Shock Invades Nursing," *Journal of Nursing Administration,* Vol. 5 (March–April 1975), pp. 27–28.

Jones, E., "Who Supports the Nurse?" *Nursing Outlook,* Vol. 10 (July 1962), pp. 476–478.

Kornfield, D., "Psychiatric View of the Intensive Care Unit," *British Medical Journal,* (January 11, 1969), pp. 108–109.

Michaels, D., "Too Much in Need of Support to Give Any?" *American Journal of Nursing,* Vol. 71 (October 1971), pp. 1932–1935.

Nash, P., "Nursing Stress," *Nursing Times,* Vol. 71 (March 1975), p. 476.

Oberst, M., "The Crisis-Prone Staff Nurse," *American Journal of Nursing,* Vol. 73 (November 1973), pp. 1917–1921.

Strauss, A., "The Intensive Care Unit: Its Characteristics and Social Relationships," *Nursing Clinics of North America,* Vol. 3, No. 1 (March 1968), pp. 7–15.

Vreeland, R., and G. L. Ellis, "Stress and the Nurse in an Intensive Care Unit," *Journal of the American Medical Association,* Vol. 208 (April 1969), pp. 332–334.

West, D., "Stresses Associated with ICU's Affect Patients, Families, Staff," *Hospitals,* Vol. 49 (December 1976), pp. 62–63.

core body systems

A. THE CARDIOVASCULAR SYSTEM
B. THE RESPIRATORY SYSTEM
C. THE RENAL SYSTEM
D. THE NERVOUS SYSTEM

MARGARET ANN BERRY, R.N., M.A., M.S.

7

normal structure and function of the cardiovascular system

anatomy and physiology of the heart

During the 70 years in the life of the average individual, the heart pumps 5 quarts of blood per minute, 75 gallons per hour, 70 barrels a day – 18 million barrels in a lifetime. The work accomplished by this organ is completely out of proportion to its size, but this fact is not so surprising when one considers the economy of size in the overall architecture of the entire body. The surprising thing is that for most people the heart presents no illness problem, and it functions normally throughout their life span. For the individual who does develop a cardiac problem, the result is much different. When a pathological condition manifests itself in this vital organ, the effects are extremely dramatic and the outcome often drastic. It is for this reason that you the reader are presently addressing yourself to the problems that arise from functional deviations of the heart. To assess, manage, and evaluate nursing problems with which you must deal, it is necessary to have a solid foundation in understanding normal structure, function, and pathogenesis of cardiac action. Nursing appropriately addresses itself to supporting the medical regimen developed for the individual patient. However, its primary concern should lie in the conservation of the patient's resources by accurately predicting when and where critical problems may present themselves which will deter the success of the medical and nursing plan and the improvement of the individual's health status. The information contained in this chapter and the one following is therefore concerned with the normal structure and function of the heart and with the pathogenic variables which lead to the development of coronary heart disease, as well as those which progressively produce more dysfunction in the circulatory system.

Humans are biopsychosocial beings, constantly faced with the necessity of interacting with their environment and all other organisms and forces within it. Although it is necessary to approach the study of structure and function in a dissective manner, every effort will be made to recall the reader to the consideration of the *gestalt* of cardiac function as it operates to maintain the individual's steady state in harmony with the environment.

As multicellular organisms evolved, two crucial problems arose: (1) providing each cellular unit with those substances needed to carry on its differentiated function, and (2) removing waste products from the immediate vicinity. In response to these fundamental demands, a circulatory system evolved along with a pumping unit—the heart. As the complexity of the organism increased, this system became further elaborated, culminating in the four-chambered heart of the mammal or class Mammalia of which man is but one species.

Although humans enjoy a terrestrial existence, their individual cells are dependent upon the ability to exchange materials across membranes which are constantly bathed in aqueous solutions. Fundamentally, then, humans are still aquatic animals at the cellular level, and their functions are controlled and mediated by the efficiency with which materials are moved to and from cells. For this reason the heart is completely dependent upon its own effectiveness as the circulatory pump to provide for its differentiated function—that of constantly moving aqueous solutions into and out of the vicinity of individual cells through a highly developed tubular system.

microstructure of cardiac muscle

In the human organism there are three kinds of contractile tissue found in various locations in the body: *striated muscle,* sometimes referred to as skeletal or voluntary muscle; *smooth* or *involuntary muscle;* and *cardiac muscle.* The cells of striated muscle have lost their distinctive cell walls and therefore are syncytial in nature. There are cross-striations which appear when the tissue is studied under the microscope. These "stripes" are due to the different optical densities of the chemical contractile elements actin and myosin. These two substances are found in all contractile tissues of the body, and the characteristic linear arrangements coupled with the cellular arrangement allow one to histologically differentiate between the three types of muscle cells.

Figure 7-1 diagrammatically shows the three types of contractile tissue. Figure 7-1A is striated muscle as just described. As shown in Fig. 7-1C, smooth muscle is made up of individual spindle-shaped cells which are densely packed into layers. When these cells are stretched, the total muscle layer is thinned out. When the contractile elements shorten, the total effect is one of thickening the muscle layer. It is easily seen that this type of contractile tissue is characteristically found surrounding the lumen of tubular structures such as gut and vessel walls. When the muscle contracts, the

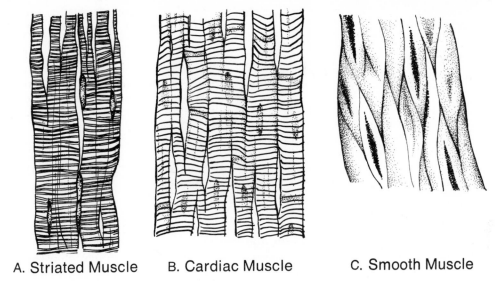

A. Striated Muscle   B. Cardiac Muscle   C. Smooth Muscle

Fig. 7-1. Histological features of the three types of contractile tissue.

diameter of the lumen is decreased and the contents are propelled along the tube in a linear fashion.

Microscopically cardiac muscle contains visible striations similar to those found in skeletal muscle. The ultrastructural pattern also resembles that of striated muscle since the cells branch and anastomose freely, as can be seen in Fig. 7-1B, and they form a three-dimensional, complex network. The elongated nuclei, like those of smooth muscle, are found deep in the interior of the cells and not adjacent to the sarcolemma. Unlike skeletal muscle, which is a morphological syncytium, cardiac muscle fibers are completely surrounded by a cell membrane. At the point where two fibers meet, the two membranes become elaborately folded into a structure known as an intercalated disk. These areas, the intercalated disks, provide strong connections among all the fibers of the cardiac muscle.

Although it was indicated that cardiac muscle is not a morphological syncytium, it functions as one. Because of the presence of the intercalated disks whose electrical potentials are extremely low, the rapid spread of excitation from cell to cell is possible. With each contractile impulse generated at the pacemaker, the spread of excitation is so rapid that there is essentially simultaneous contraction of the muscle.

Yet another difference, perhaps the most important difference between cardiac muscle and skeletal muscle cells, is that of automaticity, whereby cardiac muscle cells are capable of initiating rhythmic action potentials and thus waves of contraction without any outside humoral and/or nervous intervention.

The syncytial organization of cardiac muscle is such that there are two "lat-

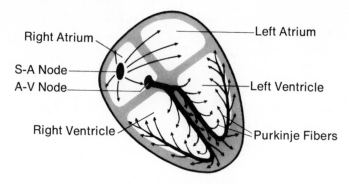

Fig. 7-2. Distribution of the Purkinje system and the location of the sinoatrial node in the human heart.

tice works"—the atrial syncytium and the ventricular syncytium. Though physically discontinuous, these two syncytia are functionally connected by the specialized conduction system. These specialized cardiac muscle fibers provide for communication of the contractile stimulus from one to the other. The Purkinje system is composed of the A-V node and the A-V bundle, which further subdivides into the right and left ventricular branches. These two branches then spread across the entire myocardium of each ventricle. The fibers then fuse with the syncytial muscle fibers so that their membranes are continuous and any impulse traveling along the membrane of a Purkinje fiber is transmitted directly to the ventricular myofibril.

Figure 7-2 is a schematic representation of the distribution of the Purkinje system and the location of the S-A node where the contractile impulse is initiated.

In summary, the microstructure of human cardiac muscle provides the knowledge necessary to understand the structural components which contribute to normal cardiac function. This microstructure orders the overall characteristics of cardiac function which result in a very efficient propulsive unit in the circulatory system.

general characteristics of the developing heart

The human heart begins its function at an extremely early age in the individual. The rhythmic contraction of cardiac muscle is initiated long before there is much form to the organ itself, to say nothing of the undifferentiated state of the body form of the whole embryo. In fact, the early heart is little more than a tube when the first wave of contraction is initiated. This innate heartbeat is referred to as a "myogenic" beat—that is, it is initiated in the muscle itself and needs no nervous stimulation for its initiation or maintenance. Once the rhythmic contractions have started they will continue without interruption until the death of the individual. Nervous stimulation may alter the rhythm and/or the rate, but the contractile characteristic of cardiac muscle resides in the biochemical properties of the chemical substances found in the tissue itself.

The structural developmental sequence of the heart is very interesting and of great importance to a discussion of those pathological conditions which arise from congenital cardiac defects. A discussion of structural development of the heart can be found in any good textbook which deals with the description of human cardiac development. For purposes of this discussion, however, it is sufficient to briefly touch on the development of the individual contractile units. The musculature of the atria develops and functions independently of the musculature of the ventricles. Timewise, this development is simultaneous. Therefore, when the myogenic beat is initiated in the atrial musculature, it occurs soon after in the ventricular lattice. The atria contract at a faster rate than do the ventricles because the muscular walls of the atria are both thinner and smaller, permitting the spread of excitation to reach all parts much more quickly. The initiation of the contraction is an electrochemical stimulus and is dependent upon changes in the membrane potential for the spread of excitation to all parts of both the atrial and ventricular musculatures.

The difference in the "natural" rates of contraction between the atrial and ventricular lattices is of prime importance when one is dealing with the effect of abnormalities in the conduction system. These differences in myogenic contractile rates are the main reason that the disruption of the normal conduction patterns in each lattice work is incompatible with life and why restoration of normal coordinated rhythmicity is absolutely essential. If the normal rhythmicity is not restored, the result is that approximately two atrial contractions occur for each ventricular contraction. The ultimate problem is one of incomplete emptying of the chambers and valvular regurgitation. When dealing with patients whose normal cardiac conduction mechanisms are disrupted, the nurse must be cognizant of the impending dangers and exigencies of the situation.

conductive and contractile characteristics of cardiac muscle

All membranes of the cells in the human body are charged—that is, they are polarized and therefore have electrical potentials. This means simply that there is a separation of charges at the membrane. In humans all cell membranes regardless of type are positively charged, there being more positively charged particles at the outer surface of the cell membrane than at the inner surface.

Figure 7-3A illustrates this "resting stage." This does not mean that there is an absence of negatively charged particles at the outer surface, nor that there is an absence of positively charged particles at the inner surface. It merely means that there is a net difference in the number and kind of charged particles at the outer surface as compared to the inner surface.

Cardiac muscle membranes are polarized, and the electrical potential can be measured, as is the situation in any of the cells in the human body. The

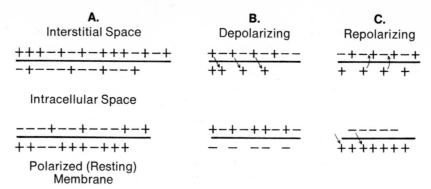

Fig. 7-3. The nature of cellular membranes in the human body.

potential results from the difference of intra- and extracellular concentrations of electrolytes. The electrolyte mainly responsible for the charge at the membrane is potassium with some contribution from sodium and chloride. When compounds of salts of the elements are dissolved in aqueous solutions, they dissociate into their charged particles called *ions*. It is through the selective control of the concentrations on either side of membranes of these ions that the electrical membrane potential is maintained.

Since the cell membrane is permeable to certain ions whose concentration gradient favors diffusion into the cell, energy must be expended to remove them from the cytoplasm and out through the cell membrane by means of a chemical carrier. The process is called "active transport." For each molecule of an ion pumped from the cell, one molecule of adenosine triphosphate (ATP) is required to provide the energy necessary to affect the chemical bond between the ion and the chemical carrier. The process of maintaining membrane potentials in living cells is an *endergonic* (energy-consuming) phenomenon.

When a stimulus is applied to the polarized cell membrane, the membrane which ordinarily is only slightly permeable to sodium permits sodium ions to diffuse rapidly into the cell. The result is a reversal of net charges; the outer surface is now more negative than positive and the membrane is said to be "depolarized" (Fig. 7-3B). As soon as the impulse moves along the membrane, the separation of charges is restored by way of the sodium pump and potassium diffusion restoring the original state or "repolarizing" the membrane (Fig. 7-3C). This method for transmitting impulses of physical, chemical, or electrical origin is not peculiar to cardiac muscle membranes, but indeed is common to all excitable membranes in the human body.

The Purkinje system is composed of very specialized cardiac muscle fibers which have the ability to depolarize and recover at a much more rapid rate than ordinary cardiac myofibril membranes. Also, the membrane of the cells of the S-A node is extremely sensitive to minute changes in electrochemical conditions in the posterior wall of the right atrium where it is situated. As a result, it initiates the impulse of depolarization leading to contraction of the atrial musculature. The impulse is passed to the A-V node by adjacent atrial cells.

The A-V node lies on the posteriomedial surface near the right atrioventricular valve (tricuspid). The membranes of the node fibers have a slower depolarization rate and thus there is a slight delay before the impulse reaches the midline bundle and spreads to the right and left ventricular branches. This delay allows the atria to completely empty their contents into the two ventricular chambers before there is any contraction of the myocardium of those chambers.

The discussion on membrane dynamics and the characteristics of the conduction of impulses in cardiac muscle readily indicates the importance of the electrolytes sodium, potassium, chloride, and calcium. Of these four, sodium plays the most obvious role in membrane action potentials. The role of potassium ions is in establishing membrane potentials. Calcium is chemically involved in the combination and release of the contractile substances of actin and myosin and membrane thresholds. The importance of understanding the separate and collective functions of these electrolytes is prerequisite to an understanding of normal cardiac function.

control of rate and rhythm of cardiac function

It was emphasized in the section on cardiac embryogenesis that cardiac muscle has a myogenic beat. The S-A node of the heart, without any outside influence, will discharge an impulse to the atrial muscular lattice 70 to 80 times per minute, while the A-V node, if not fired by the S-A node, will stimulate the ventricular lattice to contract 40 to 60 times per minute. Because the S-A node not only discharges at a faster rate than does the A-V node or the bundle fibers, but also recovers at a much more rapid rate, it controls the rhythmic discharge and resultant contractile rate of the heart. For these reasons it is called the "pacemaker." In order for the heart to function efficiently as a pump, both atria must contract simultaneously. This presents no real problem, inasmuch as the spread of excitation from the S-A node through the atrial muscle membranes to the A-V node takes only 0.08 second. There is a delay at the A-V node which is sufficient to permit complete emptying of the atrial contents into the ventricular chambers.

The rate at which the S-A node can initiate cardiac contractions does not allow the heart to change either its rate or its rhythm to meet the physiological demands of the body. The nervous innervation via the autonomic nervous system performs this function. The distribution of the parasympathetic and sympathetic nerve fibers is shown in Fig. 7-4.

The effect of sympathetic stimulation of the heart is one of increasing the rate of contraction; that of parasympathetic stimulation is a decrease in the contractile rate. Both responses are mediated by chemical mediators which are secreted by the nerve endings themselves. In the case of vagal (parasympathetic) fibers, the chemical substance is acetylcholine, and for the sympathetic fibers the substance is the familiar norepinephrine. The effects of both

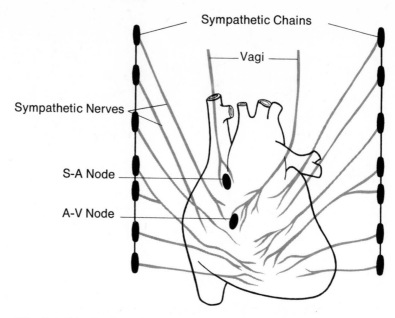

Fig. 7-4. Distribution of autonomic nerve fibers to the human heart.

substances are the result of changing the rate of depolarization in S-A cells.

It is during the spread of excitation to the ventricular walls that the value of the Purkinje system is most easily demonstrated. Both ventricles must contract simultaneously after the completion of atrial contraction. Since the Purkinje fibers conduct impulses 3 to 7 times as rapidly as cardiac muscle fibers, they contribute to the rhythmicity of cardiac function and increase the efficiency of the heart as a pump by some 25 percent.

The very quality of cardiac muscle that provides for its maximum efficiency can become the etiology of some very serious problems in rhythmicity. The five most common causes of abnormal rhythm of the heart rate are:

1. Abnormal rhythmicity in the pacemaker itself.
2. Shift of the pacemaker activity to some other site.
3. Blocks in transmission of the impulse through the heart.
4. Development of abnormal pathways of transmission.
5. Spontaneous generation of abnormal impulses while the pacemaker is still firing.

These pathological problems will be dealt with in detail throughout other sections of this book. A listing of the possibilities is sufficient at this time to point out the extreme importance for the nurse addressing herself to the care of patients with life-threatening heart disease of adequately understanding the mechanism for the establishment and control of normal rate and rhythm.

The reader will recall that the divisions of the autonomic nervous system operate in direct opposition to one another and thus provide a system of checks and balances upon each other. For example, if in response to heavy exercise the sympathetic nerve fibers serving a large leg muscle receive impulses as a result of increased local levels of carbon dioxide in the muscle itself, they then transmit the impulse to the cardiac centers in the hypothalamus of the brain. From the hypothalamus the impulse is in turn transmitted to the fibers directly connected to the cardiac muscle membranes. This action results in decreasing the time required to depolarize the membrane and causes contraction of the myofibrils. The total effect is one of increased rate of contraction of the heart, and ultimately increased circulation to the large leg muscle itself. This effect would continue indefinitely were it not for the stimulation of vagal fibers in the myocardium which would secrete acetylcholine, increasing the time necessary for repolarizing the membrane of the cardiac muscle. This increase would result in a slowing of the contractile rate and allow for a return to normal rate and rhythm.

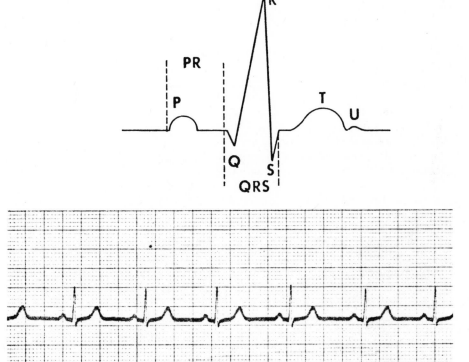

Fig. 7-5. Normal electrocardiogram tracing.

As a result of the electrochemical nature of the excitatory impulse characterizing the depolarization of the cardiac membrane, it is possible to pick up and record these action potentials from the surface of the body. As stated earlier, the membrane potentials are the result of separation of charged particles situated at the surface. As the impulse spreads and passes to all parts of the cardiac musculature, electrical currents spread into the tissues surrounding the heart. This is not a surprising fact when one recalls that the chemical composition of extracellular fluids is not different in any of the tissues of the body. A small number of these currents reach the surface of the body, and if electrodes are placed at opposite sides of the heart the potentials generated can be recorded. The reader readily recognizes this recording as an electrocardiogram. Electrocardiogram tracings are covered in detail in another chapter, and therefore it will be sufficient to emphasize that the deflection of the recording needle is the direct result of the depolarization and repolarization of the membranes of the atrial and ventricular musculatures.

Figure 7-5 (p. 81) is a schematic presentation of a normal tracing. These tracings provide a means of constant monitoring of what is happening internally to the conduction system of the heart. It is this feature of extending one's five senses to allow for internal assessment via an external means that makes the knowledge of cardiogram tracings relevant to nursing.

the cardiac cycle

In the foregoing sections the more subtle and less obvious features of cardiac function have been discussed. There are more obvious functional characteristics with which you are familiar but until now they have been ignored. Pulse, blood pressure, and heart sounds are very important indicators of cardiac function and will now be discussed in light of the characteristics which have just been presented.

When atrial contraction is completed and ventricular contraction is initiated, three events occur simultaneously. The atrioventricular valves shut to prevent the regurgitation of blood back into the relaxed atria. The leaves or "cusps" of the bicuspid and tricuspid valves close and the blood rushes against them resulting in the production of the first heart sound, "lub." At the same time, there is a surge of fluid pressure against the walls of the major arteries as a result of increased volume of blood pumped from the ventricles. This surge is felt in the peripheral circulation and is known as the *pulse.* The contractile phase or period is known as *systole,* and thus the blood pressure of this period of ventricular systole is called the *systolic pressure.* Immediately following the period of ventricular systole comes the relaxation or "refractory" period which is called *diastole.* One result of ventricular relaxation is the closing of the semilunar valves in both the systemic and pulmonary aortae to prevent backflow of blood. The closing of these valves results in the second heart sound, "dub." The fluid pressure of the blood against the arterial walls drops to its lowest level during diastole and is known as the *diastolic pressure.* Following the period of complete recovery of both lattice works, "absolute

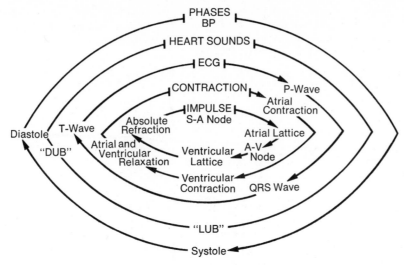

Fig. 7-6. The cardiac cycle.

refraction," this chain of events is reinitiated with a new contractile impulse being initiated at the S-A node.

The cyclical chain of events is schematically summarized in Fig. 7-6.

This scheme points out how there are several simultaneously occurring events which can be assessed at any given time. It is of the utmost importance for the nurse to be fully aware of a number of routes available to her in gathering data on the state of the patient's cardiac function at any given moment. The gathering of data from multiple sources provides her with a "set" to analyze and a base upon which she can plan her *modus operandi*.

coronary circulation

Blood supply to the myocardium is derived from the two main coronary arteries which originate from the aorta, immediately above the aortic valve. The left coronary artery supplies the major portion of the left ventricle, while the right coronary artery supplies the major portion of the right ventricle.

Shortly after its origin, the left coronary vessel branches into the anterior descending artery, which traverses the groove between the two ventricles on the anterior surface of the heart, and the circumflex artery, which passes to the left and posteriorly in the groove between the left atrium and the left ventricle. The circumflex branch may terminate before reaching the posterior side of the heart, or it may continue into the posterior groove between the left and right ventricles. The coronary circulation is referred to as *dominant left* if this branch of the left coronary artery supplies the posterior aspect of the heart, including the septum.

Eighty percent of human hearts are *dominant right*. When this situation prevails, the right coronary artery passes posteriorly and is responsible for the blood supply to the posterior side of the heart and the posterior portion of the interventricular septum.

pathogenesis of coronary heart disease

It is estimated that 95 percent of all cases of myocardial damage are due to intrinsic disease of the coronary vessels as a result of arteriosclerotic changes in the vessel walls. Arteriosclerotic changes in coronary vessels do not absolutely parallel systemic sclerotic changes and thus may be more severe than the observed peripheral alterations would indicate. The most common characteristic of the diseased vessel is the presence of patchy atheromatosis scattered in the lining of the vessels and projecting into the lumen. Because of this propensity for atherosclerotic vessel changes, it is imperative that a brief discussion of the etiology of these vascular changes be included, as well as the correlation of vascular dysfunction and its effect upon functional anatomy of the myocardium.

As vessels respond to the local physiological demands for nutrients, oxygen, and the removal of waste products, the diameter of the lumen changes in response to the sympathetic innervation of the muscularis. In effect, over long periods of time minute breaks develop in the integrity of the endothelial lining, and atheromatous plaques begin to form. These plaques contain lipid deposits and large amounts of cholesterol. Later, fibroblasts invade the plaques, resulting in the development of inelastic deposits which not only restrict the physiological response to demands but progressively can restrict the lumen of the artery. The etiology of atherosclerotic changes in the arteries in humans is almost certainly a derangement of lipid metabolism. It can involve increased lipid mobility, dietary lipid overload, and/or an error in the metabolic breakdown of lipids. It has also been demonstrated that the vessel wall has the ability to secrete cholesterol in response to the breaks in the lining of the vessels. This fact would account for the extensive atherosclerotic changes sometimes seen in individuals whose serum levels are well within normal limits.

Although sclerotic changes are usually associated with the normal aging process, there is an increasing incidence in the middle-aged affluent male in the American population. The sex differential must be taken into account, inasmuch as twice as many men die of atherosclerotic changes than do premenopausal women. This differential levels off after age 50. It would appear that estrogens protect the female from developing atherosclerotic vessel changes. There is also evidence that atheromatous plaque formation in the major vessels tends to run in families.

Certain physiological states predispose to the development of atheromatous plaques. Severe diabetes and hypothyroidism, conditions which are accompanied by hypercholesterolemia, are two examples. Another physiological etiological factor is any situation that results in diabetogenic conditions by immobilizing fat stores and increasing blood glucose by glycogen turnover and gluconeogenesis. All three of these conditions are mediated through the glucocorticoids from the adrenal cortex as a part of the general adaptive syndrome in response to stress.

Any situation which causes hyperemia, tissue damage, or hypothalamic sympathetic stimulation also causes a functional stimulation to the heart. Consequently the coronary circulation responds to permit junctional hyperemia in the myocardium. If the vessels are inelastic or are partially occluded due to atherosclerotic changes in the vessel walls, the result is myocardial ischemia in certain areas instead of hyperemia. If the coronary arteries become completely occluded by the development of a thrombus and/or plaques, then the result is ultimately necrosis of myocardial fibers. Such necrotic changes are irreversible and the damaged fibers are replaced by inelastic scar tissue. If the occlusion is sufficiently large, or is in a main artery, death results from one or a combination of the five following situations:

1. Decreased cardiac output.
2. Hemostasis in the pulmonary circulation and resultant edema.
3. Hemostasis in the systemic circulation and resultant edema.
4. Fibrillation of the heart.
5. Occasionally, rupture of the cardiac wall itself.

In conclusion, any situation that tends to elicit a sympathetic or adrenal stress response tends to contribute to the establishment of the conditions prerequisite for the development of atherosclerotic changes in the coronary circulation. If the general physical condition of the individual is one that can handle the stress and strain of daily living, the amount of atheromatous plaque development is commensurate with the age, sex, and genetic characteristics of the individual. It is when the person's physical condition is so deteriorated, or when he lives under such an increased amount of tension-producing stress, that the changes become excessive and the conditions for the development of coronary vascular disease are met. The nurse who cares for such an individual must be able to assess the current status of the environment as well as the patient's biopsychosocial state if she is to maintain the resources available for recovery and prevent further deterioration of the situation. An understanding of the multiple causal factors which lead and/or contribute to the patient's acute condition is prerequisite to planning a means of preventing further strain on an already damaged vital organ.

BIBLIOGRAPHY

Jensen, David, *The Principles of Physiology* (New York: Appleton-Century-Crofts, 1976).
Wiggers, Carl J., *The Heart,* Scientific American, Reprint No. 62, 1957.

H. L. BRAMMELL, M.D.

8 | 8

pathophysiology of heart failure

The heart is a complex structure composed of fibrous tissue, cardiac muscle, and electrical conducting tissue that has a single function: to pump blood. In order to do its job well, a good heart pump requires good functioning muscle, a good valve system, and an efficient pumping rhythm. An abnormality of sufficient severity of any component of the pump can affect its pumping efficiency and may cause the pump to fail.

reserve mechanisms of the heart — responses of the heart to stress

When the heart is stressed, several reserve mechanisms can be called upon to maintain good pumping function, i.e., to provide a cardiac output sufficient to meet the demands of the body. These are increased heart rate, dilatation, hypertrophy and increased stroke volume.

The first response is an increase in *heart rate*. This adjustment is rapid and has been experienced by everyone during periods of exercise or anxiety. Increasing the heart rate is an excellent way to quickly increase the cardiac

Supported by a Research and Training Center Grant (16-P-56815) from the Rehabilitation Services Administration, Department of Health, Education and Welfare, Washington, D.C.

output and meet the demands of the body for blood. Its utility and effectiveness, however, are functions of age, the functional state of the myocardium, and the amount of obstructive coronary artery disease, if any. The maximum heart rate which can be achieved is related to age.[1] For example, a 20-year-old will plateau at approximately 200 beats per minute at maximum effort, whereas at age 65 maximum heart rate is about 153 beats per minute. After age 25, maximum heart rate capability drops approximately 6 beats for each 5 years. There is, of course, considerable spread around these mean maximum heart rates for each age—some persons will exceed and some fail to achieve the average value. As heart rate increases, the time for diastolic ventricular filling decreases, and at high heart rates the time available for ventricular filling may be so small that filling is inadequate and cardiac output starts to fall. In addition to advancing age, the functional state of the heart muscle (how capable it is of maintaining repeated rapid contractions) and the state of the coronary circulation are important determinants of the effectiveness of heart rate as a response to stress. In persons with coronary artery disease and significant obstruction to one or more coronary arteries, a substantial increase in heart rate can be a potentially dangerous event. Coronary artery blood flow to the left ventricle takes place primarily in diastole. With increasing heart rates, decreased diastolic filling time, and increased demands of the heart for oxygen (heart rate being one of the major determinants of myocardial oxygen demand) coronary blood flow may become critical and angina pectoris, congestive failure, or occasionally myocardial infarction may be produced. Furthermore, if the heart muscle contracts poorly and cannot sustain strong contractions at moderate or rapid rates, then heart failure may follow. Heart rate, then, is an immediate response to stress that is effective in maintaining or increasing cardiac output but whose value depends on the patient's age, functional state of the myocardium, and amount of obstructive disease in the coronary arteries.

The second reserve mechanism of the heart is *dilatation*. With dilatation the muscle cell stretches. The relationship between the cardiac output (the amount of blood the heart pumps in each unit of time) and the length of the heart muscle cell at the end of diastole is expressed in the well-known Starling relationship, which states that as the end-diastolic fiber length increases, so does the cardiac output. Like heart rate, however, its usefulness is self-limiting. There is a point beyond which the stretching of the muscle cell does not lead to an increase in cardiac output but instead cardiac output falls. This is partly explained by the Laplace relationship, which states that the tension in the wall of a chamber such as the left ventricle is directly related to the pressure in that chamber and its radius. Put another way, as the radius of the chamber increases (dilatation), so does the wall tension as long as the pressure in the chamber rises or does not fall. Since wall tension is directly related to the demand of the myocardium for oxygen, it is not difficult to see that eventually the radius will dilate to such a degree that the demand of the heart for oxygen cannot be met. In this instance, dilatation has advanced to the point where it is no longer providing an increase in cardiac output and the pump has started to fail.

Third, individual cardiac muscle cells may *hypertrophy*. The process of hypertrophy requires time and is not an acute adjustment to stress. However, if the stress is applied long enough, such as with systematic or pulmonary hypertension or significant stenosis of the aortic or pulmonic valve (pressure loads), the muscle of the chamber pumping against the resistance may hypertrophy to such a degree that it effectively outgrows its blood supply and becomes ischemic. When this happens, hypertrophy ceases to be a useful compensatory mechanism and the heart's pumping ability decreases. A similar situation may occur with the imposition of a volume load on the pumping ventricle, e.g., mitral or aortic regurgitation.

A fourth reserve mechanism of the heart is to increase its *stroke volume*, the amount of blood that it ejects into the circulation with each systole. It can do this either by increasing the percentage of the end-diastolic volume ejected with each beat (increase the ejection fraction through an increase in contractility) or by increasing the amount of blood presented to the heart (increased venous return). This is commonly accomplished by the reflex increase of sympathetic nervous system activity which increases venous tone. Venous pressure is then raised and thus venous return to the heart is increased. Venous return is also increased with elevated body temperature, which shortens the time required for blood to completely circulate through the body; by recumbency, in which case the volume of blood that is held in the legs as a result of gravity is largely returned to the central circulation and presented to the heart; or by taking a deep breath, which increases intrathoracic negativity, thereby "sucking" more blood into the chest. Also, any increase in intravascular volume will increase venous return. By either an increase in ejection fraction (contractility) or venous return (volume), stroke volume and cardiac output will increase. As with other mechanisms of response to stress, increased venous return ("preload" to the physiologist) and increased contractility may not function to increase cardiac output. For example, the myocardium may be so fatigued (depressed contractility) that it cannot respond to further attempts to improve its force of contraction. Similarly, an increase in venous return may cause increased dilatation and decrease, rather than improve, cardiac output.

This simplistic review of cardiovascular responses to stress is designed to promote a basic understanding of the topic and to indicate how the responses can be overwhelmed. In addition, it will assist in generating an appreciation for approaching clinical situations, both diagnostic and therapeutic, from a physiological cause-and-effect point of view.

heart failure

When the normal cardiac reserves for responding to stress are inadequate to meet the metabolic demands of the body, the heart fails to do its job as a pump and heart failure results. Also, as stated earlier, dysfunction of any of the components of the pump may ultimately result in failure. Heart failure was defined many years ago by Lewis very simply and appropriately as "a condition in which the heart fails to discharge its contents adequately."[2] This definition is as good today as it was in the 1930s.

causes of failure

Abnormalities of the *muscle* causing ventricular failure include myocardial infarction, ventricular aneurysm, extensive myocardial fibrosis (usually from atherosclerotic coronary heart disease or prolonged hypertension), endocardial fibrosis, primary myocardial disease (cardiomyopathy), or excessive hypertrophy due to pulmonary hypertension, aortic stenosis, or systemic hypertension.

In acute myocardial infarction, myocardial rupture presents as a dramatic and often catastrophic onset of pump failure and is associated with a high mortality. Rupture usually occurs during the first eight days following infarction during the period of greatest softening of the damaged myocardium. Fortunately, myocardial rupture is a relatively rare complication of infarction. Rupture of a papillary muscle, of the interventricular septum, or of the free wall of the left ventricle may occur.

There are two papillary muscles in the left ventricle which are thumblike projections of muscle to which the restraining "guidewires" of the mitral valve, the chordae tendineae, are attached. The papillary muscle may be involved in the infarction process and very occasionally may rupture. When it does, there is a sudden loss of restraint of one of the leaflets of the mitral valve, and free mitral regurgitation occurs with each contraction of the left ventricle. This sudden profound pressure and volume load on the left atrium is reflected back through the pulmonary veins to the pulmonary vascular bed and the acute onset of symptoms of pulmonary vascular congestion is noted. This is usually manifested as severe dyspnea and frank pulmonary edema. At the bedside a loud murmur lasting throughout systole is present. Very often nothing can be done to save the patient although occasionally emergency mitral valve replacement can be successfully accomplished.

Sudden heart failure is seen occasionally in acute myocardial infarction as a result of rupture of the interventricular septum. Like rupture of the papillary muscle, septal rupture is uncommon but when it does appear is also usually noted in the first week after damage. Septal rupture is clinically characterized by chest pain, dyspnea, shock, and a rapid onset of evidence of pump failure. There is a loud murmur that lasts throughout systole at the lower left sternal border and is often accompanied by a thrill which can be felt by placing the hand over the precordium at the left sternal border. As with all myocardial ruptures, the prognosis of septal rupture is poor. However, it is possible to occasionally repair these ventricular septal defects by emergency surgery using cardiopulmonary bypass.

Ruptures of a papillary muscle and the interventricular septum are virtually indistinguishable at the bedside with both presenting as sudden onset of left ventricular failure, a new murmur and occasionally a palpable thrill. The location of the infarction is not helpful and the clinical course in each is rapidly downhill. Emergency cardiac catheterization is the only way to clearly differentiate the two.[3]

Mechanical failure of the heart seen in acute myocardial infarction is another relatively rare event and is due to rupture of the free wall of the left ventricle and the spilling of blood into the pericardial cavity. This results in acute compression of the heart or tamponade and the inability of both chambers to fill adequately. There is then very sudden pumping failure with associated shock and death. Rupture of the free wall may be preceded by or associated with a return of chest pain as the blood dissects through the necrotic myocardial wall. Sudden vascular collapse as occurs with ventricular fibrillation but with an unchanged rhythm on the electrocardiogram (electro-mechanical dissociation) suggests rupture of the ventricular free wall. As with rupture of the papillary muscle and interventricular septum, rupture of the free wall of the left ventricle carries with it an extremely poor prognosis.

Valve malfunction can lead to pump failure by causing either obstruction to outflow of the pumping chamber such as valvular aortic stenosis or pulmonary stenosis (pressure load), or the valve may be regurgitant as with mitral or aortic insufficiency which present an increased volume of blood to the left ventricle (volume load). Valve abnormalities that impose either a pressure or a volume load on one or more chambers usually are slowly progressive conditions which cause the heart to utilize its long-term defense mechanisms of dilatation and hypertrophy. Both these mechanisms can be overcome and lead to pump failure. Less commonly, an acute volume load is imposed on the heart causing a rapid onset of pump failure. Bacterial endocarditis of the aortic or mitral valves, rupture of a portion of the mitral valve apparatus (papillary muscle or chordae tendineae) or rupture of the interventricular septum is the usual cause. In these cases, initial therapy is designed to support the heart during the period of acute insult so that the long-term compensatory mechanisms can be utilized. However, if this is not successful, emergency replacement of the abnormal valve or closure of the septal defect is indicated.

Disorders of the cardiac *rhythm* can produce or contribute to failure in several ways. Bradycardia allows for increased diastolic filling and myocardial fiber stretch with an associated increase in stroke volume (Starling relationship). Cardiac output is therefore preserved. This is well tolerated in healthy persons; resting bradycardia is, in fact, a result of high levels of aerobic physical conditioning. However, in the diseased heart contractility is decreased, the useful limits of the Starling relationship are exceeded, and cardiac output may be diminished. On the other hand, with tachycardia, diastolic filling time is decreased, myocardial oxygen demand is increased and the diseased myocardium or heart with significant coronary artery disease may tolerate the burden poorly and fail or develop ischemia, injury or infarction. Furthermore, frequent premature contractions may decrease the cardiac output, a circumstance that may be poorly tolerated in a patient with marginal pump function.

responses to failure

When the heart's normal reserves are overwhelmed and failure occurs, certain physiological responses to the decrease in cardiac output are important. All of these responses represent the body's attempt to maintain a normal perfusion of vital organs. The primary acute adjustment to heart failure is an increase in sympathetic nervous system influence on the arteries, veins, and heart. This results in an increase in heart rate, an increase in venous return to the heart, and increased force of contraction; in addition, sympathetic tone helps to maintain a normal blood pressure. The price extracted for this adjustment is an increase in myocardial oxygen demand and oxygen consumption, a request that may inadequately be met in the patient with significant coronary artery obstructive disease or poor pump contractility.

As a result of the autonomic nervous changes and other factors, the blood flow to the essential organs, specifically the brain and heart, is maintained at the expense of less essential organs such as the skin, gut and kidneys. With severe congestive heart failure there is sufficient decrease in blood flow to the skeletal muscles to cause a metabolic acidosis that must be considered when a treatment program is planned.

When the kidneys sense a decreased volume of blood presented for filtration, they respond by retaining sodium and water and thereby try to do their part in increasing the central blood volume and venous return. With an increase in circulating blood volume and venous return to the heart, there is an increase in end-diastolic fiber length (dilatation) and within limits, an increase in stroke volume and cardiac output. However, with a failing heart, an increased circulatory volume may be too great a burden for the ventricle, and failure may be worsened.

In some patients with prolonged failure, remaining heart cells will hypertrophy, increasing pumping efficiency, and the clinical findings of heart failure may improve or disappear.

recognition of failure

It is useful to think of the clinical features of heart failure as coming from failure of either the left ventricle, the right ventricle, or both. When the *left ventricle* fails, its inability to discharge its contents adequately results in dilatation, increased end-diastolic volume, and increased intraventricular pressure at the end of diastole. This results in the inability of the left atrium to adequately empty its contents into the left ventricle, and pressure in the left atrium rises. This pressure rise is reflected back into the pulmonary veins which bring blood from the lungs to the left atrium. The increased pressure in the pulmonary vessels results in pulmonary vascular congestion, which is the cause of the most specific symptoms of left ventricular failure.

The symptoms of pulmonary vascular congestion are dyspnea, orthopnea, paroxysmal nocturnal dyspnea, cough, and acute pulmonary edema. Dyspnea, characterized by rapid shallow breathing and a sensation of difficulty in obtaining adequate air, is distressing to the patient. Occasionally a patient may complain of insomnia, restlessness, or weakness which is caused by the dyspnea. Orthopnea, the inability to lie flat because of dyspnea, is another common complaint of left ventricular failure related to pulmonary vascular congestion. It is important to determine if the orthopnea is truly related to heart disease or whether elevating the head to sleep is merely the patient's custom. For example, if the patient states that he sleeps on three pillows, one might hasten to believe that he is suffering from orthopnea. If, however, when asked why he sleeps on three pillows he replies that he does this because he likes to sleep at this elevation, and has done so since before he had symptomatic heart disease, the condition does not qualify as orthopnea. Paroxysmal nocturnal dyspnea (PND) is a well-known complaint characterized by the patient's awakening in the middle of the night because of intense shortness of breath. Nocturnal dyspnea is thought to be caused by a shift of fluid from the tissues into the intravascular compartment as a result of recumbency. During the day the pressure in the veins is high, especially in the dependent portions of the body, due to gravity, increased fluid volume, and increased sympathetic tone. With this increase in hydrostatic pressure, some fluid escapes into the tissue space. With recumbency, the pressure in the dependent capillaries is decreased and fluid is resorbed into the circulation. This increased volume represents an additional amount of blood which is presented to the heart to pump each minute (increased preload), and places an additional burden on an already congested pulmonary vascular bed, with acute onset of dyspnea the resultant symptom.

One symptom of pulmonary vascular congestion that is often overlooked, but which may be a dominant symptom, is an irritating cough. It may be productive but is usually dry and hacking in character. This symptom is related to congestion of bronchial mucosa and an associated increase in mucus production.

Acute pulmonary edema is the most florid clinical picture associated with pulmonary vascular congestion. It occurs when the pulmonary capillary pressure exceeds the pressure which tends to keep fluid within the vascular channels (around 30 mm. Hg). At these pressures, there is transduction of fluid into the alveoli which in turn diminishes the area available for the normal transport of oxygen into and carbon dioxide out of the blood within the pulmonary capillary bed. Acute pulmonary edema is characterized by intense dyspnea, cough, orthopnea, profound anxiety, cyanosis, sweating, noisy respirations, and very often chest pain and a pink frothy sputum from the mouth. It constitutes a genuine medical emergency and must be managed vigorously and promptly.

In addition to the symptoms which result from pulmonary vascular congestion, left ventricular failure is also associated with nonspecific symptoms which are related to decreased cardiac output. The patient may complain of weakness, fatigability, apathy, lethargy, difficulty in concentrating, memory deficit or diminished exercise tolerance. These symptoms may be present in chronic low output states and may dominate the patient's complaints. Unfortunately, these symptoms are nonspecific and are often ascribed to depression, neurosis or functional complaints. Therefore, these potentially important indicators of deteriorating pump function are often not recognized for their true value, and the patient is either inappropriately reassured or placed on a tranquilizer or mood elevating preparation. Remember, the presence of the nonspecific symptoms of low cardiac output demands a careful evaluation of the heart as well as the psyche—an examination that will yield the information which will dictate proper management.

Physical signs associated with left ventricular failure that are easily recognized at the bedside include third and fourth heart sounds and rales in the lungs. The fourth heart sound or atrial gallop is associated with and follows atrial contraction and is best heard with the bell of the stethoscope very lightly applied at the cardiac apex. The left lateral position may be required to elicit the sound. It is heard just before the first heart sound and is not always a definitive sign of congestive failure but may represent decreased compliance (increased stiffness) of the myocardium. It therefore may be an early, premonitory indication of impending failure. A fourth heart sound is common in patients with acute myocardial infarction, and likely does not have prognostic significance, but may represent incipient failure. On the other hand, a third sound or ventricular gallop is an important sign of left ventricular failure and in adults is almost never present in the absence of significant heart disease. Most physicians would agree that treatment of congestive failure is indicated upon the appearance of this sign. The third sound is heard in early diastole following the second heart sound and is associated with the period of rapid passive ventricular filling. It is also best heard with the bell of the stethoscope applied lightly at the apex, with the patient in the left lateral position, and at the end of expiration.

The fine moist rales most commonly heard at the bases of the lungs posteriorly are often recognized as evidence of left ventricular failure, as indeed they may be. Before these rales are ascribed to pump failure, the patient must be instructed to cough deeply in order to open any basilar alveoli that may be compressed as a result of recumbency, inactivity and compression from the diaphragm beneath. Rales that fail to clear after cough (post-tussic) need to be evaluated; those that clear following cough are probably clinically unimportant. It is, however, important to note that the patient may have good evidence for left ventricular failure on the basis of a history of symptoms suggesting pulmonary vascular congestion or the finding of a third heart sound at the apex and have quite clear lung fields. It is not appropriate to wait for the appearance of rales in the lungs before instituting therapy for left ventricular failure.

Since an increase in heart rate is the heart's initial response to stress, sinus tachycardia might be expected, and is often found in the examination of a patient with pump failure. Other rhythms associated with pump failure include atrial premature contractions, paroxysmal atrial tachycardia, and ventricular premature beats. Whenever a rhythm abnormality is detected, one must attempt to define the underlying pathophysiological mechanism; therapy can then be properly planned and instituted.

Other signs of left ventricular failure which may be noted in addition to a third heart sound, rales in the lungs and supraventricular rhythms include wheezing breath sounds, pulsus alternans (an alternating greater and lesser volume of the arterial pulse), a square-wave response to a standard Valsalva maneuver (see below) and Cheyne-Stokes respirations. Indeed, patients may awaken at night during respiratory height of a Cheyne-Stokes cycle, a situation that may falsely be interpreted as PND, but which may have the same pathophysiological significance. Weight gain resulting from retention of salt and water by the kidneys is a useful sign that the patient may follow at home. Daily weight should be recorded, the observation made in the morning, after voiding and before breakfast.

Radiographic examination of the chest is often helpful in making a diagnosis of heart failure. Careful evaluation of the chest x-ray may demonstrate changes in the blood vessels of the lungs which result from an increase in pulmonary venous pressure. X-ray findings may be present in the absence of rales, and careful examination of the chest film is necessary if left ventricular failure is suspected.

Failure of the *right ventricle* alone is often the result of severe underlying lung disease and such conditions as severe pulmonary hypertension (primary or secondary), stenosis of the pulmonary valve, or a massive pulmonary embolus. The right ventricle tolerates a volume load well and pure right ventricular failure is usually due to resistance to outflow (pressure load). More commonly, however, right ventricular failure is the result of failure of the left ventricle. In this situation symptoms and signs of both left and right ventricular failure are present, and the symptoms of left ventricular failure may improve as the right ventricle fails, through relief of left ventricular preload and decrease in pulmonary vascular congestion.

In contrast to left ventricular failure, in which specific symptoms can usually be related to a single underlying mechanism—pulmonary vascular congestion—the symptoms of right heart failure are not so specific and many are related to a low cardiac output. Fatigability, weakness, lethargy or difficulty in concentrating may be prominent. Heaviness of the limbs, especially the legs, an increase in abdominal girth, inability to wear previously comfortable shoes and weight gain reflect the ascites and edema associated with right ventricular failure. In addition, symptoms of the underlying pulmonary disease usually dominate complaints if failure is due to a primary pulmonary problem, usually chronic bronchitis and/or emphysema. Occasionally bronchiectasis or restrictive lung disease may be the primary pulmonary problem, but chronic bronchitis and emphysema are by far the most common pulmonary causes of right ventricular failure.

When the right ventricle decompensates, there is dilatation of the chamber, an increase in right ventricular end-diastolic volume and pressure, resistance to filling of the ventricle and a subsequent rise in right atrial pressure. This increasing pressure is in turn reflected upstream in the venae cavae and can be recognized by an increase in the jugular venous pressure. This is best evaluated by looking at the veins in the neck and noting the height of the column of blood. With the patient lying in bed and the head of the bed elevated between 30 and 60 degrees, the column of blood in the external jugular veins will be, in normal individuals, only a few millimeters above the upper border of the clavicle, if it is seen at all. When an observation of venous pressure is recorded, the height of the column of blood above the sternal angle and the elevation of the head of the bed should be included. This will then provide a useful basis for comparison of future observations.

Edema is often considered a reliable sign of heart failure, and, indeed, it is often present when the right ventricle has failed. However, it is the least reliable sign of right ventricular dysfunction. Many people, particularly the elderly, spend much of their time sitting in a chair with the legs dependent. As a result of this body position, the decreased turgor of subcutaneous tissue associated with old age, and perhaps primary venous disease such as varicosities, ankle edema may be produced which reflects these factors rather than right ventricular failure. When edema does appear related to failure of the right ventricle it is dependent in location. If the patient is up and about it will be noted primarily in the ankles and will ascend the legs as failure worsens. When the patient is put to bed the dependent portion of the body becomes the sacral area and edema should be looked for there. In addition, other signs of right ventricular failure should be present before the diagnosis is made. Dependent edema alone is inadequate documentation of the status of the right ventricle. With congestion of the liver this organ may enlarge and become tender, ascites may be present, and jaundice may be noted.

As with left ventricular failure, sinus tachycardia and the other rhythms associated with pump failure may be present. In addition, right ventricular third and fourth heart sounds are not uncommon. They are best heard at the lower left sternal border with the bell of the stethoscope applied lightly to the chest, and can be recognized by an increase in intensity with inspiration. Finally, signs of any underlying cause of right ventricular failure may be present, e.g., hyperresonance with percussion, low immobile diaphragms, decreased breath sounds, increased anteroposterior chest diameter and use of the accessory muscles of respiration in patients with severe pulmonary emphysema.

The Valsalva maneuver[4] has been used in the diagnosis of heart failure and has a long and interesting history. It is discussed here more for its general clinical interest rather than as an important diagnostic maneuver in suspected heart failure. The Valsalva maneuver has also been implicated as causing an occasional fatality either through the production of a cardiac arrhythmia or through the dislodging of venous thrombi producing massive pulmonary embolization. A standard Valsalva maneuver is produced by blowing into a mercury manometer to a pressure of 40 mm. Hg and sustaining this effort for 10 seconds. Naturally a patient does not do this on his own during the day but may closely simulate the maneuver during a prolonged effort of straining at stool. Intermittent positive pressure breathing may produce short periods of a similar type of strain as may a cough or sneeze.

In the normal response to the Valsalva maneuver there are four phases. Phase I occurs with the onset of strain at which time there is an increase in intrathoracic pressure which is transmitted to the great vessels (aorta and pulmonary artery) and leads to a rise in arterial blood pressure. During Phase II, as a later result of the increased intrathoracic pressure and limitation to venous return to the heart, there is a decrease in right atrial filling and a decrease in left ventricular stroke volume producing a fall in arterial blood pressure and pulse pressure (the difference between the systolic and diastolic pressures). This fall in pressure stimulates the receptors in the carotid sinus, aortic arch, and common carotid artery which are sensitive to pressure and which in turn cause an increase in sympathetic activity, resulting in an increase in heart rate and peripheral vasoconstriction. At the bedside, Phase II is characterized by an increase in heart rate and a fall in blood pressure.

With Phase III or release of the strain there is an increased venous return to the right heart and an increase in blood volume in the pulmonary vascular bed. This is ultimately transmitted to the left side of the heart with an associated increase in the left ventricular stroke volume as the left ventricle once again fills. Because it takes a few seconds for the pulmonary vascular bed to fill with blood before it reaches the left heart, there may be a continuous fall in cardiac output and blood pressure for 2 to 3 seconds immediately upon the release of the strain.

Phase IV is called the overshoot and is characterized by bradycardia and a rise in blood pressure over the resting observed values. This occurs because the increased left ventricular stroke volume is ejected into a constricted peripheral vascular bed. This constricted bed causes an increase in peripheral resistance and the pressure therefore rises. The pressure-sensitive receptors in the carotid body sense the higher pressure, and parasympathetic activity through the vagus nerve is stimulated, causing a reflex slowing of the heart. The overshoot period is then characterized by blood pressure that is greater than the initial resting values and by bradycardia.

In the patient with heart failure the response to the Valsalva maneuver is quite different. As the strain begins, there is a rise in intrathoracic pressure. This rise in pressure is transmitted and is noted as an increase in the peripheral arterial pressure. However, as the strain continues, there is no decrease in pressure and no increase in the heart rate. Upon release of the maneuver the blood pressure returns to the baseline values and there is no overshoot. This kind of response, in which there is only a rise in arterial pressure without any heart-rate changes and no overshoot response, has been called the square-wave response and is due to the fact that the failing myocardium with its already maximized preload will not change total stroke volume enough to decrease cardiac output further and stimulate the pressor receptors. The same kind of response is seen in patients with a significant atrial septal defect since the preload to the right ventricle remains high because of the shunt from the left to the right atrium.

A pilot study of 51 postinfarction patients designed to serially evaluate the Valsalva maneuver showed it to be an insensitive indicator of an impending acute event.[5]

management of heart failure

Heart failure may be present in varying degrees of severity. In acute myocardial infarction, heart failure has been simply and usefully classified by Killip into four classes: I — no failure; II — mild to moderate failure; III — acute pulmonary edema; and IV — cardiogenic shock.[6]

Early, moderate (Killip Class II) and chronic failure are often characterized by a third heart sound, increased heart rate (usually sinus rhythm), and possibly fine post-tussic crackling rales at the lung bases. In addition, evidence of pulmonary vascular congestion (often without pulmonary edema) is often present on the chest x-ray and arrhythmias may be present: atrial premature contractions, atrial fibrillation, atrial flutter, paroxysmal atrial tachycardia and junctional rhythms. The patient may be reasonably comfortable at rest or may have symptoms of low cardiac output or pulmonary vascular congestion. Symptoms are increased with activity.

Acute pulmonary edema (Killip Class III) is a life-threatening situation characterized by transudation of fluid from the pulmonary capillary bed into the alveolar spaces with associated extreme dyspnea and anxiety. Immediate care is required if the patient's life is to be saved.

Cardiogenic shock (Killip Class IV) is the most ominous pump failure syndrome and has the highest mortality, even with aggressive care. Cardiogenic shock is recognized clinically by a systolic blood pressure less than 80 mm. Hg (often it cannot be measured); a feeble pulse that is often rapid; pale, cool, and sweaty skin that is frequently cyanotic; restlessness, confusion and apathy. Coma is not usual. Urine output is decreased and may be absent. These manifestations of shock are a reflection of the profound inadequacy of the heart as a pump, and usually reflect a large amount of muscle damage (40 percent or more of the left ventricular mass). Some patients with significant, long-standing arterial hypertension will have manifestations of cardiogenic shock at relatively normal pressures. These people require a higher pressure to perfuse vital organs and maintain viability. Knowledge of the preceding blood pressure history is of great importance in recognizing these people. Not all clinical circumstances of cardiogenic shock are associated with an inadequate cardiac output, however. Depending on modifying circumstances, such as fever, the cardiac output may occasionally be normal or even increased.

The failure to decrease coronary care unit mortality below 10 to 15 percent is largely due to only modest improvement in the management and mortality of severe pump failure syndromes, especially cardiogenic shock.

The physiological responses to heart failure form a rational basis for treatment. The goals of the management of congestive heart failure are to reduce the work of the heart, to increase cardiac output and myocardial contractility, and to decrease retention of salt and water.

Since the heart cannot be put to complete rest to heal in the same fashion as a broken bone, the best that can be done is to put the entire patient to rest; thereby through inactivity the overall pumping demand on the heart is decreased. *Bed rest* is therefore an important part of the treatment of congestive heart failure, especially in acute and refractory stages. In addition to decreasing the overall work demands made on the heart, bed rest assists in lowering the work load by decreasing the intravascular volume through a recumbency-induced diuresis.[7] Studies of prolonged bed rest have demonstrated that within 48 to 72 hours of inactivity there is a decrease of plasma volume of 300 ml. or more. While this is not a great volume in terms of the overall intravascular fluid compartment, it does assist in decreasing the volume load that is presented to the failing heart. It therefore assists in decreasing dilatation of the heart chambers and establishing a compensated state. This effect results from stimulation of atrial stretch receptors which sense the increased volume of blood returning to the right side of the heart that would be sequestered in the lower extremities if the patient were upright. These receptors then "turn off" the production of antidiuretic hormone and a diuresis follows. By decreasing intravascular volume and therefore the amount of blood presented to the heart to pump (preload), compensation of the heart may be enhanced.

In addition to bed rest, *salt* and *water restriction* and *diuretics,* either oral or parenteral, will also decrease preload and the work of the heart.

All diuretics, regardless of the route of administration, may cause significant changes in the serum electrolytes, especially potassium and chloride. Therefore, regular determination of serum electrolytes is important in patient follow-up. This is particularly true when the patient is also receiving digitalis, because low potassium produced by diuretics predisposes to digitalis toxicity, a life-threatening but avoidable complication. Because of this possibility, potassium supplements are customarily ordered when potassium-depleting diuretics are given, especially when digitalis is given as well.

The choice of route of administration of the diuretic is largely a function of the gravity of the clinical situation: mild to moderate left ventricular failure (manifested by sinus tachycardia, post-tussic rales and a third heart sound) can usually be managed with oral preparations. On the other hand, acute pulmonary edema, a life-threatening situation, demands more drastic approaches and the parenteral route should be chosen.

Other modifiers of preload and afterload are valuable approaches to the management of acute and chronic failure states. Both pharmacological and mechanical methods are useful.

Morphine is the single most useful drug in the treatment of pulmonary edema. It achieves its primary physiological usefulness through a peripheral vasodilating effect, forming a peripheral pool of blood (bloodless phlebotomy) which decreases venous return and decreases the work of the heart. In addition, morphine allays the great anxiety associated with severe dyspnea and quiets the patient, thereby decreasing the respiratory pump mechanism for increasing venous return. Morphine also decreases arterial blood pressure and resistance, lessening the work of the heart (decreased afterload).

An even more dramatic method for decreasing preload and the work of the heart is *phlebotomy,* a procedure that is often useful in the patient with acute pulmonary edema because it immediately removes a volume of blood from the central circulation, decreases venous return and filling pressure, and provides rather prompt reversal of some basic hemodynamic problems. Phlebotomy may be bloodless (rotating tourniquets), or whole blood may be directly removed from the circulation. Tourniquets are less effective than direct removal of blood. While often helpful in managing acute pulmonary edema, phlebotomy may be dangerous in the patient who does not have an increased intravascular volume. This situation most commonly occurs in patients with acute myocardial infarction in which there is extensive muscle damage and rapid onset of pulmonary edema before the kidneys can compensate for a diminished cardiac output by sodium and water retention. Patients with normal blood volume and pulmonary edema usually have a normal-sized heart on chest x-ray. Removing a unit of blood from the circulation either by use of tourniquets or by venesection may cause a significant drop in blood pressure in these patients. On the other hand, the person with more chronic congestive heart failure with an increased intravascular volume and dilatation of the heart in association with pulmonary edema is often an excellent candidate for rotating tourniquets or venesection.

Recently, the use of *nitrates,* both acutely and chronically, has been advocated in the management of heart failure.[8] By causing peripheral vasodilatation, the heart is "unloaded" (decreased afterload) with a subsequent increase in cardiac output, decrease in pulmonary artery wedge pressure (a measurement which reflects the degree of pulmonary vascular congestion and the severity of left ventricular failure), and decrease in myocardial oxygen consumption. This form of therapy has been found useful in mild to moderate failure and acute pulmonary edema failure associated with myocardial infarction, chronic refractory left ventricular failure, and failure associated with severe mitral regurgitation. At the present time, the use of parenteral vasodilator therapy (sodium nitroprusside) requires accurate hemodynamic monitoring of arterial and pulmonary wedge pressure (arterial cannula and Swan-Ganz catheter) and use of an infusion pump to carefully titrate the dose delivered. Nitroprusside must be used with care. Long-acting nitrate therapy is usually given with isosorbide dinitrate (sublingual or oral, the former being preferred), or nitroglycerin ointment. Some patients who have received maximum benefit from other forms of therapy for left ventricular failure have been substantially improved by vasodilator treatment.

While modification of the work of the heart through decreasing preload and afterload is indicated in heart failure and at times permits avoidance of drugs which increase the force of myocardial contraction, inotropic agents remain important therapeutic tools. *Digitalis* is the primary drug for increasing contractility. This inotropic drug has a multiplicity of uses in cardiology and is also potentially one of the most dangerous, a fact recognized in 1785 by William Withering, discoverer of the pharmacological value and toxicity of digitalis (foxglove): "Foxglove when given in very large and quickly repeated doses occasions sickness, vomiting, purging, confused vision, objects appearing green or yellow, increased secretion of urine with frequent motions to part with it and sometimes inability to retain it; slow pulse even as low as 35 in a minute, cold sweats, convulsions, syncope and death."[9] In the failing heart, digitalis slows the ventricular rate and increases the force of contraction, increasing cardiac efficiency. As cardiac output increases, a greater volume of fluid is presented to the kidneys for filtration and excretion, and intravascular volume decreases.

In early failure with acute myocardial infarction, digitalis may increase the potential amount of damaged myocardium by causing increased contractility and therefore increased myocardial oxygen demand. Treatment of failure in this circumstance is probably best if preload and/or afterload are decreased through the use of diuretics and/or nitrates. Of course, if either agent causes a significant drop in central aortic pressure, coronary artery perfusion may fall and the area of damage increase. The key lesson here is that any medication has potentially ominous side effects, that a management regimen must be selected with care and with a full understanding of potential adverse effects, and that close patient monitoring is mandatory.

Cardiogenic shock unfortunately is not a completely understood situation at this time. Accordingly, the management of cardiogenic shock is generally unsatisfactory. At the very least, treatment requires administration of bicarbonate to correct the metabolic acidosis, oxygen, and agents to elevate the blood pressure. The most commonly used pressor agents at this time are dopamine, norepinephrine, and glucagon. Depending upon the pulmonary artery wedge pressure (left ventricular filling pressure) the administration of small amounts of fluid may be indicated. Mechanical life support devices such as intra-aortic balloon counterpulsation, direct ventricular assistors, or left heart bypass are occasionally used. The intra-aortic balloon assist device has been the most successful to date and has established a place in cardiac care. The general outlook for patients with cardiogenic shock is poor for both the short and the long term. Heart failure, with its accompanying symptoms of low cardiac output and/or pulmonary vascular congestion, is one of the major sources of disability in cardiovascular disease. Its recognition and pathophysiologically based management are of paramount importance if a patient's functional capacity and vocational and community viability are to be optimized and maintained.

REFERENCES

1. S. M. Fox, P. C. Gazes, and H. W. Blackburn, et al., "Exercise and Stress Testing Workshop Report," *Journal of the South Carolina Medical Association*, Vol. 65 (1969, Suppl.), p. 74.
2. T. Lewis, *Diseases of the Heart* (New York: The Macmillan Company, 1933).

3. E. A. Longo and L. S. Cohen, "Rupture of Interventricular Septum in Acute Myocardial Infarction," *American Heart Journal,* Vol. 92 (1976), p. 81.

4. W. E. Judson, J. D. Hatcher, and R. W. Wilkins, "Blood Pressure Responses to the Valsalva Maneuver in Cardiac Patients With and Without Congestive Failure," *Circulation,* Vol. 11 (1955), p. 889.

5. H. L. Brammell, unpublished observations.

6. T. Killip and J. T. Kimball, "Treatment of Myocardial Infarction in a Coronary Care Unit. A Two-Year Experience with 250 Patients," *American Journal of Cardiology,* Vol. 20 (1967), p. 457.

7. P. B. Miller, R. L. Johnson, and L. E. Lamb, "Effects of Four Weeks of Absolute Bed Rest on Circulatory Function in Man," *Aerospace Medicine,* Vol. 35 (1964), p. 1194.

8. P. L. DaLuz and J. S. Forrester, "Influence of Vasodilators Upon Function and Metabolism of Ischemic Myocardium," *American Journal of Cardiology,* Vol. 37 (1976), p. 581.

9. W. Withering, *An Account of the Foxglove and Its Medical Uses, with Practical Remarks on Dropsy and Other Diseases* (London: C. G. J. and J. Robinson, 1785).

General Reference Volume

Mason, D. T. (ed.), *Congestive Heart Failure: Mechanisms, Evaluation and Treatment* (New York: Yorke Medical Books, 1976).

ALVA R. DEGNER, R.N.
LANE D. CRADDOCK, M.D.
PHILLIP S. WOLF, M.D.

9 **6**

management modalities: cardiovascular system

cardiac monitoring

Monitoring the patient with cardiac disturbances is now accepted as routine practice. Since the first hard wire bedside monitor, modern electronics has constantly been making sophisticated advances in monitoring equipment. Remote display systems currently incorporate features such as *nonfade scopes* which keep the ECG pattern visible across the screen; *freeze* modes which allow the ECG pattern to be held for more detailed examination; *storage capability*, either by tape loops or an electronic memory, which permits retrieval of arrhythmias from 8 to 60 seconds after their occurrence; *automatic chart documentation* when the ECG recorder is activated by alarms and/or at preset intervals; *heart rate monitors* which display the rate either by meter or by digital display (the alarm system is incorporated into the heart rate monitor with adjustments for both the high and low settings); *multiparameter displays* which offer display of pressures, temperature, EEG, respirations, etc.; *computer systems* which store and analyze ECG data. The information can then be retrieved at any time to aid in diagnosis and to note trends in the patient's status.

Two types of patient monitoring equipment presently in use are hard wire devices and telemetry. Hard wire monitors require an electrical cable between the patient and the ECG display device. Telemetry simply requires the patient to carry a small battery-operated transmitter. No wire connection is needed between the patient and the ECG display device. In addition to the *transmitter*, which has a frequency similar to radio stations, telemetry systems require *receivers* which pick up and display the signal on a scope and

103

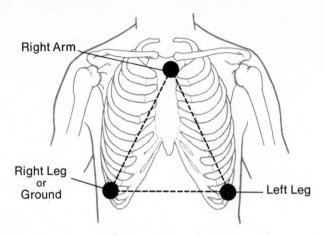

Fig. 9-1. 3-lead system when lead selection is not part of monitor.

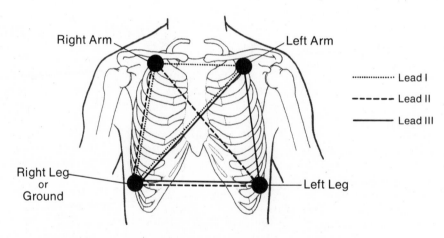

Fig. 9-2. 4-lead system when lead selection is part of monitor.

antennas which are built into the receiver and may be mounted in various areas to widen the range of signal pick-up. Mercury batteries are the power source for the transmitter, thus making it possible to avoid electrical hazards by isolating the monitoring system from potential current leakage and accidental shock.

Manufacturers of hard wire and telemetry monitoring systems provide operating instructions, which should be followed to insure proper and safe functioning of the equipment.

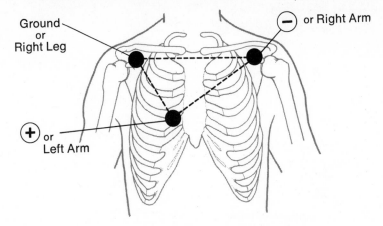

Fig. 9-3. Marriott's MCL[1]. (Use Lead I selection.)

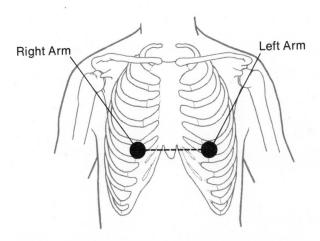

Fig. 9-4. For telemetry no ground electrode is necessary.

electrode/lead application

A high quality trace will exhibit a narrow stable baseline, absence of distortion or "noise," and sufficient amplitude of the QRS complex to properly activate the rate meters and alarm systems and to allow for identification of P waves.

Figures 9-1, 9-2, 9-3, and 9-4 show suggested lead placements.

TYPES OF ELECTRODES

Needle electrodes are placed under the skin and thus eliminate variations caused by skin resistance. However, they are traumatic and provide a source of infection because of the break in skin integrity.

Metal disk electrodes are cumbersome and restricting to the patient. Considerable artifact occurs because of the inability to seal the disk adequately to the skin.

Pregelled disposable silver- and nickle-plated electrodes are at this time the most suitable for long-term monitoring. They are the most comfortable for the patient, but if not applied properly, they are susceptible to motion and muscle artifact which can result in wandering baselines and false alarms.

SKIN PREPARATION

Proper skin preparation and application of electrodes are imperative to good monitoring.

1. Select site. Avoid bony protuberances, joints and folds in skin. Areas where muscle attaches to bone have the least motion artifact.
2. Shave excessive body hair from site.
3. Use alchohol to remove residue from oils, lotion, etc. used in patient care. Sites must be free of any oil film or residue which could affect electrode adhesion.
4. Briskly rub each site with dry gauze. The sites must be dry before electrodes are applied; solvents trapped under the electrodes are frequent causes of skin irritation.

ELECTRODE APPLICATION

1. Place electrode on the skin by tacking one edge of the adhesive area to the skin surface and then pull very gently against the tack.
2. Smooth the electrode to the skin by running your finger around the circular adhesive area. This will reduce motion artifact.

ECG monitor problem solving

Baseline But No ECG Trace

Check proper adjustment of the size (gain or sensitivity) control.
Determine if patient cable is fully inserted into ECG receptacle.
Are lead wires fully inserted into patient cable?
Are lead wires firmly attached to the electrodes?
Examine lead wires for damage.
Have patient cable checked for possible damage.
Call for service if trace is still absent.

Intermittent Trace

Is patient cable fully inserted in monitor receptacle?
Are lead wires fully inserted into patient cable?
Are lead wires firmly attached to electrodes?
Check for loose or worn lead wire connectors.
Have electrodes been applied properly?

Check each electrode for proper location and firm skin contact.
Check patient cable for possible damage.

Wandering Baseline

Is there excessive cable movement? Can be reduced by clipping cable to patient's clothing.
Is there excessive movement of patient?
Is site selection correct?
Was proper skin prep and application followed?
Check each electrode to make sure it is still moist.

Weak Signal

Is size control adjusted properly?
Were the electrodes applied properly?
Check each electrode for dried gel.
Change electrode sites. Check 12-lead ECG for lead with highest amplitude and attempt to simulate that lead.
If none of the above steps remedies the problem, the weak signal may be the patient's normal complex.

Sixty Cycle Interference

Is the monitor size control set too high?
Nearby electrical devices in use may be the cause.
Were the electrodes applied properly?
Check electrodes for dried gel.
Check for damaged lead wires and connections.

Excessive Triggering of Heart Rate Alarms

Hi-Low alarm may be set too close to patient's normal rate.
Is patient cable securely inserted into monitor receptacle?
Check for damaged lead wires and connections.
Electrode site selection, because of low amplitude, may affect waveform amplitude.
Were electrodes applied properly?
An unstable baseline or excessive cable and lead wire movement can set off alarm. Check steps to remedy the problem.

Skin Irritation

The presence of preparation materials such as alcohol and acetone or skin conditioners under the electrodes is the most frequent cause of patient skin irritation. The skin must be dry before electrode application.
Harsh skin preparation technique.
Patient sensitivity to gels, adhesives or prep solutions.
DC leakage from the monitor.

BIBLIOGRAPHY

Marriott, H., and E. Fogg, "Constant Monitoring for Cardiac Dysrhythmias," *Modern Concepts of Cardiovascular Disease*, Vol. 39 (June 1970), pp. 103-108.

Beaumont, E., "ECG Telemetry," *Nursing '74* (July 1974), pp. 27-34.

artificial cardiac pacing

Electrical stimulation of the heart was tried experimentally as early as 1819. In 1930 Hyman noted that he could inject the right atrium with a diversity of substances and restore a heartbeat. He devised an "ingenious apparatus" that he labeled an artificial pacemaker, which delivered a rhythmic charge to the heart. In 1952 Zoll demonstrated that patients with Stokes-Adams syndrome could be sustained by the administration of current directly to the chest wall. Lillehei in 1957 affixed electrodes directly to the ventricles during open-heart surgery. In the period 1958 to 1961 implantable pacemakers for treatment of complete heart block came into use in a rather extensive fashion. Over subsequent years, various improvements and refinements have been made for both short-term temporary pacing and long term permanent pacing.

indications for artificial pacing

Indications for short-term cardiac pacing include:
1. Emergency pacing for prolonged Stokes-Adams attack.
2. Myocardial infarction associated with symptomatic second- or third-degree A-V block, acute bifascicular blocks, or severe bradycardias not responsive to drug therapy.
3. In preparation for long-term pacing to improve the patient's clinical state, guard against serious arrhythmias, and allow for evaluation of the benefits of long-term pacing.
4. Coverage against the risk of cardiac arrest during the implantation of the permanent pacemaker.
5. Coverage for anesthesia and surgery in patients with a history of cardiac arrest or complete heart block.
6. Control of rate during periods of implanted pacemaker failure.
7. Treatment of complete heart block developed during cardiac surgery.
8. Overdriving the heart in order to control tachyarrhythmias or to suppress ectopic ventricular activity.

Indications for long-term pacing include:
1. Severe bradycardia or complete heart block associated with inadequate cardiac output, resulting in myocardial ischemia, congestive heart failure, or renal insufficiency.
2. Recurrent Stokes-Adams attacks.
3. Sick sinus syndrome which includes sinus bradycardia, brady-tachycardia syndrome and sinus arrest, in those who are symptomatic.

methods of pacing

The electrical stimulus can be delivered to the heart in three basic ways:
1. External—by means of an electrode placed on the chest wall.
2. Transthoracic—by implanting electrode wires into the myocardium via needles inserted through the chest wall.
3. Direct—by passing a small electrode through the venous system into the right ventricle or by attaching electrodes to the epicardial surface of the heart via a thoracotomy.

The technique for establishing the various pacing systems is described in order to give the nurse greater understanding of the procedure so that she is better prepared to assist with it and to explain it to the patient.

EXTERNAL CARDIAC PACING

After Zoll's work, external cardiac pacing became the accepted approach for treating ventricular asystole. However, this method is now largely abandoned because of its unpredictable effectiveness and is utilized only as a desperation technique in emergency situations. This approach to pacing is precluded by severe pain, skin burns, and skeletal muscle contractions resulting from the high voltage and current required. Therefore, it is unsuitable for the preventive treatment of warning arrhythmias or as long-term prophylaxis against recurrent cardiac standstill. Its single advantage is the ease and rapidity with which it can be initiated. The technique of external pacing is as follows:

1. A small metal electrode is attached to the chest wall in the left precordial area and is anchored with adhesive tape. The ground electrode is placed on the right side of the chest in a similar manner.
2. The electrodes are then attached to the power supply which may be part of the monitoring system or a separate battery pack.
3. With external pacing, the energy level of the power supply is set at the maximum level.
4. Rate should be set at 70 to 80 impulses per minute.
5. If the heart is not stimulated, initiate cardiopulmonary resuscitation immediately.

TRANSTHORACIC OR PERCUTANEOUS PACING

Wires inserted percutaneously into the wall of the right ventricle via a needle introduced through the chest wall can produce ventricular stimulation. The advantage of this method is the rapidity and ease with which pacing can be initiated and the availability of the necessary equipment. It is not suitable for long-term pacing or as a prophylaxis against warning arrhythmias. There is a small risk of coronary artery puncture and hemopericardium associated with this method. The technique of transthoracic pacing is as follows:

1. A #20 gauge spinal needle with a stylet is introduced through the anterior chest wall at the fifth or sixth left intercostal space near the sternum. The needle is advanced at a 30-degree angle toward the right second intercostal space about 5 mm. into the myocardium.
2. The stylet is removed and a stainless steel noninsulated surgical wire is advanced through the needle about 1 cm. beyond the tip.
3. The needle is removed, the electrode is withdrawn until contact is made with the endocardium, and then the electrode is connected to the negative pole of the external power source.
4. The energy level of the power supply is set at 10 to 15 milliamperes and a pacing rate of 70 to 80 impulses per minute is appropriate.

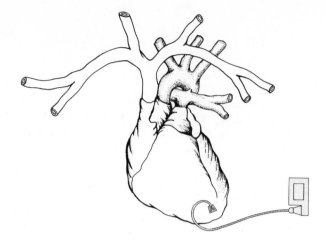

Fig. 9-5. Epicardial implantation of pacemaker electrode.

DIRECT EPICARDIAL PACING

Effective pacing can be accomplished by implanting the electrode system directly on the myocardium (Fig. 9-5). This is done under general anesthesia via a left anterolateral thoracotomy.

This method is being abandoned in favor of endocardial electrodes because it involves a thoracotomy, while the transvenous method can be done under local anesthesia. The life span for both pacemakers is approximately the same. Since the procedure involves direct visualization of the heart, there is greater operative risk, a longer hospitalization, and more postoperative complications.

Some physicians prefer this approach in children and young adults because of the possibility of yet unknown hazards of the long-term presence of an endocardial electrode and the chance of electrode displacement due to growth. This method is also utilized as a temporary adjunct after open-heart surgery. In these cases, the electrodes are sutured to the heart and brought out through the chest wall. The wires can be pulled out when they are no longer needed. The technique of epicardial pacing is as follows:

1. A thoracotomy is performed under general anesthesia.
2. The electrode tips are sutured to the apex of the right or left ventricle.
3. The wires are connected to the power pack which is implanted in a subcutaneous pouch in the axillary region or the abdominal wall.

DIRECT ENDOCARDIAL OR TRANSVENOUS PACING

Transvenous electrodes are presently the most utilized and satisfactory method of pacing. This method can be employed as a temporary or permanent measure.

The catheter electrode is introduced into a superficial vein (brachial, external jugular, femoral, or subclavian), threaded through the vena cava and right atrium, and lodged against the endocardial surface of the right ventricle. The electrical stimulus is provided by an external generator source or an implanted power supply (Fig. 9-6). The technique of temporary transvenous pacing is as follows:

1. The vein is selected and the skin area is cleansed with an antiseptic solution.

   Brachial vein — usually requires a cutdown. The patient's arm must be immobilized as the electrode can easily become dislodged. Phlebitis is a rather common complication.

   Femoral vein — involves a percutaneous puncture. The patient's mobility is markedly reduced.

   External jugular vein — a cutdown is required. It is desirable to reserve this site since it is most often used for the permanent transvenous elctrode. This site does permit patient mobility and the use of both arms (Fig. 9-7).

   Subclavian vein — a cutdown is not required and insertion is therefore more expedient. It allows for patient mobility and the use of both arms. It also results in greater catheter stability and a lesser incidence of infection and phlebitis. Complications encountered with use of this site include pneumothorax, hemothorax, subcutaneous emphysema, brachial plexus injury, septicemia, local hematoma, and air embolism (Figs. 9-8 and 9-9).

2. The puncture site is infiltrated with a local anesthetic.

3. The needle is inserted into the vein and the catheter is threaded into position in the right ventricular apex.

4. The catheter is ideally positioned under fluoroscopy but this is not always feasible. An alternate method of positioning the catheter may be accomplished by attaching the electrode to the "V" lead of the electrocardiogram machine with an alligator clamp. When the tip of the catheter is in the vena cava, the amplitude of the P wave and the QRS will be about the same. When the tip has crossed the tricuspid valve, the QRS amplitude will increase markedly. The ECG will reveal a current of injury pattern when the tip touches the endocardium (Fig. 9-10).

Use of the balloon-tipped or flow-directed catheter in conjunction with ECG monitoring generally precludes the need for fluoroscopy and is commonly placed in the critically ill patient. The balloon is partially inflated when the tip has reached the veins in the areas of the shoulder to facilitate the passage of the catheter through the venous bed to the right atrium. The balloon is then fully inflated and the catheter is advanced by allowing blood flow to carry the tip into the right ventricle. To prevent the catheter from floating into the pulmonary outflow tract, the balloon is deflated and the catheter is lodged into the ventricular apex. Either carbon dioxide or air may be used to inflate the balloon. Much caution must be exercised when using air to prevent fracture of the balloon. All air must be removed from the balloon before the catheter is removed.

(*Text continued on page 115.*)

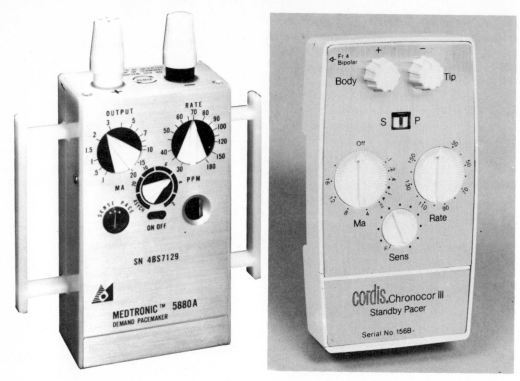

Fig. 9-6. External battery-powered pacemakers. (*Left*) Medtronic, Inc. (*Right*) Cordis Corporation.

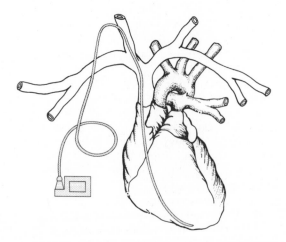

Fig. 9-7. Endocardial pacemaker electrode via jugular vein.

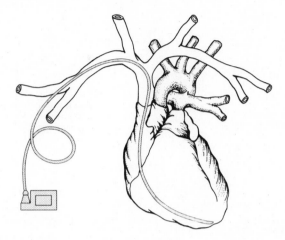

Fig. 9-8. Endocardial pacemaker electrode via right subclavian vein.

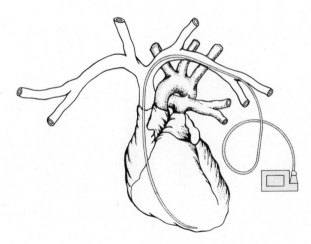

Fig. 9-9. Endocardial pacemaker electrode via left subclavian vein.

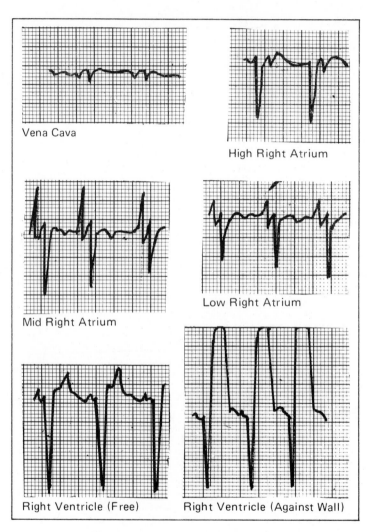

Fig. 9-10. Intracavitary ECG recording.

nursing responsibilities

Related to insertion of pacemaker:
1. The patient must be prepared by having the purpose of the pacemaker and the procedure explained.
2. If the catheter electrode is positioned by ECG, attach the limb leads to all extremities and use the V lead as the attachment for the electrode. It is vital that all equipment be grounded to prevent electrocution by current leakage passing through the catheter.
3. Establish a patent intravenous site.
4. Have a bolus of lidocaine available in case of ventricular irritability.
5. Have an isoproterenol (Isuprel) infusion available to maintain the patient until the pacemaker is ready.
6. Defibrillator should be on standby.
7. Assist in the observation of the ECG recording.

Related to postinsertion of pacemaker:

To provide an electrically safe environment:
1. The patient should be in a nonelectric bed.
2. The following sources of potentially excessive stimulation must not be used near the patient: electric radios, shavers or toothbrushes, microwave ovens, diathermy, electrocautery or electrocoagulating equipment. Battery-operated applicances may be used.
3. Keep the patient in a dry environment. Change gown and linen if wet.
4. If the pacemaker battery pack is of the type in which the terminal connectors are exposed, the battery pack must be encased in an insulated material so that current leakage from other equipment will not be delivered to the heart. Newer battery pack models have insulated connectors which encase the terminals and therefore eliminate the need for enclosing the pack in additional nonconductive material. Whenever the metal terminals of the catheter are touched, rubber gloves must be worn.
5. Disconnect the patient from the cardiac monitor prior to taking an ECG if a common ground is not available.
6. Use only electrical equipment that is properly grounded. If any doubt exists concerning the safety of any electrical equipment, do not use it until it is checked by the biomedical engineer.
7. Cover the external battery pack with a plastic cover to prevent inadvertent changing of dials.
8. If defibrillation or countershock is needed, avoid close contact with the generator.

To prevent catheter displacement:
1. Allow no direct tension on the pacemaker catheter.
2. Minimize the amount of motion allowed to an extremity where the catheter is located.
3. Secure the pacemaker battery pack to the patient.
4. Tape the pacemaker catheter to the skin securely.

To prevent infection:
    1. Keep the pacemaker dressing dry and intact. Dressings should be changed every other day, using sterile technique.

Observations and appropriate actions for pacemaker malfunction are discussed later in this chapter.

Technique for permanent implantation of a transvenous pacemaker:
    1. Local anesthesia is used at the cutdown site and the incision for the battery pack.
    2. The electrode is passed through either the jugular vein or the subclavian vein.
    3. Fluoroscopy is utilized to position the catheter in the right ventricular apex.
    4. The power pack is embedded in the axillary area and the electrodes are connected subcutaneously either over or under the clavicle. Alternate sites for the power pack are overlying the abdomen or the pectoralis major muscle.

types of pacemaker generators

Pacemakers are basically of two types: the fixed rate or asynchronous system and the demand or synchronous system.

FIXED RATE – ASYNCHRONOUS – PARASYSTOLIC

The electrical mechanism of this pacemaker discharges at a fixed rate which is independent of the electrical activity of the heart. It is not changed by any physiological parameter which might require an increased rate with subsequent increased cardiac output. The constant threat of the patient's own rhythm competing with the pacemaker makes this a very undesirable type of generator. The fixed-rate pacemaker should be used only when it is unlikely that the patient will return to normal sinus rhythm. This generator is less prone to failure because of the simplicity of its design. This mode of pacing is used in both temporary and permanent pacing (Figs. 9-11 and 9-12).

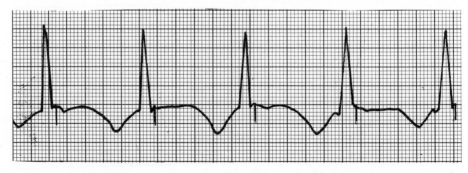

Fig. 9-11. Fixed rate pacemaker artifact with electrode in ventricle.

DEMAND—SYNCHRONOUS—NONPARASYSTOLIC

The *ventricular inhibited demand* or *"R" wave inhibited* device is stimulated only when the patient's ventricular rate falls below the preset rate of the generator. The pacemaker senses the signal of the QRS (whether from atrial conduction or ventricular extrasystoles) coming back through the electrodes and suppresses the output of the generator. It is important to obtain a stable electrode position to provide an ECG signal of sufficient amplitude to be sensed. The pacemaker can be falsely inhibited by a P or T wave (Fig. 9-13). However, improved sensing filters have reduced this hazard. In some pacemakers, the escape interval is preset at a slower rate than the automatic pacing interval. This is known as rate hysteresis (Fig. 9-14). Ventricular fibrillation due to competition is almost nonexistent. Figures 9-15 and 9-16 illustrate a demand pacemaker firing when the patient's ventricular rate falls below a preset rate.

A *ventricular triggered, "R" wave triggered, standby* or *ventricular synchronous* device senses the "QRS" (either normal or ectopic) and superimposes the pacing impulse into the absolute refractory period. The only purpose of the "QRS" triggered pacemaker stimulus is to demonstrate the sensing mechanism. If a spontaneous beat fails to occur, the pacemaker will discharge at a preset escape interval. Because the pacemaker distorts the QRS complex, problems occur in the interpretation of the ECG in certain arrhythmias and in the evaluation of acute myocardial injury.

An *atrial synchronous* or *"P" wave triggered ventricular* pacemaker has a sensing electrode located in the atrium and a stimulating electrode in the ventricle. The electrode in the atrium senses the natural P wave and, after a delay which corresponds to the normal P-R interval, the ventricle is stimulated. If a P wave fails to appear, the ventricular pacemaker will fire after a preset escape interval. The rate varies according to physiological demands. The problem with this method is that it also responds to pathological impulses and could result in rapid ventricular responses with atrial fibrillation or flutter.

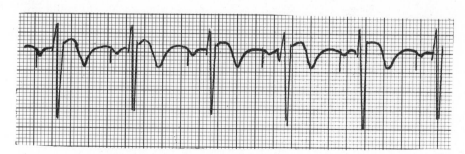

Fig. 9-12. Fixed rate pacemaker artifact with electrode in atrium.

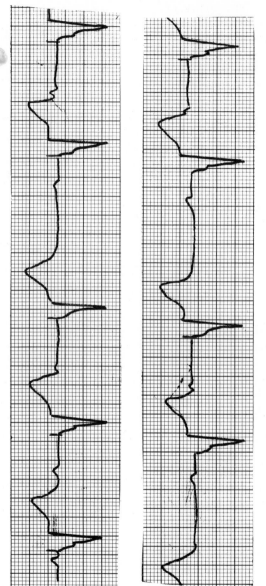
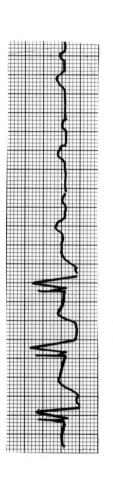

Fig. 9-13. Ventricular-inhibited pacemaker sensing T waves.

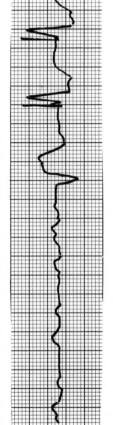

Fig. 9-14 (*top and bottom*). Pacemaker with rate hysteresis. The escape interval is longer than the automatic interval.

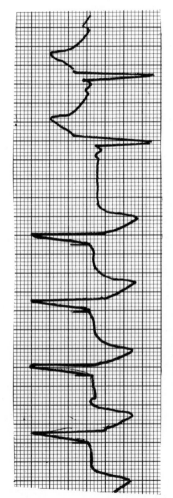

Fig. 9-15. Demand pacemaker. Last two beats are conducted normally.

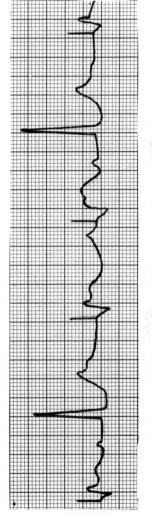

Fig. 9-16. Pacemaker fires when patient's ventricular rate falls below a preset rate.

atrial pacemakers

A *continuous sequential atrial* or *ventricular* or *biofocal demand* device has stimulating electrodes in both the atrium and ventricle which fire continuously in sequence. The sequential delay between the two stimuli is equal to the normal P-R interval. The hazards present with asynchronous pacemakers are a problem with this type of pacemaker also.

The *QRS inhibited sequential atrial and ventricular* pacemaker has a sensing and stimulating electrode in the ventricle and a stimulating electrode in the atrium. When a natural QRS is sensed, both atrial and ventricular stimuli are inhibited. If a natural QRS is not sensed, the atria and ventricles are stimulated in sequence (Fig. 9-17).

types of catheter electrodes

There are two basic electrodes. In order for electrical stimulation to occur, current must flow between two poles to create an electrical circuit. With the unipolar electrode, the negative pole is within the heart and the positive pole is accomplished by a wire suture placed in the skin on the chest wall. The bipolar electrode has both poles at the tip of the catheter about 1 cm. apart. It is felt that a bipolar electrode will continue to pace even if contact with the endocardium is lost. However, the unipolar catheter will stop pacing if this contact is lost. The unipolar catheter also causes pain at the site of the indifferent electrode.

pacing rate

The most advantageous rate for pacing will depend on the specific indications and the clinical condition of the patient. The rate should be set to the point where cardiac output is maximal (50 to 105 per minute). However, the optimal rate for achieving maximal cardiac output may not coincide with the best rate for suppressing ectopic activity. The oxygen demand of the myocardium is increased and results in angina if the rate is too fast. Also, at rapid pacing rates, inadequate ventricular filling takes place and the cardiac output is decreased. In complete heart block, the atrial rate is an index to the ventricular pacing rate necessary for adequate cardiac function. In other words, if the atrial rate is 70 per minute, the pacemaker rate should be set at 70 per minute.

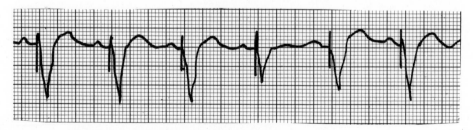

Fig. 9-17. Atrial synchronized pacemaker functioning normally.

energy of pacing

When the heart is stimulated by an electrical impulse, it either contracts completely or not at all. The lowest level of energy at which the heart will contract is called the *threshold level*. If the pacing stimulus is less than the threshold level, the heart will not contract. However, if the stimulus is greater than the threshold level, it will not improve contractility.

When the catheter is positioned and connected to the power supply, the energy-level dial is gradually increased until a QRS is noted with each stimulus. This level is called the *threshold* and is measured in milliamperes (mA).

The pacing threshold is affected by tissue excitability, electrode position, impulse duration, waveform and wave amplitude. The threshold is increased the first few days after insertion of the pacemaker due to local tissue reaction. Drugs affect the threshold in various ways. Sympathomimetic amines, adrenal steroids, and glucocorticoids decrease the threshold. Beta-adrenergic and mineralocorticoids increase the threshold. Atropine, quinidine, procainamide (Pronestyl), and lidocaine do not affect the threshold.

The relationship of extracellular to intracellular potassium concentration is important in determining the pacing threshold. When the serum potassium is elevated, the threshold is decreased, and when the extracellular potassium is decreased, the muscles become refractory to electrical stimulation.

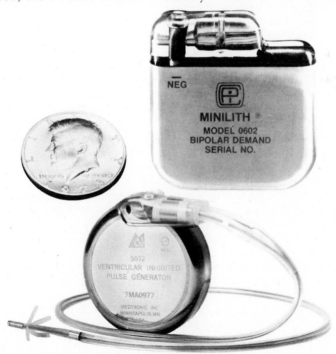

Fig. 9-18. Internal pacemaker generators. (*Top*) Cardiac Pacemakers, Inc. (*Bottom*) Medtronic, Inc.

power sources

Currently the mercury-zinc batteries are the most universal type of power source readily accessible to all. These batteries have a short life of two to four years and consequently need close follow-up observation (Fig. 9-18, p. 121).

New sources of energy are being developed and are expected to be in common usage. These new sources include lithium batteries which are expected to last four to ten years.

Pacemakers that can be recharged by holding a special device over the site of implantation are in use. At this time, the recharging requires 60 to 90 minutes per week.

Nuclear-powered batteries have been used. These batteries have a potential life of 20 years, being powered by plutonium which converts radioactive energy to heat and then to electrical energy.

Other power sources being investigated include piezoelectric materials which are crystalline structures that act by bending molecules to generate electricity. Possibly, such material could generate enough energy for pacing if attached to the heart or diaphragm. Biological batteries that utilize electrolytic interactions of body fluids and metals are also being investigated.

complications of pacing

Related to insertion or presence of the electrode within the body:
1. There is a surgical risk if the epicardial technique is used. It involves direct exposure of the heart in an often elderly, debilitated patient. In the 7.5 percent mortality, intraoperative infarction has been observed. With endocardial technique there is less than a 1 percent mortality and less morbidity.
2. Infection or phlebitis at the venous entry site.
3. Pulmonary air embolism if the patient is improperly positioned at the time of the cutdown in the neck. The patient should be flat so that a positive venous pressure exists to prevent an influx of air into the venous system.
4. Ventricular irritability due to the electrode catheter.
5. Myocardial perforation with the use of stiff electrodes. This is more common when the catheter is positioned in the apex of the heart.
6. Pericardial tamponade, although this rarely develops with small electrodes unless the patient is anticoagulated.
7. Entanglement of the electrode around the chordal structures of the tricuspid valve.
8. Large thrombi occurring at the electrode tip or in the right atrium lead to pulmonary emboli or obstructed blood flow.
9. Segments of a fractured electrode may migrate within the vascular system.
10. Electrical stimulation of noncardiac sites such as the phrenic nerve, diaphragm, intercostal muscles, or retrosternal muscles.
11. Endocarditis due to adherence of the catheter to the tricuspid valve.

Related to subcutaneous implantation of the generator:

1. Infection or hematoma.
2. Battery extrusion.
3. Muscular contractions in the region of the implantation.

Related to improper pacer function:

Malfunction of the pacemaker is due to component failure, improper interfacing between the host and the pacer system, and physiological changes within the heart. Failure of the power supply presents itself clinically either by complete cessation of pacing or by intermittent pacing. Complete cessation of pacing may occur abruptly or be preceded by a prolonged period of disordered functioning (Figs. 9-19 to 9-24).

Clinical manifestations of cessation are (1) fatigue, (2) cerebral symptoms, such as syncope, loss of memory, convulsions, (3) Stokes-Adams attack, (4) congestive heart failure, (5) sudden death. If a spontaneous heart rate is present, failure of the demand mode will not be detected unless it is specifically tested. This can be done by slowing the heart with carotid sinus massage or converting the pacemaker to a fixed rate mode by the use of a magnet.

Causes of intermittent pacing are:

1. Displaced catheter or perforation of the ventricular myocardium. (This usually occurs during the first few weeks after implantation. Pacing may vary with body position or respirations.)
2. Partially fractured electrode due to faulty insertion.
3. Changing myocardial threshold. (Threshold is affected by meals, exercise, infection, electrolyte imbalance, change in body metabolism and myocardial fibrosis.)
4. Extraneous electrical signals, as occur when the power supply is close to intense high frequency electrical fields such as microwave ovens and radio and television stations.
5. Diathermy or electrocautery.
6. Poor electrical connections within the power system such as fractured electrodes or an improper pacemaker electrode junction.
7. Competitive rhythms, which are especially hazardous with myocardial ischemia, electrolyte imbalance or hypoxic states. In these conditions, ventricular fibrillation may ensue.

If there is an alteration in the pacing rate with either an increase or decrease in the preset rate, battery depletion is most likely the cause (Fig. 9-24).

Other malfunctions include the loss of the specialized functions of the demand type systems and aberrant stimulation of the diaphragm, intercostal muscles, or abdominal muscles.

Assessment clues to pacemaker malfunction for the nurse:

1. An apical heart rate that is slower or faster than that which was preset for the pacer.
2. Development of abdominal muscle or diaphragmatic twitching (hiccoughs).
3. Appearance of a widely split second heart sound. This is suggestive of migration of the electrode from the right to the left ventricle.

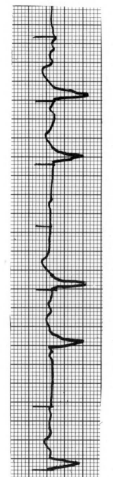

Fig. 9-19. Ventricular pacemaker which fails to capture.

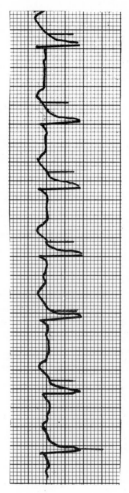

Fig. 9-20. Pacemaker fails to sense. Artifact falls on T wave and not sensing QRS.

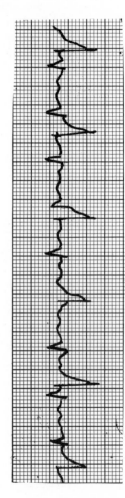

Fig. 9-21. Pacemaker malfunction: not sensing and not capturing.

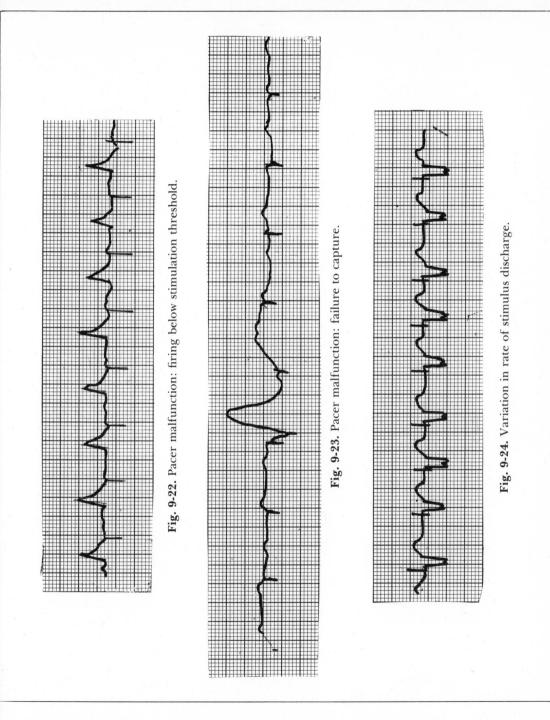

Fig. 9-22. Pacer malfunction: firing below stimulation threshold.

Fig. 9-23. Pacer malfunction: failure to capture.

Fig. 9-24. Variation in rate of stimulus discharge.

4. Absence of pacer spikes with a bradycardia. This may indicate failure or electrode breaks.
5. Alteration in pacing spike rate. This indicates battery depletion or component failure.

Suggested nursing actions for specific malfunctions:

MALFUNCTION	NURSING ACTION
No pacemaker spike and pulse is below rate the pacemaker is set for; or the pacemaker fails to capture.	1. Evaluate adequacy of patient's own rhythm. 2. Check needle on pacemaker box to see that it is fluctuating back and forth. 3. Check all possible connections. 4. Turn up mA as far as it will go *only* if an emergency exists. 5. If patient's clinical status does not improve, turn mA back to its original setting. 6. Have intravenous isoproterenol (Isuprel) on standby. *7. Take emergency measures immediately.
Pacemaker fails to sense the QRS complex; a QRS complex is followed by a pacemaker spike which may or may not cause stimulation of the QRS complex.	1. Evaluate patient's clinical status. 2. Reposition entire limb in which pacemaker is inserted or move the entire body. 3. If patient's rate is adequate, turn pacemaker off. 4. If patient's rate is inadequate, turn the sensitivity clockwise as far as it will go. If this is unsuccessful, turn the mA as high as it will go. 5. If patient's clinical status does not improve, turn the mA and rate back to their original settings. *6. Take emergency measures immediately.
Patient has hiccoughs, diaphragmatic contractions or twitching.	1. Evaluate patient's clinical status. 2. Change position of entire body.

* If defibrillation is necessary, turn off pacemaker and disconnect catheter wires from battery pack. Avoid contact between the paddles and wires.

follow-up care for the patient with an implanted pacemaker

The purpose of follow-up care is to identify malfunction before it causes symptoms and to prevent early replacement of units.

Pacemaker clinics and telephone monitors are becoming available in many areas of the country which replace the routine physician visit and add to the ease of follow-up.

Because the pacemaker power sources do not have a predictable life span, patients must be followed at regular intervals. They should be examined routinely one month postinsertion, and then every six months until 24 months postimplantation. Thereafter, they should be seen at shorter intervals. If at any time there is evidence of pacemaker malfunction, they should be seen more frequently.

An interval history should be included in the follow-up exam. If the patient has experienced any symptoms that he had prior to insertion, intermittent malfunction must be suspected.

A 12-lead ECG should be documented at each visit to determine if the QRS generated by the pacemaker has changed configuration or axis, which suggests movement of the electrode tip. If a change has occurred, an x-ray should be taken. Replacement or reposition of the tip must be considered if displacement is documented.

Gross alteration of rate (5 to 10 percent) from the first exam is indicative of battery depletion, and the unit should be replaced. Many pacemaker clinics have specialized equipment available to precisely measure the rate, amplitude, duration and contour of the impulse. X-ray pictures of the power pack have proved to be of no value, and this practice has been stopped.

patient teaching

A planned and systematic approach to teaching the patient to live with his pacemaker is a vital part of nursing care. A helpful tool in patient teaching is a progress report which is accessible to the physician and other members of the team, along with written guidelines for the nurse instructing the patient. The patient's family should also be involved in the learning process. The following outline gives general instructions for areas to include in patient teaching.

CONTENT AREAS	TEACHING POINTS
Knowledge of Condition Patient's impression	Clarify difference between heart block and heart attack
General anatomy	Make sure that patient knows where natural pacemaker is located and how artificial pacemaker functions

CONTENT AREAS	TEACHING POINTS
Reason for temporary artificial pacemaker	Describe difference between temporary and permanent pacemaker
Protection of Pacemaker	
Sturdiness of pacemaker	Explain that pacemaker is strong
Discuss patient's activities of daily living and recreational activities	Determine which activities should be avoided; instruct patient to report any activity that may have damaged pacemaker
Electrical Interference	
Inform patient of all electrical sources to be avoided	Instruct patient to have someone accompany him if he must be in proximity of potential hazards
Signs of Malfunction	
Inform patient of signs of malfunction	Discuss signs he may have experienced prior to pacemaker insertion
Dizziness	Define; differentiate between transient dizziness experienced when getting up quickly and true syncope
Shortness of breath	Stress that a notable increase may be meaningful
Chest pain	Stress importance of reporting this symptom
Pulse range	Depends on type of pacemaker and the rate at which it is set
Fluid retention and weight gain	Describe as "puffy ankles," "rings too tight," etc.
Signs of Infection	
Redness, soreness or drainage from incision	Reinforce importance of reporting these findings
Battery Replacement	
Battery lifetime	Type of battery. Expected lifetime now four years
Procedure for battery replacement	Need for hospitalization for about three days. Incision made at same site
Pulse rate change	Instruct patient to report to doctor or clinic. Stress that changes will not be abrupt if batteries need to be changed
Safety Measures	
Physician/dentist visits	Patient is to inform any physician or dentist that he sees that he has a pacemaker
Pacemaker identification card	Patient carries pacemaker identification card with him at all times. Should know brand and model of pacemaker. Knows rate of pacemaker

Specific instructions:

1. Instruct in pulse taking if possible. Patient should take pulse once a day upon awakening. If pulse is slower than set rate of fixed rate or demand, he should notify his physician.
2. Instruct patient regarding any medications he will be taking at home.
3. Passive and active range of motion exercises should be started on the affected arm 48 hours after implantation. Discuss benefits of regular exercise. Encourage patient to walk regularly but to avoid excessive fatigue.
4. Provide patient with extra copies of pacemaker warranty card. Instruct him to carry one on his person at all times.
5. Identify electrical hazards. Patient should avoid contact with questionably defective electrical equipment; avoid working directly over ignition systems and going into an area where there are high voltage radio transmitters; avoid close contact with microwave ovens. Electrical devices may be used, but use should be discontinued if light-headedness or dizziness occurs.
6. If he is to pass through an airport bomb-screening device, patient should alert the authorities because the pacemaker may set off the alarm.
7. Patient can return to work when physician permits. Talk over type of work he will do and what his job entails.
8. Patient may return to whatever degree of sexual activity he wants or tolerates.
9. Driving a car—when physician permits, usually after a month. Advise against long distance travel for at least three months.
10. Sports—as soon as physician permits. Suggest sports with a "buddy." Patient must always avoid contact sports such as football.

BIBLIOGRAPHY

Hoechst-Roussel Pharmaceuticals, Inc., "Cardiac Pacemaking," *Directions in Cardiovascular Medicine,* Vol. 9.

Lown, B., and B. Kosowsky, "Artificial Cardiac Pacemakers," *New England Journal of Medicine,* Vol. 283 (October 22, October 29, November 5, 1970), pp. 907–916, 971–977, 1023–1031.

Spence, M., and L. Lemberg, "Cardiac Pacemakers. I: Modalities of Pacing," *Heart and Lung,* Vol. 3 (September 1974), pp. 820–827.

———, "Cardiac Pacemakers. II: Indications for Pacing," *Heart and Lung,* Vol. 3 (November 1974), pp. 989–995.

———, "Cardiac Pacemakers. IV: Complications of Pacing," *Heart and Lung,* Vol. 4 (March 1975), pp. 286–295.

Vera, Z., et al., "Cardiac Pacemakers: Indications and Complications," *Heart and Lung,* Vol. 4 (May 1975), pp. 444–451.

Winslow, E., and L. Marino, "Temporary Cardiac Pacemakers," *American Journal of Nursing,* Vol. 75 (April 1975), pp. 586–591.

The author of this section wishes to acknowledge the assistance of Mrs. Doris Westra in the preparation of this manuscript and Dr. Dennis Battock for his invaluable suggestions in reviewing the manuscript.

cardiopulmonary resuscitation

definitions

Because of the dual nature of resuscitation — that is, availability (ventilation) and transport (circulation) of oxygen — the more appropriate term is *cardiopulmonary resuscitation.*

Cardiac Arrest   This means abrupt cessation of effective cardiac pumping activity resulting in cessation of circulation. There are two types only: cardiac standstill (asystole) and ventricular fibrillation (plus other forms of ineffective ventricular contraction, i.e., ventricular flutter and rarely ventricular tachycardia). The condition referred to as "profound cardiovascular collapse" will not be specifically included since its recognition and definiton are nebulous and management less specific. One form, referred to as cardiogenic shock, is included in Chapter 8.

Resuscitation   Liberally interpreted, this means the restoration of vital signs by mechanical, physiological, and pharmacological means.

The application of cardiopulmonary resuscitation is made possible by the concept of clinical versus biological death. Clinical death is defined as the absence of the vital signs, and biological death refers to irreversible cellular changes. As determined both experimentally and clinically, the interval between the two approximates four minutes.

who should be resuscitated

It is easier to say who should *not* be resusciated, and this includes individuals with known terminal illness and those who are known to have been in clinical death for longer than five minutes. Both represent situations not only where resusciation would likely prove impossible but where survival would be meaningless. All others should be regarded as candidates for resuscitation. The key here is to remember that resuscitation can always be abandoned, but it cannot be instituted after undue delay.

One additional point: the term "the very elderly" is often used to differentiate likely degrees of vitality and therefore of survival probability. On the surface of it, this is perhaps reasonable, but age alone should rarely, if ever, determine treatment. Bear in mind that, regardless of chronological age, a person who is alert and able to carry on any sort of thoughtful conversation is a candidate for resuscitation, just as you or I.

recognition

The recognition of cardiac arrest depends on the finding of signs of absence of circulation: (a) unconscious state (preceded of course by less profound states of mental obtundation), (b) pulselessness, (c) dilated pupils, and (d) minimal or absent respirations. Two things should be noted. First, the pupils require a certain amount of time to dilate; this has been estimated to be approximately 45 seconds and may be longer than 1 minute. It is therefore at times a valuable sign for pinpointing the time of cardiac arrest. Second, inadequate respiratory excursions may be noted in the early seconds of cardiac arrest, and these should not cause delay in recognition of the other signs.

Pulselessness is best determined by palpation of either the carotid or femoral arteries (the former is almost always immediately available, the latter not); less adequate is palpation of brachial or radial pulses. Determination of pulselessness should not be done by attempting to obtain a blood pressure.

An ideal situation should obtain in coronary care units or well-equipped critical care units: continuous monitoring, electronic warning signals, automatic conditioned response of a skilled team without the delay of feeling pulses, auscultating over the precordium, and the like.

the troops

An organized approach to resuscitation is essential; regardless of how it is organized or of whom it is made up, resuscitation should be approached by a team made up of trained personnel and should include nurses, physicians, electrocardiographic technicians, inhalation-therapy technicians, and individuals to transport special instruments such as defibrillators, pacemakers, and special tray sets. It should also include an administrative or secretarial member who can do the legwork, make all necessary phone calls, and perform other miscellaneous duties that are minor but necessary parts of every prolonged resuscitation attempt. We will describe a specific method geared to an institution with trained resuscitative personnel and found successful. The team includes the nurse as the primary member. The first nurse present becomes the initial captain of the team, and institutes the resuscitation attempt as outlined below. A single call, preferably by the secretary, should summon the entire team on an immediate, spontaneous basis—ECG technicians, inhalation therapy technicians, available physicians including house staff and senior staff members in the area, nurses from the appropriate intensive care unit who will immediately transport the defibrillator, monitor, and pacemaker instrument to the site of the emergency, and the nursing supervisor. The last but not least member of the team is the switchboard operator or operators, who must react immediately in alerting the entire team in preference to all other duties. A single digit on the telephone dial should be utilized to alert the switchboard; they will often know where to find key physician members of the team and can summon them individually, whereas they may otherwise not be alerted. Hospitals with house officers who carry emergency electronic communication equipment are at an advantage (obviously) and should have the best resuscitation statistics; many smaller institutions, however, may be just as successful utilizing only nursing personnel and well-trained technicians.

Although minor variations in different approaches may bring the same results, the important thing is to have a definite routine kept rigorously up-to-date (including one's own experience).

It is to be emphasized that the nursing personnel and other key nonphysician members must have sanction to act spontaneously.

steps in management

There are two situations here: that in which the patient's electrocardiogram is being continuously monitored, as in the coronary care unit, and that in an area where the patient is not under continuous monitoring, such as an ordinary hospital room or unit.

For the continuously monitored patient the arrhythmia sets the alarm, and if it is ventricular fibrillation, the patient is immediately defibrillated (without prior attempts by other means), after which a physician is summoned for evaluation.

In the unmonitored patient the nurse immediately proceeds as below:

1. A sharp blow to the precordium. This requires virtually no time and may institute a cardiac rhythm; if so, it may be all the resuscitation required.

2. Call for help. This should require one simple phrase such as "cor zero," or "red alert," together with the location, to a second individual who then places the emergency call to bring the team together.

3. Obtain adequate airway, immediately institute artificial ventilation (mouth-to-mouth).

4. External cardiac compression. The technique is simple and it is applied by standing at either side of the patient, placing the heel of one hand over the lower half of the sternum and the heel of the other hand over the first, and applying vigorous compression directly downward, depressing the sternum between 1½ and 2 inches, releasing abruptly, and maintaining this rhythm at the rate of 60 to 80 times per minute. To be effective it must be learned correctly and applied skillfully. A little attention to instructors, two hands, and a lack of timidity are all that is required.

    If a single individual must apply both ventilation and massage, it is best to give two or three quick inflations by mouth-to-mouth or other readily available means of inflating the lungs, followed by 12 to 15 external cardiac compressions. This routine may be maintained until additional members of the team arrive.

5. External countershock should be applied as soon as the instrument is available. This should be done without knowing the specific rhythm diagnosis if there is a delay in determining this. If cardiac standstill is present, the countershock will take only moments and will do no harm. If ventricular fibrillation is present, the earliest possible countershock delivered is the one most likely to be effective and should be done at a time when the rhythm may more likely be maintained.

6. A specific *diagnosis* now is required (the word *recognition* has been used up to now, not diagnosis). As mentioned earlier, this will be either cardiac standstill or ventricular fibrillation (continued in Items 10 and 11).

7. This item will be devoted to a very important member of the team: the nurse who is first available after two members are applying ventilation and massage. This individual will man the emergency cart, be responsible for preparation of drugs to be used and preparation of an intravenous infusion set (with several types of venapuncture equipment), and do whatever is necessary to see that an intravenous infusion is started, thus paving the way for drug therapy. The importance of this function underlies the continuously available venous cannula maintained in patients in critical care units.

At this point the need for an intravenous infusion is obvious and must be fulfilled by whatever route is feasible. The simplest of all is the insertion of a needle, cannula, or scalp needle into an arm vein. Failing this, the femoral vein is readily accessible and a very large cannula can easily be inserted into the largest blood vessel in the body (the inferior vena cava) by simple puncture. A cutdown on a branch of the basilic system just above the elbow crease on the medial aspect of either arm or on the external jugular vein will allow insertion of a large cannula into the superior vena cava or right atrium. The subclavian venipuncture is perhaps ideal, being readily available and easily done. In addition, it may be used for rapid infusion or withdrawal, and monitoring of CVP and O_2 saturation, and it is well tolerated for large periods of time. The internal jugular route is also excellent but is less desirable than the subclavian. The intracardiac route should be reserved for situations in which urgency takes precedence over availability of the intravenous route. This should be a rare occurrence.

8. In a patient in whom spontaneous cardiac rhythm and respiration have not resulted by this time, endotracheal intubation is required.

9. Pharmacological agents and appropriate preparations to be made ready immediately are as follows:

a. Sodium bicarbonate in a 5 percent solution IS GIVEN IN 50-cc. ALIQUOTS EVERY 5 TO 10 MINUTES AND IS THE INITIAL DRUG USED. Tromethamine (THAM) can also serve as a buffer, but has disadvantages and is used much less often than sodium bicarbonate.

It has been argued that giving sodium bicarbonate intravenously results in a rise in Pco_2 (by the reaction $HCO_3^- + H^+ \rightarrow H_2CO_3 \rightarrow H_2O + CO_2$) and an increase in osmolality. This is often the case, but there is little choice when significant acidosis is present and this is the situation in virtually all instances of cardiopulmonary arrest. Thus, consensus holds that alkalinization is important, even vital, and that increased osmolality is seldom sufficient to be a major factor.

b. Epinephrine (adrenalin) in a 1:1,000 aqueous solution.

c. Isoproterenol should be available in an intravenous preparation; 2 mg. in 250 cc. of appropriate vehicle solution is an adequate routine preparation.

d. Calcium chloride 10 percent solution.

e. Lidocaine (Xylocaine) should be prepared in an intravenous solution of varying concentration, but 1 mg./ml. is an adequate solution for initial use. This drug is used most frequently by intravenous push in 50-mg. doses.

f. A vasopressor, preferably a peripheral vasoconstrictor such as methoxamine (Vasoxyl) or phenylephrine (Neo-Synephrine, an alphamimetic) or norepinephrine (both alpha and beta stimulating) should be available in an intravenous infusion of appropriate concentration.

The critical emergency drugs given by IV push (sodium bicarbonate, epinephrine, calcium chloride, lidocaine) are all supplied in ready-to-use forms and should be readily available. Other preparations such as procainamide (Pronestyl), quinidine, diuretics such as ethacrynic acid (Edecrin) and furosemide (Lasix), mannitol, dexamethasone (Decadron), and propranolol (Inderal) should be available though not routinely prepared for immediate use. The inotropic and chronotropic agent glucagon has gained use in some situations. Its effects are less predictable and it should not be considered a routine drug. Its inotropic effect is substantial, though less than that of isoproterenol, and it has the advantage of a lesser chronotropic effect and generally induces less hyperexcitability. The catecholamine dopamine has emerged as perhaps the inotropic agent of choice. Its central inotropic effect is comparable to that of isoproterenol, but it has the advantage of augmenting renal blood flow. It has largely replaced isoproterenol and norepinephrine for enhancing perfusion pressure (although isoproterenol is still more effective as a temporary medical "pacemaker").

10. If cardiac standstill, epinephrine should be given routinely, usually 1 mg. intravenously, artificial ventilation and circulation continued; if unsuccessful, epinephrine should be repeated and the isoproterenol drip started. At this point, calcium chloride, 0.5 to 1.0 gm., is given intravenously. If no response, continued artificial ventilation and circulation, continued intravenous epinephrine injections, and insertion of a transvenous pacemaker are indicated (less often a percutaneous transthoracic pacemaker is used).

11. If ventricular fibrillation, epinephrine is given intravenously (it is important that the continuous artificial ventilation and circulation are maintained and that interruptions not exceed 5 seconds) and external countershock is given at the maximum setting of the instrument with immediate resumption of artificial circulation and ventilation. If unsuccessful, the cycle should be repeated. If ventricular fibrillation persists in spite of the above or if reversion to ventricular fibrillation occurs each time it is applied, intravenous lidocaine is given by push in 50- to 100-mg. aliquots. Procainamide, if preferred, may also be given by intravenous push, and either drug may be given by intravenous drip. Beta blocking drugs, e.g., propranolol (Inderal), may be the only effective agents here and have their prime indication in cardiac arrest. Quinidine is preferred by some, but its tendency to lower peripheral blood pressure and reduce myocardial contractility (resulting in a

diminished cardiac output should a rhythm be resumed) constitute important disadvantages. It should also be emphasized here that regardless of the initial mechanism (whether it be an irritable or a depressive phenomenon) once cardiac arrest has gained foothold with some duration it must be assumed that the heart is depressed, making the routine use of depressive drugs unwarranted. Since uneven tissue perfusion, particularly myocardial perfusion, may be a factor in perpetuating the ventricular fibrillation or standstill, a vasopressor agent of the peripheral constrictor type may be of value at this point. Digitalis and potassium chloride are rarely indicated in resuscitative attempts, their use being based on knowledge of special preexisting situations. As indicated above, depressive cardiac mechanisms are often the cause of repetitive ventricular fibrillation and paradoxically, pacing the heart (pharmacologically with isoproterenol or electronically by transvenous pacing catheter) is the treatment of choice in some cases (after resumption of rhythm, of course).

12. If above fail: (a) Pericardial tap should be performed, preferably by the subxyphoid route; although an uncommon factor in cardiac arrest it may result in dramatic recovery. (b) Consider further underlying causes subject to treatment such as pneumothorax (insertion of chest tubes); pulmonary embolism (assisted circulation, surgery); ventricular aneurysm, rupture of papillary muscle or interventricular septum (assisted circulation, surgery); subvalvular muscular aortic stenosis with extreme gradients (propranolol, reserpine, etc.). Failing these, the decision to terminate resuscitative attempts is imminent, based on CNS changes and/or the assumption of a nonviable myocardium.

postresuscitative care

If there is resumption of spontaneous cardiac activity, the situation should be thoroughly evaluated as to the clinical state, underlying causes, and complicating factors in order to determine proper management. A routine as follows has been found successful: Intravenous diuretic (e.g. furosemide 80 to 240 mg.), a steroid such as dexamethasone for its salutary effect on cerebral edema, and electrical and physiological monitoring in an intensive care unit. A portable chest x-ray and an arterial sample for determination of pH and blood gases are obtained as soon as possible following resumption of cardiac rhythm. Continuous oxygen therapy is maintained; an intravenous infusion is of course essential. Routine measurements other than continuous electrocardiographic monitoring include frequent blood pressures (ideally done by intra-arterial cannula), hourly urine volumes, frequent bedside estimates of tissue perfusion, and central venous pressure measurements through a cannula extending into the superior vena cava or right atrium connected through a stopcock to a simple water manometer.

If central nervous system damage is evident, hypothermia should be instituted immediately, additional mannitol or intravenous urea should be given, and dexamethasone for cerebral edema should be continued. Monitoring otherwise is continued as outlined above.

If oliguria or anuria is present, massive doses of furosemide should be given immediately. If there is no response to these, management as in acute renal insufficiency should be instituted.

The specific approach in the postresuscitative period will depend not only on the patient's condition at the time, but on the underlying disease process, the previous condition of the patient, and the events in the immediate postresuscitative period. More patients are being studied by catheter techniques acutely to evaluate them for emergency surgical procedures such as saphenous bypass grafts. The state of this art is changing rapidly.

complications of resuscitation

Resuscitation has come a very long way; it has changed drastically with time and undoubtedly will continue to do so. It has proven its worth beyond doubt. There are of course complications, and these include (a) injuries to sternum, costal cartilages, ribs, esophagus, stomach, liver, pleura and lung. Any one of these can be serious. (b) Another—fortunately rare—complication is the production of a live patient with permanent central nervous system damage such as to render him totally dependent. (c) There are also medical-legal considerations, which originally leaned against the attempt because of the frequency of undignified failures. This aspect should probably be ignored for the most part, since we are dealing with an earnest and reasonable approach to the treatment of sudden death in reversible situations, but it does emphasize that it should always be applied by well-trained, responsible people. The aim should be to reverse the reversible and not to inflict suffering in situations involving the irreversible. The alternative in both, of course, is death. The differentiation lies in good judgment which, as someone has said, "is difficult to learn, impossible to teach."

commonly used cardiac drugs
digoxin

Digoxin reduces the heart rate both by increasing vagal tone and by an extravagal mechanism. In normal hearts, reduction in heart rate is insignificant, but some slowing may occur in patients with heart failure who are digitalized. The decrease in heart rate in such patients appears to be secondary to an improvement in cardiac output.

Digoxin decreases conduction through the A-V junction. It is this property that makes digoxin so valuable in the management of atrial fibrillation or flutter by controlling ventricular rate.

There are two clear-cut indications for the use of digoxin: congestive heart failure and supraventricular tachyarrhythmias (atrial fibrillation, atrial flutter, atrial or junctional tachycardia). Digitalization may result in either reversion to a normal sinus rhythm or more effective control of the ventricular rate.

The most serious contraindication to the use of digoxin is, of course, the

table 9-1
antiarrhythmic drugs

DRUG	USUAL DOSES	USUAL ROUTES OF ADMINIS-TRATION	CONCENTRATIONS μg./ml.			TOXIC EFFECTS
			USUALLY EFFECTIVE	POTEN-TIALLY TOXIC		
Lidocaine	50–100 mg. bolus, followed by 1–4 mg./min.	IV	2–5	>5		Drowsiness, disorientation, paresthesias, seizures
Quinidine	200–400 mg. every 6 hr.	PO	2.5–5	>5		QRS widening 50%, diarrhea, cinchonism, thrombocytopenia, hypotension, ventricular tachyarrhythmias, syncope
	250–500 mg. every 3–4 hr. (usually 2–4 gm. but sometimes up to 8 gm./day)	PO				QRS widening 50%, hypotension, lupuslike syndrome
Procainamide	100–200 mg. every 5 min. to 1,000 mg. followed by 1–4 mg./min.	IV	4–8	>8		
Propranolol	10–40 mg. every 4–6 hr.	PO	Variable			Bradycardia, A-V block, hypotension, congestive heart failure, bronchospasm
	0.5–3 mg. every 2–3 hr.	IV				
Diphenyl-hydantoin	1 gm. loading dose, followed by 100 mg. every 6–8 hr.	PO	8–16	>16		Ataxia, nystagmus, drowsiness, hematological effects
	50 mg. every 5 min. to 500 mg.	IV				

J. Koch-Weser, "Antiarrhythmic Prophylaxis in Ambulatory Patients with Coronary Heart Disease," *Archives of Internal Medicine*, Vol. 129 (1972), pp. 763–772. Copyright 1972. American Medical Association.

presence of digitalis intoxication. Extracardiac symptoms suggestive of digitalis intoxication include anorexia, nausea, vomiting, blurred or colored vision, and fatigue. The most frequent cardiac sign of digitalis overdosage is the occurrence of PVCs. Ventricular tachycardia, ventricular fibrillation, atrial or junctional tachycardia, or second and third degree heart block are other common manifestations of digitalis overdosage.

Digitalis should *not* be used to treat sinus tachycardia except when the tachycardia is due to congestive heart failure. The drug should be used with caution in patients with hypokalemia, renal failure, hypothyroidism, severe hypoxemia or acute myocarditis due to a greater than usual risk of digitalis intoxication in such cases.

propranolol (Inderal)

Of the drugs which induce beta blockade, only propranolol is currently available in this country. It is useful in a variety of arrhythmias including atrial fibrillation and flutter, paroxysmal atrial tachycardia and junctional tachycardia. Propranolol may be used alone or as an adjunct to digoxin or quinidine. Propranolol is also useful in the management of PVCs and ventricular tachycardia. It appears to be especially helpful if the arrhythmia is due to digitalis intoxication. The oral dosage should be adjusted on an individual basis from 10 to 40 mg. every 6 hours.

Propranolol depresses cardiac output and therefore is contraindicated in patients with congestive heart failure. An exception to this statement is a patient with congestive heart failure due to an atrial tachyarrhythmia. Reducing the ventricular rate in such a patient will improve cardiac output and offset any depressant effect of this agent on the myocardium. The concurrent use of digoxin is advisable for most of these patients.

lidocaine (Xylocaine)

This drug is of great value in the management of ventricular ectopic rhythms in the critically ill. Lidocaine has the advantages of rapid effectiveness and minimal effect on cardiac contractility. An initial intravenous bolus of 50 to 100 mg. will usually suppress ectopic activity for approximately 20 minutes. Recurrence of PVCs calls for a repeat intravenous bolus followed by a sustained intravenous infusion of 1 to 4 mg. per minute. The dose is adjusted to control ventricular ectopic beats. Care is taken to avoid excessive doses which produce agitation or seizures. As a rule, lidocaine is not helpful in the management of supraventricular arrhythmias.

Since lidocaine is metabolized by the liver, the dose should be reduced when hepatic blood flow is decreased as in congestive heart failure. A-V block with a slow junctional or ventricular focus is also a contraindication to the use of lidocaine.

quinidine

This agent is both a highly effective and toxic drug. It is useful for both supraventricular and ventricular ectopic rhythms. In each case the advantages of rhythm control must be weighed against the risks of the drug.

Quinidine is nearly completely absorbed by the intestinal tract. It is less effective when given intramuscularly. The intravenous route should be used only in extreme emergencies since the toxicity of quinidine sharply increases with direct infusion.

Quinidine has the following cardiac actions:

1. It increases the effective refractory period of cardiac muscle in doses which have little effect upon the refractory period of normal pacemaker tissue.
2. It decreases myocardial excitability (ability of the ventricle to respond to a stimulus).
3. It decreases conduction in cardiac conduction tissue and cardiac muscle.
4. It decreases myocardial automaticity (the automatic rhythmic activity of the tissue).
5. Finally, it depresses myocardial contractility. In addition, quinidine is a potent vasodilator. Hence, blood pressure may fall after large doses of quinidine.

Quinidine is uniquely effective in terminating supraventricular as well as ventricular tachyarrhythmias. Because of its toxicity, it is generally used only when other agents have failed to control the arrhythmia. Patients who receive quinidine for conversion of atrial fibrillation or flutter should be digitalized first, since quinidine increases conduction through the A-V junction in low doses and may raise the ventricular rate to dangerously high levels. This effect is blocked by digoxin.

procainamide (Pronestyl)

The principle use of this agent is the management of PVCs or ventricular tachycardia not responsive to lidocaine. Procainamide is well absorbed when given orally and intramuscularly. The intravenous use is reserved for patients critically ill who have failed to respond to lidocaine. Procainamide is thought to be less effective than quinidine in controlling atrial fibrillation.

In low doses, procainamide enhances A-V conduction. Higher doses depress A-V conduction, and when A-V block is present, the drug should be used with great caution. Toxic doses widen the QRS complex, and the drug must be stopped if this finding develops.

Side effects are common. Gastrointestinal effects include nausea, vomiting, abdominal cramps and diarrhea. Another reaction mimics some features of systemic lupus erythematosus (skin rash, fever, pleuropericarditis, joint and muscle pains). The latter findings tend to occur with increasing frequency in patients who are maintained on procainamide for prolonged periods.

Depression of cardiac contractility is the most serious side effect, and is more apt to occur when procainamide is given intravenously. Those patients with preexisting heart failure and impaired renal function are most susceptible, and the dosage should be reduced in such cases.

Plasma levels provide a useful guide to therapy. The normal range is 4 to 8 micrograms per ml.

Procainamide is given in doses of 250 to 500 mg. orally every 4 to 6 hours.

When given intravenously, the drug should be infused no faster than 50 mg. per minute. Infusion is stopped if hypotension or QRS widening occurs, or when the arrhythmia is controlled.

diphenylhydantoin (Dilantin, DPH)

DPH has been in use for a variety of arrhythmias. It is perhaps most useful in the management of ventricular arrhythmias due to digitalis intoxication. DPH improves A-V conduction; thus, the drug is also useful in the management of PVCs associated with varying degrees of heart block where other antiarrhythmic agents may be more hazardous. DPH is also used in treating ventricular tachycardia from myocardial infarction or cardiac surgery, but is less potent than other currently available agents.

DPH is more effective given intravenously. It should be administered slowly due to the direct cardiac toxic effects of its diluents, propylene glycol and ethyl alcohol.

atropine

Given intravenously, atropine blocks those arrhythmias related to excessive vagal activity. These include severe sinus bradycardia, S-A block, and A-V block. Atropine is ineffective in high grades of A-V block due to extensive destruction of the conduction system. In low doses, atropine exerts a paradoxical effect and causes bradycardia and decreased A-V conduction. If these occur, a larger dose will usually produce the desired effects.

PHILLIP S. WOLF, M.D.
SHIRLEY J. HOFFMAN, R.N., B.S.
JOAN MERSCH, R.N., M.S.
CAROLYN M. HUDAK, R.N., M.S.

assessment skills for the nurse: cardiovascular system

arrhythmia recognition — cardiac arrhythmias and conduction disturbances

Disorders of the heartbeat occur in the majority of patients with acute myocardial infarction. Acute respiratory failure is a frequent cause of arrhythmias as well. The importance of rhythm disturbances in these situations differs; some lack clinical significance while others are lethal.

Arrhythmias commonly encountered in monitored patients can be recognized with a little practice. The types that occur most frequently are discussed in the following section. In dealing with these disturbances of rhythm, the nurse must appraise the patient's total clinical situation.

Understanding of arrhythmias is helped by knowledge of the conduction system. Before beginning your study of this section, you might find it helpful to review the conduction system (pp. 79–82) and the principles of electrocardiography. (See also Figs. 10–1 and 10–2.)

An arrhythmia will result when any of the following three situations exists:
1. The *rate* is too slow or too fast (the rhythm may be regular or irregular).
2. The *site* of impulse formation is abnormal (atrial fibers, fibers of the A-V junction, the His bundle or its branches, or the Purkinje fibers).
3. The *conduction* of impulses is abnormal at any point within the conduction system.

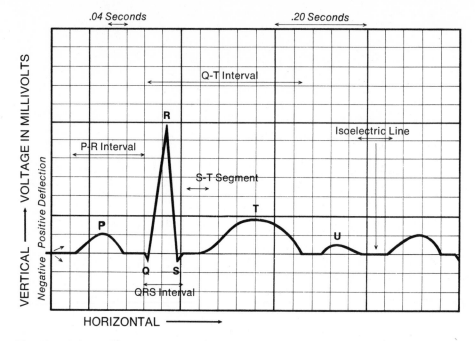

Fig. 10-1. Schematic representation of the electrical impulse as it traverses the conduction system, resulting in depolarization and repolarization of the myocardium.

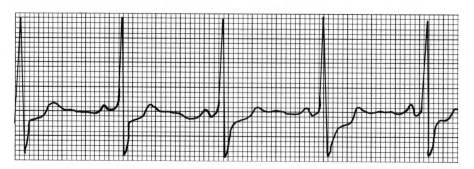

Fig. 10-2. Normal sinus rhythm. (Rate = 60 to 100 beats per minute)

In analyzing arrhythmias, it is essential to understand some of the terms commonly used. The following is a partial list of definitions:

TACHYCARDIA—A heart rate in excess of 100 per minute.

BRADYCARDIA—A heart rate under 60 per minute.

ISOELECTRIC LINE—The straight line seen when no electrical activity is occurring. The baseline of the tracing.

P WAVE—A deflection from the baseline produced by *depolarization* of the atria.

P-R INTERVAL—The time required for the impulse to travel through the atria into the first portion of the conduction system, the A-V junction. Normal limits are 0.12 to 0.2 second. The interval is measured from the beginning of the P wave to the start of the QRS complex.

QRS COMPLEX—A deflection from the baseline produced by depolarization of the ventricles. Normal duration is 0.06 to 0.08 second.

ST SEGMENT—The segment between the *end* of the QRS complex and the *beginning* of the T wave.

Q-T INTERVAL—The time required for the ventricles to depolarize and repolarize. Usual duration is 0.32 to 0.40 second. The interval is from the *beginning* of the QRS complex to the *end* of the T wave.

T WAVE—A deflection from the baseline produced by ventricular *repolarization* and normally of the same deflection as the QRS complex.

U WAVE—A small, usually positive deflection following the T wave. Its significance is uncertain, but it is typically seen with hypokalemia.

Sinus Tachycardia

DEFINITION: A rapid heart rate (100 to 180 beats per minute). The rhythm is regular but usually varies from minute to minute. The rapid rate decreases diastole more than systole.

ETIOLOGY: Sinus tachycardia may be a physiological response to any form of stress and is found in all age groups. It occurs in such diverse conditions as excitement, physical exertion, fever, anemia, hyperthyroidism and hypoxia, and with the administration of some drugs, such as atropine, isoproterenol

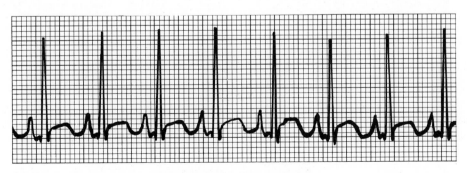

Fig. 10-3. Sinus tachycardia.

and epinephrine. Sinus tachycardia may also occur with heart disease and is often present with congestive heart failure.

Sinus tachycardia results from decreased vagal tone or increased sympathetic nervous system activity and the release of catecholamines (epinephrine and norepinephrine) by the adrenal medulla and from nerve endings in the heart.

SYMPTOMS: Ordinarily the only symptom described is a sense of "racing of the heart.". The cause of sinus tachycardia determines its prognosis, not the duration of the arrhythmia, which in and of itself is usually harmless. In persons who already have depleted cardiac reserve, ischemia, and/or congestive heart failure, the persistence of a fast rate may worsen the underlying condition.

TREATMENT: Specific measures may include sedation, digitalis (only if heart failure is present) or propranolol, if the tachycardia is due to thyrotoxicosis.

Sinus Bradycardia

DEFINITION: A heart rate of fewer than 60 per minute with impulses originating in the S-A node. Rhythm is regular but may vary from minute to minute. The duration of diastole is lengthened.

ETIOLOGY: Sinus bradycardia is common among all age groups and is present in both normal and diseased hearts. It is also seen in highly trained athletes, patients with severe pain, myxedema, or acute myocardial infarction, and as the result of medication (digitalis or reserpine).

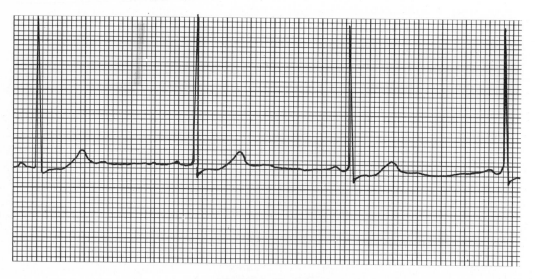

Fig. 10-4. Sinus bradycardia.

Sinus bradycardia results from excessive parasympathetic activity. Slow rates are tolerated well in persons with healthy hearts. With severe heart disease, however, the heart may not be able to compensate for a slow rate by increasing the volume of blood ejected per beat as is true of the healthy heart. In this situation, sinus bradycardia will lead to a low cardiac output. This in turn may lead to weakness (due to inadequate blood flow to the muscles), congestive heart failure, or serious ventricular arrhythmias.

TREATMENT: None is usually indicated unless symptoms are present. If the pulse is very slow and symptoms are present, appropriate measures include atropine to block the vagal effect, isoproterenol, or transvenous pacing.

Sinus Arrhythmia

DEFINITION: All impulses originate in the S-A node, but the rate of discharge varies. Some occur prematurely while others are delayed, which causes the rate to alternately increase and decrease. In young persons, the heart rate usually varies with respiration, increasing with inspiration and slowing with expiration.

ETIOLOGY: Sinus arrhythmia is usually a physiological variation in young people. It may indicate disease of the S-A node in the elderly (see section on Sick Sinus Syndrome).

TREATMENT: Usually none is necessary.

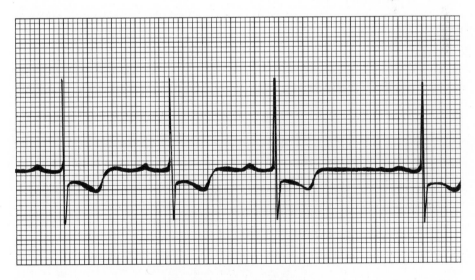

Fig. 10-5. Sinus arrhythmia.

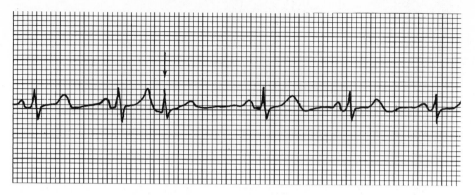

Fig. 10-6. Premature atrial contraction.

Premature Atrial Contraction (PAC)

DEFINITION: During the normal cardiac rhythm, a contraction occurs earlier than expected. The stimulus for this contraction arises from elsewhere in the atrium rather than from the S-A node. The P wave is usually visible and typically has a somewhat different form than the P wave of the sinus impulse. The QRS complex is usually of normal configuration but may appear distorted when the PAC is conducted aberrantly, or the QRS may not occur at all (PAC is blocked). A short pause, usually less than "compensatory," is present (see definition of PVC below).

ETIOLOGY: This is a common arrhythmia seen in all groups. It may occur in normal individuals and in patients with rheumatic heart disease, ischemic heart disease or hyperthyroidism.

An impulse arises in the atrial musculature from an ectopic focus, producing an atrial contraction. Usually the stimulus travels through the A-V junction and continues its normal course through the ventricles. If a PAC occurs too early it may be blocked because the A-V junction is refractory from the previous stimulus and is unable to receive the current one. In most instances, the atrial ectopic beat is followed by an incomplete compensatory pause. The patient may have the sensation of a "pause" or "skip" in rhythm.

TREATMENT: In many cases, no treatment is necessary. Mild sedation or removal of the exciting cause is indicated if the PACs are symptomatic. If they occur as a result of underlying heart disease, specific drugs such as quinidine, digitalis, or propranolol may be in order.

Supraventricular Tachycardia

DEFINITION: These tachycardias are rapid, regular rhythms. They may originate in an ectopic atrial focus (paroxysmal atrial tachycardia) or in the A-V junction (paroxysmal nodal tachycardia). These ectopic rhythms are similar in all respects except their site of origin. In almost all instances re-

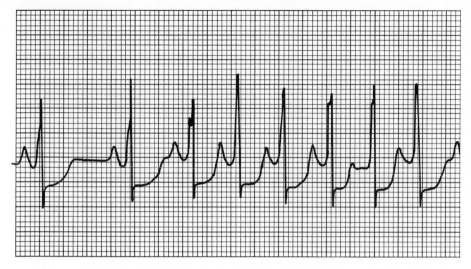

Fig. 10-7. Supraventricular tachycardia.

corded, the tachycardia begins with a premature atrial or junctional beat (as in Fig. 10–7).

SIGNIFICANT ECG CHANGES

Rate: Range, 140 to 220 beats per minute. The rhythm is regular and the paroxysms may last from a few seconds to several hours or even days.

P waves: Usually upright with atrial tachycardia and may be inverted in leads II, III and aVF when the tachycardia is of junctional origin (Fig. 10–8). If the rate is very rapid, the P wave may be buried in the QRS complex or superimposed on the T wave.

P-R interval: If seen, the P-R interval is usually shortened with junctional tachycardia and normal, shortened, or, rarely, lengthened with atrial tachycardia.

QRS complex: This is usually of normal configuration, but may be distorted if aberrant conduction is present.

ETIOLOGY: These arrhythmias occur often in adults with normal hearts and for the same reasons as PACs. When heart disease is present, such abnormalities as rheumatic heart disease, acute myocardial infarction or digitalis intoxication may serve as the background for these arrhythmias.

Atrial tachycardia is typically preceded by a PAC. The ectopic pacemaker discharges impulses to which the atrium and/or A-V junction respond, firing so rapidly that the S-A node is suppressed. Extreme regularity (in a given person the rate stays constant) is one of the hallmarks.

SYMPTOMS: Early symptoms are palpitations and light-headedness. With underlying heart disease, dyspnea, angina pectoris and congestive heart failure may occur.

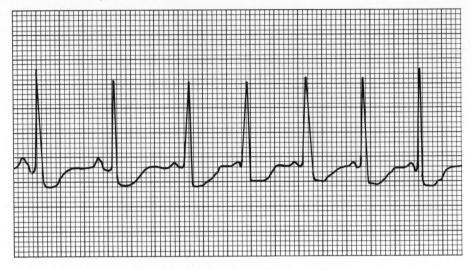

Fig. 10-8. A-V junctional tachycardia.

DIFFERENTIAL DIAGNOSIS: A supraventricular tachycardia must be differentiated from sinus tachycardia. The following points favor the diagnosis of ectopic atrial tachycardia:

1. An atrial premature beat often initiates the rhythm.
2. It begins and terminates abruptly.
3. The rate is often faster than a sinus tachycardia and tends to be more regular from minute to minute.
4. In response to a vagal maneuver, such as carotid sinus massage, the ectopic tachycardia will either be unaffected or revert to a normal sinus rhythm. Sinus tachycardia, on the other hand, will slow slightly in response to increased vagal tone.

TREATMENT: Stimulation of the vagal reflex will often terminate the paroxysms. This reflex may be elicited by brief massage on the carotid sinus (unilaterally), the Valsalva maneuver, or agents that raise the blood pressure such as phenylephrine, 1 mg. intravenously, or methoxamine, 5 to 15 mg. intravenously. If these measures are unsuccessful, antiarrhythmic drugs including digitalis, quinidine or propranolol are used. If the attack persists or if complications occur which demand more immediate action, countershock is indicated.

Atrial Flutter

DEFINITION: An ectopic atrial rhythm occurring at a rate of 250 to 350 beats per minute. The ventricular rate is usually one-half the atrial rate at the beginning of the attack. With treatment the degree of A-V block increases and the ventricular rate slows further. The rapid and regular atrial rate produces a "saw tooth" or "picket fence" appearance on the electrocardiogram. It is usual for a flutter wave to be partially concealed within the QRS complex or T wave. The QRS complex exhibits a normal configuration except when aberrant conduction is present. The QRS complexes do not follow each flutter wave since the ventricles cannot respond this rapidly.

ETIOLOGY: In the patient with atrial flutter, underlying cardiac disease is usually present, including coronary artery disease, cor pulmonale, or rheumatic heart disease. The ectopic focus becomes the dominant pacemaker and is conducted through the A-V junction into the ventricles in normal fashion. Two theories are currently favored as to the mechanism of atrial flutter. (1) A continuous impulse travels through the atrium causing a "circus" movement at a very rapid but coordinated rate, and (2) a single ectopic focus discharges rapidly. At the onset of the arrhythmia, the ventricles respond once to every two atrial impulses. Further A-V block may develop if the arrhythmia persists, and the ventricles usually respond irregularly every two to six beats. If the ventricular rate is within normal limits, the cardiac output will remain adequate. If the rate is so rapid that the chambers cannot fill adequately, hemodynamic changes occur as described in the section on supraventricular tachycardia.

When the ventricular rate is rapid, the diagnosis of atrial flutter may be difficult. Vagal maneuvers such as carotid sinus massage will often increase the degree of A-V block and allow recognition of flutter waves.

TREATMENT: If flutter is associated with a high degree of A-V block so that the ventricular rate remains within normal limits, no treatment is necessary. When the ventricular rate is rapid, prompt treatment to control the rate and/or revert the rhythm to a sinus mechanism is indicated. Digitalis is the initial drug of choice. It increases the degree of A-V block and thus controls the ventricular rate, or it may produce atrial fibrillation. Reversion to a sinus mechanism often follows. If complications occur suddenly and more immediate action is required, countershock is indicated.

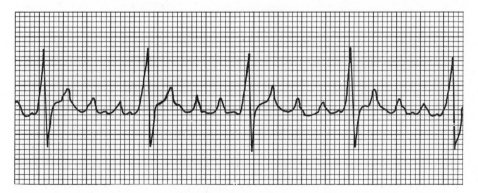

Fig. 10-9. Atrial flutter.

Atrial Fibrillation

DEFINITION: An atrial arrhythmia occurring at an extremely rapid atrial rate (400 to 600 per minute), lacking coordinated activity. The A-V junction is able to respond only partially to the rapid rate of discharge from the atria; hence, the ventricular rate is slower, irregular, and usually 140 to 170 beats per minute at the onset of the arrhythmia.

SIGNIFICANT ECG CHANGES

P waves: Absent; irregular "fibrillary" waves (an uneven pattern in the baseline of the tracing) are usually seen.

QRS complex: Complexes may appear normal or show aberrant conduction.

ETIOLOGY: Although atrial fibrillation may occur as a transient arrhythmia in healthy young people, the presence of permanent atrial fibrillation is almost always associated with underlying heart disease. One or both of the following are present in patients with permanent atrial fibrillation: atrial muscle disease and atrial distention together with disease of the S-A node. Atrial fibrillation is usually initiated by PACs. Once established, it is sustained by multiple small circulating wave fronts within the atrium. This is also known as micro re-entry.

In patients with heart disease, atrial fibrillation causes the cardiac output to fall because of (1) a rapid rate allowing less time for the ventricles to fill, and (2) loss of effective atrial contractions. Signs of another complication may arise from atrial fibrillation, that of peripheral arterial emboli. Due to the passive dilated state of the atria, thrombi can form on the atrial wall and dislodge, producing embolization. The incidence of embolization can be reduced by anticoagulation.

The nurse will note a pulse deficit with atrial fibrillation. The radial pulse is slower than the apical pulse because some systolic contractions are feeble and not palpable in the peripheral arteries.

TREATMENT: If complications develop rapidly, countershock is indicated immediately. If cardiac output remains sufficient, and the patient is not

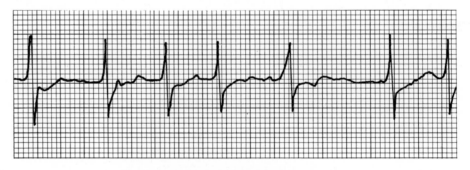

Fig. 10-10. Atrial fibrillation.

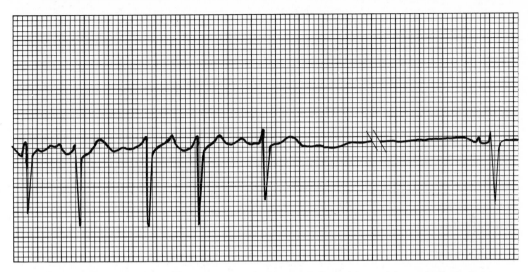

Fig. 10-11. Sick sinus syndrome. Atrial fibrillation followed by atrial standstill. A sinus escape beat is seen at the end of the strip.

hypotensive or in significant heart failure, drug therapy is usually utilized first. Digitalis is specifically useful because it increases A-V block and allows more time for diastolic filling of the ventricles. This produces more volume per stroke. The rhythm may also convert with digitalis to a normal sinus mechanism. Quinidine aids in maintenance of normal sinus rhythm.

Sick Sinus Syndrome

DEFINITION: The term refers to patients exhibiting severe degrees of sinus node depression including marked sinus bradycardia, S-A block and S-A node arrest. Often rapid atrial arrhythmias coexist, such as atrial flutter or fibrillation (the "tachycardia-bradycardia syndrome") which alternate with periods of sinus node depression.
TREATMENT: Management of this condition requires control of the rapid atrial arrhythmias with drug therapy and control of very slow heart rates as well (a permanent transvenous pacemaker).

Atrial Standstill

DEFINITION: Complete cessation of the S-A node occurs. The pacemaker shifts to a lower focus, either in the atrium, in the A-V junction, or within the Purkinje system.
ETIOLOGY: As with sick sinus syndrome; the sinus arrhythmia may occur in the elderly patient with disease of the S-A node. It is also the result of

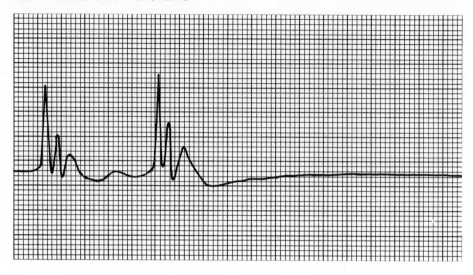

Fig. 10-12. Atrial standstill (lower pacemaker does not take over).

intoxication from quinidine, digitalis or potassium. Acute myocardial infarction may also produce atrial standstill.

SYMPTOMS: Light-headedness or fainting will occur depending on the duration of standstill. Sudden death, of course, is inevitable if a lower pacemaker does not take over.

TREATMENT: Intravenous atropine or isoproterenol is sometimes of value. Drugs that depress S-A node function such as digitalis and quinidine should be discontinued, and hyperkalemia, if present, should be managed with intravenous sodium bicarbonate or glucose and insulin mixtures. If the arrhythmia is recurrent, an artificial pacemaker is the preferred management.

A-V Junctional Premature Beats

DEFINITION: An impulse from an ectopic focus in the A-V junction or His bundle occurring earlier than the normal sinus impulse. The P waves are inverted in leads II, III and aVF and may occur before, during, or after the QRS complex.

ETIOLOGY: As with PACs, junctional premature beats may occur in normal persons or in those with underlying heart disease. The A-V junction or His bundle acts as pacemaker. The impulses pass normally through the conduction system into the ventricles producing a normal QRS. Aberrant conduction, however, may occur and lead to confusion with a PVC. It is helpful to obtain a long rhythm strip to find prematurities that are normally conducted. This may establish that the abnormal appearing beats with wide QRS complexes are atrial with aberrant conduction.

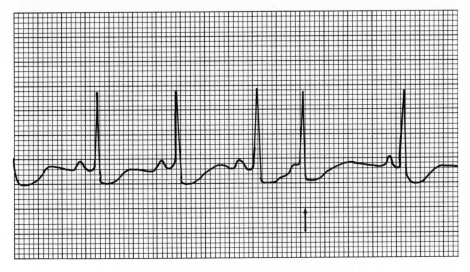

Fig. 10-13. A-V junctional premature beats.

An inverted P wave is produced when the A-V junction stimulates the atria and causes the impulse to travel upward through the atrial fibers in retrograde fashion.

TREATMENT: Identical to the management of PACs.

Premature Ventricular Contraction (PVC)

DEFINITION: A ventricular contraction originating from an ectopic focus in the Purkinje network of the ventricles, occurring earlier than the expected sinus beat. In contrast to a PAC with aberrant conduction, there is no P wave before the QRS complex. An inverted P wave may follow the PVC due to retrograde depolarization of the atria.

The QRS complex cannot be missed. It is not only premature, but is bizarre, widened, and notched, and it may be of greater amplitude. The T wave of the PVC is opposite in deflection to the QRS complex. A compensatory pause often follows the premature beat as the heart awaits the next stimulus from the S-A node. The pause is considered fully compensatory if the cycles of the normal and premature beats equal the time of two normal heart cycles.

ETIOLOGY: PVCs are the most common of all arrhythmias and can occur in any age group, with or without heart disease. They are especially common in a person with myocardial disease (ischemia, myocardial infarction, or following cardiac surgery) or with myocardial irritability (hypokalemia or digitalis intoxication).

If PVCs occur after each sinus beat, a bigeminal rhythm is present (Fig.

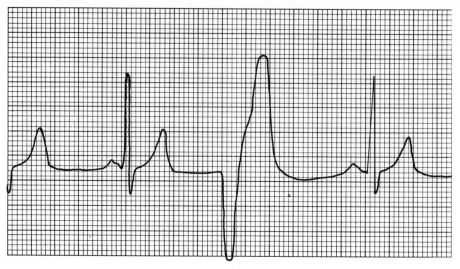

Fig. 10-14. Premature ventricular contraction.

10-15). Trigeminy is a PVC occurring after two consecutive sinus beats. When PVCs originate from different ectopic foci, they are known as *multi-focal*.

SYMPTOMS: Often PVCs are asymptomatic, but some people may experience a "thump" or "skipping" sensation. PVCs may be the earliest sign of heart disease, and when they are especially frequent or approach the apex of the T wave, they may be the forerunner of more serious arrhythmias such as ventricular tachycardia or fibrillation.

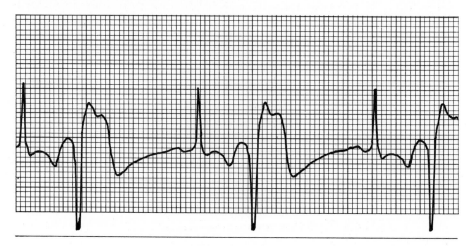

Fig. 10-15. Bigeminal rhythm.

TREATMENT: If infrequent, isolated PVCs require no treatment. Multiple, "back to back" PVCs, or PVCs falling on the apex of the T wave of the previous beat, are managed with antiarrhythmic agents, including lidocaine, procainamide, quinidine and propranolol. If the serum potassium is low, potassium replacement may correct the arrhythmia. If the arrhythmia is due to digitalis toxicity, withdrawal of the drug may correct it.

Ventricular Tachycardia

DEFINITION: The ventricular ectopic focus emits a series of rapid and regular impulses, and the ventricular contractions are dissociated from the atrial contractions.

The ventricular rate ranges from 100 to 220 beats per minute. P waves are rarely seen to superimpose on the rapid, bizarre QRS–T complexes. The QRS complex resembles that of PVCs, and the T wave, when visible, is opposite in deflection to the QRS complex. In the example shown, ventricular tachycardia terminates spontaneously, resulting in sinus rhythm. An "R on T" PVC is present in the next to last beat.

ETIOLOGY: Ventricular tachycardia is rare in adults with normal hearts, but is common (20 to 30 percent) as a complication of myocardial infarction or digitalis intoxication.

Ventricular tachycardia is thought to arise within the Purkinje network. A re-entrant mechanism is usually present causing a circulating wave front. Each completion of the wave front causes a ventricular contraction appearing as a series of PVCs. The atria continue to respond to the S-A node but

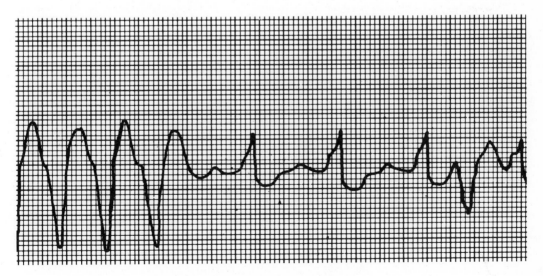

Fig. 10-16. Ventricular tachycardia.

the atria and ventricles beat independently. The rapid rate without a properly timed atrial contraction leads to decreased cardiac output.

SYMPTOMS: Palpitations, angina pectoris, weakness and fainting are frequent symptoms. Hypotension or congestive heart failure may follow due to decreased stroke volume.

TREATMENT: Lidocaine, procainamide, propranolol, quinidine or diphenylhydantoin and occasionally potassium chloride may terminate the arrhythmia. Electrical countershock is almost always effective. If the arrhythmia is due to digitalis intoxication, digitalis should be stopped and potassium given.

Accelerated Ventricular Rhythm

DEFINITION: This ectopic ventricular rhythm resembles ventricular tachycardia except that the rate is slower. The ventricular rate is between 60 and 100 beats per minute and the characteristically wide QRS complexes are identified as being of ventricular origin. Often the ventricular rate closely parallels the sinus rate.

ETIOLOGY: Typically this rhythm occurs in patients with acute myocardial infarction. Less commonly it may occur as a result of ischemia or digitalis intoxication.

TREATMENT: In most cases, no treatment is necessary because the arrhythmia terminates spontaneously in less than 30 seconds.

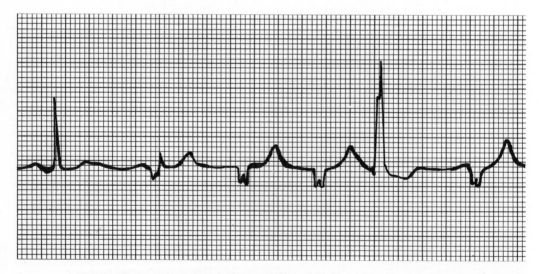

Fig. 10-17. Accelerated ventricular rhythm. The first two sinus beats are followed by a fusion beat. A ventricular focus, rate 114 per minute, takes over. Note the PVC from a different focus (third complex from end of strip).

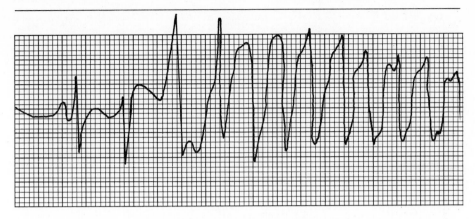

Fig. 10-18. Ventricular fibrillation.

Ventricular Fibrillation

DEFINITION: Rapid irregular and ineffectual contractions of the ventricle. The ECG shows a wavering baseline and bizarre waveforms.

ETIOLOGY: Ventricular fibrillation is favored by several causes. These include myocardial infarction, PVCs occurring at the apex of the preceding T wave (Fig. 10-18), and drugs such as digitalis or quinidine in toxic doses.

SYMPTOMS: With ventricular fibrillation, the ventricles immediately cease to expel blood, and death will occur rapidly in untreated cases. Loss of consciousness occurs within 8 to 10 seconds and a seizure may occur. No pulse is elicited, and the pupils become dilated. Clinical death is present and biological death follows in a few moments. Ventricular fibrillation is the most common basis of sudden death and is nearly always fatal if resuscitation is not immediately instituted. Rarely, ventricular fibrillation will terminate spontaneously within seconds.

TREATMENT: The best treatment is prevention. In monitored patients with multiple, consecutive, or encroaching PVCs, immediate treatment with lidocaine or procainamide will often prevent more serious ventricular rhythms. If fibrillation occurs, rapid defibrillation with DC countershock performed by the nurse in attendance is the management of choice (see the discussion of cardiopulmonary resuscitation in Chapter 9).

Sinoatrial Block

DEFINITION: The impulses originating in the S-A node occasionally fail to appear and one or more beats are totally dropped. The time interval after the blocked beat is twice as long as the interval for each normal cardiac cycle.

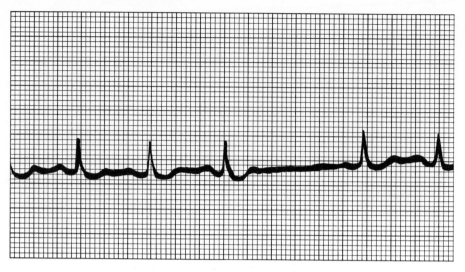

Fig. 10-19. Sinoatrial block.

ETIOLOGY: This is a rare arrhythmia which may result from excessive vagal stimulation, myocardial infarction, or digitalis intoxication. It may be a manifestation of "sick sinus syndrome."

SYMPTOMS: Symptoms of light-headedness or syncope due to prolonged standstill are common.

TREATMENT: When sinoatrial block is due to drug intoxication, the offending agent is stopped. Atropine or isoproterenol is useful, and transvenous pacing is the management of choice for permanent control of the arrhythmia.

First Degree A-V Block

DEFINITION: A delay in conduction through the A-V junction. The P-R interval exceeds the upper limit of 0.20 second in duration. In the example shown, the P-R interval is 0.30 second.

ETIOLOGY: This finding occurs in all ages and in both normal and diseased hearts. Drugs such as digitalis, quinidine and procainamide may prolong the P-R interval into the abnormal range.

The impulse originates normally in the S-A node and travels through the atria in normal sequence. The A-V junction delays the conduction for a longer than normal interval. When the impulse does pass through the A-V junction, the ventricles respond normally. This conduction disturbance is of no significance except when it is a precursor of second or third degree A-V block.

TREATMENT: None needed.

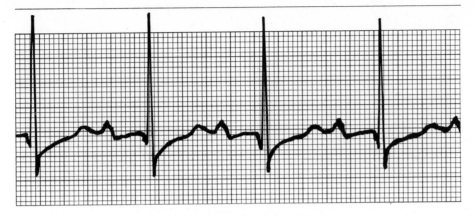

Fig. 10-20. First degree A-V block.

Second Degree Block—Mobitz I (Wenckebach)

DEFINITION: With each beat, the delay of conduction through the A-V junction is progressively increased. Eventually, the sinus impulse is completely blocked and no QRS complex occurs. In the strip shown, the blocked P wave is followed by a pause, then a paced beat.

SIGNIFICANT ECG CHANGES

   P-R interval: Progressively lengthens with each beat.

   QRS complex: Normal configuration, but progressively delayed after each P wave until one is dropped. The interval between successive QRS complexes shortens until a dropped beat occurs.

ETIOLOGY: Of the two types of second degree block, the Wenckebach

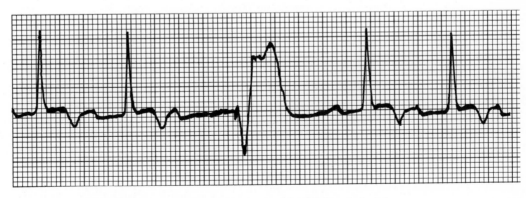

Fig. 10-21. Second degree block—Mobitz I (Wenckebach).

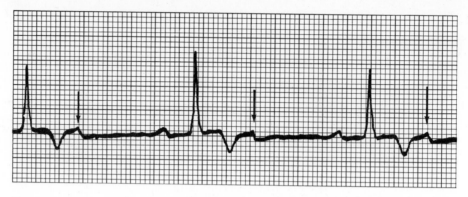

Fig. 10-22. Second degree block — Mobitz II.

phenomenon is the more common. Inferior myocardial infarction and digitalis toxicity may cause this type of second degree block.

TREATMENT: No treatment is required except to discontinue digitalis when it is the offending agent.

Second Degree Block — Mobitz II

DEFINITION: With this rhythm, some sinus impulses are conducted through the A-V junction with a constant P-R interval. Other sinus impulses are blocked completely. The ventricular rate is a fraction (1:2, 1:3, 1:4, etc.) of the atrial rate. In the strip shown, note the blocked P wave (arrow).

ETIOLOGY: Mobitz II A-V block indicates more severe impairment of A-V conduction. It is seen, for example, with acute anterior myocardial infarction, and its presence implies extensive destruction of the ventricular septum. Digitalis toxicity is not a cause.

Atrial contractions result from regular S-A impulses. Only those impulses which penetrate the A-V junction cause ventricular contractions. No symptoms occur unless the ventricular rate is so slow that cardiac output falls. This type of arrhythmia is potentially dangerous as it may progress to third degree block or ventricular standstill.

TREATMENT: Constant monitoring and observance of progression are required. Medications used include isoproterenol and epinephrine. Transvenous pacing is often indicated.

Third Degree Block (Complete A-V Block)

DEFINITION: None of the sinus impulses are conducted through the A-V junction. The atrial rate is faster than the ventricular rate. The atrial rate is usually normal and regular. The ventricular rate is regular but slower, averaging 30 to 45 beats per minute. The P-R interval is variable as in the example shown. The QRS complex is of normal configuration if it originates

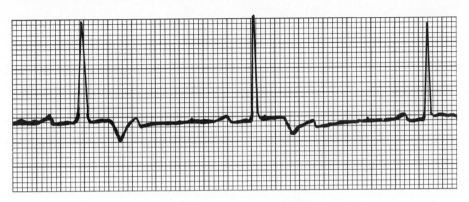

Fig. 10-23. Third degree block (complete A-V block).

in the His bundle and becomes widened if it originates from below this point.
ETIOLOGY: Occasionally complete heart block is congenital. In acquired cases, causes include degeneration of the conduction system due to advanced age, acute myocardial infarction, myocarditis, cardiac surgery, and digitalis intoxication.

With complete A-V block, the S-A node continues to pace in normal fashion but the impulse is blocked at the A-V junction. A lower cardiac pacemaker initiates the rhythm from a point distal to the A-V junction.

SYMPTOMS: If the ventricular rate is adequate to allow a normal cardiac output, the person is asymptomatic. When the rate is slow and cardiac contraction impaired from underlying heart disease, the cardiac output will fall. In the latter instance, heart failure may result and the patient may develop Adams-Stokes seizures (episodes of ventricular tachycardia, fibrillation, or cardiac standstill resulting in syncope, hypoxic seizures, coma or death). Untreated cases with symptoms carry a poor prognosis, and most such patients die within the year.

TREATMENT: Isoproterenol is the drug of choice. Temporary or permanent pacing is usually indicated. The nurse should familiarize herself with the benefits and hazards of electrical pacing (see Chapter 9).

Bundle Branch Block (BBB)

DEFINITION: A delay of conduction through the right or left bundle.
SIGNIFICANT ECG CHANGES

QRS complex: Prolonged to 0.12 second or longer. Typically, the QRS complex is notched and/or slurred with a widening of the QRS complex. With right bundle branch block, the S wave in lead I is broadened and an

R' is present in V_1. Left bundle branch block produces a positive broad deflection in lead I and a broad negative deflection in lead V_1. The T wave is wide and of opposite direction to the QRS complex.

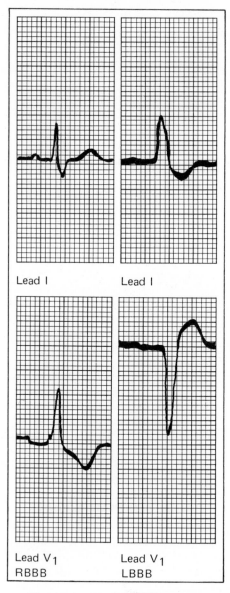

Fig. 10-24. Bundle branch block.

ETIOLOGY: The most common causes of bundle branch block are myocardial infarction, hypertension, and cardiomyopathy. It may also result from medications including procainamide and quinidine, or from hyperkalemia.

When conduction through one bundle is blocked, the impulse travels along the unaffected bundle and eventually reaches the other blocked area via the ventricular musculature. Transmission by this route is slower, and right and left ventricular contractions do not occur simultaneously. The abnormal contraction produces a wide QRS complex.

SYMPTOMS: Cardiac output is not decreased and thus the arrhythmia itself does not produce symptoms.

TREATMENT: The underlying heart disease determines treatment and prognosis.

serum electrolyte abnormalities and the electrocardiogram

The maintenance of adequate fluid and electrolyte balance assumes high priority in the care of patients in any medical, surgical, or coronary intensive care unit. Patients being treated for renal or cardiovascular diseases are especially vulnerable to electrolyte imbalances. The cure may well be worse than the disease if electrolyte abnormalities go undetected or ignored, since they frequently are caused by the treatment rather than the disease itself. Dialysis can very quickly cause major shifts in electrolytes. Certainly the often insidious drop of serum potassium levels in the digitalized cardiac patient who receives diuretics is well known.

Potassium and calcium are probably the two most important electrolytes that are concerned with proper function of the heart. They help produce normal contraction of cardiac muscle. They are also important in the propagation of the electrical impulse in the heart. Because of the latter function, excess or insufficiency of either electrolyte frequently causes changes in the electrocardiogram. The nurse who is aware of and is able to recognize these changes may well suspect electrolyte abnormalities before clinical symptoms appear or hazardous arrhythmias occur.

Hypokalemia (hypopotassemia) is probably the most frequently encountered electrolyte abnormality. It is commonly associated with vomiting, diarrhea, prolonged digitalis and diuretic therapy, and prolonged nasogastric suctioning. The alkalotic patient may also be hypokalemic. In most laboratories, normal serum potassium levels are about 3.5 to 5.0 mEq. per liter. The ECG which exhibits U waves should immediately alert the nurse to the possibility of hypokalemia in that patient (Fig. 10-25). Although the U wave is normal for many people, it is worthwhile to obtain a serum potassium level since it may be an early sign of hypokalemia. The normal U wave is often seen best in lead V_3. It is usually easily recognized, but may encroach on the

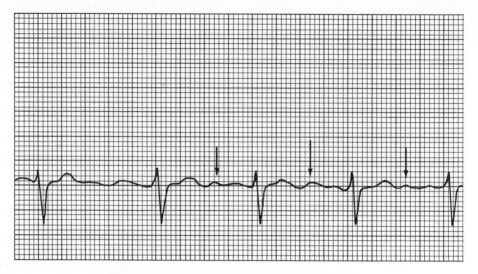

Fig. 10-25. Presence of U waves (hypokalemia).

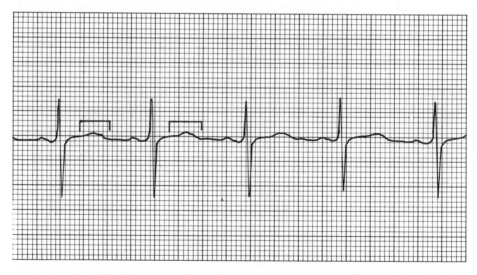

Fig. 10-26. Fusion of T and U waves (hypokalemia).

preceding T wave and go unnoticed (Fig. 10-26). The T wave may look notched or prolonged when it is hiding the U wave, giving the appearance of a prolonged Q-T interval. As potassium depletion increases, the U wave may become more prominent as the T wave becomes less so. The T wave becomes flattened and may even invert. The S-T segment tends to become depressed, somewhat resembling the effects of digitalis on the ECG. These electrocardiographic changes are not particularly well correlated with the severity of hypokalemia; however, they are good indicators of this abnormality and can be recognized by the nurse who has basic knowledge of ECG complexes. Untreated hypokalemia can produce ventricular premature contractions, atrial or junctional tachycardias, and eventually ventricular tachycardia, ventricular fibrillation, and death. The severity of the arrhythmias resulting from hypokalemia certainly points out the need for early recognition of this problem.

The U wave may also be accentuated in association with digitalis, quinidine, epinephrine, hypercalcemia, thyrotoxicosis, and exercise. The normal U wave should be upright in all leads that have upright T waves, and its polarity may be reversed in the presence of myocardial ischemia and left ventricular strain.

Hyperkalemia (hyperpotassemia) is often the result of overenthusiastic or poorly supervised treatment of hypokalemia. Sometimes early detection of hypokalemia is accomplished, treatment is instituted, and the problem is considered solved. However, if potassium supplements are not stopped or reduced when normal serum potassium levels are reached, hyperkalemia will result. Other causes of hyperkalemia include Addison's disease, acute renal failure, and acidosis. Another not infrequently seen cause of high potassium levels is the use of potassium-sparing diuretics. Triamterene (Dyrenium) is an example of this type of drug that is currently in common usage as an adjunct to the more potent diuretics. It must be remembered that these drugs not only spare potassium but may increase the potassium level of the serum.

The earliest sign of hyperkalemia on the electrocardiogram is a change in the T wave. It is usually described as tall, narrow and "peaked" or "tenting" in appearance (Fig. 10-27). The T wave height is normally not more than 5 mm. in any standard lead and not more than 10 mm. in any precordial lead. T waves may be abnormally tall in myocardial infarction and may also be found in ventricular overloading and in patients with cerebrovascular accidents.

As potassium levels rise, changes occur first in the atrial portion of the ECG complex, then in the ventricular portion. The P wave flattens and becomes wider as the result of intra-atrial block. Further potassium elevation causes progression to A-V nodal block and a prolonged P-R interval. The P wave may disappear entirely. With even higher potassium levels, the QRS begins to widen, indicating intraventricular block. If untreated, severe hyperkalemia will progress to increased widening of the QRS until ventricular fibrillation occurs at serum potassium levels of 8 to 10 mEq. per liter. In terms of arrhythmias, the patient may progress from sinus bradycardia to first degree block, through junctional rhythm, idioventricular rhythm, and ventricular tachycardia and fibrillation. Hyperkalemic changes on ECG correlate well with serum potassium levels. The T-wave changes described begin to appear at serum levels of 6 to 7 mEq. per liter; the QRS widens at

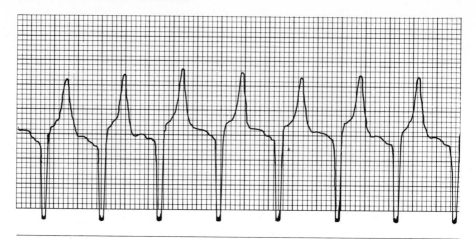

Fig. 10-27. Hyperkalemia.

8 to 9 mEq. per liter. Vigorous treatment must be instituted to reverse the condition at this point, as sudden death may occur at any time after these levels are reached.

Calcium is the second electrolyte important to normal functioning of the heart. It is thought to have an effect on linking the electrical impulse to myocardial contraction. Calcium increases cardiac contractility and is often administered intravenously to the patient who has sustained cardiac arrest in an attempt to increase the force of cardiac contraction.

Normal serum calcium is about 9 to 11 mg. percent. Hypercalcemia is often seen in patients with hyperparathyroidism, neoplastic diseases and acute osteoporosis. Hypocalcemia may occur in patients with renal failure, hypoparathyroidism and malabsorption syndromes.

The Q-T interval length is the most frequent ECG indicator of excess or insufficient calcium. It is somewhat shortened in hypercalcemia and lengthened in hypocalcemia (Figs. 10-28 and 10-29). In the hypercalcemic patient the shortening of the Q-T interval takes place especially in the portion from the beginning of the QRS to the apex of the T wave, making the beginning of the T wave an abrupt slope. U waves may also develop or be accentuated in the hypercalcemic patient. Hypocalcemia may also cause lowering and inversion of the T wave.

The Q-T interval is measured from the beginning of the QRS to the end of the T wave. The normal length of this interval varies with heart rate, sex and age and can be determined by consulting the chart of calculated normal Q-T intervals found in most texts on electrocardiography. A general guideline that can be used in clinical situations is that the Q-T interval should be less than half the preceding R-R interval when the heart rate is 65 to 90 beats per minute. The interval will normally shorten during tachycardia and lengthen during bradycardia.

Calcium abnormalities are not often seen in the cardiac patient unless there is an associated noncardiac disease. The more frequent cause of Q-T interval shortening or prolongation in the cardiac patient is the administration of cardiac drugs. Digitalis may cause a *shortened* Q-T interval. Quinidine and procainamide frequently cause *prolongation* of the Q-T interval. Drugs should always be considered when the ECG is evaluated for electrolyte abnormalities.

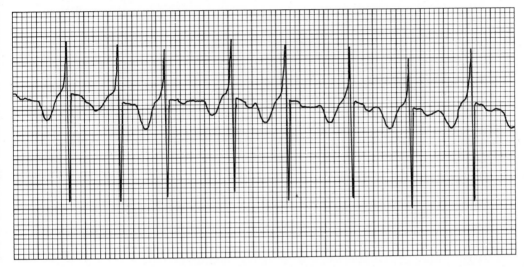

Fig. 10-28. Shortened Q-T interval (hypercalcemia).

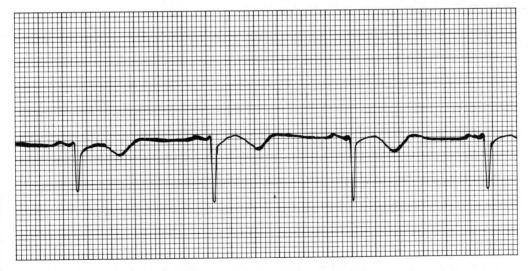

Fig. 10-29. Prolonged Q-T interval (hypocalcemia).

Arrhythmias are not commonly associated with either calcium excess or calcium insufficiency; however, too-rapid intravenous infusion of calcium salts may result in ventricular fibrillation and sudden death. The digitalized patient who receives calcium salts seems especially prone to this reaction for reasons not known.

Just as the patient who sustains myocardial infarction may not have chest pain, the patient who has electrolyte abnormalities may not exhibit any of the ECG changes described. Conversely, a patient with normal serum electrolytes may show some of these ECG changes for other reasons. None of the ECG manifestations described here even approach being diagnostic. They are of value primarily in alerting one to suspect electrolyte abnormalities. It is appropriate for the nurse, especially one who cares for the critically ill patient, to be alert to ECG changes and to interpret what is seen in the context of what is already known about that patient.

BIBLIOGRAPHY

Goldman, Mervin J., *Principles of Clinical Electrocardiography* (Los Altos, Calif.: Lange Medical Publications, 1973).

Marriott, Henry, *Practical Electrocardiography* (Baltimore: Williams and Wilkins, 1972).

Massie, Edward, and Thomas J. Walsh, *Clinical Vectorcardiography and Electrocardiography* (Chicago: Year Book Medical Publishers, 1960).

Relman, Arnold S., and John A. Kastor, *Disturbances of Potassium and Calcium Balance and their Effect on the Electrocardiogram*. Rocom.

Ritota, Michael C., *Diagnostic Electrocardiography* (Philadelphia: J. B. Lippincott, 1969).

serum enzyme studies

As the role of the nurse is expanded, there is a need for more knowledge on which to base the judgments necessary to assume new responsibilities. Knowledge of the purpose, functions and significance of laboratory values in relation to the diagnosis and prognosis of acute myocardial infarction can enhance the quality of nursing care available to patients. Armed with a basic understanding of serum enzyme determinations, the nurse can exercise judgment in their interpretation in relation to other information known about the patient. The ability to exercise this kind of judgment may well affect the clinical course or prognosis of the patient. It is certainly as important to the physical and mental well-being of these patients to rule out the presence of acute myocardial infarction as it is to confirm its existence.

Enzymes are proteins that are found in all living cells. Different enzymes are found in different kinds of cells and in varying concentrations. The function of enzymes is to serve as accelerating agents or catalysts for chemical reactions. They temporarily combine with one substance to form an enzyme substrate complex, which then breaks down to form the end products of the chemical reaction. When the enzyme has completed this task, it is liberated, unchanged, to continue functioning as a chemical catalyst.

Enzymes are produced in the cells and are released into the plasma. Overactive, diseased, or injured cells increase the release of their particular enzymes into the serum. The difference in composition and concentration of various enzymes from one kind of tissue to another (cardiac, liver, skeletal muscle, and the like) determines which serum enzyme elevations reflect damage to specific tissues. Thus serum enzyme determinations can be used to detect cell damage and to suggest where the damage has occurred.

Many studies have been done in relation to the diagnostic value of serum enzyme determinations. As sometimes happens in research, the results vary and are debated by clinical diagnosticians and pathologists alike. To further cloud the issue, enzymes are evaluated by a variety of laboratory methods and the determinations are reported in different quantitative units. This results in different "normal" ranges, which vary according to the procedures used by the particular laboratory. The nurse must become familiar with the range of normals for each enzyme as it is reported by the laboratory where she works.

Serum enzyme determinations have been helpful in the diagnosis of cardiac, hepatic, pancreatic, muscular, bone, and malignant diseases. Each of these kinds of tissue releases a particular enzyme or enzymes when diseased or damaged. Since each kind of cell contains and releases more than one enzyme, there is overlapping of enzymes from one tissue source to another. For this reason there is no one serum enzyme elevation that is diagnostic of any one disease.

The term "cardiac enzyme" is used in reference to those enzymes which occur in and are released in proportionately larger amounts from cardiac tissue. These include creatine phosphokinase (CPK), hydroxybutyric dehydrogenase (HBD), serum glutamic-oxalacetic transaminase (SGOT), and lactic dehydrogenase (LDH). Serum glutamic-pyruvic transaminase (SGPT) may show a slight increase in the presence of massive myocardial infarction, but it is more specific for liver disease. Each of these enzymes varies in its degree of specificity for myocardial disease. The relationship between acute myocardial infarction and elevated SGOT and LDH was established in the mid-1950s. CPK was added to the list of diagnostic aids in the mid-1960s. Controversy regarding their usefulness continues.

Total LDH is probably the least specific for cardiac disease of the "cardiac enzymes." It is abundant in kidney, cardiac, liver and muscle tissues and in red cells (Table 10-1). The onset of LDH elevation occurs 12 to 24 hours after tissue damage, and peak elevation, averaging about three times upper normal, is at 72 hours. Return to normal is not complete for 7 to 11 days. The fact that LDH elevation is prolonged for a week or more after myocardial infarction is often helpful in late diagnosis. Some patients do not come to the hospital until several days after their initial symptoms, so early blood specimens cannot be obtained.

Because LDH has widespread distribution in body tissues, its serum level

table 10-1
enzyme distribution in cells

SGOT	CPK	LDH (ISOENZYMES)	
Heart	Heart	Heart ⎫	
Kidney		Kidney ⎬ (Fast)	
Red cells		Red cells ⎬	
Brain	Brain	Brain ⎭	
		Lymph nodes ⎫	
		Spleen ⎬	
		Leukocytes ⎬ (Intermediate)	
Pancreas		Pancreas ⎬	
Lung		Lung ⎭	
Liver		Liver ⎫	
Skeletal muscle	Skeletal muscle	Skeletal muscle ⎬ (Slow)	
		Skin ⎭	

is elevated in a variety of diseases. In 1957 it was found that LDH could be subjected to certain procedures that separate the enzyme into five components or isoenzymes which demonstrate five zones of activity of the enzyme. Since enzyme activity is measured by its rate of acceleration of chemical reactions, these five zones range from fastest-acting to slowest-acting. The two fastest-acting isoenzymes are found in cardiac muscle, the renal cortex, erythrocytes, and the cerebrum and reflect disease or damage in these tissues. Thus if these isoenzymes are elevated in the serum of a patient who presents with chest pain but has no evidence of renal, hemolytic, or cerebral disease, myocardial infarction is the likely diagnosis. The two slowest-acting LDH isoenzymes are found in the liver, skeletal muscle, and skin. These reflect acute liver disease or hepatic congestion, muscle injuries, or dermatological disease or trauma. The intermediate isoenzyme is found in lymph nodes, spleen, leukocytes, pancreas, and lung tissue. It in turn reflects disease or damage to these tissues. These five isoenzymes, also called fractions of LDH, are numbered 1 through 5. Many laboratories report LDH_1 and LDH_2 as the faster isoenzymes and LDH_4 and LDH_5 as the slower, while others report them in reverse order. Care must be taken in reading the literature on serum enzymes to avoid the confusion caused by various methods of reporting. LDH_1 will henceforth be referred to as fastest-acting and LDH_5 as slowest-acting. Here again the nurse must be aware of how LDH isoenzymes are reported in her hospital laboratory.

The introduction of isoenzyme separation has made determination of the LDH isoenzymes one of the most specific tests for the diagnosis of myocardial infarction. Most diagnosticians consider myocardial infarction the problem when LDH_1 activity is greater than LDH_2. Both these isoenzymes have been found in the serum up to two weeks or more after infarction even though total LDH has returned to normal.

When blood specimens for LDH determinations are collected, it is essential to avoid hemolysis of the sample. Since LDH is found in erythrocytes, even slightly hemolyzed blood will show an elevation of the serum LDH. It is for this same reason that hemolysis caused by an artificial valve or by use of the cardiopulmonary bypass pump results in elevation of serum LDH.

The enzyme HBD may possibly be the same as the fast-moving cardiac isoenzyme of LDH. It correlates with the LDH fractions and therefore is frequently omitted from the commonly used series of enzymes. HBD activity is always associated with LDH activity. The serum evaluation of both enzymes after myocardial infarction is about the same, both in quantity and in duration of elevation, with only a slight time lag in HBD. In laboratories that do not have the necessary equipment for fractionating LDH isoenzymes, HBD determination can serve as an alternate for this study, although it is felt to be less specific.

CPK is the fastest-rising and fastest-falling of all the "cardiac enzymes." Onset of serum elevation is about 2 to 5 hours after infarction, with a peak elevation of five to twelve times normal, or more, by 12 to 36 hours. Serum levels may return to normal by the second or third day. This transient nature of CPK elevation following myocardial infarction can be a distinct aid to diagnosis if the patient is reached early in the acute episode. However, this frequently is not the case; the CPK rise may be missed entirely by the time the patient enters the hospital and is seen by a physician and a tentative diagnosis made. About 90 percent of patients with myocardial infarction show the early rise in serum CPK.

The CPK enzyme is second only to LDH isoenzymes in specificity for cardiac damage. CPK is found in skeletal and cardiac muscle and in brain tissue. Since red cells contain almost no CPK, slight hemolysis does not interfere with the accuracy of its determination. It is of particular value in diagnosing cardiac disease because it is not found in liver tissue as are LDH and SGOT. Hepatic congestion or disease which frequently accompanies cardiac disease will therefore not affect CPK values. CPK determination is also helpful in differentiating myocardial infarction from pulmonary embolism, which often present very similar clinical pictures. Because of the proportionately smaller amount of CPK in lung tissue, any rise with pulmonary embolism will be much smaller than the very high elevation associated with myocardial infarction. CPK values are normal in pericarditis, but an elevation occurs in myocarditis because of the cardiac muscle involvement. Recall that overactivity as well as disease or damage of tissue cells will cause release of enzymes into the serum. This should be kept in mind when CPK elevation is found in the patient who collapsed on the golf course or while skiing. Severe or prolonged exercise of the untrained "social athlete" can result in CPK elevation for up to 48 hours. Other conditions causing a rise in CPK levels include acute cerebrovascular disease, muscular dystrophy and other muscle trauma. Elevations are sometimes found following peripheral arterial embolism, repeated intramuscular injections and operative procedures. It has been reported that morphine sulfate injected intramuscularly causes a significant increase in CPK values in 25 percent of patients.

The recent discovery that CPK can be fractionated into isoenzymes is felt by many to be a great boon to the diagnosis of myocardial infarction. CPK isoenzymes are again measured by their rate of chemical reaction acceleration. They are designated as MM, the fast-acting isoenzyme found in skeletal muscle; MB, the intermediate-acting myocardial isoenzyme; and BB, the slow-acting isoenzyme found in brain tissue. Since there are so many causes for total CPK release, especially from injured skeletal muscle tissue, the ability to differentiate muscle, myocardial or brain tissue as the source of the CPK elevation can be extremely helpful. CPK-MB is reported to be up to 94 percent sensitive and 100 percent specific for myocardial infarction. CPK-MB may be elevated after acute myocardial infarction even though total CPK is not.

The CPK-MB isoenzyme is elevated in the serum for only 24 to 72 hours after its initial appearance. It is obvious that proper timing of the blood specimen is extremely important. The peak rise of CPK-MB is 16 to 24 hours after initial elevation. If the patient is not seen until 24 to 48 hours after the onset of symptoms of myocardial injury, one must rely more on the LDH isoenzymes. The rapid appearance and disappearance of the CPK-MB isoenzyme may be a positive factor in its usefulness in diagnosing the extension of an acute myocardial infarction. This can be a very difficult diagnosis to make when the resolved chest pain of myocardial infarction recurs and the initial total enzyme elevations have not yet returned to normal. Determination of CPK-MB may be especially helpful in the CCU patient when there are additional causes for total enzyme elevations such as cardioversion or defibrillation, multiple intramuscular injections for pain or vomiting, trauma due to falls secondary to arrhythmias, prolonged use of rotating tourniquets, or hypotension.

CPK-MB may also be helpful in diagnosing acute myocardial infarction in the postoperative patient. The muscle trauma incurred during surgical procedures will cause all three of the total "cardiac enzymes" to rise. In these patients, one should be able to determine whether total CPK elevation is entirely due to surgical trauma or partially due to myocardial infarction, by employing CPK isoenzymes as a specific test. Unfortunately, CPK isoenzymes are not very helpful in diagnosing myocardial infarction in the postoperative cardiac patient. Some rise in CPK-MB will occur after open heart surgery due to cardiac manipulation and cannulation.

SGOT is the last of the most frequently used "cardiac enzymes" to be discussed. Its tissue distribution is quite widespread, with large SGOT concentrations in red cells and cardiac, liver, skeletal muscle, and renal tissue. Lesser amounts are found in brain, pancreas, and lung tissue. Its widespread distribution makes it one of the least specific enzymes, second only to total LDH. Over 95 percent of patients with myocardial infarction have SGOT elevation; an infarction as little as 5 percent can cause a serum rise. SGOT falls between CPK and LDH in both degree and duration of elevation. SGOT rise begins about 6 to 8 hours after onset of an acute myocardial episode, reaches its peak in 18 to 36 hours, and returns to normal at the end of 4 to 6 days. Average elevation following myocardial infarction is five times normal, but may go much higher with an extensive infarct.

SGOT may become elevated with tachyarrhythmias with or without myocardial infarction, probably reflecting liver decompensation due to decreased perfusion. Liver damage resulting from congestive heart failure or shock due to myocardial infarction can also cause an increase in SGOT. It has been reported that about 25 percent of cardioverted patients have elevation of SGOT up to three times normal, probably due to muscle release of the enzyme. Other causes of SGOT elevation include acute liver damage after alcohol ingestion, tachyarrhythmias with a ventricular rate of over 160 per minute, shock, pericarditis, dissecting aortic aneurysm, unaccustomed vigorous exercise, trauma, cerebral infarction, acute cholecystitis, pancreatitis and certain drugs such as narcotics and anticoagulants. SGOT rises several days after pulmonary infarction. This may help to differentiate this problem from acute myocardial infarction when the time of onset of symptoms of pulmonary infarction can be determined.

As mentioned previously, the SGPT enzyme is more specific for liver disease and does not usually rise with cardiac damage. However, both SGOT and SGPT will rise if myocardial infarction is accompanied by prolonged or profound shock or severe congestive heart failure which results in liver congestion or damage. SGOT evaluation may be of particular value in the early diagnosis of reinfarction. A second infarction often cannot be read on ECG because of the changes already incurred by the first infarction. A rise in SGOT within 6 to 8 hours after an episode of chest pain will help to make the diagnosis.

One can almost always be assured that myocardial infarction has not occurred if serum enzyme levels remain normal for 36 to 48 hours after onset of symptoms. If infarct has occurred, all the enzymes should be elevated between 24 and 48 hours after symptom occurrence (Fig. 10-30). In comparing enzyme elevations, CPK rises first and highest and falls to normal first, followed by SGOT, with LDH rising last. LDH elevation is the lowest but the most prolonged. In comparing the specificity of each enzyme as an indicator of myocardial necrosis, LDH isoenzymes are most specific, followed by CPK, SGOT, and total LDH (least specific).

In general it can be said that the size of a myocardial infarction correlates fairly well with the height of the enzyme peaks and the duration of enzyme elevation, as well as with patient mortality. Some studies show that CPK elevation of ten times normal is accompanied by 50 percent mortality, while a mortality of 6 percent is shown with CPK rises of less than five times normal. It has been reported that: (1) 81 percent of ventricular arrhythmias occur in patients whose enzyme levels are more than four times normal; (2) the incidence of congestive heart failure is significantly increased in those with enzyme levels of 4 to 5 times normal; (3) patients with cardiogenic shock

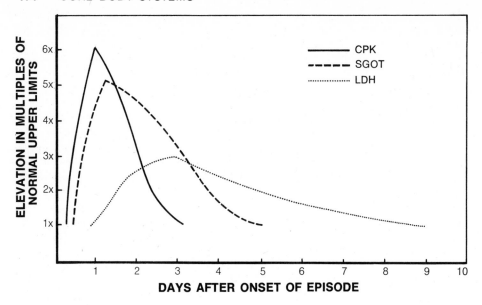

Fig. 10-30. Peak elevation and duration of serum enzymes after myocardial injury.

have enzyme increases of more than five times normal. If enzyme peak levels do indeed correlate with infarct size, they should be helpful to the nurse in anticipating those complications which are related to infarct size, as well as prognosis and ultimate rehabilitation.

There are a number of "red herrings" to be kept in mind when elevated serum enzymes are evaluated. Severe or prolonged exercise has been mentioned. Defibrillation with large amounts of voltage or repeated defibrillation may cause enzymes to rise because of the sudden severe contraction of all muscle tissues. Even one defibrillation with 400 watt-seconds may result in enzyme rise sufficient to mimic myocardial infarction. HBD, which is thought to be much like the cardiac isoenzymes of LDH and CPK, sometimes rises with liver disease. The extent of surgical trauma during operative procedures should be considered when enzyme elevations are evaluated postoperatively. Tissue damage from frequent intramuscular injections must also be remembered as a source of enzyme rises. CPK elevations of more than eight times normal have been seen after frequent injections. It is also possible to produce elevation of SGOT and SGPT with administration of salicylates, sodium warfarin (Coumadin), and other drugs that are detoxified in the liver. There may be minimal enzyme elevations after cardiac catheterization and coronary angiography, but these are mainly caused by the injection of intramuscular premedications. The introduction of catheters via arteriotomy or percutaneous routes alone does not cause significant rise of enzymes.

It is apparent from the discussion of these four enzyme studies used in diagnosing myocardial infarction that none are actually diagnostic. Many areas still remain unclear or unknown. No enzyme or enzyme fraction has yet been found to exist in cardiac muscle alone. There is much disagreement about the normal range of CPK activity. Some studies indicate that the upper limit of normal in females is about two thirds that of males, and that blacks may have higher normals than whites. Other enzymes have been found to rise with myocardial necrosis, but they are either no more specific than the ones currently used, or are technically difficult and time-consuming to measure.

As yet enzyme determinations can serve only as an adjunct to diagnosis by ECG and the patient's clinical picture. In order to be of most value they should be ordered with discretion. Consideration must be given to the length of time that has passed since the onset of symptoms, as each enzyme rises and returns to normal at different time intervals. One often finds an order for "stat" enzymes upon admission of the patient with suspected myocardial infarction to the critical care unit. The results will be useless if only an hour or two has passed since the onset of symptoms. If the patient suffered only moderate symptoms and did not come to the hospital until several days later, CPK determination is useless because the enzyme will already have returned to normal. Usually two enzyme determinations are considered more valid than one, but the gamut of enzyme tests may not be necessary.

Enzyme determinations have been of greatest value in the patient whose ECG and clinical picture are equivocal for diagnosis of myocardial infarction. Enzyme elevation may well confirm a suspected diagnosis in this case. Sometimes it is difficult or impossible to interpret infarction on ECG because of previous infarction changes, the effects of certain drugs or electrolyte imbalances, conduction defects such as bundle branch block or Wolff-Parkinson-White syndrome, arrhythmias, or a functioning pacemaker. Enzyme determination may be a distinct advantage here. If a definite diagnosis can be made by ECG, there may be no need for enzyme tests, except for academic interest.

It must be stressed that serum elevations are nonspecific in the diagnosis of myocardial infarction, and they must be considered in view of the total clinical picture. We are in a highly technical age of nursing and must not forget to look at and listen to the patient before making judgments and decisions.

BIBLIOGRAPHY

Chahine, R. A., et al., "Interpretation of Serum Enzyme Changes Following Cardiac Catheterization and Coronary Angiography," *American Heart Journal*, Vol. 87 (February 1974), pp. 170–174.

Coodley, Eugene L., "Prognostic Value of Enzymes in Myocardial Infarction," *JAMA*, Vol. 225 (August 6, 1973), pp. 597–600.

Dade Reagents, Inc., *Diagnostic Enzymology*, 1970.

Dixon, Sewell H., Jr., et al., "Recognition of Postoperative Acute Myocardial Infarction — Application of Isoenzyme Techniques," *Circulation*, Vol. 48, Suppl. 3 (July 1973), pp. 137–140.

Galen, Robert S., James A. Reiffel, and S. Raymond Gambino, "Diagnosis of Acute Myocardial Infarction—Relative Efficiency of Serum Enzymes and Isoenzyme Measurements," *JAMA,* Vol. 232 (1975), pp. 145–147.

Gesink, Melvin H., "Enzymes in the Diagnosis of Myocardial Infarction," unpublished paper, 1971.

Hurst, J. W., and R. B. Logue, *The Heart,* ed. 2 (New York: McGraw-Hill, 1970), pp. 296, 964–967.

Nevins, Michael A., et al., "Pitfalls in Interpreting Serum Creatine Phosphokinase Activity," *JAMA,* Vol. 224 (June 4, 1973), pp. 1382–1387.

Scott, B. B., A. V. Simmons, K. E. Newton, and R. B. Payne, "Interpretation of Serum Creatine Kinase in Suspected Myocardial Infarction," *British Medical Journal,* Vol. 4 (1974), pp. 691–693.

Shaft, Franklin R., Robert W. Bun, and Hedy Imfeld, "Serum Pyruvate Kinase in Acute Myocardial Infarction," *American Journal of Cardiology,* Vol. 26 (1970), pp. 143–150.

Sobel, B. E., "Serum Creatine Phosphokinase and Myocardial Infarction," *JAMA,* Vol. 229 (July 8, 1974), pp. 201–202.

Varat, M. A., and D. W. Mercer, "Cardiac Specific Creatine Phosphokinase Isoenzyme in the Diagnosis of Acute Myocardial Infarction," *Circulation,* Vol. 51 (May 1975), pp. 855–859.

Wagner, G. S., et al., "The Importance of Identification of the Myocardial-Specific Isoenzyme of Creatine Phosphokinase (MB Form) in the Diagnosis of Acute Myocardial Infarction," *Circulation,* Vol. 47 (February 1973), pp. 263–269.

Wilkinson, J. Henry, "The Diagnostic Value of LDH Isoenzymes in Clinical Medicine," *Clinical Profile,* Beckman Instruments, Inc., Vol. 1 (1968).

the significance of auscultation of the heart

Nurses throughout the country have done well in terminating and preventing lethal arrhythmias. With the development of electrocardiographic monitoring and the education of nurses in interpreting arrhythmias and initiating emergency treatment, the mortality incidence among patients with myocardial infarction has decreased. However, nurses need to improve their care of patients who develop heart failure. Of the patients who develop blatantly obvious left ventricular failure, an estimated 40 percent die.[1]

One of the earliest and frequently the only cardiac sign of congestive heart failure in the adult is the development of a third heart sound. If nurses are taught to detect the third heart sound and are aware of its clinical significance, it is possible that they could decrease the incidence of heart failure in their patients.

the characteristics of sound

Sound is a series of disturbances in matter to which the human ear is sensitive. Sound is a wave motion which has four characteristics—intensity, pitch, duration, and timbre. *Intensity* is the force of the amplitude of the vibrations. It is a physical aspect of sound, whereas loudness is a subjective aspect dependent upon (1) intensity of the sound, and (2) sensitivity of the ear. *Pitch* is the frequency of the vibrations per unit of time. The human ear is most sensitive to vibrations of 500 to 5,000 per second. Vibrations of less than 20 per second or greater than 20,000 per second cannot be heard by the human ear. *Duration* is the length of time that the sound persists. *Timbre* is a quality dependent upon overtones that accompany the fundamental tone. In other words, most fundamental vibrations have higher frequency vibrations called *overtones*. Overtones account for the difference in sound between the same note played on a piano and on a flute.[2,3]

Sound waves are initiated by vibrations. The heart sounds are produced by vascular walls, flowing blood, heart muscle, and heart valves. Sudden changes in intra-arterial pressures cause the vascular walls to vibrate, resulting in sound production. Turbulence of blood flow is produced when rapidly moving blood passes through chambers of irregular size, such as the chambers of the heart and the great vessels. When the heart muscles contract, sound waves are initiated by the contracting fibers. Sound waves are produced when the heart valves open as the blood flows through or when they close, especially with a sudden snapping of the chordae tendineae. Of the previously mentioned causes of heart sounds, the closing of the heart valves accounts for most of the sound production.[4,5]

Systole is defined as the time during which the ventricles contract. Systole begins with the beginning of the first heart sound and ends with the beginning of the second heart sound. *Diastole* is defined as the time during which the ventricles relax. Diastole begins with the beginning of the second heart sound and ends with the beginning of the next first heart sound. The cardiac cycle is determined by the cycle of the ventricles. In other words, cardiac systole and ventricular systole are synonymous.

The transmission of the heart sounds is dependent upon the position of the heart, the nature of the surrounding structures, and the position of the stethoscope in relation to the origin of the sound.[6] The stethoscope is a tool used to transmit sounds produced by the body to the ear. Sound waves that travel a shorter distance are of greater intensity; likewise, the shorter the distance the less the possibility for distortion to occur. It then follows that the shorter the tube of the stethoscope the better the transmission of sound. Convenience and comfort as well as maximum sound production must be considered.

In order to facilitate accurate auscultation, the patient should be comfortable, in a quiet room, and in a recumbent position. The bell of the stethoscope transmits low-pitched sounds best when there is an airtight seal and when the instrument is applied lightly to the chest wall. An airtight seal helps to occlude extraneous sounds. The diaphragm of the stethoscope best transmits the high-pitched sounds when it is applied with firm pressure to the chest wall.

the first heart sound

The first heart sound is produced by the asynchronous closure of the mitral and tricuspid valves. Mitral closure precedes tricuspid closure by 0.02 to 0.03 second. Such narrow splitting is generally not audible. The first heart sound is therefore composed of two separate components. The first component

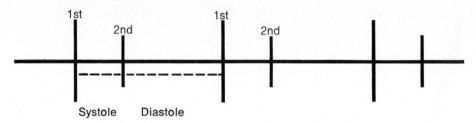

Fig. 10-31. Normal heart sounds.

of the first heart sound is the closure of the mitral valve. The second component of the first heart sound is the closure of the tricuspid valve. The first heart sound is generally best heard at the apex. It represents the beginning of ventricular systole.[7]

the second heart sound

The second heart sound is produced by the vibrations initiated by the closure of the aortic and pulmonic semilunar valves. The second heart sound, like the first heart sound, is composed of two separate components. The first component of the second heart sound is closure of the aortic valve. The second component of the second heart sound is the closure of the pulmonic valve. With inspiration, systole of the right ventricle is slightly prolonged due to increased filling of the right ventricle. With increased right ventricular filling, the pulmonary valve closes later than the aortic valve. Aortic valve sounds are generally best heard in the second intercostal space to the right of the sternum, whereas the sound produced by the pulmonic valve is generally best heard in the second left intercostal space. Splitting of the second heart sound is best heard upon inspiration with the stethoscope placed in the second intercostal space to the left of the sternum. The second heart sound represents the beginning of ventricular diastole.[8,9] See Fig. 10–31 for a graphic representation of the normal first and second heart sounds.

comparison between electrocardiogram and phonocardiogram

To facilitate understanding of the phonocardiogram, it will be compared with the electrocardiogram. The electrocardiogram is a graphic representation of the electrical activity of the heart, whereas the phonocardiogram is a recording of the sound vibrations produced by the heart.

When the sinoauricular node fires, the electical current travels through the atrial muscle to the atrioventricular node. The P wave is then written on the electrocardiogram. The electrical current then travels down the common bundle of His, right and left bundle branches, Purkinje fibers, and throughout the ventricular muscle. Following electrical stimulation of the ventricles, the latter contract. Early in ventricular systole the mitral and tricuspid valves

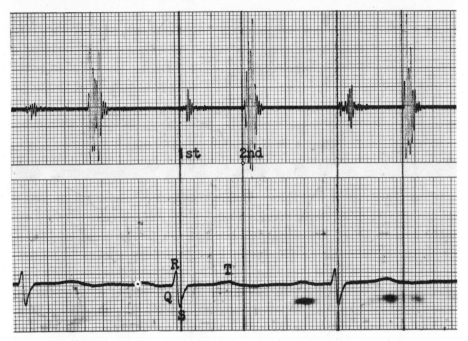

Fig. 10-32. Simultaneous recording of a phonocardiogram and an electrocardiogram.

close. This is the reason the first heart sound occurs during or following ventricular depolarization, which is represented on the electrocardiogram by the QRS complex (Fig. 10–32).

During ventricular systole, the blood is forced from the right and left ventricles into the pulmonic and aortic arteries. When the ventricles relax, the aortic and pulmonic semilunar valves close. The second heart sound represents the beginning of ventricular diastole. The second heart sound occurs after the repolarization of the ventricular muscle, which is represented by the T wave on the electrocardiogram.

the third heart sound

A third heart sound represents pathology in the adult. The third heart sound is believed to be produced by the rapid inrush of blood into a nonpliable ventricle. During ventricular diastole, the apex extends downward and the mitral valve extends upward. As the ventricle fills, the chordae tendineae become tense and partially close the mitral valve. This, along with the increasing resistance of diastole, causes a sudden decrease in blood flow. The cardiac muscle, chordae tendineae, heart valves, and blood are set into motion and are responsible for the production of sound. The third heart sound is heard after the closure of the semilunar valves, early in diastole, and best at the

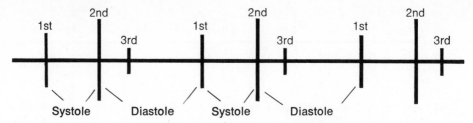

Fig. 10-33. Third heart sound.

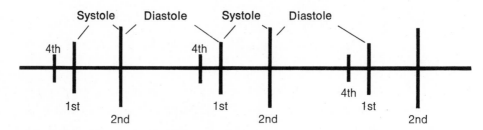

Fig. 10-34. Fourth heart sound.

apex. Most third heart sounds are of relatively low pitch, between 25 and 35 vibrations per second. They are best heard with the bell of the stethoscope applied lightly to the chest wall[10,11] (Fig. 10-33).

the fourth heart sound

The fourth heart sound, also called an atrial sound, is believed to be produced by atrial contraction that is more forceful than normal. At the end of atrial contraction, more blood is forced from the atria into the ventricle which causes a sudden increase in ventricular pressure. This increased pressure produces vibrations which cause the fourth heart sound. The fourth heart sound is therefore believed to be produced by atrial contraction and the consequent impact of the rapid inflow of blood on the ventricle. The fourth heart sound is of low pitch, heard best at the lower end of the sternum and sometimes at the apex. It has a short duration and a low frequency. It is best heard with the bell of the stethoscope.[12] Figure 10-34 shows the timing of the fourth heart sound.

gallop rhythms

Gallop rhythm is the name given to the heart sounds when they are grouped so as to mimic the cadence of galloping horses. There are three types of gallop rhythms. The protodiastolic or early diastolic gallop rhythm, also known as the ventricular gallop rhythm, is believed to be due to an exaggerated third

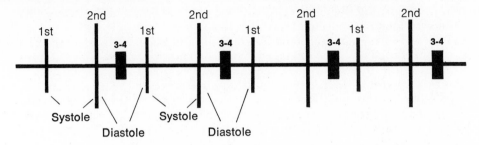

Fig. 10-35. Summation gallop.

heart sound. This rhythm is commonly heard in congestive heart failure. It is frequently the earliest sign of heart failure. Controversy still exists regarding the significance of the third sound. The ventricular gallop is generally believed to result from the rapid inflow of blood into a dilated ventricle early in diastole. The third heart sound occurs between 0.12 and 0.18 second after the second heart sound. It is of low pitch and heard best at the apex with the bell of the stethoscope.[13]

A presystolic gallop rhythm exists when the gallop sound occurs late in diastole or immediately preceding systole. The sound occurs with atrial systole and is believed to represent an accentuated atrial sound. It occurs with systolic overloading notably in hypertension, myocardial infarction, aortic stenosis, pulmonary hypertension, pulmonary stenosis, and various cardiomyopathies. It is often unaccompanied by heart failure. The presystolic or atrial gallop rhythm is low-pitched and is heard best with the bell of the stethoscope. A left atrial sound is heard best on expiration at the apex, whereas a right atrial sound is best heard on inspiration at the left border of the sternum.[14]

A summation gallop occurs because of a tachycardia so rapid that the third and fourth heart sounds combine and are heard as one[15] (Fig. 10-35).

mechanisms of heart murmurs

In order to understand the heart murmurs it is vital to understand the mechanism reponsible for the sound production. To fully understand murmur formation it is important to understand the principles of turbulence of blood flow. Blood flows most rapidly in the center of a vessel, less rapidly nearer the wall, and least rapidly immediately along the internal surface of the vessel. In other words, as blood flows through a vessel the friction along the wall of the vessel tends to slow the rate of blood flow nearest the wall. The smoother the internal surface of the vessel the less turbulence in blood flow. The slower the rate of blood flow the less chance there is for turbulence. Any irregularity in the inner surface of the vessel or change in the size of the lumen results in turbulence of blood flow and sound production. The narrower the opening the more rapid the rate of blood flow and the greater the possibility for turbulence and murmur formation.[16]

The murmurs of mitral stenosis, mitral insufficiency, aortic stenosis, and aortic insufficiency will be discussed. With the knowledge of the mechanisms which produce these murmurs, the nurse will be able to deduce the mechanisms responsible for the other murmurs not discussed. The mechanisms reponsible for the murmurs of mitral stenosis and mitral insufficiency are also responsible for the murmurs of tricuspid stenosis and tricuspid insufficiency. The only difference is that the latter murmurs occur on the right side of the heart. Likewise, the mechanisms responsible for the murmurs of aortic stenosis and aortic insufficiency are also responsible for the murmurs of pulmonary stenosis and pulmonary insufficiency. The difference is that the latter murmurs occur on the right side of the heart.

the murmur of mitral stenosis

In mitral stenosis the mitral orifice can be narrowed by inflammation and/or fibrosis of the mitral valve because of rheumatic heart disease or arteriosclerosis. A stenotic mitral valve causes an increased left atrial pressure during ventricular diastole. In ventricular diastole the left atrium contracts forcing blood through the narrowed opening. This produces turbulence of blood flow and the production of a diastolic murmur. The murmur is low-pitched and rumbling.[17]

The murmur of mitral stenosis may be a crescendo or decrescendo in configuration. It may be a crescendo in shape because the left atrium contracts progessively, the rate of blood flow increases, and the mitral valve becomes narrower. It may be a decrescendo in shape because as the ventricle fills, the left atrium empties, and the amount of blood passing through the stenotic valve decreases. The murmur therefore decreases in intensity and is a decrescendo in shape[18] (Fig. 10-36).

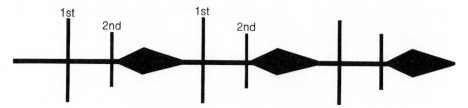

Fig. 10-36. Murmur of mitral stenosis.

the murmur of mitral insufficiency

The murmur of mitral insufficiency is heard in systole. Mitral insufficiency occurs when the mitral valve is incompetent, and the valve leaflets fail to approximate. During ventricular systole, intraventricular pressure exceeds intra-atrial pressure. With an incompetent mitral valve, the blood regurgi-

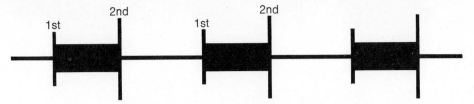

Fig. 10-37. Murmur of mitral insufficiency.

tates through the valve opening into the left atrium. This results in turbulence of blood flow and a high-pitched, blowing murmur. The murmur is systolic, heard best at the apex, and is transmitted laterally to the axillary line when the heart is enlarged. As a rule, a murmur is transmitted in the direction of the blood flow that is responsible for the turbulence. The murmur of mitral insufficiency is generally pansystolic or holosystolic[19,20] (lasting all of systole) (Fig. 10-37).

The murmur of mitral insufficiency is the murmur of myocardial infarction. In myocardial infarction, dilatation of the left ventricle occurs because of ischemia and/or necrosis. When the left ventricle is dilated, the papillary muscle tends to move away from the valve leaflets. The chordae tendineae are unable to lengthen, and the mitral leaflets are held open, preventing complete approximation. With dilatation of the left ventricle, the mitral ring dilates. The leaflets remain the same size and are unable to close the enlarged opening. When the left ventricle dilates, it loses its ability to contract and there is an associated papillary muscle dysfunction.[21]

the murmur of aortic stenosis

The murmur of aortic stenosis is heard during systole. Aortic stenosis is the result of narrowing of the aortic cusps. During ventricular systole, the pressure within the ventricle exceeds the pressure of the aorta and the blood flows out of the ventricle into the aorta. If there is thickening of the aortic cusps or narrowing of the aortic valve, the rapidly flowing blood passes through the constricted valve and causes turbulence of blood flow. The murmur is of medium pitch and has a rough or harsh sound. It is heard best over the aortic valve area, the second right intercostal space. The murmur of aortic stenosis is transmitted into the arteries of the neck, since the blood flow

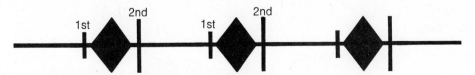

Fig. 10-38. Murmur of aortic stenosis.

responsible for the turbulence is moving in that direction. It can also be transmitted to the apex, where it may be confused with the murmur of mitral insufficiency—also a systolic murmur. The murmur of aortic stenosis occurs in systole, and it is a diamond shape. It is composed of a crescendo and a decrescendo[22,23] (Fig. 10-38, p. 183).

the murmur of aortic insufficiency

The murmur of aortic insufficiency is diastolic in time. In ventricular diastole, the intraventricular pressure is lower than the intra-aortic pressure. The aortic cusps fail to support the blood and it regurgitates into the ventricle. Turbulence of blood flow results in the formation of a high-pitched, blowing murmur. It is usually best heard in the third left intercostal space. As the pressure in the ventricle increases and the aortic pressure decreases, the turbulence of blood flow decreases. The murmur is therefore a decrescendo in shape[24,25] (Fig. 10-39).

Nurses need not distinguish the specific heart murmur; however, it is important for nurses to recognize the difference between the extra heart sounds and the murmurs. The key diagnostic sign of early congestive heart failure is the development of the third heart sound. Nurses can and should become adept at auscultating the heart. This knowledge and skill should be an integral part of the nursing assessment.

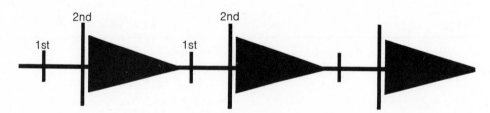

Fig. 10-39. Murmur of aortic insufficiency.

REFERENCES

1. Lawrence E. Meltzer, Faye G. Abdellah, and J. Roderick Kitchell, *Concepts and Practices of Intensive Care for Nurse Specialists* (Philadelphia: Charles Press Publishers, Inc., 1969), p. 52.
2. Abe Ravin, *Ausculatation of the Heart* (Chicago: Year Book Medical Publishers, Inc., 1967), pp. 15-17.
3. George E. Burch, *A Primer of Cardiology* (Philadelphia: Lea & Febiger, 1955), p. 97
4. Aubrey Leatham, "Auscultation of the Heart," *The Lancet* (Oct. 4, 1958), p. 703.
5. Burch, *op. cit.,* p. 98.
6. *Ibid.*
7. Leatham, *op. cit.,* pp. 703-704.
8. *Ibid.,* p. 49-52.

9. Leatham, *op. cit.*, pp. 704-706.
10. Ravin, *op. cit.*, pp. 80-83.
11. Burch, *op. cit.*, p. 108.
12. Ravin, *op. cit.*, pp. 64-67.
13. Ravin, *op. cit.*, pp. 64-68.
14. *Ibid.*, pp. 65-66.
15. *Ibid.*, pp. 84-87.
16. Burch, *op. cit.*, pp. 122-124.
17. Ravin, *op. cit.*, pp. 123-125.
18. Burch, *op, cit.*, pp. 125-127.
19. *Ibid.*, pp. 133-134.
20. Ravin, *op. cit.*, pp. 102-105.
21. *Ibid.*, p. 104.
22. *Ibid,* pp. 111-115.
23. Burch, *op. cit.*, pp. 138-140.
24. *Ibid.*, pp. 140-143.
25. Ravin, *op. cit.*, pp. 131-134.

BIBLIOGRAPHY

Burch, George E., *A Primer of Cardiology.* Philadelphia: Lea & Febiger, 1955.

Freeman, Ira M., *Physics: Principles and Insights.* New York: McGraw-Hill Book Company, 1973.

Harriston, T. R., et al., *Principles of Internal Medicine.* New York: McGraw-Hill Book Company, 1966.

Leatham, Aubrey, "Auscultation of the Heart," *The Lancet,* Oct. 4, 1958, pp. 703-708.

Marshall, Robert M., Gilbert Blount, and Edward Genton, "Acute Myocardial Infarction," *Archives of Internal Medicine,* Vol. 122 (December 1968), pp. 472-475.

Meltzer, Lawrence E., Faye G. Abdellah, and Roderick J. Kitchell, *Concepts and Practices of Intensive Care for Nurse Specialists.* Philadelphia: Charles Press Publishers, Inc., 1969.

central venous pressure

Central venous pressure refers to the pressure of blood in the right atrium or vena cava. It actually provides information about three parameters—blood volume, the effectiveness of the heart as a pump, and vascular tone. CVP is to be differentiated from a peripheral venous pressure, which may reflect only a local pressure.

Central venous pressure is measured in centimeters or millimeters of water pressure, and considerable variation exists in the range of normal values cited. Usually pressure in the right atrium is 0 to 4 cm. H_2O, while pressure in the vena cava is approximately 6 to 12 cm. H_2O. More important, it is the trend of the readings that is most significant regardless of the baseline value. The upward or downward trend of the central venous pressure, combined with clinical assessment of the patient, will determine appropriate interventions. For example, a patient's CVP may gradually rise from 6 cm.

H_2O to 8 cm. and then to 10 cm. While this may still be in the range of "normal," other parameters may indicate ensuing complications. Auscultation of breath sounds may reveal basilar rales, a third heart sound may be audible, or the pulse and respiratory rate may be increasing insidiously. In this context the trend of a gradual rise in CVP is more significant than the actual isolated value. When the nurse interprets CVP data in conjunction with her other clinical observations, she has a better understanding of their significance for that particular patient and recognizes the outcome to which her interventions must be geared. In this instance she is aware that too much fluid administration would further compromise the patient's circulatory status, and she would act accordingly to reduce this risk.

Sometimes rate of fluid administration is titrated according to the patient's CVP and urinary output. So long as the urinary output remains adequate and the CVP does not change significantly, this is an indication that the heart can accommodate the amount of fluid being administered. If the CVP begins to rise and the urine output drops, indicating a decreased cardiac output to perfuse the kidneys, circulatory overload must be suspected and either ruled out or validated in view of other clinical symptomatology.

The patient who is started on a vasopressor agent will show a rise in CVP due to the vasoconstriction produced. In this situation the blood volume is unchanged but the vascular bed has become smaller. Again, this change must be interpreted in conjunction with other information the nurse assesses about the patient. Alone a CVP value can be meaningless, but used in conjunction with other clinical data it is a valuable aid in managing and predicting the patient's clinical course.

For central venous pressure recordings a long intravenous catheter is inserted into an arm or a leg vein or the subclavian vein and threaded into position in the vena cava close to the right atrium. Occasionally the catheter may be advanced into the right atrium as indicated by rhythmic fluctuations in the pressure manometer corresponding to the patient's heartbeat. In this situation the catheter may simply be withdrawn to the point at which the pulsations cease.

Figure 10-40 illustrates a typical setup for measuring the central venous pressure. A manometer with a three-way stopcock is introduced between the fluid source and the patient's intravenous catheter. In this way three separate systems can be created by manipulating the stopcock. System 1 connects the fluid source with the patient and can be utilized for routine administration of IV fluids or as an avenue to keep the system patent. System 2 runs from the fluid source to the CVP manometer and is opened in order to raise the fluid column in the manometer prior to measuring the venous pressure. System 3 connects the patient's intravenous catheter with the manometer and it is this pathway which must be open to record the central venous pressure. Pressure in the vena cava displaces or equilibrates with the pressure exerted by the column of fluid in the manometer and the point at which the fluid level settles is recorded as the central venous pressure.

To obtain an accurate measurement, the patient should be flat, with the

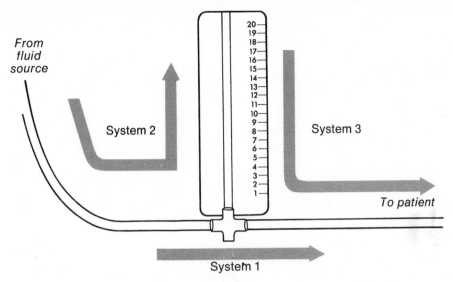

Fig. 10-40. Central venous pressure. (See text for description.)

zero point of the manometer at the same level as the right atrium. This level corresponds to the midaxillary line of the patient or can be determined by measuring approximately 5 cm. below the sternum. However, consistency is the important detail, and all readings should be taken with the patient in the same position and the zero point calculated in the same manner. If deviations from the routine procedure must be made, as when the patient cannot tolerate being flat and the reading must be taken with the patient in a semi-Fowler's position, it is valuable to note this on the patient's chart or care plan to provide for consistency in future readings. A patent system is assured when the fluid column falls freely and slight fluctuation of the fluid column is apparent. This fluctuation follows the patient's respiratory pattern and will fall on inspiration and rise on expiration due to changes in interpulmonic pressure. If the patient is being ventilated on a respirator, a false high reading will result. If possible, the respirator should be discontinued momentarily for maximum accuracy. If the patient cannot tolerate being off the respirator for even this short period, significant trends in the CVP can still be determined if consistency in taking the readings is followed.

As noted earlier, changes in central venous pressure must be interpreted in terms of the clinical picture of the patient. There are however, some situations which commonly produce an elevated CVP. These include congestive heart failure when the heart can no longer effectively handle the venous return, cardiac tamponade, a vasoconstrictive state, or states of increased blood volume such as overtransfusion or overhydration.

A low central venous pressure usually accompanies a hypovolemic state due to blood or fluid loss or drug-induced vasodilatation. Increasing the rate of fluid administration or replacing blood loss is indicated in this situation.

the significance of hemodynamic pressure monitoring

Pressure is a basic concept taught to nurses early in their education. Mathematically, pressure is defined as the product of flow and resistance. Pressure = Flow × Resistance. Initially performed by physicians, measuring blood pressure was delegated to nurses early in the 1930s. Now blood pressure is one of the "vital signs" routinely obtained, reported, and recorded by the nurse. The concept of pressure is a key parameter in patient assessment. For the critical care nurse to make important clinical decisions, the knowledge of pressure concepts must be incorporated into patient evaluation. The purpose of this section is to describe a current method of measuring heart and blood pressures; to discuss normal and abnormal hemodynamic pressures; and to assist the nurse in determining the physiological importance of these pressures.

method of measuring heart and blood pressures

Advances in medical technology have made it possible to measure pressures directly within the chambers of the heart and great vessels. This section will emphasize the necessary essentials and principles behind the method of direct pressure measurement.

Essential to direct measurement of hemodynamic pressures are catheters, a transducer, and a pressure module.

Essentials

A. *Catheters*

1. *Flow-Directed Catheter.* The development of the flow-directed (Swan-Ganz) catheter has made possible the measurement of pulmonary artery wedge (PAW) pressure at the bedside. This pressure is an index of left ventricular function. The catheter has two lumens, one for intravenous fluid to assure catheter patency and the second for the balloon (Fig. 10-41). At the tip of the radiopaque catheter is a balloon, which when inflated causes the tip of the catheter to become buoyant. If then advanced, the catheter will float in the direction of blood flow. Introduced into either a brachial or a femoral vein, it can be passed into the superior or inferior vena cava respectively. It then can be passed to the right atrium, through the tricuspid valve into the right ventricle, through the pulmonary valve into the pulmonary artery. And, if advanced further, the catheter will obstruct forward blood flow which allows *left* heart pressures to be reflected through the catheter tip. Because of the catheter size, it obstructs forward flow in a small pulmonary artery.

Right atrial (RA), right ventricular (RV), and pulmonary artery (PA)

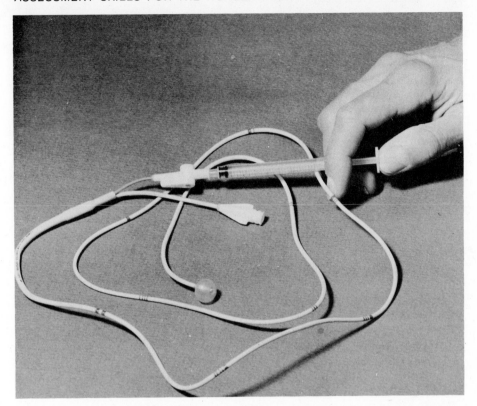

Fig. 10-41. Flow-directed catheter.

pressures give precise information on heart valve function and circulatory volume. The value of the flow-directed catheter lies in the fact that left ventricular function can be determined by inserting a catheter into the right side of the heart. This procedure has fewer risks and is simpler to perform than measuring left ventricular pressures directly.

2. *Arterial Catheter.* The ability to measure arterial pressures directly has been available for a longer time. A simple catheter inserted into an artery suffices. Directly measuring arterial pressure affords the nurse precise blood pressure readings and easy access to arterial blood samples. In addition, it saves the patient from numerous arterial punctures.

B. *Transducer.* The transducer is the second essential component for measuring pressure. It is an electrical device which converts one form of energy into another. Specifically, it senses mechanical energy—pressure— and converts it into electrical energy—the waveform. The pressures generated by myocardial contraction and relaxation are reflected through the lumen of the catheter to the transducer, where the pressure is converted to an electrical waveform. For the waveform to have meaning, two conditions must be met, a zeroing condition and a calibrating condition.

For accurate pressure measurement, the transducer must be placed at a standard level in relation to patient position — mid-chest suffices as a reference level. To meet the zeroing condition, the transducer must be set at an arbitrarily assigned zero value pressure. This can be done by opening the transducer to room air or atmospheric pressure (760 mm. Hg at sea level) and assigning that pressure zero value in mm. Hg (0 mm. Hg). The second necessary condition for the transducer is the calibrating condition. That is, the amplitude of the electrical signal (height of the waveform) must be assigned a value in millimeters of mercury pressure. The transducer is calibrated when a numerical value in mm. Hg pressure is assigned to each centimeter of waveform amplitude. For instance, 1 cm. = 4 mm. Hg or 1 cm. = 20 mm. Hg.

C. *Pressure Module.* The pressure module allows the transducer to be zeroed and calibrated, and allows the pressure waveform to be displayed on an oscilloscope or paper tracing. Different pressure modules and transducers require varying techniques for zeroing and calibrating. Though the technical procedure changes according to specific equipment, the principles for zeroing and calibrating are the same.

Preparation for Pressure Measurement

Prepare for pressure measurement by: (A) gathering supplies and (B) assembling supplies.

A. Gather supplies
   1. Intravenous fluid in a plastic bag
   2. Heparin (1 cc./1,000 units) and syringe
   3. Pressure bag
   4. IV tubing (15 gtt./cc.)
   5. Pressure valve (C.S.F. ®Intraflo, Continuous Flush System)*
   6. Three 3-way stopcocks (2 plain, 1 with Luer-lock)
   7. IV extension tubing
   8. Transducer
   9. Pressure module

B. Assemble supplies
   1. Heparinize the IV solution in the plastic bag by adding 1 unit of heparin per cc. IV fluid. Label solution.
   2. Connect the IV tubing to the IV solution in the plastic bag (Fig. 10-42).
   3. Place the IV solution bag in the pressure bag and inflate to 300 mm. Hg pressure.
   4. Connect the IV tubing to the IV port of the pressure valve.
   5. Connect the 3-way stopcock with Luer-lock to the pressure valve port which is at the same end as the IV port.
   6. Attach transducer to stopcock, Step 5.

---

* Sorenson Research Company, Salt Lake City, Utah.

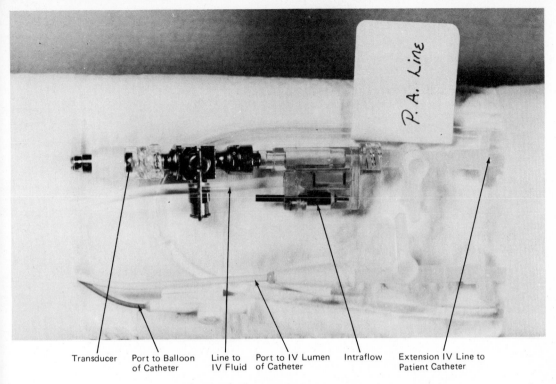

| Transducer | Port to Balloon of Catheter | Line to IV Fluid | Port to IV Lumen of Catheter | Intraflow | Extension IV Line to Patient Catheter |

Fig. 10-42. Arterial line set-up.

7. Fill dome of transducer with IV fluid (fluid without air bubbles must fill dome for accurate pressure measurement).
8. Attach a 3-way stopcock to the distal port of the pressure valve.
9. Connect IV extension tubing to the stopcock, Step 8.
10. Attach a 3-way stopcock to the other end of the IV extension tubing.
11. Flush the line with IV fluid and connect it to the patient's flow-directed or arterial catheter. The assembled set-up is shown in Fig. 10-43.

Pressure Measurement

Following are the steps for pressure measurement:
1. Flush line with IV fluid.
2. Open stopcock attached to transducer to room air.
   a. Zero transducer.
   b. Calibrate transducer.
3. Open stopcock attached to transducer to patient pressure.
4. Assess quality of waveform.
5. Measure and record pressures.

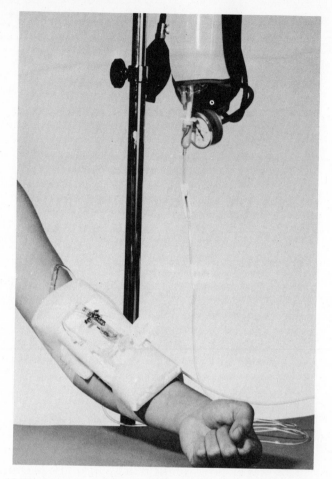

Fig. 10-43. Assembled set-up for monitoring hemodynamic pressures.

6. Flush line with IV fluid.
7. Adjust treatment according to pressure values.

normal pressure values

It is paramount for the critical care nurse to understand the physiological mechanisms producing normal pressure in order to knowledgeably care for the patient requiring invasive pressure monitoring. A systematic approach to waveform analysis is essential. One such approach is to:

1. Review the mechanical events of the heart and the normal pressures,
2. Learn the normal waveform characteristics, and

3. Correlate the electrical and mechanical events of the heart.
In the following section this approach will be employed to analyze normal pressure tracings. Under the subheading Waveform Interpretation, the mechanical events, waveform characteristics, and normal pressure values will be discussed. The correlation between electrical and mechanical events will be discussed under the subheading Comparison of Electrocardiogram with Waveform. The following abbreviations will be used throughout:

right atrial—RA
right ventricular—RV
right ventricular end diastolic pressure—RVEDP
pulmonary artery—PA
pulmonary artery diastolic—PAd
pulmonary artery wedge—PAW
left atrial—LA
left ventricular—LV
left ventricular end diastolic pressure—LVEDP
aortic—Ao
mean arterial pressure—MAP

Although the most frequently monitored pressures in the acute care setting are pulmonary artery, pulmonary artery wedge, and arterial, this section will discuss normal pressure values within all chambers of the heart and great vessels, emphasizing the process of waveform analysis.

right atrial pressure

Visualize the catheter tip in the right atrium. The pressure created during right atrial systole, contraction, is greater than during right atrial diastole, relaxation. During right atrial systole, the tricuspid valve will open when RA pressure exceeds RV pressure. When the RV contracts, the tricuspid valve will be closed. The pulmonary artery cusps will open when the RV pressure exceeds the pressure in the pulmonary artery.

An RA pressure tracing appears as shown in Fig. 10-44.

Waveform Interpretation The right atrial waveform has three positive waves: *a*, *c*, and *v*. The *a*-wave represents right atrial systole. The *v*-wave represents right atrial diastole. Following RA systole, the tricuspid valve closes, the RA is filling with blood, and the RV is beginning to contract. At this point, the pressure within the RA briefly increases because the force of RV contraction causes the tricuspid valve to balloon into the right atrium, producing the *c*-wave. Thus the *c*-wave is caused by the closed tricuspid valve's pushing into the right atrium during right atrial diastole. Sometimes the *c*-wave is superimposed on the *a*-wave and is not distinguishable, or it appears as a notch in the *a*-wave.

The right atrial pressure tracing has three negative waves or descents: *x*, *x'*, and *y*. The descents are of less significance and will be briefly mentioned here. The *x* descent follows the *a*-wave and represents right atrial relaxation. The *x'* descent follows the *c*-wave and represents atrioventricular movement during ventricular contraction. The *y* descent follows the *v*-wave and represents passive right atrial emptying immediately after opening of the tricuspid valve just before right atrial systole.

The right atrium is a low-pressure chamber; the significant right atrial pressure is the mean or midpoint between the systolic and diastolic pressures. Normal right atrial mean ($\overline{\text{RA}}$) pressure is < 6 mm. Hg.

Comparison of Electrocardiogram with Waveform   The electrical energy of the heart is demonstrated by the electrocardiogram; the mechanical energy is demonstrated by the pressure waveform. The electrical events precede and cause the mechanical events. On the ECG (Fig. 10-44), the P wave represents the discharge of electrical current from the sinoatrial node. Following electrical activation, the atria contract. In comparing the ECG and the pressure waveform, the P wave on the ECG precedes the *a*-wave, atrial systole, on the pressure tracing. The QRS complex represents ventricular depolarization, and it precedes ventricular systole. While the right ventricle is contracting, the right atrium is relaxing. Thus, on the ECG, the QRS complex will precede the *v*-wave on the RA pressure tracing. The *v*-wave frequently extends beyond the T wave which demonstrates ventricular repolarization on the ECG. If the *c*-wave is visible, it will occur between the *a*- and *v*-waves, and it will occur immediately after the QRS complex. Early in ventricular systole, the pressure within the ventricle pushes the closed tricuspid valve into the right atria causing a slight increase in RA pressure, demonstrated by the *c*-wave on the RA pressure tracing.

right ventricular pressure

Again, visualize the flow-directed catheter in the right atrium. By inflating the balloon at the tip of the catheter, the catheter tip will become buoyant. The catheter will tend to float in the direction of blood flow. If it is advanced, the slack in the line will allow the catheter to float through the open tricuspid valve into the ventricle. At this point, Fig. 10-45 shows how the right ventricular waveform would be seen on the oscilloscope.

Waveform Interpretation   In order to identify the specific mechanical events causing the RV waveform configuration, arbitrary letters *a* through *e* have been assigned to simplify the discussion. The initial rapid rise in the right ventricular waveform represents isovolumetric contraction, *a*. That is, the tricuspid and pulmonary valves are closed, and the volume of blood within the RV remains constant while the pressure increases. When RV pressure exceeds PA pressure, the pulmonary valve opens, *b*. Blood is then ejected from the RV into the pulmonary artery. Maximum RV systolic pressure is presented by point *c* on the waveform. The pulmonary valve closes, and the RV pressure rapidly decreases. The tricuspid valve opens, and the RV passively fills with blood from the right atrium. Point *d* represents right atrial contraction, with *e* representing right ventricular end diastole. Note that the right ventricular pressure waveform goes below baseline. It is generally characteristic of both right and left ventricular waveforms to return to or to go below baseline. Significant right ventricular pressures are systolic and end diastolic. Right ventricular systolic pressure is < 30 mm. Hg and end diastolic pressure is < 5 mm. Hg.

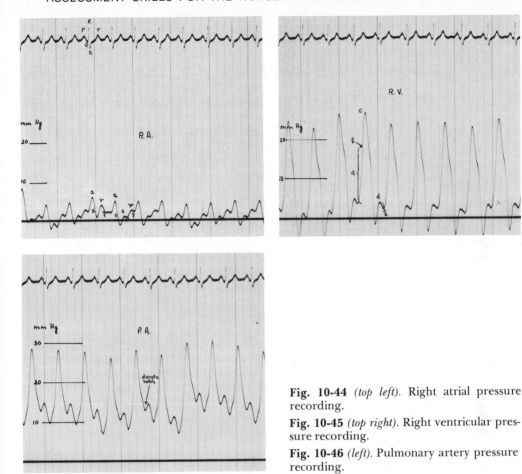

Fig. 10-44 *(top left)*. Right atrial pressure recording.

Fig. 10-45 *(top right)*. Right ventricular pressure recording.

Fig. 10-46 *(left)*. Pulmonary artery pressure recording.

Comparison of Electrocardiogram with Waveform   The P wave on the electrocardiogram generally precedes two positive deflections on the RV waveform. Following electrical activation of the atrium (P wave), the tricuspid valve opens, and the RV passively fills with blood, causing an increase in RV diastolic pressure. The second positive deflection is caused when the atrium contracts, *d,* emptying the RA more completely which increases RV diastolic pressure. Ventricular depolarization demonstrated by the QRS complex on the ECG precedes ventricular contraction causing a rapid increase in the RV pressure wave. Following the electrical event of ventricular depolarization, the mechanical event of isovolumetric contraction occurs. During ventricular repolarization (T wave on the ECG), maximum ejection, reduced ejection, pulmonic valve closure, and rapid decrease in pressure occur.

Sometimes a slight increase in pressure can be seen following reduced ejection on the downward slope of the right ventricular tracing. Immediately after closure of the pulmonic valve, the pressure in the right ventricle increases slightly as the column of blood behind the closed valve pushes toward the ventricular chamber.

pulmonary artery pressure

To float the catheter from the right ventricle into the pulmonary artery, the balloon is inflated and the catheter is advanced. The PA pressure tracing is as shown in Fig. 10-46 (p. 195).

Waveform Interpretation   The rapid rise in the pulmonary artery waveform represents right ventricular ejection. The dicrotic notch in the downward slope corresponds with pulmonary valve closure. Note that the PA waveform always has a positive pressure; at no time does the pressure wave fall to zero or reach baseline. Normal pulmonary artery pressures are systolic < 30 mm. Hg, diastolic < 10 mm. Hg, and mean < 20 mm. Hg.

Under normal conditions, the mean pulmonary artery ($\overline{\text{PA}}$) pressure will be closer to diastolic pressure than to systolic pressure. This pressure is not a true mathematical mean because systolic pressure is sustained approximately one third of the cardiac cycle, whereas, diastole lasts about two thirds of the cycle. The diastolic pressure, therefore, contributes more in determining the $\overline{\text{PA}}$. As heart rate increases, systole changes little, but diastole is shortened; likewise, as heart rate slows, systole changes minimally, but diastole is prolonged. Thus, as heart rate increases, diastole contributes less to the mean value, whereas, as heart rate decreases, diastolic pressure contributes more to the mean pressure value.

Comparison of Electrocardiogram with Waveform   Immediately after ventricular depolarization (QRS complex) ventricular ejection occurs. As the ventricle contracts, blood is ejected into the pulmonary artery causing the rapid rise in pulmonary artery pressure. Maximum PA pressure is reached during ventricular repolarization (T wave). Closure of the pulmonary valve, dicrotic notch, corresponds with the end of ventricular repolarization.

pulmonary artery wedge pressure

A flow-directed catheter in the pulmonary artery can be wedged in the pulmonary capillary bed by advancing the catheter or by inflating the balloon (Fig. 10-47). When forward blood flow is prevented, the catheter is wedged. The pulmonary artery wedge (PAW) pressure reflects left heart pressures. That is, it reflects left atrial mean and left ventricular end diastolic pressure. When the catheter is advanced from the PA to the PAW position, the waveform configuration will change as shown in Fig. 10-48.

Waveform Interpretation   The pulmonary artery wedge tracing has an *a*-wave and a *v*-wave. The *a*-wave reflects left atrial contraction and, in addition, left ventricular relaxation. The *v*-wave reflects left atrial relaxation and left ventricular contraction. Mean pulmonary artery wedge pressure is < 12 mm. Hg.

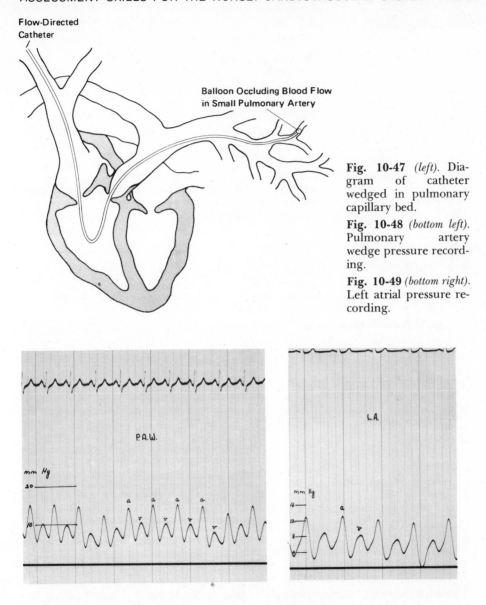

Flow-Directed
Catheter

Balloon Occluding Blood Flow
in Small Pulmonary Artery

Fig. 10-47 *(left)*. Diagram of catheter wedged in pulmonary capillary bed.

Fig. 10-48 *(bottom left)*. Pulmonary artery wedge pressure recording.

Fig. 10-49 *(bottom right)*. Left atrial pressure recording.

Comparison of Electrocardiogram with Waveform   The ·P wave on the ECG will precede the *a*-wave on the PAW tracing. On the ECG, the QRS complex will precede the *v*-wave of the pressure recording. Note that the QRS precedes both the *a*-wave and the *v*-wave because of delay in pulmonary artery wedge pressure transmission (Fig. 10-48).

left atrial pressure

The left atrial pressure is rarely measured in the critical care setting. It is, however, measured in the cardiac catheterization laboratory. A special catheter, one which can be passed transseptally from the right atrium to the left atrium, is used. The left atrial pressure is shown in Fig. 10-49 (p. 197).

Waveform Interpretation   The LA pressure tracing has the same characteristics as the PAW pressure tracing. It has an *a*-wave and a *v*-wave. The *a*-wave corresponds with left atrial contraction, whereas, the *v*-wave corresponds with left atrial relaxation. A *c*-wave is not generally seen on an LA pressure tracing; however, it may be seen as the *c*-wave on the RA pressure tracing. Left atrial mean (LA) pressure is < 12 mm. Hg.

Comparison of Electrocardiogram with Waveform   The P wave precedes the *a*-wave since the electrical events precede and cause the mechanical events; likewise, the QRS complex precedes the *v*-wave.

left ventricular pressure

The configuration of the left ventricular pressure waveform is comparable to that of the right ventricular waveform. The significant difference is the pressure which each ventricle can generate. A left ventricular pressure tracing appears as shown in Fig. 10-50.

Waveform Interpretation   Again, arbitrary letters have been assigned to various points in the waveform for ease of discussion. Interval *a* represents left ventricular isovolumetric contraction. As the pressure within the left ventricle exceeds the pressure in the aorta, the aortic valve is forced open, point *b*. Maximum ejection pressure is shown by *c*. The point at which the aortic valve closes, *d*, is followed by a rapid decrease in LV pressure. Opening of the mitral valve, *e*, allows passive left ventricular filling; and *f* demonstrates the increases in LV pressure because of LA contraction. Point *g* represents left ventricular end diastolic pressure.

Left ventricular end diastolic pressure is an indication of left ventricular function. It is not customary to measure LV pressures directly; therefore, the flow-directed catheter is used. The value of this catheter lies in the following relationships (≈ means "is approximately equal to"):

$$\text{PAd} \approx \overline{\text{PAW}}$$
$$\overline{\text{PAW}} \approx \overline{\text{LA}}$$
$$\overline{\text{LA}} \approx \text{LVEDP}$$

The normal, significant left ventricular pressures are systolic < 140 mm. Hg and end diastolic < 12 mm. Hg.

Comparison of Electrocardiogram with Waveform   Following atrial depolarization, P wave, the mitral valve opens causing a slight increase in pressure, *e* on the pressure recording. Left atrial contraction, *f*, causes a second positive wave during ventricular diastole. The QRS complex precedes the systolic component of the left ventricular waveform. As the ventricles repolarize, maximum LV pressure, *c*, is attained. The dicrotic notch represents aortic valve closure, *d*, and occurs at the end of repolarization.

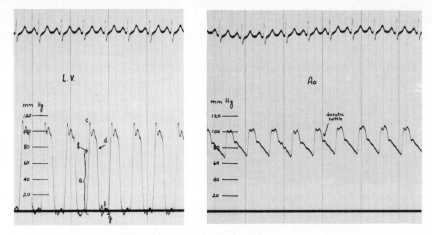

Fig. 10-50 (*left*). Left ventricular pressure recording.
Fig. 10-51 (*right*). Aortic pressure recording.

arterial wave pressure

Radial or femoral arteries are common sites for arterial lines. The arterial pressure waveform has the same configuration as that of the pulmonary artery. The primary difference is that the systemic arteries support greater pressures than the pulmonary artery.

Waveform Interpretation When LV systolic pressure exceeds aortic pressure, the aortic valve opens. On the arterial pressure tracing, this is the point at which the pressure rapidly rises. On the LV pressure tracing, it is point *b*, the end of isovolumetric contraction. The rapid rise in arterial pressure occurs after LV ejection. An arterial line measuring pressure within the aorta will have a systolic pressure rise at the time of ventricular contraction; however, a line measuring radial artery pressure will have a delayed pressure rise because the artery is more distal to the left ventricle. Even though the line is in a distal artery, the dicrotic notch which indicates aortic valve closure can generally be seen (Fig. 10-51). Arterial pressures are systolic < 140 mm. Hg, diastolic < 90 mm. Hg, and mean 70-90 mm. Hg.

Comparison of Electrocardiogram with Waveform The rapid rise in arterial pressure follows electrical depolarization of the ventricles, QRS complex. The more distal the artery is to the left ventricle, the greater the delay in systolic pressure rise. For instance, the time interval between the QRS complex and a radial artery pressure waveform will be greater than between the QRS complex and an aortic pressure tracing. The dicrotic notch occurs at the end of ventricular repolarization, T wave.

abnormal pressure values

Before proceeding, the importance of understanding the normal mechanisms of hemodynamic pressures will be emphasized. In the previous discussion of normal pressures, the following components and pressures were identified as important:

CHAMBER OR VESSEL	SIGNIFICANT COMPONENTS OF WAVEFORM	SIGNIFICANT PRESSURE
RA	*a*-wave	$\overline{\text{RA}}$ (<6 mm. Hg)
	c-wave	
	v-wave	
RV	systole	RV systole (<30 mm. Hg)
	end diastole	RV end diastole (<5 mm. Hg)
PA	systole	PA systole (<30 mm. Hg)
	diastole	PA diastole (<10 mm. Hg)
		$\overline{\text{PA}}$ (<20 mm. Hg)
PAW	*a*-wave	$\overline{\text{PAW}}$ (<12 mm. Hg)
	v-wave	
LA	*a*-wave	$\overline{\text{LA}}$ (<12 mm. Hg)
	v-wave	
LV	systole	LV systole (<140 mm. Hg)
	end diastole	LV end diastole (<12 mm. Hg)
Ao	systole	systole (<140 mm. Hg)
	diastole	diastole (<90 mm. Hg)
		$\overline{\text{Ao}}$ or MAP (70–90 mm. Hg)

The nurse who has a working knowledge of the normal hemodynamic pressures will be able to identify and interpret the abnormal pressures. She is at ease with the systematic approach to waveform analysis. Feeling confident with her knowledge, she automatically considers:
 1. The mechanical events of the heart and the normal pressures,
 2. The characteristics of each waveform, and
 3. The correlation between the electrical and mechanical events of the heart.
It then follows that the nurse can learn to:
 1. Identify the abnormal component(s),
 2. Identify the mechanical events which cause and which affect the abnormal portion of the waveform,
 3. Enumerate the possible physiological reasons,
 4. Review the goals of treatment, and
 5. Evaluate the effectiveness of treatment.
It is not within the realm of this section to address steps 4 and 5 but they are mentioned here because they, too, are necessary steps for the nurse to take in

order to assure sound clinical decisions. Steps 1 through 3 outline the approach used in this section to analyze abnormal hemodynamic pressures. Under the subheadings, the components of each waveform will be discussed. The process for determining abnormal pressures will be emphasized.

right atrial waveform abnormalities

Normal $\overline{RA}$ pressure is < 6 mm. Hg. Mean right atrial pressure is equivalent to central venous pressure. A catheter in the right atrium reflects systemic venous pressure; in addition, it reflects pressures beyond the right atrial chamber. Problems which affect systemic venous resistance, pulmonary vascular resistance, tricuspid or pulmonary valves, or myocardial contraction or relaxation will be reflected by changes in $\overline{RA}$ pressure. Both increased vascular tone and hypervolemia elevate systemic venous pressure and, likewise, increase $\overline{RA}$ pressure, whereas, loss of systemic venous tone and hypovolemia would decrease $\overline{RA}$ pressure. Pulmonary vascular resistance is increased in pulmonary hypertension, and as the right ventricle fails, the $\overline{RA}$ pressure would increase. Valvular problems, notably tricuspid stenosis and tricuspid insufficiency, elevate $\overline{RA}$ pressure. Problems which affect the ability of the myocardium to contract and relax include right heart failure, constrictive pericarditis, and pericardial tamponade, all of which elevate $\overline{RA}$ pressure.

a-**Wave Changes**   On a right atrial pressure tracing, the *a*-wave represents right atrial contraction and follows the P wave when compared to the electrocardiogram. The electrical impulse which causes atrial depolarization, the P wave on the ECG, initiates atrial contraction. In cardiac arrhythmias such as atrial fibrillation and junctional rhythms, there are no P waves, no organized atrial contraction, and, therefore, no *a*-wave on a right atrial tracing.

When the right atrium must generate increased systolic pressure in order to eject blood into the right ventricle, the *a*-wave would be elevated. In tricuspid stenosis, the right atrioventricular valve is narrowed, and the right atrium must contract with greater force to squeeze blood through the stenotic opening. Conditions beyond the right atrial chamber which cause increased pressure will be reflected in an elevated *a*-wave. For instance, right ventricular hypertrophy causes the right ventricle to contract with greater force which, in turn, causes the right atrial *a*-wave to have a higher pressure than normal. Such conditions include pulmonary stenosis and pulmonary hypertension.

Pathological conditions which cause changes in myocardial tissue itself or prevent the heart muscle from relaxing completely would elevate the ventricular filling pressure, and thus cause the *a*-wave to be elevated. When fibrotic changes occur in the myocardium, as in constrictive pericarditis, the elevated right ventricular diastolic pressure would be reflected in the RA pressure tracing by an elevated *a*-wave.

Cardiac tamponade occurs when fluid collects under pressure in the cardiac sac between the visceral and parietal pericardium. With fluid filling this space, the heart muscle is restricted and prevented from filling normally.

Fluid compressing the myocardium during ventricular diastole causes an elevated *a*-wave on the RA pressure tracing. Severe cases of both constrictive pericarditis and pericardial tamponade cause pressure changes in all chambers of the heart. These two conditions elevate RA, LA, RVED, and LVED pressures.

v-**Wave Changes**   The *v*-wave on a right atrial pressure tracing corresponds with right atrial filling and right ventricular systole. It occurs after the T wave and precedes the P wave when compared to the electrocardiogram. On a right atrial tracing, the *v*-wave will be elevated in conditions which cause an increase in right atrial filling pressure. For example, in tricuspid insufficiency, the tricuspid valve is incompetent. The valve remains open, when, under normal conditions, it should be closed. With the tricuspid valve open during right ventricular contraction, blood regurgitates from the RV into the RA causing an increased *v*-wave.

c-**Wave Changes**   A normal variant of the RA pressure tracing can demonstrate the absence of a *c*-wave or a *c*-wave superimposed on the *a*-wave. Since the *c*-wave occurs because of the ballooning of the closed tricuspid valve into the RA during RV contraction, it is not seen in the pressure tracing of a patient with tricuspid insufficiency. No *c*-wave is seen because the valve leaflets do not close and cannot bulge into the RA causing a slight pressure increase.

right ventricular waveform abnormalities

Normal significant RV pressures are systolic < 30 mm. Hg and end diastolic < 5 mm. Hg. Abnormal RV pressures are seen in right ventricular failure, pulmonary stenosis, pulmonary insufficiency, and pulmonary hypertension. Eventually, untreated left ventricular failure would cause right ventricular pressures to be elevated; however, other signs and symptoms would be obvious to the nurse before the RV pressures become elevated.

Right Ventricular Systolic Changes   Right ventricular systolic pressures would be elevated in conditions which require greater force to eject the blood. For example, in pulmonary stenosis the RV must generate enough pressure to overcome the resistance caused by the narrowed pulmonary valve. Pulmonary hypertension is a common cause of elevated right ventricular systolic pressure and usually occurs because of LV failure.

Right Ventricular End Diastolic Changes   Under normal conditions the pulmonary valve is closed during right ventricular diastole. The right ventricle fills with blood only from the RA, and the RV end diastolic pressure is < 5 mm. Hg. When the pulmonary valve is incompetent, blood regurgitates through the opened pulmonary cusps from the PA into the right ventricle. In severe cases of pulmonary insufficiency, the additional blood volume because of regurgitant flow causes an elevated right ventricular end diastolic pressure.

Right Ventricular Systolic and End Diastolic Changes   Initially, in right ventricular failure the RV tracing would show a decreased systolic and an increased end diastolic pressure. As the failure increases, systolic pressure would decrease, the body's compensatory mechanisms would fail, and cardiac output would decline. Thus, the RV systolic pressure may be low or within normal limits, but the end diastolic pressure would remain elevated, indicating decreased right ventricular output because of reduced ventricular contractile force. In this situation, a larger volume of blood remains in the ventricle at the end of diastole.

Pulmonary hypertension elevates the right ventricular systolic and end diastolic pressures. The more severe the pulmonary hypertension, the greater the RV pressures. Eventually the right ventricle fails, at which point the pressures vary according to the pressure changes seen in right ventricular failure.

pulmonary artery waveform abnormalities

Normal pulmonary artery pressure values are systolic < 30 mm. Hg, diastolic < 10 mm. Hg, and mean < 20 mm. Hg. The pulmonary artery diastolic (PAd) pressure is an approximation of the mean pulmonary artery wedge (PAW) pressure which reflects mean left atrial (LA) pressure which indicates left ventricular function. For this reason, the PAd is the most significant pulmonary artery pressure. The exception occurs in pulmonary hypertension which causes elevated pulmonary artery systolic, diastolic, and mean pressures but a normal pulmonary artery wedge pressure. Pulmonary artery pressures are elevated in pulmonary vascular disease, mitral stenosis, and left ventricular failure.

Pulmonary Artery Diastolic Changes In the absence of pulmonary vascular disease, pulmonary artery diastolic pressures accurately reflect pressures in the left chambers of the heart. Conditions which require increased left atrial systolic pressures increase pulmonary artery pressure values. For example, the left atrial systolic, *a*-wave, pressure would be elevated if the mitral valve was narrowed. This increase in LA *a*-wave pressure would be reflected in the pulmonary system. The pulmonary artery diastolic pressure would be abnormally high because the LA must contract with greater force to eject the blood through the stenotic mitral valve. Thus, in mitral stenosis, the PAd pressure would be elevated. In the presence of mitral stenosis, a simultaneous PA and LV pressure tracing would demonstrate a pressure difference between the PAd and the LVEDP. Recall the following:

$$PAd \approx \overline{PAW}$$
$$\overline{PAW} \approx \overline{LA}$$
$$\overline{LA} \approx LVEDP$$

Normally, all of these pressures do not vary more than 1 to 3 mm. Hg. When the difference among these pressures is > 1 to 3 mm. Hg, pathology exists.

Pulmonary Artery Systolic and Diastolic Changes Left ventricular failure is reflected in the PA tracing by an elevation of all pressures. Early in left ventricular failure, the loss of LV compliance causes the LVEDP to be elevated. The heart rate increases in an attempt to compensate for the decreased force of left ventricular contraction. With the increase in heart rate, diastole is shortened and there is less time for ventricular filling. With decreased ventricular filling time and loss of compliance, the blood volume ejected from the LV is less, and cardiac output falls. Left ventricular systolic pressure decreases as the LV compliance decreases. Concurrently, the LVEDP increases because of the increased blood volume remaining in the ventricle. This cycle is reflected in the PA, and eventually causes the PA pressures to be elevated.

pulmonary artery wedge abnormalities

Pulmonary artery wedge pressure is < 12 mm. Hg. It reflects left ventricular function. The catheter is wedged in the pulmonary capillary bed, pressures from the right heart are blocked, and only pressures forward to the catheter are sensed. Pulmonary artery wedge pressures are elevated in mitral stenosis, mitral insufficiency, and left ventricular failure. When aortic stenosis and aortic insufficiency are severe, the elevated left ventricular pressures are also reflected in the PAW tracing.

a-**Wave Changes**   The *a*-wave of the PAW tracing corresponds with left atrial systole, and will therefore be elevated in conditions which elevate left atrial systolic pressure. Left atrial systolic pressure is elevated in mitral stenosis. This increase in LA systolic pressure will cause the *a*-wave of the PAW pressure to be elevated.

v-**Wave Changes**   The *v*-wave on the PAW pressure tracing reflects left atrial filling and left ventricular contraction. Conditions which cause the LA diastolic pressure to be elevated will cause the PAW *v*-wave to be elevated. In mitral regurgitation, the LA diastolic pressure is increased because of blood regurgitation from the LV, through the incompetent mitral leaflets. This additional volume of blood in the LA during LA relaxation elevates the *v*-wave on the PAW tracing.

a-**Wave and** *v*-**Wave Changes**   Both *a*-waves and *v*-waves will be elevated on the PAW tracing in left ventricular failure. The myocardium loses elasticity, compliance, and its ability to contract. In early left ventricular failure, the LVEDP is elevated. The heart rate increases to compensate for the decreased force of contraction. Diastole is shortened, less blood is ejected, more blood remains in the ventricle, and the LVEDP increases. An elevated *a*-wave on the PAW tracing reflects this increase in pressure. The *v*-wave pressure would likewise decrease, reflecting the decrease in left ventricular pressure. The PAW pressure is elevated since it is an approximation of the left ventricular end diastolic pressure.

The abnormal pressures discussed heretofore are pressures with which the critical care nurse will become familiar. These pressure abnormalities were discussed in detail so that the nurse will have the understanding necessary to make sound clinical judgments in caring for the patients who require invasive monitoring. The following abnormal pressure tracings are ones commonly seen in the cardiac catheterization laboratory rather than the acute care setting.

left atrial waveform abnormalities

Mean left atrial pressure is < 12 mm. Hg. The *a*-waves and *v*-waves of the LA pressure tracing are elevated in the same pathological conditions which cause the PAW waveforms to be elevated. Since they are elevated for the same reasons that were previously discussed, the rationale will not be reiterated.

left ventricular and aortic waveform abnormalities

The left ventricular and aortic pressures will be discussed together since most frequently the pressures are measured simultaneously. Normal left ventricular pressures are systolic < 140 mm. Hg and end diastolic < 12 mm. Hg. Normal aortic pressures are systolic < 140 mm. Hg, diastolic < 90 mm. Hg, and mean 70 to 90 mm. Hg. Left ventricular and aortic systolic pressures are equal. Differences between these pressures indicate a gradient across the aortic valve and demonstrate pathology. The diagnosis of aortic valvular problems is made by a composite patient examination which includes palpation, auscultation, phonocardiogram, and catheterization.

left ventricular and aortic systolic pressure differences

In the presence of aortic stenosis, the left ventricle must contract with greater force to overcome resistance caused by the narrowed orifice. Left ventricular systolic pressure would be elevated; however, aortic systolic pressure would be within normal limits. The millimeters of mercury pressure difference between these two systolic values demonstrates the pressure gradient across the aortic valve. As the degree of stenosis increases, the left ventricle would require increasing pressure in order to eject blood out the aortic valve and maintain cardiac output. A simultaneous LV and Ao pressure tracing would demonstrate: (1) systolic pressure differences between the left ventricle and aorta, and (2) a slowly rising initial aortic systolic upstroke. The obstructed aortic valve prevents the normal rapid ejection of blood from the left ventricle into the aorta causing the delayed pressure rise. Study the pressure tracing shown in Fig. 10-52.

left ventricular and aortic diastolic pressure changes

In aortic insufficiency, blood regurgitates from the aorta into the left ventricle during diastole, which elevates the LVEDP. As the aortic valve deteriorates, the aortic diastolic pressure decreases, which increases the pulse pressure. The characteristics of aortic insufficiency on a simultaneous LV and Ao pressure tracing are the following: (1) an elevated LVEDP, (2) a pulse pressure < 100 mm. Hg, and (3) no dicrotic notch on the aortic pressure waveform. Since the dicrotic notch is caused by aortic valve closure which does not occur in aortic regurgitation, no dicrotic notch is seen. Study the pressure tracing shown in Fig. 10-53.

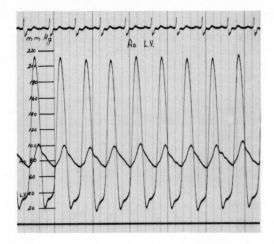

Fig. 10-52. Simultaneous aortic and left ventricular pressure recordings from patient with aortic stenosis.

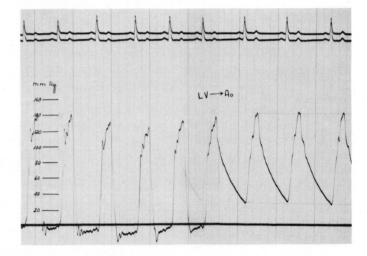

Fig. 10-53. Left ventricular pressure recording with catheter pull-back to aorta in patient with aortic insufficiency. Note that the LVEDP is not elevated in this patient at rest.

nonphysiological waveform changes

When changes occur in waveform configurations, one way to identify the problem is to consider possible causes. Begin by checking with the patient to ascertain if the problem is with the hardware. Affirming no patient change in status, start the equipment check; i.e.: Are the electrical plugs secure in the outlet? Is the power on? Finding no problem, proceed to the transducer. The transducer needs to be covered with fluid; air cannot be in the dome of the transducer. All connections must be secure. Stopcocks connecting lines must be turned correctly to (1) zero and calibrate the transducer, (2) measure patient pressures, and (3) aspirate blood samples. Continue the problem identification search until the cause is found. Then proceed with the problem-solving process.

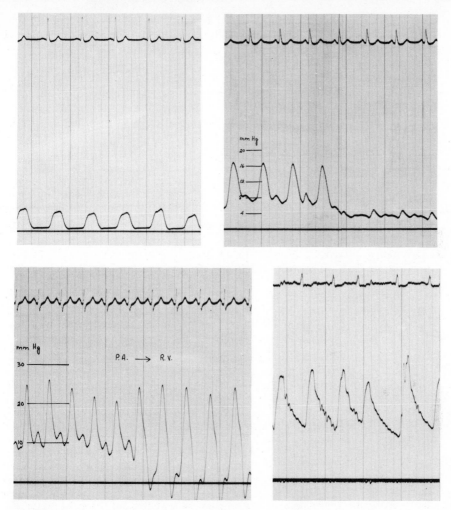

Fig. 10-54 *(top left)*. Damped pressure waveform.

Fig. 10-55 *(top right)*. Pulmonary artery and pulmonary artery wedge pressure recording.

Fig. 10-56 *(bottom left)*. Pulmonary artery pressure recording with catheter pull-back to right ventricle.

Fig. 10-57 *(bottom right)*. Aortic pressure recording demonstrating catheter fling.

A waveform which becomes flattened is said to be damped. Figure 10-54 shows a damped waveform.

Damped waveforms occur when there is air in the fluid line, when IV flow rate decreases and blood stasis occurs, when a fibrin clot is at the catheter tip, or when the catheter adheres to the vessel wall. A damped waveform indicates that air needs to be evacuated from the line, the line needs to be flushed with heparinized saline, or the line tip needs to be rotated or moved slightly. To flush the line, use the pressure valve or a bolus of 10 cc. heparinized saline.

The flow-directed catheter can become wedged in the pulmonary capillary bed by (1) inflating the balloon or (2) advancing the catheter into the pulmonary artery. When the catheter goes from the PA into the PAW position, the waveform on the oscilloscope will change and appear as shown in Fig. 10-55 (p. 207).

Noting a tracing such as in Fig. 10-55 or seeing a PAW waveform on the oscilloscope, the nurse would first consider that the catheter balloon may be inflated and second, that the catheter tip may have floated into the wedge position. Pulmonary infarction has occurred when the flow-directed catheter was unintentionally in the wedge position. Because of this danger, the catheter balloon must be deflated and/or the catheter must be withdrawn into the PA immediately.

Occasionally, the Swan-Ganz catheter floats from the PA to the RV. The pattern on the oscilloscope would change from the PA to the RV waveform as shown in Fig. 10-56 (p. 207).

To correct this situation, inflate the balloon with air and allow the catheter to float from the RV into the PA.

The pressure tracing shown in Fig. 10-57 (p. 207) demonstrates catheter fling.

Catheter fling is caused when the catheter can move laterally in the vessel. It produces spiked waves, distorting the waveform configuration and pressure values. To remedy the problem, add IV extension tubing between the patient line and the pressure valve.

nursing considerations

The Nurse-Patient Relationship   The nurse who desires to care for the patient requiring hemodynamic pressure monitoring must know normal physiology, normal pressure values, the reasons for abnormal pressures, and problem-solving procedures. It is essential for the nurse to be at ease with the technical and theoretical components of invasive monitoring in order to work with each patient as an individual and to establish a therapeutic nurse-patient relationship. Nurses have the responsibility to create an environment in which the patient is free to ask questions, express concerns, participate in patient care and decision making, and relate to family and friends. Some patients requiring invasive monitoring are severely weakened by their cardiac problem, whereas others are stronger and more troubled by the activity restriction imposed because of the lines. These patients have individual concerns, but they also have common concerns and potential problems which the nurse can alleviate, prevent, or correct.

Patient fear and anxiety are allayed by the nurse who is confident in her knowledge, skill, and problem-solving abilities. This nurse is free to listen to the patient's fears and concerns and to watch for nonverbal cues which need to be clarified. A caring attitude includes an explanation of the routines and reasons for them. Family members should be included in this education process. Both patient and family members need to realize that the nurse cares for the patient as a whole individual and that the technical equipment assists the nurse in monitoring parameters necessary for optimal care.

Prevention of Problems Patients need instruction to exercise the extremities where the lines are inserted. Exercising the fingers and toes and contracting and relaxing arm and leg muscles will promote circulation in the extremity. Most patients requiring invasive monitoring have compromised circulation. Inactivity further adds to this problem. Patients unable to exercise extremities need to have routine passive exercises done for them.

The presence of a catheter in a vessel increases the likelihood of inflammation leading to the development of phlebitis. The catheter site should be looked at several times daily for early signs of inflammation, i.e., tenderness, changes in local temperature, redness, and swelling. The dressing should be changed every eight hours; the insertion site is cleansed with soap and water, and antiseptic ointment, sponges, and tape are applied in a secure but comfortable manner. The previously pictured method for securing the lines and transducers on a short armboard recommended for patient safety and nurse convenience is shown again in Fig. 10-58.

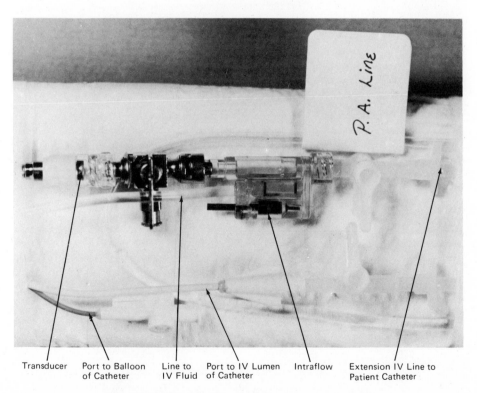

| Transducer | Port to Balloon of Catheter | Line to IV Fluid | Port to IV Lumen of Catheter | Intraflow | Extension IV Line to Patient Catheter |

Fig. 10-58. Pressure lines mounted on armboard.

Individuals confined to bed rest for several days need to consciously take slow, deep breaths, using their abdominal muscles. Reminding the patient to breathe in this manner 10 times an hour while awake will expand the alveoli and prevent atelectasis. Although when pressures are recorded the patient is generally in the supine position, he/she should be encouraged to rest on either side between pressure readings.

closure

Pressure is an essential concept for the critical care nurse to understand because it affects all body systems. Along with basic knowledge of the body systems, the critical care nurse must possess a questioning mind and a caring spirit. An inquisitive nurse will formulate her questions in a methodical, scientific manner, seek answers, and find new questions. The analytical approach to patient care fosters improved patient care. The critical care nurse is well named because a caring spirit makes the nurse's efforts complete by combining the science and art of nursing intervention.

MARGARET ANN BERRY, R.N., M.A., M.S.

11

normal structure and function of the respiratory system

All reactions in higher living organisms which release energy to the overall system are combustion reactions. That is, the reaction requires oxygen in some step along the way to eventually break down certain chemical compounds to give energy, carbon dioxide, and water. Organisms living in an aquatic environment extract oxygen from the water, while other organisms, including humans, must have some method of removing oxygen from the air and transporting it to the cells where it is used. At the same time carbon dioxide, an end product of the combustion reactions, must be transported back to the atmosphere. Humans have the ability to store energy compounds but must have a constant source of oxygen to maintain life. Perhaps the most basic of all human needs is the need for air, and one of the most critical subsystems of the organism is the respiratory system. Because of the respiratory system's dependency upon the cardiovascular system, the latter also occupies a position of extreme critical importance. At times it is most difficult to establish priorities between these two subsystems, and it is probably more accurate to consider them as being equally critical to the dynamic stability of the human organism.

Respiration means literally the movement of oxygen from the atmosphere to the cells and the return of carbon dioxide from the cells to the environment. As such, then, the total process can be divided into four major phases.

1. Pulmonary ventilation—actual flow of air in and out between the atmosphere and the alveoli of the lung.

211

2. Diffusion of oxygen and carbon dioxide between the alveoli and the blood.
3. Transport of oxygen and carbon dioxide in the blood and body fluids to and from the cells.
4. Regulation of ventilation by control mechanisms of the body with regard to rate, rhythm, and depth.

functional anatomy of the respiratory system

The basic components of the respiratory system are the nose and the nasal cavity, the mouth and the pharyngeal cavity, the nasopharynx, the trachea, the primary and secondary bronchi, the bronchioles, the alveolar ducts, the alveoli, and the functional respiratory membrane in the alveolar sac. For further detail it is recommended that the reader review the anatomical characteristics of these various structures by using standard textbooks and audiovisual materials.

mechanics of respiration

The downward and upward movement of the diaphragm, which lengthens and shortens the chest cavity, combined with the elevation and depression of the ribs, which increases and decreases the anteroposterior diameter of the cavity, causes the expansion and contraction of the lungs. It is estimated that about 70 percent of the expansion and contraction of the lungs is accomplished by the change in anteroposterior measurement and about 30 percent by the change in length due to movement of the diaphragm.

respiratory pressures

The lungs—two air-filled spongy structures—are attached to the body only at their hila and thus the outer surfaces have no attachment. However, the membrane lining the interpleural space constantly absorbs fluid or gas which enters this area creating a partial vacuum. This phenomenon holds the visceral pleura of the lungs tightly against the parietal pleura of the chest wall. As the volume of the chest cavity is increased by the muscles of inspiration, the lungs also enlarge; as it is decreased during expiration, they likewise become smaller. The two pleurae slide over one another with each inspiration and expiration, lubricated by the few millimeters of tissue fluid containing proteins in the intrapleural space.

Because of the foregoing reasons, with each normal inspiration the pressure within the alveolar sacs, the intra-alveolar pressure, becomes slightly negative (−3 mm. Hg) with regard to the atmosphere. This slightly negative pressure sucks air into the alveolar sacs through the respiratory passage.

During normal expiration and resultant compression of the lungs, the intra-alveolar pressure builds to about +3 mm. Hg and forces air out of the respiratory passages. During maximum respiratory efforts, the intra-alveolar pressure can vary from −80 mm. Hg during inspiration to +100 mm. Hg during expiration.

The lungs continually tend to collapse. Two factors are responsible for this phenomenon. First of all there are many elastic fibers contained within the lung tissue itself which are constantly attempting to shorten. The second and more important factor contributing to this tendency to collapse is the high surface tension of the fluid lining the alveoli. A lipoprotein substance call "surfactant" is constantly secreted by the epithelial alveolar lining which decreases the surface tension of the fluids of the respiratory passages seven- to fourteenfold. The absence of the ability to secrete surfactant in the newborn is called *hyaline membrane disease* or *respiratory distress syndrome.*

No single factor or phenomenon is responsible for the body's ability to maintain inflated functional lungs; rather it is the combination of all of these factors.

compliance of the lungs and thorax

As can be seen from the preceding discussion, both the lungs and the thorax itself have elastic characteristics and thus exhibit expansibility. This expansibility is called *compliance,* and is expressed as the volume increase in the lung for each unit increase in intra-alveolar pressure. Normal total pulmonary compliance, i.e., both lungs and thorax, is 0.13 liter per centimeter of water pressure. Or every time alveolar pressure is increased by an amount necessary to raise a column of water one centimeter in height, the lungs expand 130 ml. in volume.

Conditions or situations which destroy lung tissue, cause it to become fibrotic, produce pulmonary edema, block alveoli, or in any way impede lung expansion and expansibility of the thoracic cage reduce pulmonary compliance and decrease the efficiency of meeting the need for oxygen to carry on the necessary functional activities of the total organism.

It is extremely important to emphasize that when the lungs are expanded and contracted through the action of the respiratory muscles, energy is required for the muscular activity involved.

In addition to this "work," energy is also required to overcome two other factors which tend to prevent expansion of the lungs. They are (1) nonelastic tissue resistance, and (2) airway resistance, meaning that energy is required to rearrange the large molecules of viscous tissues of the lung itself so that they slip past one another during respiratory movements. In the presence of tissue edema, the lungs lose much of their elastic qualities, and increased viscosity of the tissues and fluids increases the nonelastic resistance. Thus the "work" of breathing is increased and the energy expended to accomplish the task is also greatly increased.

Under normal conditions the airway resistance is low and the amount of energy required to move air along the passages is only slight. When the airway becomes obstructed, such as in obstructive emphysema, asthma, or diphtheria, then airway resistance is greatly increased and the energy required simply to move air in and out is greatly increased.

pulmonary volumes and capacities

The preceding sections have discussed the factors that contribute to pulmonary ventilation, but have said nothing about the volume of air moved with each respiratory cycle. Under certain conditions such as exercise or forced expiration or inspiration, the actual volume of air will vary and the events of pulmonary ventilation become difficult to describe. Consequently, to facilitate the discussion of the events of pulmonary ventilation, the air in the lung has been defined in terms of four volumes and capacities.

The four respiratory volumes when added together result in the maximum volume to which the lung can be expanded. There is a difference between males and females in all pulmonary volumes and capacities. They are approximately 20 to 25 percent lower in females. Obviously, general body size and the amount of physical development also affect these measurements.

The volume of air moved in and out with each normal respiration is called *tidal volume* and is about 500 ml. in normal young males. If the individual forces inspiration over and beyond tidal volume, it amounts to about 3,000 ml. and is called the *inspiratory reserve volume.* Conversely, the *expiratory reserve volume* is the volume of a forced expiration following the normal tidal expiration and amounts to about 1,100 ml. The *residual volume* is the volume of air remaining following forced expiration. This volume can only be measured by indirect spirometry while the others can be measured directly.

When one studies the actual moment-to-moment events of the pulmonary cycle, it is sometimes more convenient to consider some volumes in combination with others. These various combinations are known as the *four pulmonary capacities.* The first we will consider is the *inspiratory capacity*, which is equal to the tidal volume plus the inspiratory reserve volume. This is about 3,500 ml. and is that amount of air which, when starting from normal expiratory level, the individual can forcibly inspire. The second capacity, the *functional residual capacity*, is the sum of the expiratory reserve volume and the residual volume. It is the amount of air remaining in the lungs at the end of normal expiration, about 2,300 ml.

The *vital capacity* is the summation of the inspiratory reserve volume, the tidal volume and the expiratory reserve volume. Stated another way, it is the maximum amount of air that can be forcibly expired following a forced maximal inspiration. This volume is about 4,500 ml. in a normal male.

Last is *total lung capacity.* This is equal to the volume to which the lungs can be expanded with greatest inspiratory effort. The volume of the capacity is about 5,800 ml.

Two major factors determine the amounts of the above-mentioned volumes: *body size* and *position when measured.* Collectively, the various volumes and capacities give a picture of respiratory efficiency and pulmonary compliance.

A very important factor of respiratory function is the rate of alveolar air renewed with each cycle, or *alveolar ventilation.* Obviously, per minute alveolar ventilation is less than the minute respiratory volume (tidal volume × respiratory rate) because a large amount of the air inspired goes to fill respiratory passages whose membranes are essentially incapable of gaseous exchange with the blood. This dead-space volume is about 150 ml. in young adult males and is affected by activity and the physiological state of the individual. In normal individuals it is all the space except the alveoli. In individuals with nonfunctional alveoli, abnormal pulmonary ventilation, or abnormal pulmonary circulation, the dead space increases and pulmonary efficiency is reduced.

About 2,300 ml. of air remains in the lung at the end of expiration. With each new breath about 350 ml. of new air is brought into the alveoli and mixed with the volume remaining from the last cycle, thus only about one seventh of the total volume. The normal alveolar ventilation rate is about 4,300 ml. per minute. At this rate the alveolar gases are replaced by new air about every 23 seconds. The slow turnover rate prevents rapid fluctuations in concentration in the alveoli with each breath.

diffusion of gases through the pulmonary membrane

The pulmonary membrane in humans is made up of all the surfaces in the respiratory wall that are thin enough to permit the exchange of gases between the lungs and the blood. The total area of this membrane in the average normal adult male is about 60 square meters, or about the size of a moderate-sized classroom. It is 0.2 to 0.4 micron thick, or less than the thickness of the average red blood cell. These two outstanding features combine to allow large quantities of gases to diffuse across the pulmonary membrane in a very short period of time.

The air that is taken into the respiratory passages is a mixture of primarily nitrogen and oxygen (99.5 percent) and a small amount of carbon dioxide and water vapor (0.5 percent). The molecules of the various gases behave as in solution and exhibit Brownian movement. Thus a mixture of gases such as air has all molecular species evenly distributed throughout the given volume. Because of this constant molecular bombardment the volume of gases exerts pressure against the walls of the container. This pressure can be defined as the force with which a gas or mixture of gases attempts to move from the confines of the present environment. Therefore each of the components of a mixture such as air will account for part of the total pressure of the entire mixture. Consequently, if we take 100 volumes of air and place them in a container under 1 atmosphere of pressure (760 mm. Hg), by analysis we would find that nitrogen makes up 79 of the 100 volumes and oxygen makes up 21 volumes, or 79 and 21 percent concentration respectively.

Both these gases are contained at 760 mm. Hg pressure in this container. If we now take the same volume of nitrogen and move it to a container of the same volume and allow to expand until it completely fills all of the volume (100 percent) we will observe that the pressure in the second con-

tainer drops from 760 to 600 mm. Hg. If we do the same thing with the 21
volumes of oxygen and allow them to expand to 100 percent of the volume,
we observe that the pressure in the third container drops from 760 to 160
mm. Hg. We conclude then that in the original container the *part* of the
total pressure due to nitrogen was 600 mm. Hg and the *part* due to oxygen
was 160 mm. Hg. This pressure of nitrogen is called the *partial pressure* of
nitrogen (P_{N_2}) and that of oxygen the *partial pressure* of oxygen (P_{O_2}). The
partial pressure of a gas in a given volume is the force it exerts against the
walls of the container. If the walls of the container are permeable, like the
pulmonary membrane, then the penetrating or diffusing power of a gas is
directly proportional to its partial pressure.

It is extremely important to point out that atmospheric air differs from
alveolar air in partial pressures of the components. The comparative concentrations of each are as follows:

GAS	ATMOSPHERIC AIR, PERCENT	ALVEOLAR AIR, PERCENT
N_2	78.62	74.90
O_2	20.84	13.60
CO_2	0.04	5.30
H_2	0.50	6.20
	100.00	100.00

The difference between atmospheric air and alveolar air is in the increased
concentration of carbon dioxide and water in alveolar air. The reasons for
these differences are twofold. First, the air is humidified as it is inspired by
the moisture of the epithelial lining of the respiratory tract. At normal body
temperature water vapor has a partial pressure of 47 mm. Hg and mixes
with and dilutes the other gases, decreasing their partial pressures.

Second, molecules in a given volume of gas behave like molecules in a
solution and diffuse from an area of high concentration to one of lower
concentration.

The factors that govern the rate of diffusion of the gases through the pulmonary membrane are as follows. First, the greater the pressure difference
on either side of the membrane the faster the rate of diffusion. Second, the
larger the area of the pulmonary membrane the larger the quantity of gas
that can diffuse across the membrane in a given period of time. The thinner
the membrane the more rapidly do gases diffuse through it to the compartment on the opposite side. Finally, the diffusion coefficient is directly proportional to the solubility of the gas in the fluid of the pulmonary membrane
and inversely proportional to molecular size. Therefore, small molecules

that are highly soluble diffuse more rapidly than do large molecular gases that are less soluble. The diffusion coefficients are as follows:

Oxygen	1
Carbon dioxide	20.3
Nitrogen	0.53

These three gases are very similar to each other with regard to molecular size but have quite different solubilities in the fluids of the pulmonary membrane. It is these differences that account for the difference in the rate of diffusion of the gases through the pulmonary membrane.

transport of oxygen and carbon dioxide through the tissues

As oxygen diffuses from the lungs to the blood, a small portion of it becomes dissolved in the plasma and cell fluids but more than 60 times as much combines immediately with hemoglobin and is carried to the tissues. Here the oxygen is used by the cells, and carbon dioxide is formed. As the carbon dioxide diffuses into the interstitial fluids, about 5 percent is dissolved in the blood and the remainder diffuses into the red blood cells where one of two things occurs: (1) carbon dioxide either combines with water to form carbonic acid and then reacts with the acid base buffer and is transported as the bicarbonate ion, or (2) a small portion of the carbon dioxide combines with hemoglobin at a different bonding site than oxygen and is transported as carbaminohemoglobin.

Nitrogen diffuses from the alveolus into the blood, but because there is no carrier mechanism and under standard conditions nitrogen has only slight solubility in tissue fluid, it quickly establishes an equilibrium state on either side of the membrane and thus is essentially inert.

The relative partial pressure (mm. Hg) in the various compartments is as summarized below.

GAS	ATMOSPHERIC AIR	ALVEOLAR AIR	VENOUS BLOOD	ARTERIAL BLOOD
P_{O_2}	159	104	40	100
P_{CO_2}	0.15	40	45	40
P_{N_2}	597	569	569	569

It can readily be seen that concentration gradients are established that then foster the diffusion of these gases in the direction which is physiologically advantageous. Figure 11-1 summarizes the events of gaseous diffusion through pulmonary membrane and transport to and from the tissues.

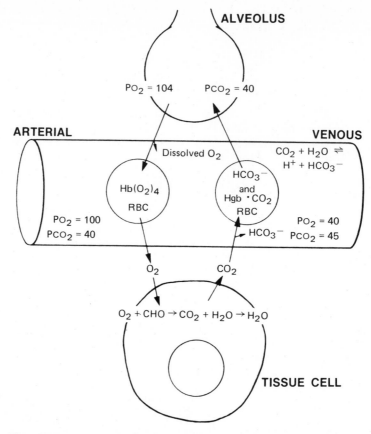

Fig. 11-1. Gaseous diffusion through pulmonary membrane in respiration.

regulation of respiration

The basic rhythm of respiration is controlled by the interaction of inspiratory and expiratory neurons of the respiratory center in the brain stem. This center receives stimuli from spinal cord, cortical, and midbrain areas of the brain and from the vagus and glossopharyngeal nerves which cause reflex excitation or depression of the respiratory center. It sends motor impulses to the spinal cord and nerves that serve the muscles of respiration and via the phrenic nerve—a special nerve innervating the diaphragm. Located throughout the lung tissue itself are many nerve endings which when the lungs are distended send inhibitory impulses via the vagus nerve to the inspiratory neurons of the respiratory center. This response to lung distention is called the *Hering-Breuer reflex.* Its function is to prevent overinflation and aid the respiratory center in maintaining the basic rhythm of respiration.

Regardless of the continuity of the basic respiratory rhythm, the rate and depth of respiration vary tremendously in response to physiological demands in the body. Four factors serve to affect the rate and depth of respiration: carbon dioxide concentrations, hydrogen-ion concentration, oxygen concentration, and exercise.

The most powerful stimulus for the respiratory center is the carbon dioxide content of the blood and tissue fluids of the body. When the carbon dioxide level rises above normal, both inspiratory and expiratory neurons are stimulated and thus both rate and depth of respiration are increased. Approximately one half of the effect of carbon dioxide on respiration is due to its direct effect on the respiratory neurons themselves. The other half is due to the indirect effect of carbon dioxide in the cerebrospinal fluid. As carbon dioxide diffuses into the cerebrospinal fluid, it combines with water to form carbonic acid which then dissociates to hydrogen and bicarbonate ions. This familiar reaction is represented by the following equation:

$$CO_2 + H_2O \rightleftarrows H_2CO_3 \rightleftarrows H^+ + HCO_3^-$$

The increased hydrogen-ion concentration directly stimulates the neurons of the respiratory center as the fluid bathes the sides of the brain stem.

The respiratory system's response to carbon dioxide concentrations is extremely important because it is the main pathway for regulating carbon dioxide levels in body fluids. Should carbon dioxide accumulate in the tissues and fluids of the body, all chemical reactions of the body are essentially inhibited. If the carbon dioxide level drops too low, alkalosis develops which is also incompatible with life.

Hydrogen-ion concentration, as implied in the previous section, is the second most powerful influence on alveolar ventilation. In the equation showing carbon dioxide combining with water in body fluids, it is noted that the reactions are reversible. Therefore, if there is an accumulation of hydrogen-ion concentration (a low pH tending toward acidemia), the center neurons respond, increasing the rate of respiration, which drives the reaction to the left and lowers the hydrogen-ion concentration. If the hydrogen-ion concentration is low (high pH tending toward alkalemia) alveolar ventilation is depressed and the reaction is driven to the right. This response of the respiratory system in conjunction with the kidneys to a large extent controls the acid-base balance of the body.

Although normally hemoglobin is almost completely saturated with oxygen, the body does have chemoreceptors located in the carotid bodies in the neck and in the aortic arch which monitor blood oxygen levels. These receptors are sensitive to oxygen diffusion, and the respiratory center is stimulated via the vagus and glossopharyngeal nerves. The chemoreceptor mechanism is not as powerful a respiratory stimulus as either carbon dioxide or hydrogen-ion concentration.

The rate and depth of respiration are directly proportional to the amount of work done during exercise. It is not the chemical factors that appear to cause increased rate and depth of respiration during exercise, except secondarily. The primary cause of increased respiration during exercise is the simultaneous stimulation (by the cerebral cortex) of the muscle exercised and of the sensory pathway from the cord that stimulates the respiratory center.

JOSEPH O. BROUGHTON, M.D.

pathophysiology of the respiratory system

A broad definition of the function of the respiratory system is (1) to provide adequate oxygenation to all body tissues, and (2) to eliminate excess CO_2 gas produced by the tissues. Performance of these functions requires not only normally functioning lungs and thorax, but also a normally functioning medullary respiratory center and cardiovascular system, normally functioning aortic and carotid chemoreceptors, and a normal amount of functioning hemoglobin. Malfunction of any of these components can cause respiratory failure—inadequate oxygenation of the tissues, inadequate elimination of CO_2 gas, or both. Since hypoxemia and hypercapnia are the essence of respiratory failure, they deserve special attention.

Normal function of the lungs and thorax may be impaired by various disease processes. These pulmonary diseases are often placed in two main categories: (1) airway obstructions, and (2) restrictive defects. The obstructive diseases seen most commonly are chronic bronchitis, asthma, and emphysema. Frequent subjection to irritants, allergens, and infections can cause gradual but definite tissue changes. In chronic bronchitis and asthma the airways may be obstructed by mucosal edema, increased mucus in the lumen, and presumably by spasms of the muscle encircling the bronchi and bronchioles. In chronic bronchitis there may also be an increased number of mucus glands, and in emphysema there may be loss of support for the walls of the airways so that they collapse rapidly on expiration, like a wet straw.

Rarer causes of airway obstructions are aspirated foreign bodies (most often in children), bronchial or tracheal stenosis from scarring (often from a previous tracheostomy), intrabronchial tumors, occasionally silicosis, tuberculosis, and other granulomatous diseases and sometimes the frothy, bubbly secretions of severe pulmonary edema. Upper-airway obstruction from large tonsils and adenoids has on occasion been the cause of respiratory failure in children.

On pulmonary function tests, obstructive diseases are manifested by slowing of expiratory flow ratio; i.e., reduced FEV_1, FEV/VC ratio of less than 75 percent, and reduced FEF 25-75 percent (MMEF). If severe, obstructive diseases usually cause hypoxemia and hypercapnia.

Although many conditions can cause restrictive pulmonary problems, obstructive problems are more common. Restrictive refers to any situation which makes it difficult to expand the lungs. Diffuse interstitial pulmonary fibrosis, either idiopathic or associated with sarcoid, causes fibrosis inside the lung. The stiffness or noncompliance of the tissue restricts lung expansion. Fibrosis outside the lung as in pleural thickening or fibrosis can also make it difficult to expand the lungs, and is therefore a restrictive process.

Abdominal distention and/or abdominal pain can limit movement of the diaphragm, thereby restricting lung expansion. Failure of the left ventricle results in pulmonary vascular congestion, another restrictive process. Skeletal abnormalities such as kyphoscoliosis and ankylosing spondylitis as well as neuromuscular disorders such as Guillain-Barré syndrome also restrict chest expansion.

On pulmonary function tests, restrictive problems are reflected by low vital capacity and reductions in all other lung volumes. They do not often cause blood gas abnormalities unless they are associated with another abnormality; i.e., diffusion (gas transport) problems. When restriction to lung expansion is caused by interstitial fibrosis, there is usually interference with transport of oxygen from the alveoli into the bloodstream, and this is reflected by a low Po_2. If the diffusion problem is severe, there may be hypoxemia at rest but if the condition is mild or moderate, the Po_2 at rest is usually normal and exercise is required to demonstrate the hypoxemia. With exercise, blood flows through the lung faster than at rest, so blood may not remain in the pulmonary capillaries long enough to pick up oxygen if the oxygen is delayed in getting into the capillaries because of a diffusion problem.

Pulmonary edema is another cause of diffusion problems. It may take longer for oxygen to diffuse from the alveoli through alveolar edema, through the interstitial edema and into the capillary. In other conditions such as emphysema there may be a diffusion abnormality because of a lack of alveoli and/or pulmonary capillaries, thus less opportunity for gas transport.

If the Po_2 is normal, 97 percent of the oxygen-carrying capacity of hemoglobin is used. Even though the Po_2 may rise as high as five times normal when a person breathes 100 percent oxygen, the hemoglobin can carry only 3 percent more oxygen.

There are certain disease states in which the hemoglobin is abnormal and carries either more or less oxygen for a given Po_2 than does normal hemoglobin. When a certain type of hemoglobin carries less oxygen than normal at a given Po_2, it is the same as having the oxyhemoglobin dissociation curve shifted to the right.

When hemoglobin does not carry its full amount of oxygen, it assumes a blue or dark color. Generally cyanosis is recognized when there are 5 gm. or more of hemoglobin that is not saturated with oxygen. (Occasionally because of hypoxemia the body may make too many red blood cells [RBC] and too much hemoglobin.) When there is more than the usual amount of hemoglobin and when the circulation moves the RBC slowly, more unsaturated hemoglobin is present, so that cyanosis is more apparent. Sometimes, then, cyanosis may be present—particularly in the extremities—when the arterial oxygen concentration is normal, if there is an excess of hemoglobin or reduction in blood flow. Much more common is the opposite situation in which arterial oxygen concentration is low but no cyanosis is recognizable. If one relies on cyanosis to diagnose significant hypoxemia, many instances of hypoxemia will be missed completely and others will be discovered late. Cyanosis is especially hard to diagnose in anemic patients. In spite of the unreliability of cyanosis as an early indicator of hypoxia, many nevertheless continue to rely on the absence of cyanosis to indicate adequate oxygenation, to the detriment of the patient. Hypoxia may be caused by hypoventilation, diffusion problems, living at high altitudes, right-to-left shunts, and ventilation/perfusion mismatching.

Conditions which cause just hypoxemia may be even less obvious than those associated with hypoxemia and hypercapnia. A pulmonary embolus may cause or intensify hypoxemia. Other causes of chest pain, such as fractured ribs, may cause decreased expansion of part of the lung and lead to hypoxemia. Probably the most common cause of hypoxemia is ventilation/perfusion inequality ($\dot{V}/\dot{Q}$ problems) or more simply stated, mismatching of ventilation and perfusion. If any area of the lung is underventilated, for instance, because its bronchus is partially obstructed by a mucus plug with that part of the lung still receiving its normal blood supply, then there is relatively too little ventilation for the amount of perfusion (blood flow); this situation might be represented as $\dot{v}/\dot{Q}$ as compared to the normal $\dot{V}/\dot{Q}$. The blood to this part of the lung does not have the opportunity to pick up its full quota of oxygen because of the reduction in ventilation. If the bronchus to an area of the lung were completely obstructed yet with the perfusion remaining normal, it would represent a right-to-left shunt; i.e., unsaturated venous blood would flow from the right ventricle through the lungs without picking up any oxygen, would mix with blood from other parts of the lungs, and would then be pumped by the left ventricle into the systemic circulation.

Incidentally, just the opposite type of $\dot{V}/\dot{Q}$ problem may occur yet may not cause hypoxemia. For instance, the pulmonary artery to part of the lung might be occluded but the ventilation to that part of the lung might be maintained and there would therefore be excessive ventilation in respect to perfusion, which could be represented as $\dot{V}/q$. This is called *wasted ventilation*. This condition does not necessarily cause serious problems but is often associated with excessive work of breathing.

Usually the lung reflexly reduces ventilation to match reduced perfusion, and vice versa. However, in some disease states these reflex changes do not occur. For instance, in patients who have severe pathology in the upper abdomen such as pancreatitis, or who have just undergone gastric surgery or cholecystectomy, pain or tight bandages may prevent the diaphragm from descending normally with inspiration, thereby reducing ventilation in the lung bases. Sometimes the chest x-ray shows atelectasis or sometimes just a high diaphragm, but underventilation may occur without noticeable x-ray changes. If perfusion remains normal, some blood flows through under-ventilated bases without becoming oxygenated, so that the systemic arterial blood shows hypoxemia. As mentioned above, this type of reduced ventila-tion in relation to perfusion in some lung areas can occur in many different diseases and is probably the most common cause of hypoxemia. It occurs in many ill patients who would not be expected to have respiratory failure — patients with shock, GI bleeding, heart failure — in fact, in almost any patient sick enough to be in the ICU or CCU.

Diffusion problems usually occur with interstitial lung disease such as diffuse interstitial pulmonary fibrosis and metastatic carcinoma spreading through the lymphatics of the lung in the interstitial spaces (between alveoli). Diffusion problems also may occur in pulmonary edema in which edema fluid is found in the interstitial space, and often in the alveoli as well. With diffusion problems the Po_2 may be normal at rest, but with exercise the Po_2 falls; in more severe diffusion problems the Po_2 may be low even at rest. Generally the patient with a diffusion problem hyperventilates in an effort to move adequate amounts of oxygen from the alveoli through the widened interstitial space into the capillary blood. As a result of this hyperventilation, the Pco_2 is lowered. Usually in diffusion problems there is no difficulty in getting air through the airways. In severe pulmonary edema, however, because of the frothy, bubbly secretions occluding the airways, there may be enough obstruc-tion to airflow to cause a rise in Pco_2. In summary, diffusion problems show hypoxemia first only with exercise and later even at rest. The hyperventila-tion necessary to keep Po_2 up causes a low Pco_2. Only in severe problems such as severe pulmonary edema is the Pco_2 elevated.

Living at high altitudes, even with normal ventilation, is associated with hypoxemia because the inspired oxygen concentration is low. The hypoxemia usually leads to hyperventilation in an effort by the body to raise the Po_2, and the hyperventilation causes a low Pco_2. For instance, the normal Pco_2 in Denver is 36 mm. Hg as compared to the normal at sea level of 40 mm. Hg.

Right-to-left shunts which may occur with ventricular septal defects, for example, are associated with hypoxemia because part of the blood from the right heart which is destined to be oxygenated in the lungs bypasses the lungs and is shunted directly into the systemic arterial circulation. The result-ing systemic arterial hypoxemia may lead to hyperventilation and therefore low Pco_2. Occasionally right-to-left shunting occurs through abnormal vas-cular channels in the lung.

Hypoventilation from any cause leads to hypoxemia *and hypercapnia.* The hypoventilation is most frequently associated with airway obstruction such as emphysema or chronic bronchitis, or even the obstruction due to the frothy secretions which occur in severe pulmonary edema. Hypoventilation also may occur with a variety of neurological problems such as myasthenia gravis, Guillain-Barré syndrome, and polio. Hypoventilation may occur with some head injuries or with oversedation. Rarely hypoventilation may be caused by restrictive pulmonary problems such as large pleural effusion, immobile chest with ankylosing spondylitis, and so forth.

The hypoventilation that occurs with airway obstruction may be due to retained secretions, airway narrowing due to edema or swelling of the mucosal lining, bronchospasm, or airway collapse. Increase in secretions is due to increase in output of the goblet cells and submucosal glands. The submucosal glands are stimulated to produce mucus by the vagus nerve and local irritants in the tracheobronchial tree; the goblet cells are stimulated to produce mucus mainly by local irritants.

In many diseases of the respiratory tract such as asthma and bronchitis there is edema of the mucosal lining. Treating bronchospasm without treating the associated mucosal edema is treating only half of the problem, so we should usually combine an inhaled vasoconstrictor with an inhaled bronchodilator. In conditions such as emphysema there is often a rapid collapse of the trachea and bronchi during expiration which causes airway obstruction during expiration.

Hypoxemia caused by hypoventilation is accompanied by hypercapnia, but hypoxemia due to any of the other causes is usually associated with hyperventilation and therefore low P_{CO_2}.

Therefore when hypoxemia is associated with a high P_{CO_2} it generally means that hypoxemia is due to hypoventilation. When hypoxemia is associated with a low or normal P_{CO_2} it may be caused by diffusion problems, $\dot{V}/\dot{Q}$ mismatching, right-to-left shunting, or living at high altitude. The latter is obvious. Diffusion problems usually respond by a return of arterial oxygen concentrations to normal with low-to-moderate amounts of supplemental oxygen, while $\dot{V}/\dot{Q}$ mismatching and shunts usually require high levels of O_2 to bring the arterial oxygen concentrations to normal, and even then the arterial oxygen sometimes does not return to normal.

Hypercapnia (also called *hypercarbia*) is easier to explain. It always means alveolar hypoventilation. The most common causes of hypoventilation are mentioned above. Hypoventilation (and therefore hypercapnia) of limited degree may also be due to compensation of nonrespiratory alkalosis. With more significant hypoventilation, however, there is hypoxemia which is a strong stimulus to ventilation. This hypoxemia, then, increases ventilation and therefore prevents severe hypoventilation from occurring in compensation for nonrespiratory alkalosis.

There is only one cause of hypercapnia—hypoventilation. There are several causes of hypoxemia, one of which is hypoventilation. Therefore hypercapnia is a better reflector of hypoventilation than hypoxemia.

The work of breathing is often increased in diseases in which the lungs fail, and this increased work of breathing may be due to reduced compliance, increased airway resistance, or both. Reduced compliance occurs in restrictive conditions such as diffuse interstitial pulmonary fibrosis or conditions in which there is reduced surfactant—adult and newborn respiratory distress syndromes. Increased airway resistance occurs with anything that causes airway obstruction as listed above. In both increased airway resistance and reduced compliance, increased pressure is required to deliver a normal tidal volume. This is easily recognized in patients on ventilators. Increased airway resistance is noted by an initial high pressure which then falls to a lower level, and increase in compliance is noted by a sustained high pressure.

respiratory failure

Arbitrary values for defining when respiratory failure is present have been proposed. Respiratory failure is said to be present when the P_{O_2} falls below 50 mm. Hg (O_2 saturation below 85 percent) or when P_{CO_2} rises above 50 mm. Hg. Numbers, though, are not the perfect way to diagnose a complicated situation like respiratory failure. Some persons are in mild respiratory failure even before the P_{O_2} falls below 50 mm. Hg or before the P_{CO_2} rises above 50 mm. Hg. Others who have increased P_{CO_2} and/or decreased P_{O_2} are in a stable state, often still working, because they have adapted to the abnormal blood gases. In spite of these exceptions, *blood gases* are by far the best means of detecting respiratory failure.

It is easy to understand how respiratory failure occurs in one of the airway obstructive deseases—i.e., emphysema, chronic bronchitis, or asthma. A very important fact is that these diseases account for fewer than half of the cases of respiratory failure that occur in a general hospital.

It is most important to be able to diagnose respiratory failure at an early stage when treatment is most likely to be successful. Even more desirable is the recognition of *impending* respiratory failure. This can be accomplished by (1) knowing the setting in which respiratory failure is most likely to occur, (2) being aware that there are many nonspecific signs and symptoms which are indicators of early or impending respiratory failure, and (3) being inquisitive enough to obtain *arterial blood gases* when the question of respiratory failure enters your mind. (See the discussion of blood gases in Chapter 14.)

settings

Drugs such as sedatives, tranquilizers, sleeping pills, or analgesics—and rarely, alcohol—may cause depression of respiratory drive and may allow the P_{CO_2} to rise significantly while the patient is under the influence of the drug. Once the effect of the drug is gone, the remaining elevation of P_{CO_2} is often enough to cause continuing respiratory depression. It is important to remember that a small rise in P_{CO_2} is a large stimulus to breathing, but that larger rises in P_{CO_2} can cause depression of the respiratory center resulting in hypoventilation. Other brain functions may also be depressed. If the P_{CO_2} is already elevated enough to cause respiratory depression, the carotid chemoreceptors may sense hypoxemia and respond to this last remaining stimulus to breathing. If oxygen is administered because the patient is cyanotic or appears to have labored breathing, the final stimulus to respiration, hypoxemia, may be removed, causing the patient to have even less ventilation. Such a patient who has respiratory center depression due to drugs, a significantly elevated P_{CO_2}, or both, when given enough O_2 to reduce his respiratory drive may no longer appear cyanotic and as he ventilates less he may no longer appear to be laboring to breathe. In fact, he may become quieter and go to sleep. It is extremely important to recognize the set of circumstances mentioned above, for it happens daily in chronic airway obstruction patients in hospitals across the country. Usually if low flows (2 to 3 liters per minute) of oxygen or low percentages (24 to 28 percent) of oxygen are given—just enough O_2 to raise P_{O_2} to 60 mm. Hg—the hypoxic ventilatory drive will not be significantly reduced.

Often respiratory failure is misdiagnosed as congestive heart failure, as a stroke, or as "pneumonia occurring in a patient with a lousy personality." Usually the personality improves as the pneumonia clears, yet the diagnosis of respiratory failure was never made.

The patient who is semiconscious and flaccid in all extremities may be said to have a "stroke" when in reality there is no localizing finding of a cerebral thrombosis or hemorrhage, and instead hypoxia and hypercapnia cause the impaired consciousness and impaired motor function. Unless someone has a high degree of suspicion, the patient may die of respiratory failure masquerading as a stroke. On the other hand, it is certainly possible for a patient with a typical stroke to retain enough secretions in his respiratory tract to develop respiratory failure.

Most common are the patients with obvious right-sided congestive heart failure. The cause of right-sided congestive heart failure—lung failure—often goes unrecognized. Fortunately, many of these patients improve just with treatment of the heart failure, but they would improve more if respiratory failure and its cause were recognized and treated.

It is easy to recognize the respiratory distress present in a patient with asthma, but it is often difficult to tell when the patient is in real danger. The physical exam can be misleading. Occasionally, in asthma, little or no wheezing is heard because there is virtually no air exchange. The patient may appear to be making normal respiratory movements, though labored, yet in fact be exchanging very little air. The earliest blood gas abnormality in an asthmatic is hypoxemia. The hypoxemia may be worsened by treatment with the usual bronchodilators, even though the wheezing is decreasing. The worsening hypoxemia is probably due to changing $\dot{V}/\dot{Q}$ relationships. The hypoxemia causes hyperventilation which in turn causes hypocapnia. In spite of attempts at hyperventilation, if the asthma becomes more severe with increasing airway obstruction, the P_{CO_2} rises to normal. As the situation worsens even mild elevations of P_{CO_2} combined with the hypoxemia (if the patient has not been treated with O_2) signify severe asthma. In asthma slight elevation of P_{CO_2} signifies impending crisis, while similar elevations of P_{CO_2} in chronic bronchitis or emphysema have much less significance. As in other respiratory problems, the best indicators are arterial blood gases, but the interpretation of blood gases must be related to the clinical situation.

Usually some additional insult occurs in patients with chronic airway obstruction (CAO) which either (1) increases airway obstruction or (2) reduces respiratory drive. Both of these cause hypoventilation and result in an increase in P_{CO_2} and a decrease in P_{O_2}. The additional insult which causes the patient with CAO to develop respiratory failure may be (1) infection such as pneumonia or acute bronchitis (*Hemophilus influenzae* and *Diplococcus pneumoniae* are the most common organisms in outpatients), (2) pulmonary embolus, (3) congestive heart failure or fluid overload, and (4) increasing bronchospasm.

Often the patient with CAO is getting by with only marginal lung function, and even minor insults tip him over into frank respiratory failure. Such an insult may be an infectious process leading to bronchial mucosal edema, increased mucus production, bronchospasm, increased airway obstruction, and worsening hypercapnia and hypoxemia.

nonspecific signs and symptoms

There are also a number of situations in which anyone can recognize respiratory failure; i.e., patients with cardiac arrest, those with drug overdose or head injury who stop breathing, and those with cyanosis and labored breathing. However, in many patients the presence of respiratory failure may not be so obvious. The signs and symptoms may be nonspecific and manifested as lethargy, irritability, headaches, confusion (sometimes intermittent), vagueness, facetiousness, jerky motions, and asterixis (flapping tremor of hand). Other less specific manifestations may be sweating, mydriasis, tachycardia, hypotension, anorexia, impaired motor function, impaired judgment, and coma.

Respiratory failure occurs in a variety of clinical settings and is associated with a variety of signs and symptoms. One must be exceedingly astute to recognize respiratory failure every time it occurs, and perhaps all that can be expected is that one should learn to develop a high index of suspicion regarding the existence of respiratory failure and be eager to obtain arterial blood gases when a suspicion of respiratory failure exists.

The treatment of respiratory failure is designed to raise the P_{O_2} to normal and/or reduce the P_{CO_2} to normal. Usually this can be accomplished by initially supplying supplemental oxygen and treating the factors which are causing the altered physiology; for example, bronchospasm, infection, mucosal edema, and retained secretions. This treatment, if instituted early enough, usually allows the patient to increase his own ventilation so that in most cases of respiratory failure ventilators are not required. It is most important for the patient to receive adequate oxygen—just enough to raise his P_{O_2} to about 60 mm. Hg while the other treatment is being instituted. Raising the P_{O_2} to 60 will help to prevent secondary problems such as the development of heart failure or worsening coma. Hypoxemia can cause death in minutes, but it takes hours or days for hypercapnia to become marked enough to cause death.

PATRICIA K. BRANNIN, R.N., M.S.N., A.A.R.T.
MARY SUSAN KUDLA, R.N., M.S.

13 13

management modalities: respiratory system

The continuing growth of critical care nursing challenges the nurse to expand her scope to meet the needs of this rapidly advancing specialty. Increased accountability for nursing practice demands continual development of the knowledge base from which the critical care nurse operates. It is the purpose of this chapter to enable the nurse to enhance her knowledge of the respiratory system and its acute disorders. This chapter is presented to assist the reader to recall knowledge of normal pulmonary functions and apply it to abnormal situations when she is assessing, applying and evaluating therapeutic modalities. Patient observation and recognition of the signs of pulmonary insufficiency—tachypnea, tachycardia, diaphoresis and anxiety—are the keys to recognizing abnormal pulmonary function. The ability of the clinician to anticipate, recognize and intervene to treat pulmonary disorders may modify and/or prevent common lung disorders.

atelectasis

Atelectasis can be defined as a diminution of volume or collapse of lung units.[1] Several etiological factors may precipitate atelectasis. Reabsorption atelectasis occurs when communications between the alveoli and trachea are obstructed, e.g., by plugging of a bronchus with mucus. The alveolar gas is rapidly absorbed into the circulation and due to the obstruction cannot be replenished, so that alveolar collapse ensues. Passive atelectasis occurs when air and/or fluid in the pleural space prevent normal alveolar filling. Compression atelectasis occurs in the presence of a space occupying lesion such as a pulmonary mass.[2] Atelectasis may also occur in patches which may be caused by mucus plugging or altered compliance in the atelectatic area.[3]

Atelectasis results in a pathological shunting of blood from the right side of the heart to the left resulting in desaturation of blood entering the systemic circulation. The degree of shunt present depends upon the severity of the atelectasis. In the normal lung there is a small amount of unoxygenated blood entering the systemic circulation. Contributing to the normal shunt are those vessels whose venous outflow bypasses pulmonary capillaries. Shunting is increased by atelectasis because blood flow passes through the pulmonary capillaries that are in contact with nonventilated alveoli (Fig. 13-1).

Signs and symptoms vary with the severity of atelectasis and degree of shunt present. With severe shunts (i.e., large areas of atelectasis) cyanosis may become evident. Arterial blood gases will reflect the degree of hypoxemia as well as the adequacy of alveolar ventilation. There is frequently roentgenographic evidence of atelectasis. In compression atelectasis there is roentgenographic evidence of air and/or fluid collection in the pleural space resulting in atelectasis. All the roentgen signs are based on diminished volume of the affected lobe or segment.[4] Cyanosis may become evident as atelectasis increases. Large areas of atelectasis may cause a shift of the mediastinal structures toward the affected side which may be demonstrated roentgenographically. Auscultatory examination reveals decreased breath sounds over the atelectatic lung. There may be diminished chest expansion of the affected side. The patient may complain of shortness of breath (s.o.b.), dyspnea on exertion (d.o.e.), and weakness. He may have tachypnea, tachycardia, fever, anxiety, restlessness and confusion.

Treatment is based upon the etiology of the atelectasis. Meticulous bronchial hygiene (see discussion, p. 241), mobilization of the patient when appropriate and administration of oxygen in pharmacological doses comprise the basic framework of therapy.

pneumonia

Pneumonia is an inflammatory process in which alveolar gas is replaced by cellular material. The etiology may be viral, bacterial, fungal, protozoan, rickettsial or due to hypersensitivity, resulting in the primary presenting illness. Pneumonia may also result from aspiration.

The signs and symptoms will depend on the location and extent of involvement (i.e., segmental or lobar) and etiology of the pneumonia. Subjective findings include dyspnea, tachypnea, pleuritic chest pain, fever, chills, hemoptysis and cough productive of rusty or purulent sputum. Objective findings include fever, splinting of involved hemithorax, hypoxemia, percussion dullness, coarse inspiratory rales and diminished breath sounds over the involved area.

Anatomical Shunt (Q̇S anat.)

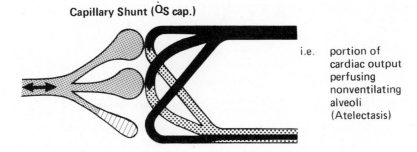

i.e. portion of cardiac output bypassing pulmonary capillaries

Capillary Shunt (Q̇S cap.)

i.e. portion of cardiac output perfusing nonventilating alveoli (Atelectasis)

Physiological Shunt (Q̇S phys.)

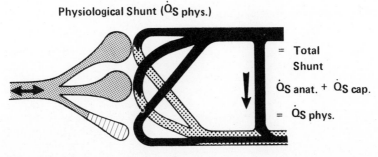

= Total Shunt

Q̇S anat. + Q̇S cap.

= Q̇S phys.

Fig. 13-1. Subdivisions of the physiological shunt. (From H. H. Bendixen et al., *Respiratory Care*, St. Louis, C. V. Mosby, 1965, p. 13)

Treatment of pneumonia is dependent upon etiology, as shown in Table 13-1. Observation of the patient for tachycardia, tachypnea, diaphoresis, restlessness and confusion (signs of hypoxemia), increased sputum production and increased splinting is essential in determination of progression/regres-

table 13-1
antibiotic therapy in pulmonary disease

PULMONARY COMPLICATION	ANTIBIOTIC	DOSAGE
Pneumococcal pneumonia with or without COLD	Penicillin	600,000 U procaine penicillin IM q12h (a blood level of 0.02 mg./ml. 12 hours after start of drug is adequate to kill organism) or IV prep: aqueous penicillin 400,000-600,000 units IV q3-4h
Staphylococcal pneumonia (production of enzymes that destroy lung tissue)	Antistaphylococcal agents: Nafcillin Methicillin Cloxacillin Penicillin	1-2 gm. IV q4h
Klebsiella pneumonia (gram negative): a very severe pneumonia with high mortality rate; seen more commonly in chronic/debilitated states	Gentamicin	Dosage will be related to renal function (i.e., creatinine clearance); commonly, 3-5 mg./kg./24 hours. Aim to achieve a trough blood level not less than 1.5 mg./ml. and a peak level not over 10 mg./ml.
Pseudomonas pneumonia (gram negative)	Tobramycin	3-5 mg./kg./24 hours, producing blood levels of 2.5 mg./ml. in presence of normal renal function
	Gentamicin	3-5 mg./kg./24 hours (see Klebsiella pneumonia, above)
Hemophilus influenza	Ampicillin	2.0-6.0 gm./24 hours, increasing to 8-12 gm./24 hours for serious infections
	Chloramphenicol	3.0-4.0 gm./24 hours PO (50-100 mg./kg./24 hours)

A complete discussion of antibiotic therapy related to pulmonary disease and/or complications is beyond the scope of this chapter.

James Good, M.D., Pulmonary Fellow, University of Colorado Medical Center, lecture, "Antibiotic Therapy" (November 1976).

sion of the process. Careful attention must be directed to improving ventilation through adequate pain medication followed by bronchial hygiene.

Complications of pneumonia include abscess formation, pleural effusion, empyema, bacteremia and septicemia. Superinfection may occur as a complication of pharmacological treatment.

pleural effusion

The pleural space is a potential space between the visceral and parietal pleura that line the lungs and interior chest wall. This space normally contains a small amount of fluid. Excess fluid may accumulate in neoplastic, thromboembolic, cardiovascular and infectious disease processes. This is due to at least one of four basic mechanisms:[5]

1. Increased pressure in subpleural capillaries and/or lymphatics
2. Decreased colloid osmotic pressure of the blood
3. Increased intrapleural negative pressure
4. Inflammatory or neoplastic involvement of the pleura.

Subjective findings include shortness of breath and pleuritic chest pain, depending on the amount of fluid accumulation. Objective findings include tachypnea and hypoxemia if ventilation is impaired, dullness to percussion and decreased breath sounds over the involved area.

Removal of the pleural effusion by thoracentesis and/or chest tubes is palliative treatment. Major treatment is that directed toward the underlying cause.

Empyema is a collection of purulent material in the pleural space secondary to an inflammatory process of the mediastinum, lung, esophagus or subdiaphragmatic space. The symptom complex may include shortness of breath and pleuritic chest pain. A major objective finding is continued fever during antibiotic administration. Other findings include those of pleural effusion. Treatment consists of rigorous antibiotic therapy and chest tube drainage (see discussion of chest tubes, p. 246). A serious complication of empyema is irreversible fibrotic changes that compromise pulmonary ventilation, due to trapping of the lung on the involved side.

bronchospasm

Bronchospasm implies a narrowing of the airways resulting in increased airway resistance which can be caused by a variety of mechanisms. These include: (1) inhalation of toxic or irritating substances such as smoke, pollens, dust or noxious gases; (2) bronchitis; (3) severe coughing episodes; (4) extreme cold and (5) exercise. Although bronchospasm is usually associated with asthma, these mechanisms may precipitate bronchospasm in anyone.

Signs and symptoms vary with the degree of bronchospasm. The patient may complain of shortness of breath associated with wheezing respirations. Further findings include tachycardia, tachypnea, retractions, restlessness, anxiety, inspiratory/expiratory wheezing, hypoxemia, hypercapnia, cyanosis and coughing. One must be aware that a decrease in wheezing does not necessarily mean decreased bronchospasm, but rather progression of airway narrowing and markedly decreased ventilation.

Treatment is directed at removing the cause of bronchospasm and initiating bronchodilator therapy (Table 13-2). The patient must be observed for increasing bronchospasm and deteriorating pulmonary function manifested by a rising P_{CO_2}.

(Text continued on p. 237.)

table 13-2
pulmonary drugs and their sites of action

Sites of Drug Actions

1. Receptors of Smooth Muscle—Airways

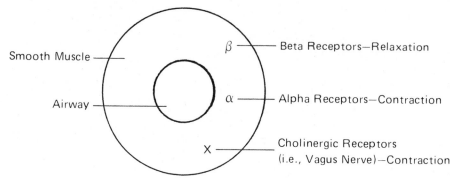

Smooth Muscle

Airway

β —— Beta Receptors—Relaxation

α —— Alpha Receptors—Contraction

X —— Cholinergic Receptors
(i.e., Vagus Nerve)—Contraction

2. Cellular Metabolism

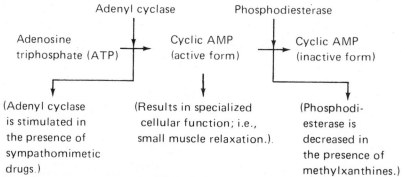

Adenyl cyclase   Phosphodiesterase

Adenosine   Cyclic AMP   Cyclic AMP
triphosphate (ATP)   (active form)   (inactive form)

(Adenyl cyclase   (Results in specialized   (Phosphodi-
is stimulated in   cellular function; i.e.,   esterase is
the presence of   small muscle relaxation.)   decreased in
sympathomimetic   the presence of
drugs.)   methylxanthines.)

Cyclic AMP is one of the intermediaries of cellular metabolism in the sequence of energy production. It is present in almost all cell membranes and is influenced by a variety of agents, such as hormones and drugs.

3. Mast Cells

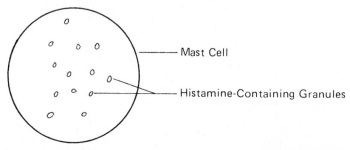

—— Mast Cell

—— Histamine-Containing Granules

Mast cells with histamine-containing granules are abundant in allergic asthmatics.

PULMONARY DRUGS	ACTION	DOSAGE	SIDE EFFECTS
1. *Bronchodilators*			
Methylxan-thines	↓ phosphodiester-ase with ↑ cyclic AMP (active form)	IV: loading — 5 mg./kg.; maintenance — 0.9 mg./kg. PO: aminophyl-line — 1200 mg./24 hrs; oxtriphyl-line (Choledyl) — 1600 mg./24 hrs. NB: Dosages adjusted to maintain serum theophylline levels 10-20 mcg./ml.	Nausea Vomiting Nervousness Arrhythmias Seizures
Sympathomi-metics	Beta (β) stimu-lants		Relatively few side effects with recom-mended dosages
Isoetharine (Bronkosol)	Stimulates adenyl cyclase with ↑ cyclic AMP (active form)	Delivered via nebulizer — either hand-powered or IPPB 0.5 cc. with sterile water or normal saline (1:3 conc.) q4h	Tachycardia Palpitations Nausea Headache Changes in blood pressure Nervousness
Terbutaline (Brethine)	Stimulates adenyl cyclase with ↑ cyclic AMP (active form)	5 mg. PO q8h; 0.25 mg. SC not to exceed 0.5 mg. q4h	↑ Heart rate ⎫ Usually Nervousness ⎪ transient Tremor ⎬ and do not Palpitations ⎪ require Dizziness ⎭ treatment
Metaproter-enol (Alupent, Metaprel)	Stimulates adenyl cyclase with ↑ cyclic AMP (active form)	Metered dose device: 0.65 mg./metered dose; 20 mg. PO TID	Tachycardia Hypertension Palpitations Nervousness Tremor Nausea and vomiting

table 13-2 *(continued)*

PULMONARY DRUGS	ACTION	DOSAGE	SIDE EFFECTS
2. *Steroids*	Stimulate adenylate cyclase with ↑ cyclic 3′, 5′— AMP; may facilitate utilization of β stimulants; anti-inflammatory agents		
Prednisone		Variable; eg., 40-60 mg. PO initially and decreasing according to PFT and eosinophil counts (in patients with ↑ Eos 2° to allergin mediated responses)	Formation of glucose from body protein→ ↑ blood sugar Depletion of bone calcium—osteoporosis Increase in fat production Impairment of immunologic response Reduction of inflammatory response Increase in gastric acidity Elevation of blood pressure Acne
Methyl-prednisolone (Solu-Medrol)		Variable; e.g., 100 mg. IV and repeat with one-fourth original dose q6h	Same as for prednisone
Beclomethasone (Vanceril)	Virtually same as above except it is an inhaled preparation with high topical effect on the airways and low systemic activity	Inhalation device; 2 inhalations (100 mcg.) QID	Oral candidiasis Mild oropharyngeal symptoms—discomfort and dryness of throat

PULMONARY DRUGS	ACTION	DOSAGE	SIDE EFFECTS
3. *Cromolyn sodium* (Aarane, Intal)	Prophylactic bronchospasmolytic in allergic asthma; *not* useful in acute bronchospasm; probably strengthens mast cell membrane preventing release of histamine and therefore decreases bronchospasm in the allergic asthmatic	1 capsule via inhaler device QID	Maculopapular rash Urticaria Cough and/or bronchospasm

H. D. Waite, M.D., Chief of Critical Care Medicine, General Rose Memorial Hospital, lecture, "Pulmonary Drugs" (November 1976).

chronic obstructive lung disease (COLD)

The common lung complications discussed above are potentially reversible causes of respiratory insufficiency, but several disease entities result in chronic obstructive lung disease (COLD). These include chronic bronchitis, emphysema and asthma. COLD is a national health problem second only to heart disease, and it is the most common cause of respiratory insufficiency.

chronic bronchitis

Chronic infection and/or irritation of the bronchi may result in bronchitis. The mucus-secreting glands of the tracheobronchial tree become thickened and encroach on the diameter of the airway lumen. In addition there is increased mucus production in peripheral airways. By far the most common cause is tobacco (Fig. 13-2).

The two most common bacterial organisms isolated from the secretions of the chronic bronchitic are *Hemophilus influenzae* and pneumococcus. Exacerbation of chronic bronchitis with resultant respiratory insufficiency most often results from an acute bacterial inflammation of the bronchial tree. An essential prophylactic measure in preventing an acute inflammatory process is rigorous bronchial hygiene to promote clearance of secretions that provide an ideal medium for bacterial growth in the peripheral airways. In contrast to emphysema, chronic bronchitis may have a reversible component if the source of chronic infection and/or irritation is treated.

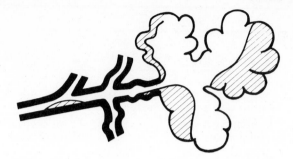

Fig. 13-2. Bronchitis. Inflammation, thickening → narrowing of airways. Lined areas indicate secretions.

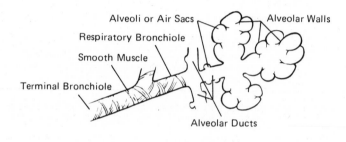

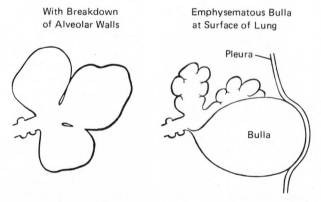

Fig. 13-3. Emphysema. Airway showing normal primary lobule *(top)* and emphysematous lobule *(bottom)*. (From American Lung Association, *Introduction to Lung Diseases*, ed. 6, 1975, p. 71)

emphysema

Emphysema is an anatomical alteration of the terminal air spaces, the acini, where exchange of oxygen and carbon dioxide takes place. Emphysema is an irreversible abnormal dilatation of the acinus accompanied by destructive changes of acinar walls with resultant loss of lung elastic recoil.[6] The destructive process resulting in airway obstruction develops insidiously. In contrast to the chronic bronchitic, patients with emphysema usually have mild chronic hypoxemia because destruction of acinar walls is accompanied by destruction of corresponding vasculature. The ratio of ventilated to perfused lung tissue remains stable (Fig. 13-3).

The majority of patients with COLD will have a mixture of chronic bronchitis and emphysema rather than "pure" bronchitis or emphysema (Table 13-3).

table 13-3
COLD: features that distinguish bronchitis and emphysema

FEATURES	BRONCHITIS	EMPHYSEMA
Clinical Exam		
History	Often recurrent chest infections	Frequently only insidious dyspnea
Chest exam	Noisy chest, slight over-distention	Quiet chest, marked over-distention
Sputum	Frequently copious and purulent	Usually scanty and mucoid
Chronic cor pulmonale	Common	Infrequent
Physiological Tests		
Chronic hypoxemia	Often severe	Usually mild
Chronic hypercapnia	Common	Unusual
Pulmonary hypertension	Often severe	Usually mild
Cardiac output	Normal	Often low
Therapeutic Modalities		
Bronchial hygiene	Very important for clearance of secretions	Less important unless patient has respiratory infection

Adapted from B. Burrows et al., *Respiratory Insufficiency*, Chicago, Year Book Medical Publishers, 1975.

asthma

In comparison to emphysema and, to a lesser extent, chronic bronchitis, asthma is a reversible obstructive lung disease in which hyperreactive bronchial airways respond to a variety of irritating stimuli (e.g., allergens, infections, exercise, and emotional factors) by widespread narrowing and subsequent bronchospasm.[7] Figure 13-4 illustrates a series of events that may become a vicious cycle resulting in life-threatening status asthmaticus unless bronchospasm is controlled.

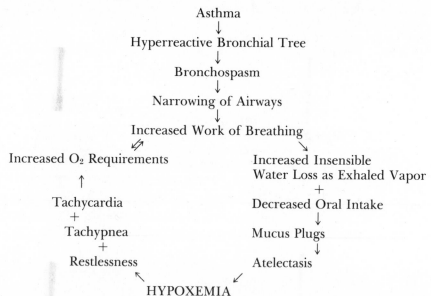

Spontaneous remission of bronchospasm may occur; however, use of bronchodilating agents (see Table 13-2) in addition to rigorous bronchial hygiene is the usual mode of treatment. The potential severity of an asthma attack is frequently minimized by these means.

According to Petty (1975), status asthmaticus is defined as "unrelenting acute wheezing dyspnea not responsive to oral, inhaled or subcutaneous sympathomimetic amines or connectional doses of oral or rectal methylxanthines."[8] The patient manifests a dramatic picture of acute anxiety, marked labored breathing, tachycardia or diaphoresis. Deterioration of pulmonary function results in alveolar hypoventilation with subsequent hypoxemia, hypercapnia and acidemia. A rising P_{CO_2} in a patient with an acute asthmatic attack is often the first objective indication of status asthmaticus.

Multiple therapeutic modalities must be instituted. All patients in status asthmaticus demonstrate hypoxemia and require oxygen therapy. Dehydration usually exists and requires correction. Pharmacological agents consist of methylxanthines, sympathomimetic amines and corticosteroids. If pul-

Bronchiole Obstructed on Expiration by:

1. Muscle Spasm

2. Swelling of Mucosa

3. Thick Secretions

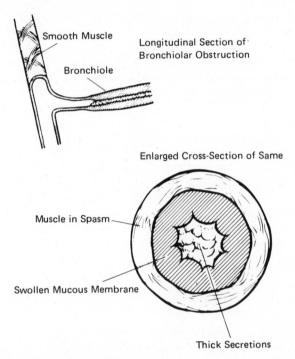

Smooth Muscle

Longitudinal Section of
Bronchiolar Obstruction

Bronchiole

Enlarged Cross-Section of Same

Muscle in Spasm

Swollen Mucous Membrane

Thick Secretions

Fig. 13-4. Pathophysiological changes in bronchial asthma. (From American Lung Association, *Introduction to Lung Diseases,* ed. 6, 1975, p. 63)

monary function cannot be improved and respiratory failure ensues, the patient may require intubation and assisted ventilation.

bronchial hygiene

Bronchial hygiene consists of any one or a combination of the following measures: aerosol therapy, deep breathing, coughing and postural drainage. The therapeutic goals of bronchial hygiene are removal of secretions, improved ventilation and oxygenation. Specific bronchial hygiene is dependent on existing pulmonary dysfunction.

intermittent positive pressure breathing (IPPB)

IPPB treatments are used for improved administration and deposition of aerosols. Successful IPPB treatments will be determined by the patient's position, ventilatory pattern and ability to cooperate and follow instructions. An adequate ventilatory pattern during an IPPB treatment consists of a deep inspiration aimed at increasing normal tidal volume two to three times. The patient is then instructed to hold his breath briefly to provide greater depth and deposition of aerosolized medication, water or saline. Exhalation should take twice as long as inspiration, resulting in complete exhalation. Contraindications of IPPB therapy may include pneumothorax, active pulmonary tuberculosis in which infection or hemoptysis is hazardous, and hemoptysis. Caution should be taken in the use of IPPB treatment immediately following lung resection because of potential bronchial leakage.

The use and value of IPPB therapy have become controversial issues.

inhaled moisture

The primary purposes of inhaled moisture are hydration of normal mucociliary clearance mechanisms and liquefaction of secretions. Adequate systemic hydration is essential for optimum results of inhaled moisture. The most important aspect of inhaled moisture therapy is active deep breathing by the patient followed by brief breath holding to allow deposition of aerosolized particles and slow, complete exhalation. Potential hazards that may exist include bronchospasm in patients with hyperreactive airways and infection from contaminated equipment. The ultimate success of inhaled moisture therapy will depend upon clearance of secretions with forceful rigorous coughing.

effective cough

An effective cough is an essential prerequisite for clearance of secretions. Various techniques are available to assist the patient in achieving an effective cough, e.g., a maximal exhalation followed by a maximal inspiration followed by a forceful cough. Gentle pressure to the trachea above the manubrial notch may be used to stimulate cough production in the comatose or uncooperative patient.

chest physiotherapy

Inadequate clearance of secretions dictates the need for chest physiotherapy. Chest physiotherapy includes utilization of gravity to aid flow of secretions to a point where they can be expectorated with forceful coughing maneuvers or reached with a suction catheter. The effectiveness of positioning may be augmented by chest percussion.[9] (Figure 13-5 demonstrates the positions.)

Modification or contraindication of chest physiotherapy may be necessary in the following: increased intracranial pressure, intravascular bleeds, cervical cord trauma, instable vertebral fractures, chest and abdominal trauma, hiatal hernia, obesity, osteoporosis and orthopedic appliances.

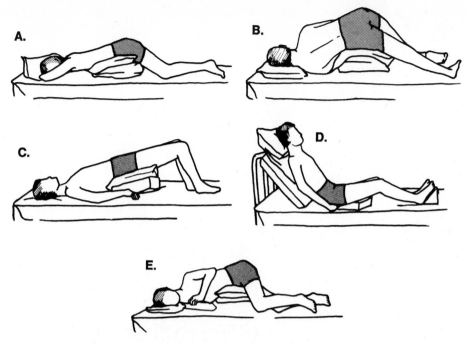

Fig. 13-5. Positions used in lung drainage. A. Face-lying—hips elevated 16-18 inches on pillows, making a 30-45 degree angle. Purpose: to drain the posterior lower lobes. B. Lying on the left side—hips elevated 16-18 inches on pillows. Purpose: to drain the right lateral lower lung segments. C. Back lying—hips elevated 16-18 inches on pillows. Purpose: to drain the anterior lower lung segments. D. Sitting upright or semireclining—to drain the upper lung field and allow more forceful coughing. E. Lying on the right side—hips elevated on pillows forming a 30-45 degree angle. Purpose: to drain the left lower lobes.

The need for and effectiveness of various modalities of bronchial hygiene must be evaluated frequently.

The preceding discussion is not intended as a specific instructional guide for bronchial hygiene. Techniques in delivery of bronchial hygiene are paramount in the prevention and treatment of pulmonary complications. The reader is referred to the bibliography for further references.

pulmonary emboli

Pulmonary emboli may occur as a complication of many medical conditions which predispose to venous thrombosis, e.g., postoperative states, prolonged bed rest and trauma. Deep venous thrombosis, particularly in the lower extremities, is the main predisposing factor for pulmonary emboli.

Both pulmonary and hemodynamic changes occur as a result of occlusion of a pulmonary artery by an embolus. Alveoli are ventilated but not perfused, thereby producing areas of ineffective ventilation, i.e., increased respiratory dead space (Fig. 13-6).

Pneumoconstriction resulting from a lack of carbon dioxide normally present in pulmonary arterial blood shifts ventilation from the underperfused alveoli. The decrease in pulmonary blood flow due to an embolus results in deficient nutrients for surfactant production, ultimately resulting in atelectasis. The severity of hemodynamic changes depends on the size of the embolus. Increased pulmonary vascular resistance occurs, which, if pulmonary blood flow remains constant, may result in right ventricular failure.[10] Pulmonary embolus may resolve or infrequently may lead to death of tissue, i.e., pulmonary infarction.

The symptom complex of a pulmonary embolus depends upon its size. Dyspnea, one of the most frequent complaints, is often out of proportion to the physical findings. Tachypnea and tachycardia may be present in varying degrees. Mild fever may exist although leukocytosis is rare.[11] It should be noted that pleuritic chest pain and hemoptysis are associated with pulmonary infarction rather than with pulmonary embolus. Massive pulmonary embolization results in a more dramatic clinical manifestation of acute illness. The patient develops pronounced tachypnea, usually with cyanosis, tachycardia, restlessness, confusion and hypotension. The resulting shock state produces concomitant changes of decreased urinary output and cold clammy skin.

A suspected pulmonary embolus may be confirmed by radioactive lung scanning and pulmonary angiography. Treatment is anticoagulation and correction of predisposing causes of venous thrombosis. Anticoagulant therapy is administered by various ways in different institutions. The nurse must be aware that multiple drug interactions may occur with use of anticoagulant therapy.

hemo/pneumothorax

A pneumothorax occurs when air enters the pleural space between the visceral and parietal pleurae. Blood in this location is called a hemothorax. There are two types of pneumothorax. A spontaneous pneumothorax may result from the rupture of a subpleural alveolar cyst or an emphysematous bleb. The signs and symptoms will vary with the size of the pneumothorax and may range from mild shortness of breath to chest pain and signs of increasing respiratory distress. Physical examination reveals decreased breath sounds and decreased respiratory movement on the affected side. The diagnosis is confirmed by roentgenography.

Chest trauma, IPPB, positive end expiratory pressure (PEEP), cardiopulmonary resuscitation, thoracic and high abdominal surgery and thora-

Anatomical Deadspace (V_D anat.)

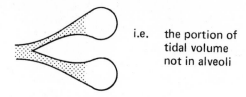

i.e.   the portion of
tidal volume
not in alveoli

Alveolar Deadspace (V_D alv.)

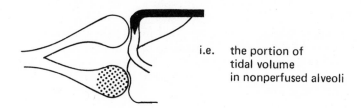

i.e.   the portion of
tidal volume
in nonperfused alveoli

Physiological Deadspace (V_D phys.)

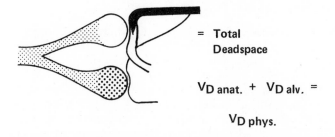

= **Total**
Deadspace

V_D anat. + V_D alv. =

V_D phys.

Fig. 13-6. Subdivisions of physiological dead space.
Only that part of the volume of ventilation which enters perfused alveoli is effective in blood-gas exchange and is labelled as alveolar ventilation. The remainder is wasted or dead space ventilation. Total ventilation may be subdivided accordingly.

Total ventilation (V) − Alveolar ventilation (V_A) = Dead space ventilation (V_D)

This division applies equally to minute ventilation and to the individual tidal volumes. Dividing by the respiratory frequency we get:

Tidal volume (V_T) − Alveolar tidal volume = Physiological dead space ($V_{D_{phys.}}$)

(From H. H. Bendixen et al., *Respiratory Care*, St Louis, C. V. Mosby, 1965, p. 17) centesis may precipitate an iatrogenic pneumo- and/or hemothorax.[12] A pneumothorax, regardless of etiology, becomes life threatening as tension in the pleural space occurs. When a tension pneumothorax develops the tear in lung bronchus or chest wall acts as a one-way valve which allows air to enter the pleural space on inspiration, but not escape on expiration. If it is not immediately recognized and treated, massive atelectasis will result. In addition, the mediastinal structures are displaced toward the unaffected side and tracheal deviation may be especially prominent. This mediastinal shift will result in a decreased venous return, decreased cardiac output and ultimately death. Clinically, the patient manifests severe respiratory distress. Agitation, cyanosis and tachypnea are severe. Tachycardia and the initial increase in blood pressure are followed by hypotension as cardiac output decreases. The diagnosis is based on the clinical manifestations as well as the clinical setting; any patient who is being ventilated and suddenly develops acute respiratory distress during ventilation evidenced by markedly increased inspiratory pressures is a prime candidate for a tension pneumothorax. Treatment must be immediate. A 16- to 18-gauge needle inserted into the second, third, or fourth intercostal space at the midclavicular line on the affected side will relieve the pressure. Once this has been accomplished a chest tube should be inserted and underwater seal drainage instituted to prevent any further development of tension.

underwater seal drainage

It is important to recall several principles to understand underwater seal drainage. There is normally negative (less than atmospheric) pressure in the pleural space which ranges from minus 5 to 3 centimeters of water during expiration.[13] The development of negative pressure during inspiration allows air to enter the lungs. As the extrapulmonary and atmospheric pressures equalize, active inspiration ceases, and passive exhalation occurs. When the integrity of the pleural space is disrupted, the air and/or fluid that accumulates prevents the development of negative pressure necessary for normal ventilation. Chest drains and underwater seal drainage are used to restore the physiological integrity of the pleural space. A chest tube (drain) inserted into the pleural space will remove air and/or fluid. The underwater seal drainage to which the chest tube is connected prevents backflow into the pleural space (Fig. 13-7).

A glass rod under water in a bottle establishes negative pressure in the water seal system. The depth of the rod in the water determines the degree of negative pressure. A basic law of physics states that gases and fluids move from areas of greater pressure to areas of lesser pressure. Therefore, the air and/or fluid disrupting the normal pressures in the pleural space will drain into the chest bottle in an attempt to equalize the more negative pressure of the underwater seal drainage system. The air vent in the chest bottle allows the drained air to escape, preventing pressure buildup in the bottle.

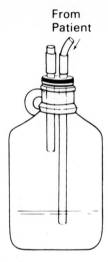

Fig. 13-7. One-bottle system underwater seal drainage.

Larger amounts of blood or fluid draining from the pleural space necessitate modification of the underwater seal system. A second bottle may be added to accommodate large amounts of fluid (Fig. 13-8).

Suction may be added to the system if the air leak into the pleural space

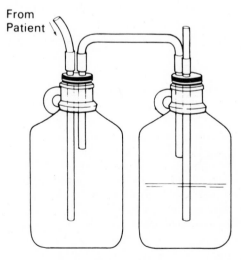

Fig. 13-8. Two-bottle system underwater seal drainage.

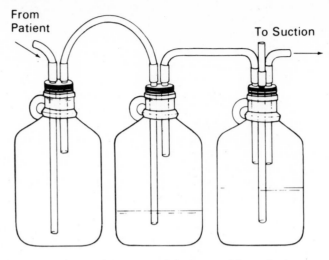

From
Patient

To Suction

Fig. 13-9. Underwater seal drainage with suctioning.

accumulates faster than the system can remove it (Fig. 13-9). A single self-contained underwater seal drainage unit which has the capacity to function as a two- or three-bottle system with suction has been developed.

The system must remain patent. Malfunction of the chest tube and/or underwater seal drainage system may result in inadequate removal of air and/or fluid from the pleural space. Occlusion of the system at any point may result in the development of a tension pneumothorax. The life-threatening seriousness of a tension pneumothorax has led to the consensus that clamping of chest tubes for more than a few seconds is a dangerous practice.[14]

nonpulmonary respiratory complications

Patients who have surgery, notably high abdominal thoracic and low abdominal resection, are especially susceptible to respiratory embarrassment. The mechanism of pulmonary compromise is a restrictive entity in which there is a reduction of vital capacity thus resulting in a limited ventilatory reserve. The major restrictive insult occurs sometime in the first 24 hours postoperatively.[15] Patients without complications gradually resume their preoperative ventilatory status.

Postoperative pulmonary complications may be avoided or minimized by adequate preoperative cardiopulmonary evaluation by the critical care nurse. The nurse may thereby institute those measures which are directed toward monitoring pulmonary status and providing modalities aimed toward improving vital capacity.

Appropriate administration of narcotics and sedatives is a necessary adjunct to pulmonary care. The use of these drugs must be guided by the patient's clinical status. The aim of pharmacological therapy is to minimize pain so that the patient will tolerate respiratory therapy and other therapeutic modalities. On the other hand, overzealous use of sedatives and narcotics may result in respiratory depression and acute respiratory failure.

The patient with a sedative or narcotic overdosage presents with respiratory insufficiency. The severity of the respiratory insufficiency is dependent upon the specific drug(s), amount ingested, time of ingestion and rate of metabolism of the drug(s). Factors which may alter drug effects include multiple drug ingestion, hepatic or renal function abnormalities, and preexisting pulmonary disease, e.g., COLD. Care of patients with drug overdose is guided by this information as well as by the knowledge that patients with certain types of drug ingestion (e.g., glutethimide) may show a fluctuation in level of consciousness. This presents a problem in the maintenance of an adequate airway. It must not be assumed that a patient who at one time appears alert and able to maintain his airway will continue to do so.

There are also drugs which in normal pharmacological doses can cause neuromuscular blockade with resultant respiratory paralysis, e.g., kanamycin, gentamycin, streptomycin, neomycin and polymyxin B.

Disease states and/or trauma involving the neuromuscular system may affect pulmonary function. The degree of dysfunction will depend upon the extent of respiratory muscle involvement. In certain neurological diseases the gag and cough reflexes may be diminished resulting in aspiration of food, fluid and/or secretions. The aspirated contents can cause atelectasis and pneumonia which, if not recognized, will lead to progressive respiratory failure. As impairment of respiratory muscles progresses there is a resultant decrease in vital capacity. Taking serial measurements of the vital capacity is an important method of assessing adequacy of pulmonary function. This assessment can be done quite readily by the nurse. Cardinal signs of respiratory embarrassment, pulmonary function measurements and arterial blood gas analysis must be correlated with the clinical status of the patient. Long-term management of a patient with a neuromuscular disorder includes maintenance of a patent airway, rigorous clearance of secretions, treatment of infections, maximum mobilization of the patient and ventilatory assistance when indicated.

Several entities restrict chest wall expansion with resultant compromised pulmonary function, e.g., kyphoscoliosis, rheumatoid spondylitis, scleroderma, pectus excavatum, and use of orthopedic appliances such as spica casts. These patients may, in a stable environment, have normal pulmonary function. A crisis such as trauma or a major medical illness such as drug overdose may precipitate severe respiratory impairment. In the management of these patients the nurse must utilize those measures which maximize ventilation and minimize pulmonary complications.

acute respiratory failure

Acute respiratory failure (ARF) may be defined as respiratory dysfunction of such a degree that gas exchange is no longer adequate to maintain normal arterial blood gases.[16] Quantitatively, ARF may be defined as a $Po_2 < 50$ mm. Hg with or without a $Pco_2 > 50$ mm. Hg[17] (Fig. 13-10).

ARF may result from a variety of insults including pneumonia, atelectasis and pneumothorax. Neuromuscular disease, drugs, toxins and trauma may also lead to acute respiratory failure.

The key to treatment of ARF is anticipation of its subsequent development in the face of a precipitating event. Management of the patient in the presence of ARF is twofold: (1) establishment of adequate arterial oxygenation thereby providing adequate tissue perfusion and (2) amelioration of the underlying cause(s) of ARF.

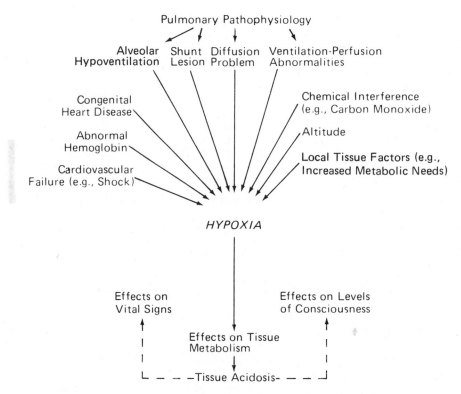

Fig. 13-10. Hypoxia: mechanisms and effects. (From P. Brannin, "Oxygen Therapy and Measures of Bronchial Hygiene," *Nursing Clinics of North America,* Vol. 9, No. 1, 1974, p. 111)

patient management

Rigorous bronchial hygiene and carefully monitored oxygen therapy may eliminate the need for an artificial airway and/or ventilatory support. When these measures fail to provide adequate oxygenation and removal of carbon dioxide, an artificial airway and/or ventilatory support become mandatory.

artificial airway

Artificial airways have a threefold purpose: (1) establishment of an airway, (2) with the cuff inflated, protection of the airway, (3) provision of continuous ventilatory assistance. Artificial airways require knowledgeable and aggressive nursing care to maintain the patency of the airway and maximize therapeutic effects while minimizing damage to the patient's natural airway. The selection of the appropriate artificial airway is most important. Any artificial airway will increase airway resistance; therefore it is essential that the largest tube possible be utilized for intubation. The cuff on the endotracheal or tracheostomy tube must be low compliance (soft) thereby minimizing barotrauma to the trachea, vocal cords and subglottic area. The competency of the cuff must be established prior to intubation. Approximately 10 cc. of air is injected into the cuff prior to use.

Once an artificial airway is placed it must be in the proper location and remain so. In order to properly ascertain tube placement the cuff must be inflated. Anterior and lateral auscultation of the chest bilaterally aids in evaluation of tube position. It must be remembered that breath sounds can be transmitted to the nonventilated or inadequately ventilated lung field. The final analysis of tube placement must depend on roentgenography. Because of normal airway anatomy, endotracheal tubes have a tendency to enter the right main stem bronchus. Chest radiographs should be ordered immediately after tube placement. Evaluation of tube placement should be ongoing, since endotracheal and tracheostomy tubes may become dislodged during routine care.

Proper securement of an endotracheal or tracheostomy tube must insure airway patency, proper alignment, and stability of the tube, and should minimize pressure at the insertion site. Immobility of the tube minimizes the riding, slipping, and twisting of the tube, which, unless prevented, injure tissue with which it comes in contact (Fig. 13-11).

It should be noted that an endotracheal tube is a round tube that is inserted through an elliptical opening, the vocal cords. Therefore a pathway is established for continual flow of oropharyngeal secretions and flora which become potential pathogens to the lower respiratory tract. Use of minimal air leak technique reduces the flow of secretions and flora.

Appropriate inflation of a cuff on an artificial airway is based on the following rationale: (1) it protects the airway in the presence of copious secretions; (2) it establishes a seal necessary for ventilatory support. An inflated cuff requires only that amount of air necessary to achieve a minimal air leak. A minimal air leak may be achieved and ascertained by the application of positive pressure (ventilator or self-inflating bag) to the patient's airway,

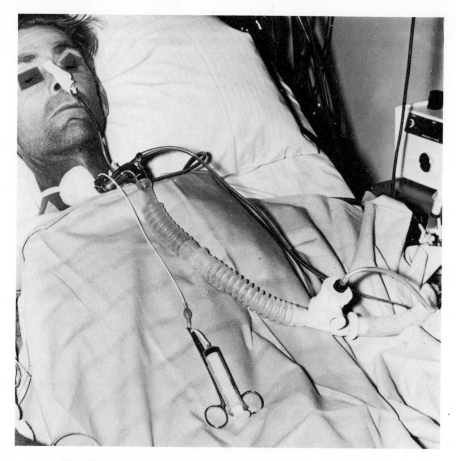

Fig. 13-11. Proper alignment for securing endotracheal tubing.

during which time air is injected into the cuff until no leak is heard over the trachea or felt over the mouth or nose. Once this is achieved, $\frac{1}{2}$ to 1 cc. of air is removed and a minimal air leak is therefore achieved. This method of cuff inflation minimizes airway trauma due to excessive cuff pressures. *It has been proven that periodic deflation of a cuff of an endotracheal or tracheostomy tube is of no value in minimizing tracheal damage.*[18] Intelligent rationale for cuff deflation is based on (1) the presence and amount of upper airway secretions, (2) continuous ventilatory support and (3) the patient's ability to protect his airway. The purpose of cuff deflation is to remove pooled secretions that have accumulated above the cuff which may seed the upper airway with potentially pathogenic bacterial growth. The frequency of cuff deflation is dictated by individual patient needs. Cuff deflation should be performed while positive pressure is applied during inspiration. This establishes retrograde flow of secretions into the oropharynx where rapid removal of these secretions is achieved by suctioning. The minimal air leak is then quickly reestablished to provide adequate ventilation and protection of the airway.

suctioning

The presence of an artificial tube impairs the patient's normal clearing mechanism, the cough, as well as increases production of secretions due to the presence of a foreign object.[19] Suctioning therefore becomes paramount to remove secretions and maintain patency. The need for suctioning is determined by visual observation of secretions and, more importantly, by chest auscultation to determine the presence of secretions or mucus plugs in major airways. The authors recommend the following suctioning procedure:

1. Hyperoxygenate the patient with 100 percent oxygen via a bag or with the ventilator (this can be done while the nurse is preparing for suctioning).
2. Assemble the following equipment:
   a. atraumatic sterile catheter
   b. glove
   c. sterile irrigation container
   d. sterile normal saline
   e. syringe containing sterile normal saline for tracheal irrigation when indicated.
3. Once the above two steps have been completed, a sterile catheter is quickly but gently inserted as far as possible into the artificial airway without application of suction. It is then withdrawn 1 to 2 cm. and intermittent suction is applied as the catheter is simultaneously rotated and removed. The aspiration should not exceed 8 to 10 seconds. Prolonged aspiration can lead to severe hypoxemia, changes in pulmonary pressure and volume and ultimately cardiac arrest.[20]
4. Reestablish ventilatory assistance, allowing the patient to receive 3 to 5 breaths before the procedure is repeated.

It should be noted that patients not on ventilators also need to be hyperoxygenated. The patient should be instructed to take deep breaths while connected to a 100 percent oxygen source. Patients incapable of taking a deep breath should be assisted by a positive pressure device. If secretions are tenacious, 3 to 5 cc. of sterile normal saline may be injected into the artificial airway. Secretions should be monitored for amount, consistency, odor and color, and the observations recorded. Changes in any of these characteristics may necessitate changes in therapy. Laboratory analysis of secretions must be performed, based on patient assessment and response to existing therapy.

humidification

An artificial airway excludes normal physiological airway humidification. Therefore, artificial humidification is essential for maintenance of airway patency and clearance of secretions. Determination of adequate airway humidification is based upon the consistency and amount of secretions as well as condensation visible in the oxygen tubing leading to the patient. The humidification devices attached to oxygen therapy equipment often become media for bacterial growth. Appropriate care should therefore be taken in the maintenance of all oxygen therapy equipment. Policies should be established to monitor, via culture, the presence of organisms.

ventilators

When ventilatory support is required, the nurse must be aware of the degree of hypoxemia present, the percentage of oxygen required and the underlying cause and subsequent management of ARF.

It is not the intent of this chapter to give technical information regarding ventilator function but to provide the nurse with an appreciation for the ventilator as an adjunct to patient management. It is necessary that a nurse caring for a patient who requires ventilatory support be able to evaluate the patient in terms of the adequacy of support. One of the most useful tools of evaluation is the pressure gauge on the ventilator which indicates lung compliance. Airway compliance may be altered by a variety of factors such as secretions, mucus plugs, pulmonary edema, pneumothorax and fibrotic changes. Such alterations result in an increase in the amount of pressure required to deliver a given volume. Baseline information must be obtained and recorded for comparison of pressure readings so that such readings are meaningful. Alterations in airway compliance indicated by pressure changes on the ventilator may require alteration and/or modification of therapy.

The presence or absence of a respiratory therapy department does not alter the nurse's responsibility for the care of a patient on a ventilator. The nurse must be able to assess the adequacy of ventilator function, interpret the alarm system, and troubleshoot the machine in the event of malfunction. No patient should ever be placed on a respirator without another means of ventilation readily available in case of mechanical failure of the respirator.[21] Ventilatory assistance does not negate the need for continued monitoring of the patient for signs of ARF, but actually increases the need for rigorous assessment and aggressive pulmonary care. Ventilatory assistance in a sense buys time for the patient, and the amount we buy for a given patient is a direct reflection of the adequacy of management.

adult respiratory distress syndrome

Adult respiratory distress syndrome (ARDS) is a distinct clinical syndrome of diverse etiology which manifests identical pathology regardless of the causative factor(s). Some precipitating factors are near drowning, fat emboli, sepsis, pancreatitis, pulmonary emboli, aspiration, hemorrhage and trauma of any kind which may occur 10 to 96 hours prior to the onset of ARDS. The pathological changes occurring within the pulmonary system result from the lungs' response to stress occurring anywhere in the body. These changes include release of enzymes, decreased surfactant production resulting in atelectasis and altered permeability of the alveolar capillary membrane leading to severe V̇/Q̇ abnormalities which ultimately result in refractory hypoxemia. An altered a-c membrane permits indiscriminate exudation of fluid into the alveoli, necessitating careful fluid management of the patient with ARDS.[22]

Main clinical manifestations include extreme dyspnea, tachypnea, refractory cyanosis and loss of lung compliance. There may be minimal auscultatory findings with a normal x-ray early in the course of ARDS. Later x-ray findings reveal the typical "white out" pattern of ARDS. Arterial blood gas analysis may reveal initial hypoxemia with or without hypercarbia.

Treatment is twofold: (1) maintenance of adequate ventilation and oxy-

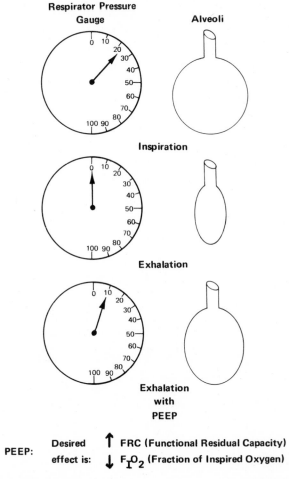

Fig. 13-12. With PEEP, the alveoli have more gas remaining after exhalation for O_2/CO_2 exchange to take place.

genation during the critical period of severe hypoxemia and (2) reversal of the etiological factors that initially caused the respiratory distress to occur.[23]

Adequate ventilation and oxygenation are provided by a mechanical ventilator to which positive end expiratory pressure (PEEP) may be added. Positive end expiratory pressure is maintained in the alveoli throughout the entire respiratory cycle thereby preventing or minimizing alveolar collapse at the end of expiration (Fig. 13-12, p. 255). The goal of continuous PEEP is improved oxygenation with subsequent decrease in inspired oxygen concentration needed to correct life-threatening hypoxemia.

Positive end expiratory pressure may alter intrathoracic pressures so that venous return and ultimately cardiac output are decreased. Careful monitoring of the patient's blood pressure, pulse, urine output and sensorium is necessary. Positive end expiratory pressure may also increase the patient's susceptibility to developing a pneumothorax and, more significantly, a tension pneumothorax. Anticipation of such an occurrence and immediate intervention will minimize the deleterious effects of pneumothorax.

Continuous clinical observation of the patient's response to ventilatory therapy is essential. Arterial blood gas determinations and measurement of vital signs guide oxygen therapy and application of PEEP. The altered alveolar capillary permeability renders the patient with ARDS susceptible to dangerous fluid overload. Transudation of fluid into the alveoli impairs adequate ventilation. Fluid therapy must be carefully monitored with respect to the patient's ventilatory and hemodynamic status.

The patient's response to therapy and ultimate recovery are dependent upon the rapidity and adequacy of treatment of the ARDS syndrome and its precipitating and etiological factor(s).

flail chest

Trauma to the thorax resulting in a flail chest is caused by the disruption of the normally semirigid structure of the chest cage from fracture of three or more adjoining ribs in one or more places, rib fracture(s) with costochondral separation or sternal fractures. Wherever fractures occur, that segment loses continuity with the remaining intact chest wall and subsequent paradoxical movement occurs. During paradoxical ventilation, as the intact chest expands, the injured "flail" segment is depressed thereby limiting the amount of negative intrathoracic pressure needed to move air into the lungs. During expiration the flail segment bulges outward, thus interfering with exhalation. The degree of ventilatory impairment that results from a flail chest is proportional to the extent of injury. The occurrence of concomitant hemo/pneumothorax further impairs ventilation. During inspiration, the intrapleural pressures on the unaffected side are greater, thus displacing the mediastinum toward it. Conversely, during expiration the negative pressure on the unaffected side is less than on the affected side and the mediastinum shifts toward the affected side. This phenomenon, known as mediastinal flutter, further impairs ventilation as well as cardiac output. Normally venous return to the right heart is enhanced during inspiration. Reduced intrapleural negative pressure during inspiration impairs circulating dynamics, thus decreasing venous return to the heart, right atrial filling and ultimately cardiac output.

Frequent patient assessment, including anterior and posterior visual inspection of chest movement, is essential for evaluation and intervention in the treatment of a patient with a flail chest. Treatment is directed toward improvement of ventilation and oxygenation as well as stabilization of the chest wall. The increased ventilatory effort that is needed for adequate ventilation is difficult for the patient to maintain because of the pain caused by injury. A mechanically controlled volume ventilator which will enhance chest wall stability and improve alveolar ventilation is the treatment of choice. Ventilatory support is needed for approximately 14 to 21 days or until the chest is adequately stabilized. A hemothorax or pneumothorax is treated by chest tubes, underwater seal drainage and surgical intervention when repair of structural damage is necessary. Chest tubes with underwater seal drainage systems are usually maintained during the entire time the patient needs ventilatory assistance to manage not only the initial hemo/penumothorax, but any which occur as a complication during positive pressure mechanical ventilation.

summary

Three phases of lung function—ventilation, diffusion and perfusion—exist simultaneously to provide oxygenation and removal of carbon dioxide from tissues. Pulmonary and nonpulmonary pathophysiological states may exist and interfere with normal function at any one of these three levels. The critical care nurse must have a thorough understanding of normal lung function and be able to assess the patient's respiratory status, to anticipate compromised lung function, and to intervene appropriately.

REFERENCES

1. B. Burrows et al., *Respiratory Insufficiency* (Chicago: Year Book Medical Publishers, 1975), p. 118.
2. R. Fraser et al., *Diagnosis of Diseases of the Chest,* Vol. 1 (Philadelphia: W. B. Saunders, 1970), pp. 196-239.
3. Burrows, op. cit., p. 119.
4. B. Felson et al., *Principles of Chest Roentgenology* (Philadelphia: W. B. Saunders, 1965), p. 127.
5. Burrows, op. cit., p. 116.
6. W. Thurlbeck, "Chronic Bronchitis and Emphysema," *Basics of RD* (New York: American Thoracic Society, 1974), p. 3.
7. W. Thurlbeck, *Chronic Airflow Obstruction in Lung Disease* (Philadelphia: W. B. Saunders, 1976), p. 386.

8. T. Petty, "Status Asthmaticus," lecture given at Pulmonary Medicine Course, March 11–14, 1975, Continuing Medical Education, University of Colorado School of Medicine.

9. P. Brannin, "Oxygen Therapy and Measures of Bronchial Hygiene," *Nursing Clinics of North America,* Vol. 9, No. 1 (1974), pp. 116-121.

10. K. Moser, "Diagnostic Measures in Pulmonary Embolism," *Basics of RD* (New York: American Thoracic Society, 1975), p. 1.

11. J. Fitzmaurice et al., "Current Concepts of Pulmonary Embolism: Implications for Nursing Practice," *Heart and Lung,* Vol. 3, No. 2 (March–April 1974), pp. 210–211.

12. H. Bendixen, "Pneumothorax," *Critical Care Medicine,* M. Weil and H. Shubin, eds. (John W. Kolen, 1974), p. 28.

13. L. Kersten, "Chest Tube Drainage System – Indications and Principles of Operation," *Heart and Lung,* Vol. 3, No. 1 (January–February 1974), p. 97.

14. C. Morgan et al., "The Care and Feeding of Chest Tubes," *American Journal of Nursing,* Vol. 72, No. 2 (February 1972), p. 307.

15. B. Shapiro et al., *Clinical Application of Respiratory Care* (Chicago: Year Book Medical Publishers, 1975), pp. 362-363.

16. Burrows, op. cit., p. 91.

17. Brannin, op. cit., p. 111.

18. L. Bryant et al., "Reappraisal of the Chest Injury from Cuffed Tracheostomy Tubes," *Journal of the American Medical Association,* Vol. 215, No. 4 (January 25, 1971), pp. 624-628.

19. M. Kudla, "The Care of the Patient with Respiratory Insufficiency," *Nursing Clinics of North America,* Vol. 8, No. 1 (March 1973), p. 184.

20. Ibid., p. 184.

21. Ibid., p. 185.

22. T. Petty, "Management of the Adult Respiratory Distress Syndrome," lecture given at Pulmonary Medicine Course, March 11–14, 1975, Continuing Medical Education, University of Colorado Medical Center.

23. Ibid.

The authors wish to acknowledge the assistance of Dr. Marvin Schwarz, Chief of Pulmonary Medicine, V.A. Hospital, Denver, in the preparation of this manuscript.

JANET KERKMAN, R.N., A.R.I.T., E.M.T.

intubation: a new role for critical care nurses in cardiopulmonary emergencies

The prompt use of endotracheal intubation in treating a cardiac arrest or pulmonary emergency is thought by some to improve the patient's chances of survival. Others feel that the establishment of ventilatory support with intubation is not necessary in cardiopulmonary resuscitation.

Intubation during cardiopulmonary emergencies from whatever cause provides an open airway allowing controlled ventilation with a self-inflating bag supplied with oxygen. Aspiration of vomitus often occurs when the stomach becomes distended with air while ventilation with a resuscitation bag and mask alone is carried out for a prolonged interval. Endotracheal intubation isolates the trachea from the gastrointestinal tract, thus preventing the catastrophe of aspiration. This section is written in support of the use of endotracheal intubation in these cases.

When the critical patient is first seen he should receive a few breaths with oropharyngeal airway, mask, and self-inflating bag connected to oxygen. Then, when further resuscitation is still needed, rapid and skillful intubation should be performed. However, care should be taken not to waste time in unsuccessful attempts at intubation by inexperienced personnel. Care must also be exercised in avoiding use of oropharyngeal airways that are too long and may stimulate vomiting in patients with full stomachs.

need for experienced personnel

The ideal method for handling cardiopulmonary emergencies in a general hospital is to have a physician skilled in endotracheal intubation and well versed in the physiology and pharmacology of cardiopulmonary emergencies available 24 hours a day, 7 days a week. In most hospitals this is essentially impossible.

This fact has led to the creation of a new role for nurses. Well-motivated, intelligent nurses can be trained to provide respiratory support in cardiopulmonary emergencies on a 24-hour basis during the absence of a well-qualified physician. This plan extends the concept of the critical care nurse who has learned to take responsibility for observation and interpretation of signs and symptoms of impending cardiopulmonary emergencies. Now the carefully trained critical care nurse can participate in the continuous delivery of critical care, not only in the recognition of cardiopulmonary emergencies but also in their management in the absence of a physician.

an approach to cardiopulmonary emergencies

All too frequently chaos develops when a cardiopulmonary emergency occurs. This problem has been solved in one community hospital as follows:

The chief of staff appointed a committee for planning appropriate management of "Cor Zero" (the code word used to alert the hospital team to the existence of a cardiopulmonary emergency) cases, consisting of one physician from each specialty including internal medicine, surgery, orthopedics, and anesthesiology. The committee proposed a team approach by allied medical personnel and developed a detailed protocol for this purpose. The protocol specified objectives, identified members, and described the responsibilities of the team. Specific actions to be taken by the team were as follows.

1. Nursing specialists trained in cardiopulmonary resuscitation direct the Cor Zero. A coronary care nurse is the team leader. The pulmonary nurse specialist performs pulmonary resuscitation and endotracheal intubation when indicated. When the attending physician is present, he may direct the cardiopulmonary resuscitation or he may ask the nurse specialist team to continue to direct and carry out the procedures. All other physicians not well versed in cardiopulmonary resuscitation

are expected to leave the procedure in the hands of the nurse specialist team.

2. The nurse leader may ask for and supervise assistance from other allied medical personnel, for cardiac massage, the drawing of blood, the administration of drugs, the starting of IVs or the acting as recorders of events.

3. The parent Cor Zero committee of physicians takes full responsibility for the actions of the cardiopulmonary resuscitation team.

4. The leader may ask for assistance from physicians who may be present.

5. The team continues resuscitation until directed to stop by the attending physician, by a member of the Cor Zero committee, or by any qualified physician who is at the scene.

6. All nursing specialists assigned to the cardiopulmonary resuscitation team are required to meet once a month for a critical review of their performance by physicians especially qualified in the management of cardiopulmonary disease.

7. Any criticisms of the cardiopulmonary team must be submitted in writing to the parent committee.

Three matters of paramount importance deserve special comment.

A. In most hospitals, especially those with limited house staff or none at all, physicians trained and experienced in cardiopulmonary resuscitation are not available during many hours of each day. Many specialized and otherwise well-qualified physicians have had only an occasional exposure to cardiopulmonary emergencies. When physicians not familiar with cardiopulmonary emergencies answer a Cor Zero without previous plan or organization, chaos is common. To have modern coronary care and critical care units without a plan to provide effective cardiopulmonary resuscitation on a 24-hour basis tends to defeat the purpose of such units.

B. The concept had to be developed that nurse specialists could act on the orders of physicians and be under their supervision without their physical presence. This concept and protocol were approved by the Colorado State Board of Medical Examiners as not in conflict with the Colorado Medical Practice Act.

C. Cardiopulmonary resuscitation, including endotracheal intubation, performed by the nurse specialist *in the absence of a physician* is highly justified and logical when the gravity of the situation is considered. For the patient who has suffered a cardiopulmonary catastrophe, death is imminent, if not inevitable. Immediate and precise efforts at resuscitation including cardiac massage, defibrillation, endotracheal intubation, respiratory support, and intravenous drugs are potentially lifesaving.

recognizing and managing cardiopulmonary emergencies

Cardiopulmonary emergencies often arise in a variety of clinical situations without previous warning. The nurse must be aware of these many and varied clinical situations in which such catastrophic events frequently occur.

In the coronary care unit the patient who develops complications such as arrhythmias, hypotension, and congestive heart failure, or has a recurrence of chest pain, is the most likely candidate for a cardiopulmonary catastrophe. Similar situations may occur with patients in the emergency room, intensive care unit, recovery room, or even on a general medical or surgical unit. Cardiopulmonary emergencies and the need for intubation often occur without warning and are abruptly announced by apnea. In other situations the need for intubation and assisted or controlled ventilation may be recognized only by arterial blood gas analysis—sometimes the sole means of recognizing serious life-threatening hypercarbia or hypoxemia.

The nurse should be aware that hypercarbia and hypoxemia have many *non*specific manifestations such as restlessness, confusion, irritability, and somnolence. She should be alert to the patient's clinical appearance, noting the degree of respiratory distress, level of consciousness, excursion of the thorax and abdomen, skin color, and temperature along with the classical vital signs.

An understanding with the attending physician regarding the nurse's use of arterial blood gas analysis in evaluating seriously ill patients is of paramount importance. Permission to collect arterial blood in seriously ill patients is usually quite easy to obtain if the physician realizes that the nursing personnel have been trained in recognizing the clinical indications of impending respiratory failure, in the technique of arterial puncture, and in the interpretation of the arterial blood gas analysis.

training for endotracheal intubation

Endotracheal intubation is a skill that can be attained by physicians or paramedical personnel who possess proper knowledge of the anatomy, have received expert instruction, and are given an opportunity to practice the newfound skill. A limiting factor for a nurse to maintain the skill of endotracheal intubation, once it has been perfected, is having enough opportunities to use the technique.

It is not the purpose of this chapter to discuss the specific technique of endotracheal intubation, which has been described completely elsewhere. The critical care nurse who is assigned the responsibility of emergency endotracheal intubation must have expert instruction, accomplished through training with an experienced anesthesiologist who must believe that training of the critical care nurse is of vital importance. The nurse, under the supervision of an anesthesiologist, goes to the operating room and gains experience in endotracheal intubation on anesthetized, relaxed patients who are in need of such management. Only after mastering the technique under these ideal conditions is she ready to begin handling emergency situations. To maintain this skill the nurse needs to have opportunities to use the techniques frequently, or she must return to the operating suite at regular intervals to improve her proficiency under a physician's supervision. The use of cadavers and/or dummy models provides only limited and inadequate experience for training in endotracheal intubation.

With such training as described above a group of nurse specialists have achieved a greater than 85 percent success rate in emergency endotracheal intubations.

equipment

The availability of proper equipment and an understanding of its purpose are essential. A standardized set of intubation equipment should be instantly

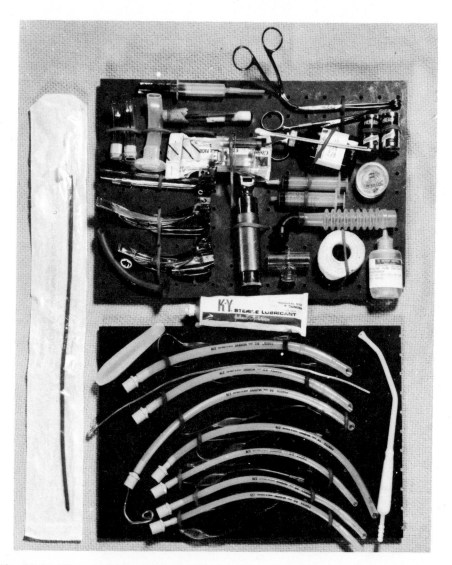

Fig. 13-13. Two sections of pegboard are cut to fit inside an attaché case. Rubber tubing is utilized to secure standardized intubation equipment to the pegboard.

available at all times. Attaché cases can be easily adapted using pegboard and rubber tubing to secure the equipment for convenient checking and rapid use (Figs. 13-13 and 13-14).

Laryngoscopes must be available in various sizes and have either straight or curved blades. Individual preference seems to be the basis for choice between the straight blade which picks up the epiglottis directly and the curved blade which inserts into the glossoepiglottic groove (above the epiglottis) and indirectly lifts the epiglottis from the laryngeal opening. Some experts consider the curved blade of greater benefit in avoiding trauma to the subepiglottic mucosa and providing more room for insertion of the tube. A #3 or #4 curved blade is adequate for most medium-size to large adults. A #1 or #2 curved blade is adequate for children from age three months to nine years; smaller straight blades are available for newborn and premature

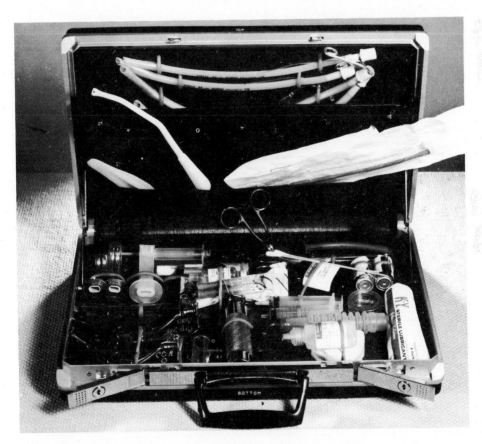

Fig. 13-14. Pegboards holding standardized intubation equipment are placed in an attaché case. The middle divider in the case separates the intubation tubes from the other equipment.

infants. Both straight and curved blades in adult and pediatric sizes should be a part of each emergency intubation setup. Fresh batteries to insure brightly lighted laryngoscopic bulbs are a crucial requirement.

Various types of intubation tubes are available. The Portex polyvinyl chloride disposable tubes with the large cylindrical cuff are excellent. These cuffs are reliable since they are used only once. The firmness of this tube is a desirable aid in intubation. Multiple use rubber tubes are also available in French sizes. Standardized 15-mm. adapters allowing a tube of any kind to be attached to a self-inflating bag unit or respirator are mandatory. French gauge tubes between sizes F32 and F36 for adult females and between sizes F34 and F40 for adult males will be utilized most frequently. In our experience, Portex tubes between sizes 6 and 7 mm. ID. for adult males will be utilized most frequently.

A good rule of thumb for children is as follows: The age of the child in years + 18 equals the French size required. Experienced anesthesiologists state that a tube which fits through the nares will most likely pass through the vocal cords. Preparation of two tubes, one of the estimated size and one of a size smaller, is a good procedure to follow.

Stylets are often placed inside tubes as an aide to insertion. Stylets should be firm, curved at one end, and long enough to bend easily over the adapter end of the endotracheal tube. Inserting the stylets and curving the endotracheal tube often aid in guiding the tube to the glottic opening. The upward curve of the tube aids in entering the glottic opening rather than the esophagus. The stylets should be pulled back approximately ½ inch from the end of the tube to prevent trauma. Bending the proximal end of the stylet over the adapter on the endotracheal tube stabilizes the position of the stylet and aids in removal. A stylet may easily perforate the trachea if not stabilized in this manner.

Suction catheters must be immediately available and should be of two types. The Yankauer pharyngeal suction tip is handy for cleaning the oropharynx, while a Teflon-coated plastic catheter is used for evacuation of secretions from the endotracheal tube. The Yankauer suction tip is rigid, allowing it to be easily introduced and manipulated in the oral cavity. The Teflon-coated plastic suction catheter does not stick to the endotracheal tube and is of adequate length for deep suctioning. Other equipment included in the attaché cases are anesthetic water-soluble jelly for lubrication of the endotracheal tube, a 10-cc. syringe for inflation of the tracheal cuff, a rubber-sheathed forceps to prevent air leak from the cuff, one-inch tape, and tincture of benzoin.

Immediate evaluation of tube placement is achieved by observing equal chest expansion and by auscultation of both sides of the chest for equal breath sounds, indicating equal ventilation of both lungs. Decreased breath sounds on the left usually indicate intubation of the right main stem bronchus and inadequate ventilation of the left lung. Intubation of the right main stem bronchus is a common error and occurs easily because it is more vertical in position. A chest x-ray should be obtained to accurately define the placement of the tube as soon as the patient's condition permits. This is ordered by the nurse according to protocol.

Securing the tube in proper position is mandatory for adequate ventilation and to prevent accidental extubation. Not infrequently, as patients arouse, they may become combative, and wrist restraints as well as sedation with drugs such as diazepam (Valium) may become necessary. Applying tincture of benzoin to each cheek and to the upper lip insures good adhesion of the tape. Secure the tube by using one-inch tape beginning on the skin beneath the ear lobe encircling the tube, crossing the upper lip, and continuing down beneath the opposite ear lobe. Lower jaw motion and/or secretions do not loosen the tube when it is taped in this manner.

An oral-pharyngeal airway is inserted into the oral cavity. It can be taped to the endotracheal tube to secure good positioning. The oral-pharyngeal airway prevents the patient from biting on the endotracheal tube and obstructing his ventilation. It also provides a route for oral suctioning.

The self-inflating bag connected to oxygen is the ideal way to ventilate the patient via an endotracheal tube during the initial phase of cardiopulmonary resuscitation until he can be moved to a critical care unit where a mechanical respirator can be applied for continued ventilatory support. Using the self-inflating bag, one can match the patient's respirations breath for breath, easily coordinate respirations with cardiac massage, and provide whatever volume is needed to ventilate the patient.

Important points to remember when utilizing the self-inflating bag attached to the endotracheal tube are the following:

1. If the patient has spontaneous efforts, it may be wise to follow and assist these at certain times. At other times the patient's rate and pattern may be inappropriate and controlled ventilation must be accomplished.
2. Hyperventilation in patients with chronic airway obstruction having a P_{CO_2} above 50 should be avoided. Excessive ventilation may lower the P_{CO_2} too rapidly, causing seizures, hypotension, and/or cardiac arrythmias.
3. Care must be taken in adding oxygen to the self-inflating bag. The valves on some bags may lock in the inspiratory position with oxygen flow rates of as low as 5 to 10 liters per minute. The locked valve prevents patient exhalation. A locked valve should be suspected when each inspiration requires greater pressure on the bag. The bag should be immediately removed from the endotracheal tube to allow the patient to exhale the trapped air.

Inserting a nasogastric tube after intubation is valuable in evacuating air and other stomach contents. Subsequent abdominal distention and possible vomiting with aspiration are thus avoided.

attitude

A discussion of such a new and controversial responsibility as intubation by the nurse specialist deserves some comment. Troublesome attitudes regarding these new responsibilities and functions of the nurse originate both from other nurses and from physicians.

Taking responsibility for techniques that deal with life-and-death situations is a new concept for nurses. We are in the early stages of developing such concepts. Consequently, many nurses are hesitant to take on duties which involve such responsibilities. Proper support from supervising physicians and hospital administration is necessary for the nurse to have enough confidence to proceed with her training. Having physicians who are eager and willing to train nurses in these skills is also important. A positive attitude by the nurse with regard to her new role in performing intubation during cardiopulmonary emergencies is a prime requirement for success. Subjective feelings concerning the patient, his condition, his family, and her own state of self-confidence are very real experiences. The nurse will have to recognize and explore such feelings before facing these tasks. The ability to become objective during cardiopulmonary emergencies and to utilize the knowledge she does possess is necessary for a successful intubation. She will also have to face up to and deal with failure.

Attitude is important in the training situation as well. This type of training is new for the nurse. For the first time she may be using cadavers of patients who have not survived cardiopulmonary resuscitation. Nurses who are not used to such an experience may feel that this is "practicing" on a patient and depriving him of his final dignity. Receiving instruction from a physician in a technique which has been the responsibility only of physicians is another new experience. Approaching these new challenges with a positive attitude is the only way the nurse can achieve success.

As the nurse is asked to take on more responsibility, especially to assume roles that heretofore have been handled by physicians, she should expect to meet resistance. The nurse must remember that anyone who has pioneered in the field of medicine has always met resistance. Only when these new programs gain wider acceptance will she find that physicians, administration, and allied medical personnel will acknowledge the value of such programs. As with any new project, the nurse must proceed with a positive attitude, physician supervision and direction, and close adherence to principle and protocol.

summary

This section was designed to describe one new facet of the critical care nurse in cardiopulmonary resuscitation. Since cardiopulmonary emergencies occur in a wide variety of clinical settings, the need for immediate cardiopulmonary resuscitation can arise at all times in any hospital. In community hospitals physicians expert in endotracheal intubation are often not available when needed. To manage cardiopulmonary resuscitation properly it has naturally evolved that a critical care nurse can and should be expert in pulmonary resuscitation and be able to intubate when indicated. Through physician supervision and guidance by a protocol with expert training by anesthesiologists, critical care nurses have successfully acquired this new technique.

A description of the manner in which one community hospital approached these problems has been given along with discussions of how the pulmonary nurse must plan and organize for cardiopulmonary emergencies.

BIBLIOGRAPHY

Bigelow, D. B., R. L. Petty, D. G. Ashbaugh, B. E. Levine, M. Nett, and S. Tyler, "Acute Respiratory Failure (Experiences of a Respiratory Care Unit)," *Medical Clinics of North America*, Vol. 51, No. 2 (March 1967), p. 323.

Fillmore, S. J., M. Shapiro, and T. Killip, "Serial Blood Gas Studies During Cardiopulmonary Resuscitation," *Annals of Medicine*, Vol. 72 (1970), p. 465.

Garvin, J. P., W. B. Neptune, L. W. Pratt, and P. Safar, "Saving the Asphyxiating Patient," *Patient Care*, June 15, 1971, p. 22.

Grace, W. J., "Intensive Care—What Are We Talking About?" *Heart and Lung*, Vol. 1 (1972), p. 187.

Lissauer, W. S., and D. B. Bigelow, Cardiopulmonary Resuscitation, A New Role for Nurses. To be published.

Milstein, B. B., *Cardiac Arrest and Resuscitation* (Chicago: Year Book Medical Publishers, 1963), pp. 121-128.

Safar, P., and D. F. Proctor, *Respiratory Therapy* (Philadelphia: F. A. Davis Company, 1965), pp. 29-92.

Sitzman, J. E., "Nursing Management of the Acutely Ill Respiratory Patient," *Heart and Lung*, Vol. 1, No. 2 (March–April 1972), p. 207.

Talmage, E. A., "House Officer Training for Cardiovascular Resuscitation," *Guthrie Clinical Bulletin*, Vol. 41 (1971), p. 40.

Votteri, B. A., "Hand-Operated Emergency Ventilation Devices," *Heart and Lung*, Vol. 1, No. 2 (March–April, 1972), p. 277.

JOSEPH O. BROUGHTON, M.D.

14 14

assessment skills for the nurse: respiratory system

understanding blood gases

Blood gases are obtained in a variety of clinical situations, but they are obtained for two major reasons: (1) to determine if the patient is well oxygenated, and (2) to determine the acid-base status of the patient, concentrating on either the respiratory component, the metabolic (nonrespiratory) component, or most often, both respiratory and metabolic components of a patient's acid-base status. In the following discussion, the term *nonrespiratory* will be used interchangeably with the term *metabolic*.

Most often blood gases are measured on arterial blood rather than on venous blood for two reasons.

1. Studying arterial blood is a good way to sample a mixture of blood that has come from various parts of the body. Blood obtained from a vein in an extremity gives information mostly about that extremity and can be quite misleading if the metabolism in the extremity differs from the metabolism of the body as a whole, as it often does. This difference is accentuated if the extremity is cold or underperfused as in a patient in shock, if the patient has done local exercise with the extremity such as opening and closing his fist, if there is local infection in the extremity, etc. Sometimes blood is sampled through a central venous catheter (CVP catheter) in hopes of getting mixed venous blood, but even in the superior vena cava or right atrium where a CVP catheter

ends there is usually incomplete mixing of venous blood from various parts of the body. For complete mixing of the blood, one would have to obtain a blood sample from the pulmonary artery through a Swan-Ganz catheter, for example; and even then one would not get information about how well the lungs are oxygenating the blood.

2. The second reason for selecting arterial blood is that it gives the added information of how well the lungs are oxygenating the blood. Oxygen measurements of mixed venous blood can tell if the tissues are getting oxygenated, but cannot separate the contribution of the heart from that of the lungs. In other words, if the mixed venous blood oxygen is low it means that either heart or lungs or both are at fault. So if mixed venous blood has a low oxygen concentration, it means either (a) that the lungs have not oxygenated the arterial blood well and that when the tissues extract their usual amount of oxygen from arterial blood, the resulting venous blood has a low oxygen concentration, or (b) that the heart is not circulating the blood well so that it is taking blood a long time to circulate through the tissues. The tissues, therefore, must extract more than the usual amount of oxygen from each cardiac cycle since the blood is flowing slowly. This produces a low venous O_2 concentration. If it is known that the arterial oxygen concentration is normal (indicating that the lungs are doing their job), but the mixed venous oxygen concentration is low, then one can infer that the heart and circulation are failing.

One advantage of using mixed venous blood instead of arterial blood is that if the oxygen concentration in mixed venous blood is normal, one can infer that the tissues are receiving enough oxygen — that is, both ventilation and circulation are adequate.

oxygen

There are three ways to measure oxygen in blood: (1) the number of ml. of oxygen carried by 100 ml. of blood, (2) the P_{O_2} or pressure exerted by oxygen dissolved in the plasma, and (3) the oxygen saturation of hemoglobin, which is a measure of the percentage of oxygen that hemoglobin is carrying related to the total amount the hemoglobin could carry, or

$$O_2 \text{ Sat} = \frac{\text{Amount of oxygen that hemoglobin is carrying}}{\text{Maximum amount of oxygen that hemoglobin can carry}} \times 100$$

The first of these three methods is the easiest to understand but the most difficult to measure, so it is not used routinely. The latter two methods which are used routinely are more understandable when compared to the first method in Table 14-1. Each gram of hemoglobin in 100 ml. of blood can carry a maximum of 1.34 ml. of oxygen, so if a patient has 15 gm.Hgb./100 ml. blood, then each 100 ml. of blood can carry 15 × 1.34 cc. or 20.1 cc. of oxygen. If hemoglobin is only 97 percent saturated (carrying 97 percent of the total it is able to carry), then it carries 97 percent of 20.1 ml. or 19.4 ml.

The table reminds us that the majority of oxygen carried by the blood is

table 14-1
how oxygen is carried in blood

Dissolved in plasma .... 0.3 ml./100 ml. blood ....Reflected by P_{O_2} 90 mm. Hg
Combined with Hgb. .....19.4 ml./100 ml. blood ....Reflected by O_2 Sat Hgb. 97%
Total in whole blood.......19.7 ml./100 ml. blood

carried by hemoglobin, and that a very small amount is dissolved in plasma. The percent saturation of hemoglobin with oxygen, then, gives a close estimate of the total amount of oxygen carried in blood. The P_{O_2} measurement, however, tells only of the pressure exerted by the small amount of oxygen that is dissolved in plasma. P_{O_2} is widely used and is valuable because P_{O_2} (pressure of oxygen dissolved in plasma) and O_2 Sat of Hgb. (which is closely related to the total oxygen content of whole blood) are related to each other in a definite fashion and the relationship has been charted—the oxyhemoglobin dissociation curve (Fig. 14-1). When the P_{O_2} in plasma is high, Hgb. carries much oxygen. When the P_{O_2} is low, Hgb. carries less oxygen. Once this relationship is known, P_{O_2} is just as valuable as a measurement of total O_2 content or the percentage of oxygen that hemoglobin is carrying. The relationship between P_{O_2} and O_2 saturation of hemoglobin is not a linear one, so that for a given rise or fall in P_{O_2} there is not always the same amount of rise or fall in O_2 saturation of hemoglobin. Instead, for very low P_{O_2}, a rise in P_{O_2} is associated with a more rapid rise in O_2 saturation; and for P_{O_2} in the normal range or higher, a rise in P_{O_2} is associated with a very small rise in O_2 saturation. This relationship is much easier to understand if one looks at the oxygen dissociation curve for hemoglobin. In simple terms, the dissociation curve indicates that in environments where the P_{O_2} is high, such as the capillaries of the lungs, hemoglobin combines with and carries a high percentage of the total oxygen it could carry; in environments where the P_{O_2} is low, such as the capillaries in the tissues, hemoglobin carries a lower percentage of the total oxygen it could carry, having given up the difference in oxygen for use by the tissues.

The dissociation curve presented applies only to normal conditions. In the presence of acidosis or fever, the entire dissociation curve is shifted to the right, so that for a given oxygen saturation the P_{O_2} is greater than usual, and more oxygen is available for the tissues. In the presence of alkalosis, hemoglobin is more stingy and for a given oxygen saturation, the P_{O_2} is lower than usual. Certain abnormal types of hemoglobin may shift the dissociation curve to the right or the left, and the presence of certain compounds such as 2,3 diphosphoglycerate (2,3 DPG) may also shift the dissociation curve. 2,3 DPG in excess amounts shifts the curve to the right, thereby making more oxygen available to the tissues for a given O_2 Sat of Hgb., for 2,3 DPG decreases the affinity of hemoglobin for oxygen.

One should always relate the oxygen content of blood to the FIO_2 (the fractional percentage of oxygen in the inspired air). For instance, an O_2 saturation of Hgb. of 96 percent is normal if the patient is breathing room air

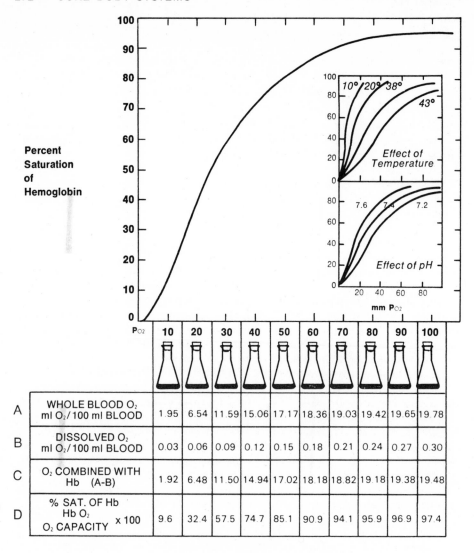

Fig. 14-1. HbO₂ dissociation curves. The large graph shows a single dissociation curve, applicable when the pH of the blood is 7.40 and temperature 38° C. The blood O₂ tension and saturation of patients with CO₂ retention, acidosis, alkalosis, fever, or hypothermia will not fit this curve because the curve shifts to the right when temperature, pH, or Pco₂ is changed. Effects on the HbO₂ dissociation curve of change in temperature and in pH are shown in the smaller graphs. (From J. H. Comroe, *Physiology of Respiration*, ed. 2. Copyright © 1974 by Year Book Medical Publishers, Inc., Chicago. Used by permission.)

which has an FIO_2 of 21, but is quite abnormal if the FIO_2 is —40. Some hospitals formally measure the A-a oxygen gradient (the difference between Po_2 in alveolar air and Po_2 in arterial blood), but much the same information can be obtained if one compares the Pao_2 or O_2 Sat of Hgb. to the FIO_2.

Normal values for blood gases are given in Table 14-2. Following this the main emphasis will concern acid-base interpretation (Table 14-3).

table 14-2
normal blood gas values

	ARTERIAL BLOOD	MIXED VENOUS BLOOD
pH	7.40 (7.35–7.45)	7.36 (7.31–7.41)
Po_2	80–100 mm. Hg	35–40 mm. Hg
O_2 Sat	95% or greater	70–75%
Pco_2	35–45 mm. Hg	41–51 mm. Hg
HCO_3	22–26 mEq./L.	22–26 mEq./L.
Base excess (B.E.)	—2–+2	—2–+2

Note that in Table 14-2 only three measurements—Po_2, O_2 saturation, and Pco_2—are actually measurements of gases. However, all should be determined in blood gas analyses. It is imperative that a measure of the nonrespiratory (or metabolic) component be included, and actual HCO_3 and base excess are the most useful. Many other terms may be given on a blood gas report, but the nurse needs to be concerned only with the ones listed in Table 14-2.

Older persons have values for Po_2 and O_2 saturation near the lower part of the normal range, and younger people tend to have high normal values.

Normal values for mixed venous blood are more variable than for arterial blood but representative normals are given in Table 14-2. There is not enough difference in normal values of HCO_3 and base excess between arterial and mixed venous blood to warrant remembering a different set of values for venous blood.

An acid is any substance that can donate a hydrogen ion, H^+. H^+ can be thought of as the most important part of an acid substance.

table 14-3
definitions

Acid: A substance that can donate hydrogen ions, H^+. Example:
$$H_2CO_3 \longrightarrow H^+ + HCO_3^-$$
(acid)

Base: A substance that can accept hydrogen ions, H^+.
All bases are alkaline substances. Examples:
$$OH^- \quad + \quad H^+ \longrightarrow H_2O$$
$$HCO_3^- \quad + \quad H^+ \longrightarrow H_2CO_3$$
(bases)

Many substances may include H in their chemical structure, but some cannot donate the H because it is too tightly bound. Only those substances that can give up their H$^+$ are acids.

Bases are substances that can accept or combine with H$^+$. The terms *base* and *alkali* are used interchangeably.

Each of the acid-base parameters (Table 14-4) will now be discussed in more detail.

table 14-4
acid-base parameters

pH measurement = Only way to tell if body is too acid or too alkaline
Acidemia = Acid condition of the blood — pH < 7.35
Alkalemia = Alkaline condition of the blood — pH > 7.45
Acidosis = Process causing acidemia
Alkalosis = Process causing alkalemia

The pH measurement is the only way to tell if the body is too acid or too alkaline. Low pH numbers (below 7.35) indicate an acid state, and high pH numbers (above 7.45) indicate an alkaline state.

If the numbers are lower than 7.35, there is acidemia, and if higher than 7.45, alkalemia. Acid*emia* refers to a condition in which the *blood* is too acid. Acid*osis* refers to the *process* in the patient which causes the acidemia, and the adjective for the process would be acid*otic*. Alkal*osis* refers to the *process* in the patient which causes the alkal*emia*, and the adjective for this process is alkal*otic*.

This much time has been spent in defining the terms because later it will be seen that in a patient there may be more than one process occurring at a time. For instance, if both an acidosis and an alkalosis are occurring at once, then the pH will tell us which is the stronger of the two processes. The pH will be below 7.35 if the acidosis is the stronger, above 7.45 if the alkalosis is the stronger and between 7.35 and 7.45 if the acidosis and alkalosis are of nearly equal strength. So the pH value of blood represents an average of the acidoses and alkaloses which may be occurring. This will be explained in more detail later in the chapter.

the respiratory parameter: PCO$_2$

The PCO_2 refers to the pressure or tension exerted by dissolved CO_2 gas in the blood (Table 14-5). The PCO_2 is influenced *only* by respiratory causes although this is an oversimplification; still remember that PCO_2 *is influenced only by the lungs*.

Where does the CO_2 come from? It is present only in very tiny amounts in the air we breathe. It comes indirectly from foods we eat. As a result of metabolism for the production of energy, foods are converted by the body tissues to water and CO_2 gas. When the pressure of CO_2 in the cells exceeds 40 mm. Hg (the normal arterial value), the CO_2 spills over from the cells

table 14-5
P_{CO_2}, the respiratory parameter

P_{CO_2} = Pressure (tension) of dissolved CO_2 gas in blood
P_{CO_2} — Influenced only by respiratory causes

$$\text{Food} \xrightarrow[\text{by body}]{\text{converted}} H_2O + CO_2 + \text{energy}$$

$$CO_2 + H_2O \rightleftharpoons H_2CO_3 \rightleftharpoons HCO_3^- + H^+$$

Normal P_{CO_2} = normal ventilation
High P_{CO_2} = hypoventilation
Low P_{CO_2} = hyperventilation

---

into the plasma. In plasma, CO_2 may combine with H_2O to form H_2CO_3 (carbonic acid), but there is actually 800 times as much CO_2 in dissolved gas in plasma as is converted to H_2CO_3.

You should consider CO_2 gas an acid substance because when it combines with water, an acid is formed — carbonic acid, H_2CO_3.

H_2CO_3 dissociates into hydrogen ion, H^+ and biocarbonate HCO_3^-. Much of the H^+ forms a loose association with the plasma proteins (is buffered), thus reducing the free H^+. The body has to get rid of the waste product, CO_2, and can do so in two ways:

1. The less important way is by converting the CO_2 gas to carbonic acid, H_2CO_3, which dissociates to H^+ and HCO_3^-. The H^+ can be excreted by the kidneys mainly in the form of NH_4^+, and HCO_3^- can also be excreted by the kidneys.
2. A much more important way is to have the lungs get rid of the CO_2.

Getting rid of CO_2 gas, then, is one of the main functions of the lungs, and a very important relationship exists between the amount of ventilation and the amount of P_{CO_2} in blood. If the P_{CO_2} in blood (i.e., the dissolved CO_2 gas in blood) is too high, it means that the lungs are not providing enough ventilation. This is called *hypoventilation.* Hypoventilation can thus be detected by finding high levels of P_{CO_2} in the blood. If the P_{CO_2} is too low, there is excessive ventilation by the lungs, or *hyperventilation,* and if the P_{CO_2} is normal, there is exactly the right amount of ventilation. This relationship between P_{CO_2} in blood and amount of ventilation is very important, P_{CO_2} being much more important than P_{O_2} in judging whether there is normal ventilation, hyperventilation, or hypoventilation, for there are other factors (such as shunting, diffusion abnormalities, etc.) which lower the P_{O_2} without reducing ventilation.

As seen in Table 14-6, there are only two abnormal conditions associated with abnormalities in P_{CO_2}: respiratory acidosis (high P_{CO_2}) and respiratory alkalosis (low P_{CO_2}).

The causes of respiratory acidosis (high P_{CO_2}) are (1) obstructive lung disease (mainly chronic bronchitis, emphysema and occasionally asthma), (2) oversedation, head trauma, anesthesia, and other causes of reduced function of the respiratory center, (3) neuromuscular disorders such as

table 14-6
respiratory abnormalities

PARAMETER	CONDITION	MECHANISM
$\uparrow P_{CO_2}$	Respiratory acidosis	Decreased elimination by lungs of CO_2 gas (Hypoventilation)
$\downarrow P_{CO_2}$	Respiratory alkalosis	Increased elimination by lungs of CO_2 gas (Hyperventilation)

table 14-7
causes of respiratory acidosis ($\uparrow P_{CO_2}$)

1. Obstructive lung disease
2. Oversedation and other causes of reduced function of the respiratory center (even with normal lungs)
3. Neuromuscular disorders
4. Hypoventilation with mechanical ventilator
5. Other causes of hypoventilation

myasthenia gravis or the Guillain-Barré syndrome, (4) hypoventilation with a mechanical ventilator, and (5) other rarer causes of hypoventilation (such as the Pickwickian syndrome). It should be noted that *respiratory* acidosis may occur even with normal lungs if the respiratory center is depressed.

The term *respiratory acidosis* means elevated P_{CO_2} due to hypoventilation.

The causes of respiratory alkalosis (low P_{CO_2}) are hypoxia, nervousness, anxiety, pulmonary emboli, pulmonary fibrosis, pregnancy, hyperventilation with mechanical ventilator, and other causes of hyperventilation.

The term *respiratory alkalosis* means low P_{CO_2} due to hyperventilation.

table 14-8
causes of respiratory alkalosis ($\downarrow P_{CO_2}$)

1. Hypoxia
2. Nervousness and anxiety
3. Pulmonary embolus, fibrosis, etc.
4. Pregnancy
5. Hyperventilation with mechanical ventilator
6. Other causes of hyperventilation

the nonrespiratory (metabolic) parameters: HCO_3^- and base excess

Bicarbonate and base excess are influenced *only* by nonrespiratory causes, not by respiratory causes. Again, this is a simplification, but a very important fact to remember—*bicarbonate and base excess are influenced only by nonrespiratory processes.* We can define a *metabolic process* for our purposes as anything other than respiratory causes that affects the patient's acid-base status. Examples of common metabolic (nonrespiratory) processes would be diabetic acidosis and uremia. When a nonrespiratory process leads to the accumulation of acids in the body or losses of bicarbonate, bicarbonate values drop below the normal range and base excess values become negative. On the other hand, when a nonrespiratory process causes loss of acid or accumulation of excess bicarbonate, bicarbonate values rise above normal and base excess values become positive. Base excess may be thought of as representing an excess of bicarbonate or other base. Bicarbonate, then, is base — or in other words, an alkaline substance. The term *base excess* refers principally to bicarbonate but also to the other bases in blood (mainly plasma proteins and hemoglobin).

As seen in Table 14-9, there are only two abnormal conditions associated with abnormalities in HCO_3^- or base excess: nonrespiratory alkalosis and nonrespiratory acidosis. (Nonvolatile acid is any acid other than Pco_2–H_2CO_3.)

table 14-9
nonrespiratory abnormalities

PARAMETER	CONDITION	MECHANISM
↑ HCO_3^- or ↑ B.E.	Nonrespiratory (metabolic) alkalosis	1. Nonvolatile acid is lost, or 2. HCO_3^- is gained
↓ HCO_3^- or ↓ B.E.	Nonrespiratory (metabolic) acidosis	1. Nonvolatile acid is added (using up HCO_3^-) or 2. HCO_3^- is lost

The causes of nonrespiratory (metabolic) alkalosis (increased HCO_3^-) are: (1) diuretic therapy with mercurial diuretics, ethacrynic acid, furosemide, and thiazide diuretics, (2) Cushing's disease, (3) treatment with corticosteriods, for example, prednisone or cortisone, (4) aldosteronism, (5) loss of acid-containing fluid from the upper GI tract as by nasogastric suction or vomit-

table 14-10
causes of nonrespiratory (metabolic) alkalosis (↑ HCO_3^-)

1. Diuretic Rx — mercurial, ethacrynic acid (Edecrin), furosemide (Lasix), thiazides
2. Cushing's disease
3. Rx with corticosteroids (prednisone, cortisone, etc.)
4. Primary aldosteronism

Augmented renal excretion of H^+, K^+, and Cl^-

5. Fluid losses from upper GI tract — vomiting or N-G tube causing loss of acid
6. Relief of chronic hypercapnia

ing (this loss of acid from the stomach leaves the body with a relative excess of alkali) and (6) relief of chronic hypercapnia. It will take the body several days to correct its compensation (accumulation of excess HCO_3^-) for hypercapnia after the hypercapnia is suddenly relieved.

The first four causes listed are due to excessive acid and potassium and chloride excretion by the kidneys. Usually, replacing potassium and chloride allows the kidneys to stop excreting acid, thus correcting the metabolic alkalosis. Treatment with two other diuretics, spironolactone (Aldactone) and triamterene (Dyrenium), does not cause metabolic alkalosis.

The following is an explanation of the relationship between hypokalemia (low K^+), hypochloremia (low Cl^-) and metabolic alkalosis. Normally in the kidney Na^+ and Cl^- pass from the blood into the urine at the glomerulus. Further along in the tubules of the kidney this Na^+, which is in the urine, must be reabsorbed from the urine into the kidney tubule cells and then into the blood.

Because Na^+ has a positive charge ($+$), when it is reabsorbed into the cells, the Na^+ must either:

1. Be reabsorbed with something that has a negative charge ($-$) like Cl^- or

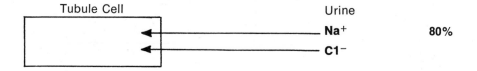

2. Enter the tubule cell in exchange for something else that has a positive charge, like K^+ or H^+ (which passes from the tubule cell to the urine).

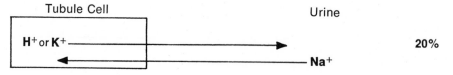

Fig. 14-2. Low Cl^- and low K^+ can cause metabolic alkalosis.

Normally, 80 percent of the Na^+ is reabsorbed while accompanied by Cl^- and 20 percent is exchanged for K^+ or H^+.

When there is hypochloremia ($\downarrow Cl^-$), the amount of Na^+ that is reabsorbed in the company of Cl^- is reduced and more Na^+ must be exchanged for K^+ or H^+. When Na^+ is exchanged for K^+ and H^+, the loss of H^+ represents a loss of acid, leaving the patient alkalotic — therefore a hypochloremic alkalosis.

When Na^+ is exchanged for K^+ and H^+, only a small amount of K^+ is available, and when this is used up the patient becomes hypokalemic and H^+ is lost. The loss of H^+ is a loss of acid, leaving the patient with an alkalosis — hypokalemic alkalosis.

A rare cause of nonrespiratory alkalosis, which unfortunately is not reflected by an elevated bicarbonate in the blood, is the intravenous infusion of phenytoin (Dilantin) which has a very alkaline pH. Infusion of this alkaline substance causes a short-lived alkalemia not associated with elevated HCO_3^-.

The causes of nonrespiratory (metabolic) acidosis (low HCO_3^-) can be divided into those causes in which there is an increase in the unmeasured anions and those causes in which there is no such increase (Table 14-11). Unmeasured anions are acids that accumulate in certain diseases or poisonings. If one subtracts the sum of HCO_3^- and Cl^- concentration from Na^+ concentration and finds a difference greater than 15, there is said to be an increase in unmeasured anions. Conditions causing this are diabetic ketoacidosis, alcoholic ketoacidosis, poisonings (salicylate, ethylene glycol, methyl alcohol, paraldehyde), lactic acidosis, renal failure and intravenous hyperalimentation. In these cases there is accumulation of or ingestion of an unusual acid. Conditions that cause a metabolic acidosis without an increase in unmeasured anions are diarrhea, drainage of pancreatic juice, ureterosigmoidostomy, treatment with acetazolamide (Diamox), renal tubular acidosis, and treatment with ammonium chloride. In most of these latter conditions there is a deficit of bicarbonate, leaving relatively too much acid.

table 14-11
causes of nonrespiratory (metabolic) acidosis (↓ HCO_3^-)

WITH INCREASE IN UNMEASURED ANIONS	WITHOUT INCREASE IN UNMEASURED ANIONS
Diabetic ketoacidosis	Diarrhea
Alcoholic ketoacidosis	Drainage of pancreatic juice
Poisonings	Ureterosigmoidostomy
Salicylate	Rx with acetazolamide (Diamox)
Ethylene glycol	Rx with NH_4Cl
Methyl alcohol	Renal tubular acidosis
Paraldehyde (rarely)	
Lactic acidosis	
Renal failure	
Intravenous alimentation	

In all of the conditions in the left-hand column there is an accumulation of an abnormal acid substance in blood which then reacts with and uses up some of the usual amount of bicarbonate, leaving the patient with reduced levels of bicarbonate and also of base excess.

One of the most important causes of nonrespiratory acidosis is lactic acidosis. Whenever body tissues do not have enough oxygen they lose their ability to metabolize lactic acid which then accumulates in the blood. This lactic acid then combines with some of the normal amount of bicarbonate, using up the bicarbonate. In a cardiac arrest, we customarily administer bicarbonate, about 1 ampul (44 mEq.) every 5 minutes, to resupply the bicarbonate which is used up by combining with lactic acid. Other conditions besides cardiac arrest which may be associated with lactic acidosis are shock, severe heart failure and severe hypoxemia.

The metabolic acidosis resulting from intravenous hyperalimentation is caused when the synthetic amino acid mixtures contain an excess of cationic amino acids in relation to other organic anions.

To review (Table 14-12), P_{CO_2} is the respiratory parameter, is a gas, is an acid, and is regulated by the lungs. HCO_3^- and base excess are nonrespiratory parameters, occur in solution, are bases (alkaline substances), and are reguated mainly by the kidneys (not by the lungs).

table 14-12

P_{CO_2} – Respiratory Parameter
  Gas
  Acid
  Regulated by the lungs
HCO_3^- or Base Excess – Nonrespiratory Parameter
  Solution
  Base
  Regulated mainly by the kidneys

Where does the CO_2 content fit in this scheme? Determination of electrolytes consists of Na^+, K^+, Cl^-, and CO_2. In this case CO_2 is an abbreviation for CO_2 content; if the term CO_2 CONTENT were used it would improve understanding. Note that in conversation CO_2 is sometimes used to mean CO_2 content (mainly bicarbonate) and sometimes to mean CO_2 GAS. This double use of the term CO_2 is one of the main reasons understanding acid-base problems is hard. Use the terms CO_2 CONTENT and CO_2 GAS to avoid confusion.

Table 14-13 shows that CO_2 content is made up mainly of bicarbonate (HCO_3^-) and to a lesser extent, dissolved CO_2 gas. The normal value of CO_2 content, 25.2 mEq./L., consists of 24 mEq./L. of HCO_3^- and 1.2 mEq./L. of dissolved CO_2 gas. The 1.2 mEq./L. of dissolved CO_2 gas is expressed in different terminology, so P_{CO_2} of 40 mm. Hg equals 1.2 mEq./L. To convert from mm. Hg to mEq./L., the conversion factor is 0.03, so 40 mm. Hg $\times$ 0.03 = 1.2 mEq./L.

table 14-13

HCO_3^-	24 mEq./L.
Dissolved CO_2 gas	1.2 mEq./L. = 40 mm. Hg P_{CO_2}
CO_2 content	25.2 mEq./L.

In Table 14-14 you will note that the ratio of HCO_3^- to P_{CO_2} is 24:1.2 or 20:1. The body always tries to keep this ratio of HCO_3^- to P_{CO_2} stable at 20:1. That is, the ratio of alkali (HCO_3^-) to acid (P_{CO_2}) is normally 20:1. As long as the ratio remains 20:1, the pH remains normal. If bicarbonate (HCO_3^-) or base excess increases, there is alkalosis causing the pH to rise. If HCO_3^- or

table 14-14

$$\frac{\text{HCO}_3^- \ (\text{base})}{\text{P}_{\text{CO}_2} \ (\text{acid})} = \frac{24 \ \text{mEq./L.}}{1.2 \ \text{mEq./L.}} = \frac{20}{1}$$

base excess falls, there is acidosis and the pH falls. IF THE pH CHANGE IS DUE MAINLY TO CHANGE IN BICARBONATE (OR BASE EXCESS), IT IS SAID TO BE DUE TO NONRESPIRATORY (METABOLIC) CAUSES.

Just the opposite happens with P_{CO_2} which, remember, is an acid substance. If the P_{CO_2} rises, there is an acidosis causing the pH to fall. If the P_{CO_2} falls, there is an alkalosis and the pH rises. IF THE pH CHANGE IS DUE MAINLY TO CHANGES IN P_{CO_2}, IT IS SAID TO BE DUE TO RESPIRATORY CAUSES.

As seen in Table 14-15, acid-base abnormalities can be separated into just four categories to make understanding them easier. First they are divided by pH into either alkalemia or acidemia. Next they are subdivided into either nonrespiratory (metabolic) or respiratory causes. This is the procedure one uses in interpreting acid base abnormalities.

table 14-15
causes of alkalemia and acidemia

TYPES		PRIMARY ABNORMALITY
Alkalemia (high pH)	Nonrespiratory (metabolic)	↑ HCO_3^-
	Respiratory	↓ P_{CO_2}
Acidemia (low pH)	Nonrespiratory (metabolic)	↓ HCO_3^-
	Respiratory	↑ P_{CO_2}

For example, if pH is high there is an alkalemia. There may be two types of alkalemia: (1) nonrespiratory, in which the primary abnormality is due to an increase in bicarbonate (example, a person who has taken too much bicarbonate or baking soda), and (2) respiratory, in which the primary abnormality is hyperventilation with loss of CO_2 gas. CO_2 gas is an acid substance; when CO_2 gas is lost (due to hyperventilation) an alkalosis occurs. (An example would be a nervous person having a hyperventilation attack.)

If the pH is low, there is an acidemia, and there are just two types of acidemia: (1) nonrespiratory, in which the primary abnormality is loss of

HCO_3^-, usually due to reaction with excessive metabolic acids (an example is diabetic acidosis in which ketoacids accumulate; these acids then react with the normal amount of HCO_3^-, using up HCO_3^- and leaving HCO_3^- and base excess levels low) and (2) respiratory, in which there is an accumulation of CO_2 gas (high P_{CO_2}) which, you remember, is an acid substance (an example is a patient with acute respiratory failure who *hypo*ventilates because his airways are obstructed by mucus). In respiratory acidosis there is an accumulation of volatile acid — CO_2 gas, but in nonrespiratory acidosis the acids which accumulate are not gases.

There are two ways in which an abnormal pH may be returned toward normal: (1) compensation, and (2) correction (Table 14-16). In *compensation*, the system not primarily affected is responsible for returning the pH toward normal. For example, if there is respiratory acidosis (high P_{CO_2}) the kidneys *compensate* by retaining bicarbonate to return the ratio of HCO_3^- to P_{CO_2} to 20:1, for when the ratio is 20:1, the pH is normal.

table 14-16
compensation vs. correction of acid-base abnormalities

In both: Abnormal pH is returned toward normal.
Compensation: Abnormal pH is returned toward normal BY ALTERING THE COMPONENT NOT PRIMARILY AFFECTED, i.e., if P_{CO_2} is high, HCO_3^- is retained to compensate.
Correction: Abnormal pH is returned toward normal BY ALTERING THE COMPONENT PRIMARILY AFFECTED, i.e., if P_{CO_2} is high, P_{CO_2} is lowered, correcting the abnormality.

In *correction*, the system primarily affected is repaired, returning the pH toward normal. For example, if there is respiratory acidosis (high P_{CO_2}) vigorous bronchial hygiene may improve ventilation and lower P_{CO_2} returning the pH toward normal. In most cases, we as physicians, nurses, and paramedical persons are more interested in correcting the abnormality than in helping the body to compensate. In both compensation and correction the pH is returned toward normal. The body tries hard to maintain a normal pH, for the various enzyme systems in all organs function correctly only when the pH is normal.

Next we will discuss how the body compensates for the various acid-base abnormalities. Remember, the body compensates for abnormalities by trying to return the ratio of HCO_3^- to P_{CO_2} to 20:1, for if this ratio is 20:1, the pH is normal. If the primary process is respiratory, then the compensating system is metabolic, and vice versa. When the lungs compensate for a nonrespiratory abnormality, compensation occurs in hours, but the kidneys take 2 to 4 days to compensate for a respiratory abnormality.

In the following four examples the first column lists normal values for the parameters listed in the second column. The uncompensated state is listed in the third column, and the last column demonstrates how compensation takes place. The primary abnormality is enclosed in a box.

table 14-17
compensation for respiratory acidosis

NORMAL		ABNORMAL	COMPENSATED
24	HCO_3^-, mEq./L.	24	36
1.2	PCO_2, mEq./L.	1.8	1.8
40	PCO_2, mm. Hg	60	60
20:1	ratio	13:1	20:1
7.40	pH	7.23	7.40

In primary respiratory acidosis, characterized by elevated levels of PCO_2 (an acid) the system at fault is the respiratory system, and compensation occurs through metabolic process. To compensate, the kidneys excrete more acid and excrete less HCO_3^-, thus allowing levels of HCO_3^- to rise, returning the ratio of HCO_3^- to PCO_2 toward 20:1 and therefore returning pH toward normal.

If the PCO_2 is high (respiratory acidosis) but the pH is normal it means that the kidneys have had time to retain HCO_3^- to compensate for the elevated PCO_2 and that the process is not acute (has been present at least a few days to give the kidneys time to compensate).

table 14-18
compensation for respiratory alkalosis

NORMAL		ABNORMAL	COMPENSATED
0	B.E.	+2.5	−5
24	HCO_3^-, mEq./L.	24	18
1.2	PCO_2, mEq./L.	0.9	0.9
40	PCO_2, mm. Hg	30	30
20:1	ratio	27:1	20:1
7.40	pH	7.52	7.40

In primary respiratory alkalosis, characterized by low PCO_2, compensation occurs through metabolic means. The kidneys compensate by excreting HCO_3^- thus returning the ratio of HCO_3^- to PCO_2 back toward 20:1, and this compensation by the kidneys takes 2 to 3 days.

In primary nonrespiratory acidosis, the major abnormality is low HCO_3^- or base excess. In most cases excess acids such as ketoacids in diabetic ketoacidosis have reacted with the normal amounts of HCO_3^- using up some of the HCO_3^- and leaving a low level of HCO_3^-. The body compensates by hyperventilating, thus lowering the PCO_2 so that the ratio of HCO_3^- to PCO_2 returns toward 20:1. Because the compensating system is the lungs, compensa-

table 14-19
compensation for nonrespiratory acidosis

NORMAL			ABNORMAL	COMPENSATED
0	B.E.		-17	-10
24	HCO_3^-, mEq./L.		12	12
1.2	P_{CO_2}, mEq./L.		1.2	0.6
40	P_{CO_2}, mm. Hg		40	20
20:1	ratio		10:1	20:1
7.40	pH		7.11	7.40

tion can occur in hours. However, if the nonrespiratory acidosis is severe, the lungs may not be able to blow off enough CO_2 gas to compensate fully.

table 14-20
compensation for nonrespiratory alkalosis

NORMAL			ABNORMAL	COMPENSATED
0	B.E.		$+13$	$+9$
24	HCO_3^-, mEq./L.		36	36
1.2	P_{CO_2}, mEq./L.		1.2	1.8
40	P_{CO_2}, mm. Hg		40	60
20:1	ratio		30:1	20:1
7.40	pH		7.57	7.40

If the primary disturbance is nonrespiratory alkalosis (i.e., presence of excess HCO_3^-), the body compensates with the respiratory system by hypoventilating so that P_{CO_2} rises and the ratio of HCO_3^- to P_{CO_2} is returned toward the normal of 20:1, therefore returning the pH to normal.

In this instance respiratory compensation is by hypoventilation, and this occurs over one or several hours. Hypoventilation allows P_{CO_2} to rise only to a maximum of 50 to 60 mm. Hg before other stimuli of ventilation such as hypoxia take over to prevent further hypoventilation. In compensating for one abnormality, high HCO_3^-, the body creates another abnormality, high P_{CO_2}, but in doing so brings the ratio of HCO_3^- to P_{CO_2} to 20:1, allowing the pH to return to normal in spite of two abnormalities. These two abnormalities balance each other.

It is important to realize that in each of these situations the body's compensation is only an effort to return the pH to normal, and the primary abnormality is not corrected. The physician's definitive treatment is aimed at correcting the primary abnormality.

For instance, if the primary problem is excess HCO_3^- (nonrespiratory alkalosis), treatment is directed toward getting rid of excess HCO_3^- rather than just allowing P_{CO_2} to rise and normalize the ratio. Excess HCO_3^- can be corrected by giving the patient acetazolamide (Diamox) to make his kidneys excrete more HCO_3^-, or more commonly by giving KCl to allow the kidneys to excrete K^+ and Cl^- rather than acids. Sometimes ammonium chloride (NH_4Cl), arginine monohydrochloride or even hydrochloric acid (HCl) is given to react with the excessive HCO_3^-, thereby correcting the metabolic alkalosis.

Respiratory alkalosis (low P_{CO_2}) is treated by getting the patient to stop hyperventilating.

Nonrespiratory acidosis, where excess acids have used up HCO_3^- or HCO_3^- has been lost, is treated by supplying HCO_3^- in the form $NaHCO_3^-$ orally or intravenously while also treating the cause of acid accumulation or HCO_3^- loss. Multiplying the body weight (in kilograms) by the deficiency of HCO_3^- (in mEq./L.) by 0.3 gives a rough guide to the amount of $NaHCO_3^-$ (in mEq.) that should be administered. Thus a 100-kg. patient with an HCO_3^- of 14 would be given 300 mEq. of $NaHCO_3^-$, or

$$(24 - 14 = 10 \times .3 \times 100 = 300)$$

Respiratory acidosis (high P_{CO_2}) is treated by increasing ventilation enabling the lungs to get rid of the CO_2. Although *overtreatment* may occur, *overcompensation* by the body usually does not occur. In fact, complete compensation seldom occurs, so that instead of the ratio returning to 20:1 it returns to nearly 20:1 and pH instead of returning to 7.40 returns almost to this point.

It is the fact that the pH usually does not return completely to 7.40 that allows us in some cases to decide just from blood gas values which is the primary process and which is the compensating process. We first look at the pH to see which side of 7.40 it is on. Even though it is in normal range, pH is usually either above or below 7.40. If above 7.40, the primary process is alkalosis. For example:

pH   7.42
P_{CO_2} 52 mm. Hg................Respiratory acidosis
HCO_3^- 33 mEq./L.................Metabolic alkalosis

Which is the primary process, respiratory acidosis or metabolic alkalosis? Since the pH, though normal, is tending toward alkalemia, the primary process is probably alkalemia. So this is a metabolic alkalosis with nearly complete compensation. Often it is clinically obvious which is the primary abnormality, but sometimes this is not clinically apparent.

It must be pointed out that there may be more than one *primary* acid-base abnormality; so, if there is both a respiratory and a nonrespiratory acid-base abnormality, instead of one compensating for the other, both may be acidoses or both alkaloses in which case the pH abnormality is more marked than if either of the abnormalities were present alone.

Here is an example of blood gases to interpret:

pH	7.24
P_{CO_2}	38 mm. Hg
HCO_3^-	15.5 mEq./L.
B.E.	−11

Coronary care nurses deciphering an arrhythmia are taught to first find the P wave, and in trying to interpret an acid-base abnormality, one must look first at the pH to see if there is an alkalemia or an acidemia. Here we have an acidemia for the pH is low. Next look at the P_{CO_2} to see if there is a respiratory abnormality. Here there is no abnormality, for the P_{CO_2} is normal. Next, look at either HCO_3^- or base excess to see if there is a metabolic abnormality. Here the HCO_3^- and the base excess are low indicating a metabolic acidosis. So we have an acidemia caused by a metabolic acidosis.

Next is a tougher example:

pH	7.20
P_{CO_2}	55 mm. Hg
HCO_3^-	20.5 mEq./L.
B.E.	−8

First, look at the pH to see if there is an alkalemia or an acidemia. Here the pH is low indicating an acidemia. Does the P_{CO_2} indicate a respiratory abnormality? Yes, P_{CO_2} is high, indicating respiratory acidosis. Does the HCO_3^- or B.E. indicate a nonrespiratory abnormality? Yes, HCO_3^- and base excess are low, indicating nonrespiratory (metabolic) acidosis. Therefore, this is an acidemia caused by combined respiratory and metabolic acidoses.

refinements and use of nomogram

The foregoing is all that is necessary to solve most acid-base problems. Some experts feel that the use of confidence limits is a big help or even a necessity in solving acid-base problems. This concept will be briefly discussed below and may help to explain some of the intricacies of acid-base problems. The use of a nomogram will also be presented.

Some of the statements made above are true most of the time but not all of the time. For instance, because of the equation, $CO_2 + H_2O \rightleftarrows HCO_3^- + H^+$ it can be seen that elevations of P_{CO_2} will raise the HCO_3^- just because of the chemical reaction. Later—several days later—the HCO_3^- is elevated further because the kidneys excrete less HCO_3^- in an effort to compensate.

Ninety-five percent confidence limits have been compiled so that if the primary problem is chronic respiratory acidosis (chronic hypercapnia), for instance, one can look up the level of HCO_3^- that would be expected in 95 percent of the cases of chronic hypercapnia.

Consider the example where the pH is 7.1, P_{CO_2} 80 mm. Hg, and HCO_3^- 24 mEq./L. One might first say there is a respiratory acidosis and no nonrespiratory problem, but if one looks at the nomogram showing the confidence limits, one learns that in acute hypercapnia of this degree the HCO_3^- should be higher than 24 mEq./L. and in chronic hypercapnia the HCO_3^- should be much higher; therefore, a concomitant nonrespiratory (metabolic) acidosis must be present in addition to the respiratory acidosis, and this nonrespiratory acidosis has lowered the HCO_3^- below what would otherwise be expected. Without using the 95 percent confidence limits or without consulting the nomogram, one may occasionally miss the less obvious combined acid-base problems. Use of base excess instead of HCO_3^- as the nonrespiratory parameter usually allows recognition of even the less obvious combined acid-base problems.

The area labeled A in Fig. 14-3 represents the 95 percent confidence limits for normal men exposed to various levels of CO_2 gas for 30 to 90 minutes. The area labeled B represents the 95 percent confidence limits for

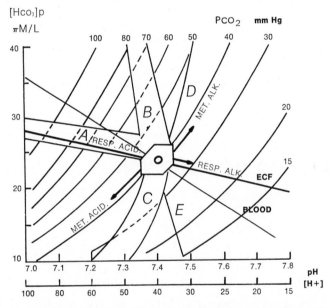

Fig. 14-3. pH−[HCO_3^-[$_p$ diagram. The PCO_2 isobars are shown as curved lines. The straight lines labeled blood and ECF represent the CO_2 equilibration curves of normal whole blood buffer value (β) = 30 and of in vivo extracellular fluid (ECF), β = 12. Area labeled A represents 95 percent confidence limits of normal men exposed to acute hypercapnia. Area B represents 95 percent confidence limits for patients with stable chronic hypercapnia (physiologically compensated respiratory acidosis). Area C represents 95 percent confidence limits for relatively stable metabolic acidosis (physiologically compensated metabolic acidosis). Line D represents mean response to metabolic alkalosis. Line E represents maximum compensation observed in chronic hypocapnia. Defined areas are often not useful in diagnosis of transient acid-base states. (From Collier et al., "Use of extracellular base excess in diagnosis of acidbase disorders," *Chest*, Vol. 61, February Supplement, 1972, pp. 6–10)

patients with chronic elevations of P_{CO_2} stable for at least 1 week and presumably representing maximum compensation. The region between areas A and B represents respiratory acidosis with area A showing least compensation and area B showing maximum compensation.

Ninety-five percent confidence limits for acute and chronic hypocapnia— i.e., uncompensated and maximally compensated respiratory alkalosis—are not available, but the area in the right lower quadrant of the figure represents acute (uncompensated) hypocapnia (respiratory alkalosis) and line E represents the maximum compensation in a group of patients with chronic hypocapnia (respiratory alkalosis).

The area labeled C represents 95 percent confidence limits for completely compensated nonrespiratory (metabolic) acidosis. The area to the left of C represents less than completely compensated nonrespiratory acidosis.

Line D represents maximal compensation for chronic nonrespiratory (metabolic) alkalosis and less than full compensation is represented by the area to the right of line D.

Further use of the pH–HCO_3^- diagram is explained in the article by Collier (see bibliography). Again it must be emphasized that most acid-base problems can be solved without use of the nomogram or confidence limits, but some feel that the nomogram makes understanding acid-base problems easier and that the use of 95 percent confidence limits is essential in recognizing all aspects of acid-base problems.

procedure for drawing blood for arterial blood gas analysis

A. Equipment
1. 5-cc. or 10-cc. glass syringe
2. 10-cc. bottle of heparin, 1000 units/cc. (reusable)
3. #21, #22 needle or even #25 disposable needle (#25 works best for radial artery)
4. Cork
5. Alcohol swab
6. Container of ice (emesis basis or cardboard milkshake cup)
7. Request slip on which to write patient's clinical status, etc. including name, date, time, whether receiving O_2, and if so how much and by what route, whether in shock, recent bicarbonate Rx, etc. If on continuous ventilation: tidal volume, respiratory frequency, and inspired oxygen concentration (FIO_2).

B. Technique
1. Call the lab to notify them you plan to draw a blood gas sample so that they can be calibrating equipment for 15 to 30 minutes.
2. Patients should be in steady state for at least 15 minutes (no recent IPPB, change in inspired O_2, exercise, etc.).

3. Brachial artery is generally preferred though radial may be used. Femoral artery sometimes must be used in hypotensive patients.

4. Elbow is hyperextended and arm is externally rotated (very important to have elbow *completely straight*—usually a folded towel or pillow under the elbow accomplishes this).

5. 1 cc. of heparin is aspirated into the syringe, barrel of the syringe is wet with heparin, and then the excess heparin is discarded through the needle, being careful that the hub of the needle is left full of heparin and there are no bubbles.

6. Brachial or radial artery is located by palpation with index and long fingers, and point of maximum impulse is found.

7. Needle is inserted into the area of maximum pulsation with the syringe and needle approximately perpendicular to the skin.

8. Often the needle goes completely through both sides of the artery and only upon slowly withdrawing the needle does the blood gush up into the syringe.

9. The only way to be certain that arterial blood is obtained is the fact that the blood pumps up into the syringe under its own power. (If one has to aspirate blood by pulling on the plunger of syringe—as is sometimes required with a tighter fitting plastic syringe—it is impossible to be positive that blood is arterial.) *The blood gas results do not allow one to determine whether blood is arterial or venous.* If one suspects that blood may be venous, then draw another sample of obviously venous blood and compare the two samples. If the two samples are similar, then the first sample also was venous, but if the Po_2 and O_2 saturation on the second (obviously venous) sample are significantly lower than the first sample, then the first sample is probably arterial.

10. After 5 to 10 cc. of blood is obtained, the needle is withdrawn and the assistant puts constant pressure on site of arterial puncture for at least 5 minutes. (If the patient is anticoagulated, longer period of pressure may be required.) Even if attempt is unsuccessful, pressure must be applied.

11. Any air bubbles should be squirted out of the syringe and needle immediately, for these can change the blood gas values. The needle is then stuck into a cork, and the syringe is shaken to ensure that the blood mixes with the heparin.

12. Corked syringe and needle are labeled and immediately placed into ice or ice water, then taken to the lab.

13. Minimal analyses required are (a) pH; (b) Pco_2 (by direct electrode or Astrup tonometer technique); (c) Po_2; and (d) Hgb. Base excess and actual bicarbonate should be calculated (standard bicarbonate may be substituted for actual bicarbonate). Other calculated values such as buffer base should not be reported, for they just tend to be confusing.

14. *Other:* (a) If O_2 saturation is also measured, this provides a cross-check for accuracy of the Po_2 (use Po_2 and pH to calculate O_2

saturation on blood gas slide rule and see if this calculated O_2 saturation agrees with the measured O_2 saturation; (b) If CO_2 content is also measured, this provides a cross-check for accuracy of P_{CO_2}. (Use P_{CO_2} and pH to calculate CO_2 content on blood gas slide rule and see if this calculated CO_2 content agrees with the measured CO_2 content.)

15. Results should be reported back to the unit on the same request slip that includes the patient's status as listed in A-7 above so that results of blood gases can be related to clinical condition. (If all information is not on the same slip, it becomes impossible to interpret data hours, days or weeks later.)

16. The technician performing analysis should report any suspicion that results are not reliable. For instance:
    a. If syringe comes to her with air bubbles in it.
    b. If she introduces air into the sample inadvertently.
    c. If calculated O_2 saturation and measured O_2 saturation do not agree.
    d. If calculated CO_2 content and measured CO_2 content do not agree.
    e. If equipment does not appear to be functioning correctly.

oxygen

The normal values for oxygen in arterial blood in Denver or any other place above sea level are lower than those at sea level because there is progressively lower P_{O_2} in the ambient air as one ascends (Table 14-21).

table 14-21
arterial blood O_2

	DENVER	SEA LEVEL
Oxygen content	18.9 cc. O_2/100 cc. of blood	19.7
P_{O_2}	70 mm. Hg (range 65–75)	> 80 mm. Hg
O_2 Saturation of Hgb	93% (range 92–94%)	> 95%

In mixed venous blood the normal values for oxygen may be slightly lower in Denver than at sea level, but not enough lower to warrant remembering a second set of values (Table 14-22).

table 14-22
mixed venous blood O_2

Oxygen content	14–16 cc. O_2/100 cc. of blood
P_{O_2}	35–40 mm. Hg
O_2 Saturation of Hgb	70–75%

Oxygen content refers to the total amount of oxygen that is present in blood in any form. Oxygen is carried in blood just two ways: (1) dissolved in the plasma, and (2) combined with hemoglobin. By far the larger amount of oxygen is carried in combination with hemoglobin, and a very small amount is dissolved in plasma (Tables 14-23 and 14-24). Oxygen is not very soluble in plasma or water, so only a very small amount can dissolve in plasma. Oxygen content and O_2 saturation of hemoglobin are indicators of the *amount* of oxygen in blood or in the red blood cells respectively.

table 14-23
how oxygen is carried in blood (Denver)

	ARTERIAL	MIXED VENOUS
Dissolved in plasma	0.2 cc. O_2/100 cc. blood	0.1 cc. O_2/100 cc. blood
Combined with Hgb.	18.7 cc. O_2/100 cc. blood	14.0 cc. O_2/100 cc. blood
Total oxygen content	18.9 cc. O_2/100 cc. blood	14.1 cc. O_2/100 cc. blood

table 14-24
how oxygen is carried in blood (sea level)

	ARTERIAL	MIXED VENOUS
Dissolved in plasma	0.3 cc. O_2/100 cc. blood	0.1 cc. O_2/100 cc. blood
Combined with Hgb.	19.4 cc. O_2/100 cc. blood	15.4 cc. O_2/100 cc. blood
Total oxygen content	19.7 cc. O_2/100 cc. blood	15.5 cc. O_2/100 cc. blood

The oxygen that is combined with hemoglobin exerts no pressure, but the oxygen that is dissolved in plasma exerts a pressure or tension. The pressure or tension of O_2 dissolved in plasma can be readily measured and is known as Po_2. We shall soon see that there is a close relationship between the pressure exerted by dissolved O_2 and the amount of oxygen carried by hemoglobin. It should be made quite clear, though, *that Po_2 is a measure of the pressure or tension exerted by dissolved oxygen, and Po_2 is not a measure of the amount of oxygen in blood.*

An explanation of Po_2 must start with an explanation of barometric pressure. Barometric pressure may be thought of as the weight of the atmosphere or the pressure exerted by the atmosphere. We are not conscious of the weight or pressure exerted on us by the atmosphere, partly because the atmosphere is made up of gases. If we dive into water we are much more aware of the weight or pressure exerted on us by the water, and this pressure increases as we dive deeper because there is progressively more water above us. Just as in water, the deeper we are in the atmosphere the higher the barometric pressure. So, at the top of Pike's Peak (elevation 14,110 feet above sea level) we are near the top of the atmosphere and the barometric pressure is lower—425 mm. Hg. Denver and the cities of Colorado and Wyoming are between these two extremes; the average barometric pressure in Denver is 625 mm. Hg. (Of course, as weather fronts approach, the barometric pressure may fluctuate slightly even though the elevation is constant.) With high-pressure weather fronts, the barometric pressure may increase by 10 to 15 mm. Hg, and with low-pressure fronts the barometric pressure may fall by 10 to 15 mm. Hg. In blood gas laboratories a barometer is necessary for determining the barometric pressure each day.

If one takes a bottle in which a vacuum has been created and inverts this bottle in a pan of water, when the cork is removed from the bottle the water in the pan will rise in the bottle (Fig. 14-4). The force that makes the water rise in the bottle is the difference between the barometric pressure exerted on the pan and the absence of barometric pressure in the vacuum bottle.

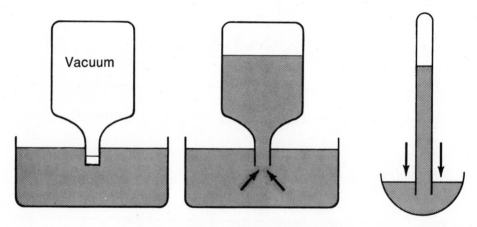

Fig. 14-4. Effects of barometric pressure.

If we substitute a long tube for the bottle, create a vacuum in the tube, and invert the tube in a container of mercury instead of a pan of water, we have a barometer. Since the vacuum in the tube remains constant, the only factor influencing how high mercury rises in the tube is the barometric pressure (or weight of the atmosphere) pressing down on the mercury in the container.

Table 14-25 is a simplified explanation of why the arterial Po_2 in Denver is about 70 mm. Hg and at sea level about 95 mm. Hg.

It should be pointed out that the percentage of O_2 in the atmosphere is 21 percent (actually 20.93) everywhere in the atmosphere and that changes in Po_2 with altitude are due to changes in barometric pressure with altitude and not due to changes in percentage of oxygen present.

table 14-25
comparison of Po₂ at sea level and Denver

AT SEA LEVEL	AT DENVER	REMARKS
760	625 mm. Hg	Average barometric pressure
− 47	− 45 mm. Hg	Water vapor pressure at body temperature (subtracted because in the body this pressure is exerted by water vapor)
713	578 mm. Hg	Corrected barometric pressure (in body or completely humidified air at body temperature)
× 21%	× 21%	Percent of oxygen in the atmosphere
150 mm. Hg	121 mm. Hg	Po₂ in air that is completely humidified
− 40	− 36	Pco₂ − pressure exerted by CO₂ in alveolus
110 mm. Hg	85 mm. Hg	Po₂ in alveolus
− 10 mm. Hg	− 10 mm. Hg	Gradient for diffusion of O₂ from alveolus into capillary
100 mm. Hg	75 mm. Hg	Po₂ in capillary blood in lungs
− 5 mm. Hg	− 5 mm. Hg	Due to venous shunting
95 mm. Hg	70 mm. Hg	Po₂ in arterial blood

The percent saturation of hemoglobin is defined as the amount of O_2 that hemoglobin *is* carrying compared to the amount of O_2 that hemoglobin *can* carry, expressed as a percentage:

$$\text{Percent } O_2 \text{ saturation of Hgb.} = \frac{\text{Amount } O_2 \text{ Hgb. is carrying}}{\text{Amount } O_2 \text{ Hgb. can carry}} \times 100$$

Since the amount of O_2 that Hgb. can carry is a constant,
1.34 cc. of O_2 per gm. of Hgb. × % saturation of Hgb.
= cc. of O_2 that Hgb. is carrying
(It should be noted that there are rare abnormal types of hemoglobin that cannot carry 1.34 cc. of O_2 per gm. There are also rare situations in which normal Hgb. has been poisoned so that it cannot carry 1.34 cc. of O_2 per gm. − sulfhemoglobin or methemoglobin, for example.)

In 100 cc. of blood $\left\{ \begin{array}{l} \text{1 gm. of Hgb. can carry 1.34 cc. of } O_2 \\ \text{15 gm. of Hgb. can carry } 15 \times 1.34 \text{ cc. of } O_2 \end{array} \right.$

In arterial blood in Denver if O_2 saturation of Hgb. is 93 percent (i.e., Hgb. *is* carrying 93 percent of the total amount of O_2 it *can* carry), then 93 percent of 20.1 cc. equals 18.7 cc. of O_2 carried by Hgb. in Denver. At sea level, arterial O_2 saturation of Hgb. is 97 percent, so Hgb. is carrying 97 percent of 20.1 cc. or 19.4 cc. of oxygen.

The major factor which determines how much O_2 Hgb. *is* carrying is the P_{O_2} that the Hgb. is exposed to. At high P_{O_2} Hgb. carries more O_2; at low P_{O_2} Hgb. carries less O_2. The exact relationship between the amount of O_2 that Hgb. is carrying and the P_{O_2} is shown by the oxyhemoglobin dissociation curve, Fig. 14-5.

There are four pulmonary reasons why arterial blood may not be carrying the normal amount of oxygen (Fig. 14-5).

1. Alveolar hypoventilation (associated with high P_{CO_2})
2. Diffusion defect (alveolar capillary block)
3. Right-to-left shunt (in lung or chest)
4. Mismatching of ventilation and blood flow in the lungs. (Blood goes by alveoli that are not ventilated or underventilated. This blood, as it passes through the lungs, picks up little or no oxygen. This blood then returns to the heart and is pumped out in the arteries to the body, therefore causing arterial blood to have less than the normal amount of oxygen.)

associated with low or normal P_{CO_2}

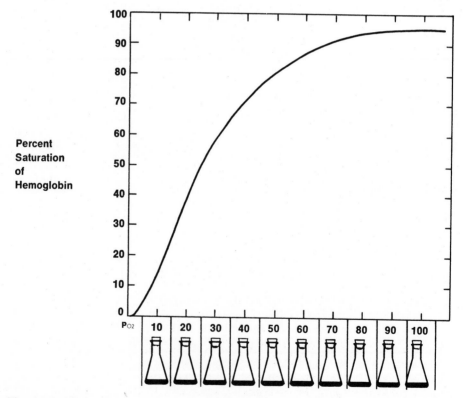

Fig. 14-5. HbO$_2$ dissociation curve. (Adapted from J. H. Comroe, *Physiology of Respiration*, ed. 2, Chicago, Year Book Medical Publishers, 1974)

The amount of oxygen that is transported to the tissues is more important than the Po_2. The Po_2 is a measure of intensity or pressure due to oxygen, and oxygen content is a measure of amount of oxygen.

Oxygen transport to the tissues = Arterial O_2 content $\times$ Cardiac output

The oxygen transported to the tissues depends on (1) the amount of oxygen in arterial blood (arterial O_2 content), and (2) the ability of the heart to pump this blood containing oxygen around to the tissues.

The arterial O_2 content depends in turn on (1) how well the lungs are able to get oxygen from air into the blood, and (2) a normal amount of functioning hemoglobin to carry the oxygen.

In summary,

Oxygenation of the tissue	depends on:	I. Arterial O_2 content, which depends on 1. Lungs' ability to get O_2 into blood 2. Ability of hemo-globin to hold enough O_2	and	II. Cardiac output (circulation)

The pulmonary causes of tissue hypoxia have already been mentioned.

The nonpulmonary causes of tissue hypoxia are (1) reduced blood flow to the tissues (reduced cardiac output); (2) anemia—not enough hemoglobin to carry O_2; (3) nonfunctioning hemoglobin—enough hemoglobin but hemoglobin that exists cannot carry O_2 because it has been "poisoned"; and (4) right-to-left cardiac shunts—most frequently seen in cyanotic congenital heart disease.

1. Reduced blood flow to the tissues (reduced cardiac output) might be caused by:
   a. Myocardial infarction
   b. Abnormal cardiac rhythm
   c. Reduced cardiac function (other causes): congestive heart failure, dilatation of heart, valvular heart lesion, etc.
   d. Hypovolemia (intimately related to anemia)
2. Anemia: 1 gm. of Hgb. carries 1.34 cc. O_2 and normally there are 15 gm. of Hgb. to carry 15×1.34 cc. O_2 or 20.1 cc. of O_2. If there is anemia so that only 7.5 gm. of Hgb. are present, then 7.5×1.34 cc. $O_2 = 10$ cc. of O_2 are all that can be carried; if anemia is milder (between 7.5 and 15 gm. Hgb.) more O_2 can be carried; if anemia is more severe (less than 7.5 gm. of Hgb.) even less O_2 can be carried. Usually the body compensates for anemia by having the heart circulate faster the lesser amount of hemoglobin that is present.
3. Nonfunctioning hemoglobin: A few rare conditions exist in which there might be a normal amount of hemoglobin, but even this normal amount

cannot function because it has been poisoned. Some examples of this are:
a. Carbon monoxide poisoning
b. Methemoglobinemia
c. Sulfhemoglobinemia

In each of these situations something (carbon monoxide, for example) has combined with hemoglobin, making it hard for oxygen to combine with and be carried by this hemoglobin.

4. In right-to-left cardiac shunts, oxygen gets through the lungs normally into the bloodstream, there is enough functioning hemoglobin to carry the oxygen, and the heart is strong enough to circulate the oxygenated blood. However, some venous blood that never passes through the lungs is *shunted* into the systemic arterial system, and the combination of oxygenated blood plus mixed venous unoxygenated blood is carried through the arteries to the tissues, supplying them with less oxygen than they need.

The patient who is hypoxemic compensates for hypoxia in the following ways: (1) tachypnea (rapid breathing), (2) tachycardia (rapid heartbeat), and (3) erythrocytosis (high hemoglobin and hematocrit). The tachypnea and tachycardia represent extra energy expenditure by the patient. Erythrocytosis simply means increased production of red blood cells by the hypoxic patient's bone marrow in an attempt to get more O_2 to the tissues. If the fault is lack of enough red blood cells, this is useful. But if the fault is in getting enough O_2 through the lungs, increasing the number of red blood cells helps little or not at all. The hypoxemic patient tries all these means of compensating for hypoxemia and often all of them together are inadequate. Hypoxia often leads to pulmonary hypertension (high blood pressure in the arteries of the lungs), and this can lead to strain or failure of the right side of the heart.

If oxygen is administered to the patient to treat his hypoxemia, tachypnea and tachycardia do not occur, no erythrocytosis occurs, and pulmonary hypertension usually goes away. Complete compensation is possible with oxygen treatment, but sometimes is not possible with patient compensation. It can be seen that supplemental oxygen is rational treatment for the patient with hypoxemia, but long-term continuous oxygen is usually reserved for the patient who when completely stable has a Po_2 below 50 mm. Hg (O_2 saturation below 85 percent) and who also has one or more of the following: (1) right heart failure which is difficult to manage with digitalis and diuretics, (2) significant secondary erythrocytosis, and/or (3) a progressive downhill course with weight loss and progressive muscle wasting.

Often such a patient responds to nocturnal oxygen (oxygen for 8 hours at night), or if the patient is living at a high altitude a move to a lower altitude may make supplemental oxygen unnecessary.

Oxygen treatment may lead to CO_2 retention if the O_2 is not carefully controlled.

There are two major reflex stimuli to breathing: (1) CO_2 retention (hypercapnic stimulus to breathe), and (2) low Po_2 (hypoxic stimulus to breathe).

Small elevations of P_{CO_2} are a major stimulus to breathing. Increasing the P_{CO_2} by 4 mm. Hg can cause a 100-percent increase in ventilation. Large elevations in P_{CO_2} reduce the amount of ventilation. In patients with significant elevation of P_{CO_2}, hypoxemia may be the most important stimulus to breathe. If a patient who no longer has a hypercapnic stimulus to breathing is treated with oxygen, thereby eliminating the hypoxic stimulus to breathe, he may breathe even less, significantly worsening his condition. It has become apparent that giving a controlled amount of oxygen—just enough to raise the arterial P_{O_2} to approximately 60 mm. Hg—allows the patient to benefit from the oxygen and usually does not reduce ventilation.

It should be clear that oxygen therapy, though often given in a haphazard fashion, requires just as much understanding and precision in dosage as any other form of drug therapy.

BIBLIOGRAPHY

Collier, Clarence R., Jack D. Hackney, and John G. Mohler, "Use of Extracellular Base Excess in Diagnosis of Acid-Base Disorders; A Conceptual Approach," *Chest*, Vol. 61 (February 1972), Supplemental, pp. 65-105.

Comroe, Julius H., Jr., *Physiology of Respiration* (Chicago: Year Book Medical Publishers, 1965).

Filley, Giles, *Acid Base and Blood Gas Regulation* (Philadelphia: Lea & Febiger, 1971).

Murray, John F., *The Normal Lung* (Philadelphia: W. B. Saunders, 1976).

Schwartz, William B., "Disturbances of Acid-Base Equilibrium," in Paul B. Beeson and Walsh McDermott, eds., *Textbook of Medicine*, 14th ed. (Philadelphia: W. B. Saunders 1975), pp. 1589-1599.

Snider, Gordon L., "Interpretation of the Arterial Oxygen and Carbon Dioxide Partial Pressures," *Chest*, Vol. 63 (May 1973), pp. 801-806.

Thomas, Henry M., et al., "The Oxyhemoglobin Dissociation Curve in Health and Disease," *American Journal of Medicine*, Vol. 57 (September 1974), pp. 331-348.

Winters, Robert W., Knud Engel, and Ralph B. Dell, *Acid-Base Physiology in Medicine*, 2nd ed. (Cleveland: The London Company of Cleveland and the Radiometer A/S of Copenhagen, 1969).

chest physical diagnosis

There is increasing recognition that nurses can contribute significantly to the care of patients with respiratory problems by performing chest physical examinations on these patients. This examination allows the nurse an opportunity to establish a "baseline" of information and provides a framework to detect some of the rapid changes in the patient's condition. Since the nurse is with the patient more frequently than the physician is, it makes sense for the nurse to detect the patient's changing condition rather than the physician, who visits the patient only once or twice a day, or even daily chest x-rays.

Sometimes a chest examination by the nurse is the quickest and most reliable assessment of the situation. In the following example, the patient, a 69-year-old hypertensive man, fainted in the shower and fell, breaking five ribs on the left side. When he recovered consciousness it was clear that he had had a CVA (cerebrovascular accident) with left-side hemiparesis. He did well until the third day of hospitalization, when he developed respiratory distress. The working diagnosis was congestive heart failure, but the nurse was able to convince those in attendance that the breath sounds and thoracic movement on the left side—which everyone agreed were depressed due to rib fractures—were more depressed than they had been previously. A chest x-ray, showing atelectasis of the entire left lung, confirmed her observations. The x-ray showed the lung returned to normal the next day after tracheostomy, vigorous bronchial hygiene, and tracheal suction. This is just one example of many in which the nurse's ability to do a competent chest physical examination led to improved patient care.

Physical diagnosis of the chest includes four examinations: (1) inspection, or looking at the patient (Fig. 14-6), (2) palpation, or feeling the patient, (3) percussion, or thumping on the patient, and (4) auscultation, or listening to the patient's chest with a stethoscope.

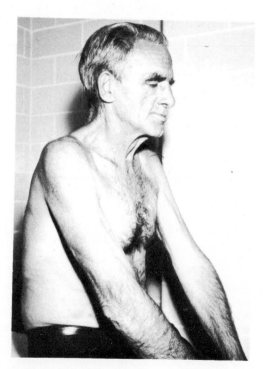

Fig. 14-6. Frequently observe the patient's overall aspect.

inspection

In inspecting the patient, one of the factors we are most interested in is the presence or absence of cyanosis. Cyanosis is notoriously hard to detect when the patient is anemic, and the patient who is polycythemic may have cyanosis in his extremities even when he has a normal oxygen tension. We generally differentiate between *peripheral* and *central* cyanosis; peripheral cyanosis occurs in the extremities or on the tip of the nose or ears, even with normal oxygen tensions, when there is diminished blood flow to these areas, particularly if they are cold or dependent (Fig. 14-7). Central cyanosis, as noted on the tongue or lips (Fig. 14-8), has a much greater significance; it means the patient actually has a low oxygen tension. The presence or absence of labored breathing is an obvious sign that we look for; we are particularly interested in knowing if the patient is using the accessory muscles of respiration. Sometimes the number of words a patient can say before having to gasp for another breath is a good measure of the amount of labored breathing. In looking at the patient we are interested in determining whether there is an increase in the AP (anteroposterior) diameter of the chest—i.e., an increase in the size of the chest from front to back. This is often due to overexpansion of the

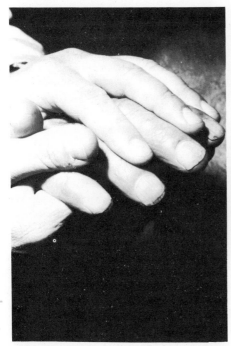

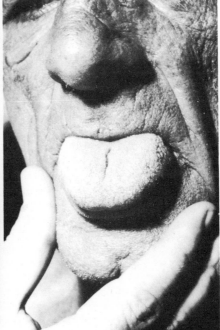

Fig. 14-7. Feel the patient's extremities and assess their temperature.

Fig. 14-8. Examine the tongue and lips for cyanosis.

lungs from obstructive lung disease, but an increase in AP diameter may also be present in a patient who has kyphosis (forward curvature of the spine). Chest deformities and scars are important in helping us to determine the reason for respiratory distress. For instance, a scar may be our first indication that the patient has had part of his lung removed. A chest deformity such as kyphoscoliosis may indicate why the patient has respiratory distress. It is also quite important to notice the patient's posture, for patients with obstructive lung disease often sit and prop themselves up on outstretched arms, or lean forward with their elbows on a desk in an effort to elevate their clavicles, thereby giving them a slightly greater ability to expand their chests.

In inspecting the patient, we are interested in the position of the trachea (Fig. 14-9). Is the trachea in the midline as it should be, or deviated to one side or the other? A pleural effusion or a tension pneumothorax usually deviates the trachea away from the diseased side. On the other hand, atelectasis often pulls the trachea toward the diseased side. The respiratory rate is an important parameter to follow; it should be counted over at least a 15-second period, rather than just estimated. Often the respiratory rate is recorded as 20 breaths/minute, which frequently means the rate was estimated rather than counted. The depth of respiration is often as meaningful as is the respiratory rate. For instance, if a patient were breathing 40 times/minute, one might think he had severe respiratory problems, but if he was breathing quite deeply 40 times/minute, it might mean that he had Kussmaul respirations due to diabetic acidosis or other acidosis. However, if the respirations were shallow at a rate of 40 times/minute, it might mean he had severe respiratory distress from obstructive lung disease, restrictive lung disease, or other pulmonary problems. The duration of inspiration versus the duration of expiration is important in determining whether or not there is airway obstruction. In patients with any of the obstructive lung diseases, expiration is prolonged, requiring more than one and one-half times as long for expiration as for inspiration.

We are quite interested in general chest expansion in examining a patient; normally we expect about a 3-inch expansion from maximum expiration to maximum inspiration (Fig. 14-10). Ankylosing spondylitis, or Marie-Strumpell arthritis, is one condition in which general chest expansion is limited. We compare the expansion of the upper chest to that of the lower chest and use of the diaphragm to see if the patient with obstructive lung disease is concentrating on expanding his lower chest and using his diaphragm properly. We look at the expansion of one side of the chest versus the other side, realizing that atelectasis, especially atelectasis caused by a mucus plug, may cause unilateral diminished chest expansion. A pulmonary embolus, pneumonia, pleural effusion, pneumothorax, or any other cause of chest pain, such as fractured ribs, may lead to diminished chest expansion. An endotracheal or nasotracheal tube inserted too far, so that it extends beyond the trachea into one of the main stem bronchi (usually the right), is a serious and frequent cause of diminished expansion of one side of the chest. When the tube slips into the right main stem bronchus the left lung is not expanded,

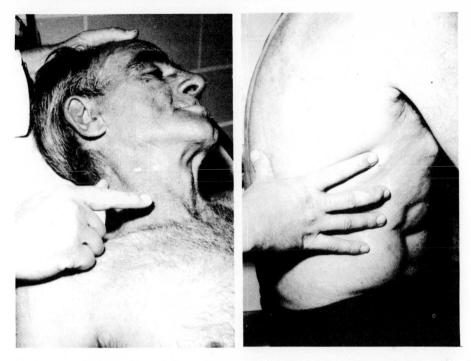

Fig. 14-9. Note the position of the trachea. **Fig. 14-10.** Note the general chest expansion.

and the patient usually develops hypoxemia and atelectasis on the left side. Fortunately the nurse who is aware of this potential problem usually recognizes it. The presence of intercostal retractions, i.e., sucking in of the muscles and skin between the ribs during inspiration, usually means that the patient is making a larger effort at inspiration than normal. Usually this signifies that the lungs are less compliant (stiffer) than usual. The effectiveness and frequency of a patient's cough are important to note, as are sputum characteristics such as amount, color, and consistency.

palpation

Palpation of the chest is done with the heel of the hand flat against the patient's chest (Fig. 14-11). Often we are determining whether tactile fremitus is present. We do this by having the patient speak, particularly asking him to say "ninety-nine." Normally, when a patient speaks, or says a word such as "ninety-nine," a vibration is felt by the hand on the outside of the chest. This is similar to the vibration one feels when putting one's hand on the chest of a cat when the cat is purring. In normal patients tactile fremitus is present. It may be diminished or absent when there is something which comes between the patient's lung and the hand on the chest wall. For instance, when

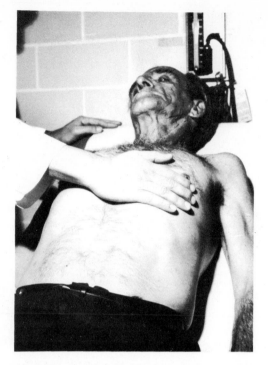

Fig. 14-11. In palpation, place the heel of your hand flat against the patient's chest.

there is a pleural effusion, thickened pleura, or pneumothorax, either it is impossible to feel this vibration or the vibration is diminished. When the patient has atelectasis due to an occluded airway, the vibration also cannot be felt. Tactile fremitus is slightly increased in conditions of consolidation, but detection of this slight increase may be difficult. Just by palpating over the patient's chest with quiet breathing, one may sometimes feel palpable rhonchi which are due to mucus moving in large airways.

percussion

In percussing a patient's chest (Fig. 14-12), one must use a finger which is pressed flat against the patient's chest; this finger is struck over the knuckle by the end of a finger from the opposite hand. Normally the chest has a resonant or hollow percussion note. In diseases in which there is increased air in the chest or lungs, such as pneumothorax or emphysema, there may be hyperresonant (even more drumlike) percussion notes. Hyperresonant percussion notes, however, are sometimes hard to detect. More important is a dull or flat percussion note such as is heard when one percusses over a

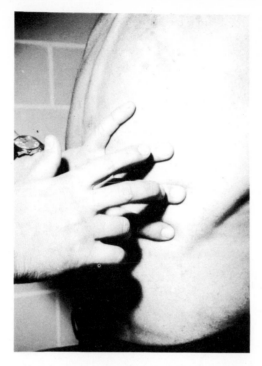

Fig. 14-12. In percussion, press a finger flat against the patient's chest or back and strike this finger over the knuckle with the end of a finger from the opposite hand.

part of the body which contains no air. A dull or flat percussion note is heard when the lung underneath the examining hand has atelectasis, pneumonia, pleural effusion, thickened pleura, or a mass lesion. A dull or flat percussion note is also heard when one is percussing over the heart.

auscultation

In auscultation, one generally uses the diaphragm of the stethoscope and presses this firmly against the chest wall (Fig. 14-13). It is important to listen to the intensity or loudness of breath sounds, and to realize that normally there is a fourfold increase in loudness of breath sounds when a patient takes a maximum deep breath as opposed to quiet breathing. The intensity of the breath sounds may be diminished due to decreased airflow through the airways or due to increased insulation between the lungs and the stethoscope. In airway obstruction, such as chronic obstructive pulmonary disease or atelectasis, the breath sound intensity is diminished. With shallow breathing there is diminished air movement through the airways and the breath sounds are also not as loud. With restricted movement of the thorax or diaphragm, there may be diminished breath sounds in the area of restricted movement. In

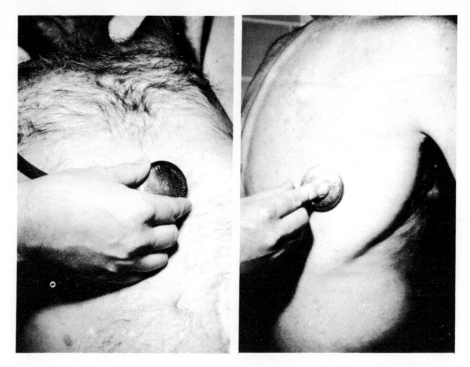

Fig. 14-13. In auscultation press the stethoscope firmly against the chest wall (*left*) or the back (*right*).

pleural thickening, pleural effusion, pneumothorax, and obesity there is an abnormal substance (fibrous tissue, fluid, air, or fat) between the stethoscope and the underlying lung; this substance insulates the breath sounds from the stethoscope, making the breath sounds seem less loud. Generally, there are three types of sounds which are heard in the normal chest: (1) vesicular breath sounds which are heard in the periphery of the normal lung, (2) bronchial breath sounds which are heard over the trachea, and (3) bronchovesicular breath sounds which are heard in most areas of the lung near the major airways. *Bronchial breath sounds* are high-pitched, seem to be close to the ear, are loud, and there is a pause between inspiration and expiration. *Vesicular breath sounds* are of lower pitch, having a rustling quality, and there is no noticeable pause between inspiration and expiration. *Bronchovesicular breath sounds* represent a sound halfway between the other two types of breath sounds. Bronchial breathing, in addition to being heard over the trachea of the normal person, is also heard in any situation where there is consolidation—for instance, pneumonia. *Bronchial breathing* is also heard above a pleural effusion where the normal lung is compressed. Wherever there is bronchial breathing, there may also be two other associated changes: (1) "E to A" changes, and (2) whispered pectoriloquy. An *E to A change* merely means that when one listens with a stethoscope and the patient says "E," what one hears is actually an A sound rather than an E sound. This occurs where there is consolidation. *Whispered pectoriloquy* is the presence of a loud volume as heard through the stethoscope when the patient whispers. For bronchial breathing and these two associated changes to be present there must be either: (1) an open airway and compressed alveoli, or (2) alveoli in which the air has been replaced by fluid.

Extra sounds which are heard with auscultation include rales, rhonchi, wheezes, and rubs. *Rales* are divided into three categories: fine, medium, and coarse. Fine rales are also called *crepitant rales,* and are produced in the small airways in patients with diseases such as pneumonia and heart failure. Medium rales are sounds produced in the medium airways and occur later in pneumonia, heart failure, and pulmonary edema. Coarse rales, also called *rhonchi,* are continuous, bubbling, gurgling, or rattling sounds, often musical and usually coming from the large airways. Extra sounds such as wheezing mean there is airway narrowing. This may be caused by asthma, foreign bodies, mucus in the airways, stenosis, etc. If the wheeze is heard only in expiration it is called a *wheeze;* if the wheezing sound occurs in both inspiration and expiration, it is usually due to retained secretions and is best called a *rhonchus.* A *friction rub* is heard when there is pleural disease such as a pulmonary embolus, peripheral pneumonia, or pleurisy, and is often difficult to tell from a rhonchus. If the abnormal noise clears when the patient coughs, it usually means that it was a rhonchus rather than a friction rub.

Certainly, critical care nurses and respiratory nurse therapists and, hopefully, unit nurses and inhalation therapy technicians should learn to participate in chest physical diagnosis so that they can detect changes in the patient's condition as soon as they occur, rather than waiting for the physician's visit once or twice a day, or depending on a daily chest x-ray.

checklist of findings

In this section the abnormal physical findings which might be seen in a variety of diseases are presented.

Bronchitis

Occasional increased respiratory rate
Occasional use of accessory muscles
Occasional intercostal retraction
Prolonged expiratory phase (often)
Increased AP diameter of the chest (often)
Decreased motion of the diaphragm (often)
Decreased intensity of breath sounds
Fine, medium, and coarse rales (rhonchi)
Wheezes (often)
Often coarse rales (rhonchi) and wheezes clear after cough

Pneumothorax
  Increased respiratory rate
  Trachea deviated to side of pneumothorax
  Occasional cyanosis
  Decreased movement of chest on side of pneumothorax (splinting)
  Hyperresonance (unreliable sign)
  Decreased breath sounds
  Decreased tactile fremitus and decreased vocal fremitus (the
    most reliable signs)
Emphysema
  Increased respiratory rate (often)
  Use of accessory muscles (neck)
  Intercostal retractions
  Propped up on outstretched arms
  Prolonged expiratory phase
  Increased AP diameter
  Decreased chest expansion
  Decreased motion of diaphragm
  Hyperresonance to percussion
  Decreased intensity (loudness) of breath sounds
  Little or no increase in loudness of breath sounds with deep breath
  Fine rales at bases (often)
  Occasional wheeze
Pneumonia
  Increased respiratory rate
  Occasional cyanosis
  Decreased expansion (splinting) (often)
  Increased fremitus (tactile and vocal)
  Occasional palpable rhonchi—usually are removed by coughing
    or suctioning
  Dullness to percussion
  Bronchial breathing, whispered pectoriloquy, and E to A changes
    (usual if consolidation is extensive)
  Fine or medium rales
  Occasional coarse rales (rhonchi)—clear with cough or
    suctioning, usually
  Occasional pleural friction rub
Atelectasis
  Increased respiratory rate
  Increased pulse
  Cyanosis (often)
  Trachea deviated to side of atelectasis
  Decreased chest expansion on side of atelectasis (splinting)
  Decreased fremitus (tactile and vocal)
  Dull or flat percussion note
  Decreased breath sounds
  Occasional rales

Pleural effusion
    Occasional increase in respiratory rate
    Trachea deviated away from side of effusion
    Decreased fremitus (tactile and vocal)
    Decreased breath sounds
    Above effusion
        Bronchial breathing   ⎫ due to compressed
        E to A changes   ⎬ lungs with open
        Whispered pectoriloquy ⎭ airway
    Friction rub — after fluid is removed and visceral pleura
      rubs against parietal pleura
Large mass lesion (tumor)
    Dullness over tumor
    Fine rales (often)
    Decreased breath sounds if airway is occluded
    Bronchial breathing, E to A changes, and whispered
      pectoriloquy if airway is open
    Occasional pleural friction rub
Subcutaneous emphysema
    Crackling sounds similar to rales that come from air outside
      the chest in the soft tissue
Pulmonary edema (congestive heart failure)
    Increased respiratory rate
    Cyanosis (often)
    Use of accessory muscles (usually)
    Apprehension
    Sitting upright (often)
    Increased fremitus (due to interstitial edema)
    Dull percussion note (due to interstitial edema)
    Bronchovesicular sounds (due to interstitial edema often
      obscured later by rales)
    Fine rales → medium rales later
    Occcasional coarse rales (rhonchi)
    Occasional wheezing
Pulmonary interstitial fibrosis
    Increased respiratory rate (often)
    Intercostal retractions
    Cyanosis (late)
    High-pitched, fine, and medium rales
    Occasional bronchovesicular breathing

MARGARET ANN BERRY, R.N., M.A., M.S.

normal structure and function of the renal system

normal function of the kidney

The regulation and concentration of solutes in the extracellular fluid of the body is the primary function of the kidney. This is accomplished by removing waste products of metabolism and excess concentrations of constituents and by conserving these substances which are present in normal or low quantities. Figure 15-1 is a schematic representation of the general macro- and microscopic structure of the kidney.

Urine, the end product of kidney function, is formed from the blood by the *nephron* and flows from the nephrons through *collecting tubules* to the *pelvis* of the kidney. From here it leaves the kidney itself via the *ureters* and flows into the *urinary bladder.* Each kidney in humans contains about one million nephrons, all of which function identically, and thus kidney function can be explained by describing the function of one nephron.

Figure 15-2 is a composite drawing of a functional nephron. Each nephron is made up of two major components; the *glomerulus* where water and solutes are filtered from the blood, and the *tubules* which reabsorb essential materials from the filtrate and permit waste substances and unneeded materials to remain in the filtrate and flow into the renal pelvis as urine.

For purposes of further describing these two major divisions of the nephron a more schematic diagram appears in Fig. 15-3.

The *glomerulus* consists of a tuft of capillaries fed by the *afferent arteriole,* drained by the *efferent arteriole,* and surrounded by *Bowman's capsule.* Fluid

309

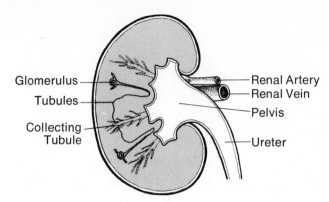

Glomerulus
Tubules
Collecting Tubule

Renal Artery
Renal Vein
Pelvis
Ureter

Fig. 15-1. General characteristics of kidney structure. Note that the glomerulus is in the cortex of the kidney while the proximal, distal, and collecting tubules are in the medulla.

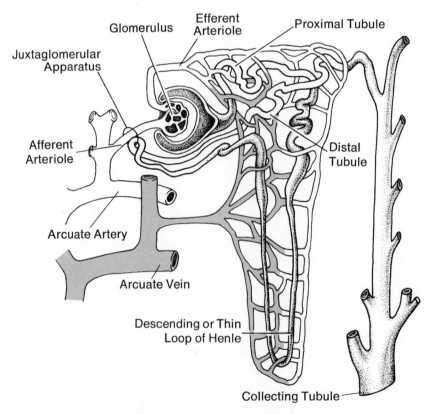

Glomerulus
Efferent Arteriole
Proximal Tubule
Juxtaglomerular Apparatus
Afferent Arteriole
Arcuate Artery
Arcuate Vein
Descending or Thin Loop of Henle
Distal Tubule
Collecting Tubule

Fig. 15-2. The nephron. (From A. C. Guyton, *Function of the Human Body*, Philadelphia, W. B. Saunders, 1969, p. 196)

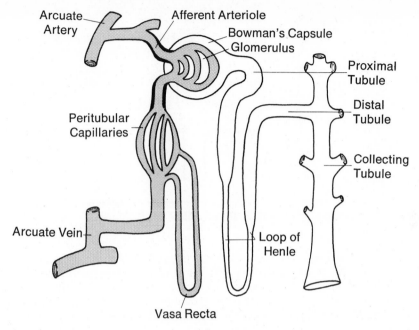

Fig. 15-3. Schematic representation of the nephron. (From A. C. Guyton, *Function of the Human Body,* Philadelphia, W. B. Saunders, 1969)

which is filtered from the capillaries into this capsule then flows into the tubular system. The first section is called the *proximal tubule;* the second, the *loop of Henle;* the third, the *distal tubule,* and last, the *collecting tubule.*

Most of the water and electrolytes are reabsorbed into the blood in the *peritubular capillaries* and the *vasa recta* while the end products of metabolism pass into the urine.

the glomerular membrane and filtration pressure

The *glomerular membrane* is composed of all the membranes of the tuft capillaries. Like other capillary membranes it is essentially impermeable to plasma protein. The difference in permeability lies in its increased permeability to water and small molecular solutes. However, the glomerular membrane follows the same principles of fluid dynamics that are applicable to any other capillary membranes. That is, the effective movement of materials out of the capillary and into the capsule is a function of the difference in fluid and osmotic pressure on either side of the membrane. Another distinguishing characteristic of the glomerulus is the increased fluid pressure (70 mm. Hg) in the tuft as compared to low fluid pressure (10 to 20 mm. Hg) found in other capillaries. This high fluid pressure (e.g., blood pressure) causes fluid to constantly leak out of the tuft and into Bowman's capsule. Figure 15-4 illustrates these principles.

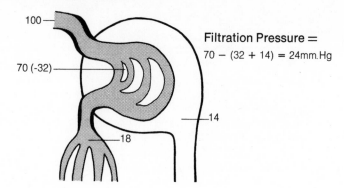

Filtration Pressure =
70 − (32 + 14) = 24 mm.Hg

Fig. 15-4. Normal fluid pressures at various points in the nephron. (From A. C. Guyton, *Function of the Human Body*, Philadelphia, W. B. Saunders, 1969, p. 197)

The reader will recall that the effective filtration pressure in the glomerular membrane is the result of the net difference in pressure on either side of the membrane. That is, if the pressure tending to push material out of the capillary is 70 mm. Hg and the osmotic pressure of the blood holding fluid in the capillary is 32 mm. Hg, the total force pushing fluid out is 38 mm. Hg. At the same time, the filtrate formed exerts fluid pressure against the membrane attempting to push fluid back into the capillary. In the normally functioning nephron, this is about 14 mm. Hg. Thus the net filtration pressure is 24 mm. Hg.

glomerular filtration rate

The rate at which fluid flows from the glomerulus into Bowman's capsule is called the *glomerular filtration rate.* This rate is directly proportional to the net filtration pressure, which means that any factor effecting a change in any one of the pressures on either side of the membrane will affect the glomerular filtration rate. For example, an increase in blood pressure in the afferent arteriole, a decrease in osmotic pressure in the blood, or a decrease in fluid pressure in Bowman's capsule would all result in an *increased* glomerular filtration rate. It is easily seen how the formation rate of glomerular filtrate acts as a regulatory mechanism for blood pressure. An increased blood pressure causes an increase in filtrate formation, decreasing the fluid volume of the blood which then lowers arterial blood pressure. As a result of low arterial pressure, the nephron decreases its function, thus permitting blood fluid volume to build up until it exceeds normal values again and initiates the whole process again.

the glomerular filtrate

Glomerular filtrate, produced in Bowman's capsule, is an ultrafiltrate of plasma. That is, it contains all but the protein fraction of the plasma. A very small amount of plasma proteins (ca. 0.03 percent) does enter the glomerular filtrate, but is extremely small when compared to their concentration in the plasma (ca. 7 percent). The kidneys form about 125 ml. of glomerular filtrate per minute. This results in about 180 liters of filtrate per day, about 4.5 times the total amount of fluid in the entire body. A quick glance at these statistics illustrates the tremendous effectiveness of the kidneys in maintaining normal body fluids and their constitutents.

The glomerular filtrate produced in Bowman's capsule of the nephron enters the tubular system where nearly all but 1 liter of the 180 liters formed is reabsorbed into the blood. As seen in Fig. 15-3, the peritubular capillaries are found in close proximity to the tubules as they loop into the medullary portion of the kidney. In tubular reabsorption substances in the tubular fluid are first moved from the tubule lumen into the interstitial fluid and then into the peritubular capillaries. Reabsorption of materials across the tubular epithelium is accomplished by *active reabsorption, diffusion,* and *osmosis.*

active reabsorption

Active reabsorption is very similar to active transport of materials across cell membranes. It means the transport of materials through the epithelial cells of the kidney tubule and into the interstitial spaces, by the involvement of special chemical carriers and the expenditure of energy. From the intercellular space the materials diffuse into the peritubular capillary. Materials reabsorbed in this fashion include glucose, amino acids, proteins, uric acid, and most of the electrolytes (e.g., Na^+, K^+, Mg^{++}, Ca^{++}, HCO_3^-, Cl^-). Active processes for glucose, amino acids, and proteins are extremely efficient so that nearly all of these substances are reabsorbed in the proximal tubules and the urine is virtually devoid of any of them. The reabsorption of electrolytes, however, is variable according to the concentration required in the extracellular fluid of the body and is regulated by a special mechanism. Therefore, when an electrolyte is present in excessive amounts in the extracellular fluid of the body, very little of it is absorbed from the tubules. When there is a depleted amount in the extracellular fluid, nearly all will be reabsorbed. This *selective* reabsorption of essential materials is the mechanism by which the kidney controls the concentration of electrolytes in the body.

The electrolyte that is actively reabsorbed to the greatest extent is sodium. Approximately 1,200 gm. of this substance is reabsorbed daily. This represents nearly three fourths of the active reabsorption of all materials from the glomerular filtrate. Therefore, sodium serves as a good example of the mechanism of active reabsorption. Figure 15-5 demonstrates the mechanism of the active reabsorption of sodium.

The tubular cells of the proximal tubules are serrated on the luminal side and the cell membrane of this *brush border* is extremely permeable to the sodium ion. Because of this, the sodium ion rapidly diffuses down its concentration gradient. The membranes facing the interstitial spaces are impermeable to sodium, and it is actively pumped out of the cell and into the peritubular space. The active transport at the base membrane is most likely

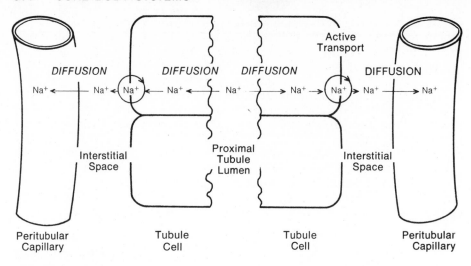

Fig. 15-5. Movement of Na⁺ by active reabsorption and diffusion. Sodium moves from the proximal tubule into the tubular cell by diffusion. From there it moves by active transport to the interstitial space, where it diffuses into the peritubular capillary; thereafter it flows back into the general circulation.

similar to that proposed for active transport in any cell membrane. That is, the sodium ion becomes chemically bound to a carrier dissolved in the cell membrane. The combination of sodium and its carrier diffuses across the membrane where the carrier releases the sodium into the peritubular fluid in the interstitial space. The high-energy compound adenosine triphosphate (ATP), which is transformed to adenosine diphosphate, supplies the energy for the carrier. The necessary enzymes for the reaction are also located in the base membrane.

As stated earlier, the active reabsorption of other substances occurs in the same manner, each having its own specific carrier and enzymes which catalyze the reactions. The importance of the active reabsorption mechanism lies in the fact that it regulates the absorption of materials even when the concentration gradient favors no removal of materials from the tubular filtrate. Because of this the metabolism of the tubular cells is commensurate with the energy requirements needed for transforming the potential energy of nutrients into chemical energy for reabsorption.

diffusion and osmosis

Diffusion and osmosis also play an important role in the reabsorption of other materials from the glomerular filtrate, especially water. *Diffusion* is the random movement of molecules in a liquid or gas and is caused by the kinetic movement of all molecules in the liquid or gas. Since there are pores in the epithelial membranes of the tubules, certain materials such as water can diffuse through them and into the renal interstitial spaces following their concentration gradients.

The principal method of reabsorption of water, however, is by osmosis. *Osmosis* is the net diffusion in one direction of permeable substances, caused by the presence of larger concentrations of nonpermeants on one side of the membrane than on the other. Thus the active transport of relatively impermeant (i.e., nondiffusable) substances, such as electrolytes, glucose, and amino acids, decreases their concentrations in the tubular filtrate, which increases them in the peritubular interstitial spaces. As this continues, an osmotic gradient for water develops and the water diffuses through the membrane. As a result, the initial phenomenon is one of active reabsorption of osmotically active substances with osmotic reabsorption of water simply following in its wake.

Some materials, such as the end products of metabolism like urea, are undesirable in body fluids. Urea diffuses through the pores at a much slower rate than water. In fact, it diffuses several hundred times less easily. As a consequence, only about 50 percent of the urea in the tubular filtrate diffuses into the interstitial spaces and the remainder is excreted in the urine. Sulphates, phosphates, creatinine, nitrates, and phenols—all end products of metabolism—are removed in the same manner. If these substances are permitted to accumulate, they produce toxic effects on cells of the body and slow down essential metabolic reactions.

A certain few substances are actively secreted from the tubular capillaries into the tubules. This phenomenon, presumed to be the reverse of active reabsorption, requires energy and a carrier mechanism. Penicillin, iodopyracet (Diodrast), and phenolsulfonphthalein are removed in this fashion; however, normally only potassium and hydrogen ion regulation is maintained by this method.

clearance

From the foregoing discussion a very important concept in renal function emerges—that of *clearance*. Each time that a small fraction of plasma filters through the glomerular membrane, the resulting filtrate passes down the tubules and reabsorption occurs, and a large proportion of unwanted metabolic end products is left behind in the urine. The blood is "cleared" of these substances. Indeed, of each 125 ml. of glomerular filtrate formed per minute, 60 ml. leaves its urea behind in the fluid within the tubules. Stated another way, 60 ml. of plasma is cleared of urea each minute in normally functioning kidneys. In the same way 125 ml. of plasma is cleared of creatinine, 12 ml. of uric acid, 12 ml. of potassium, 25 ml. of sulfate, 25 ml. of phosphate, etc., each minute. It is possible to calculate renal clearance by simultaneously sampling urine and plasma. By dividing the quantity of substance found in each millimeter of plasma into the quantity found in the urine, the milliliters cleared per minute can be calculated. This method is used as one means of testing kidney function.

regulatory mechanisms

It is apparent that kidney function is important in the regulation of (1) electrolyte concentration, (2) osmotic pressure, and (3) both the pH and the volume of the extracellular fluids (i.e., blood and interstitial fluid) of the body. As pointed out in the section on respiration, the kidney functions in conjunction with the respiratory system in the regulation of pH. The mechanisms by which materials are filtered, reabsorbed, and secreted have also just been discussed. It is important now to look at the special mechanisms which regulate these processes for certain molecules.

Nearly 90 percent of all positively charged ions in the extracellular fluids of the body are sodium ions. Only moderate changes in concentration of this ion can affect transmission of nerve impulses, strength of cardiac contraction, endocrine and exocrine secretory processes, and secretory processes and function of the brain. Consequently the extracellular concentration is finely regulated so as not to vary more than ±5 mEq. around a mean of 142 mEq. per liter. Figure 15-6 summarizes the overall mechanism for sodium ion regulation and the main secondary effect of regulating potassium concentration as well.

In the face of decreased extracellular concentration of sodium, the kidney releases *renin,* an enzyme which converts a plasma protein in the blood to *angiotensin I.* A converting enzyme found in pulmonary tissue changes angiotensin I to *angiotensin II.* Angiotensin II increases the secretion of *aldosterone,* a hormone of the adrenal cortex. The decreased extracellular Na^+ concentration is believed to cause the increase of aldosterone directly. In addition to causing increased aldosterone secretion, angiotensin II is also a potent vasopressor and thus also increases glomerular filtration. Aldosterone increases the rate of reabsorption of sodium in the tubules, exchanging a sodium for a potassium. This occurs primarily in the distal convoluted tubules, thereby finely regulating the extracellular levels of both sodium and potassium.

A backup mechanism for potassium regulation is also found in renal function. If there are high levels of potassium in the face of normal sodium levels, the distal tubules and collecting ducts actively secrete (reverse of active reabsorption) potassium back into the urine. Similar specific reabsorption mechanisms appear to exist for divalent ions such as calcium, magnesium, and phosphates.

The regulation of the monovalent anions, chloride and bicarbonate, is secondary to sodium-ion regulation. As the positively charged cation, sodium, is reabsorbed, a negatively charged ion follows to maintain electroneutrality. Whether the negative ion is bicarbonate or chloride is dependent upon the regulation of pH in conjunction with the respiratory system.

The regulation of fluid volume by the kidney resides in the mechanisms for concentrating and diluting urine. The *countercurrent mechanism* is responsible for the kidney's ability to concentrate urine. Anatomically the kidney can be divided into two major regions, the *cortex,* where the glomeruli and the proximal and distal tubules are located, and the *medulla*. The loop of Henle extends deep into the medulla, and the collecting tubules pass through it before emptying into the renal pelvis. Referring to Figs. 15-2 and 15-3, notice that the peritubular capillaries extend into the medulla forming long loops called *vasa recta* which empty into the renal veins in the cortex. As discussed earlier, sodium is actively reabsorbed from the filtrate into the interstitial spaces. It finally reaches concentrations that are three to four times normal. The reduced rate of flow as well as the anatomical arrangement of the vasa recta prevents the blood from carrying away large amounts of sodium. This is accomplished in the following manner: Blood flows downward in the vasa recta and sodium diffuses rapidly into the blood from the interstitial fluid until it reaches the bottom of the loop where the concentration reaches levels that are approximately three times normal. As the blood flows back up toward the cortex, sodium diffuses back into the peritubular fluid, conserving

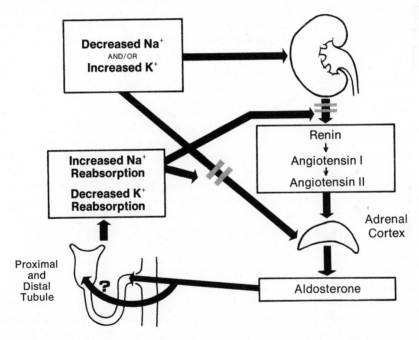

Fig. 15-6. Regulation of Na^+ and K^+ concentrations in extracellular fluids. All conditions in boxes occur in extracellular fluid. "//" equals negative feedback mechanism with ↑ Na^+ and ↓ K^+. When sodium reaches normal levels in the extracellular fluid, negative feedback occurs. Aldosterone is no longer stimulated by the low sodium level. Renin is no longer released by the kidney, and therefore Angiotensin II is not available to stimulate the adrenal cortex to produce aldosterone. Because of these negative feedback mechanisms, the level of aldosterone falls and as a result Na^+ is no longer being reabsorbed in exchange for K^+ in the distal tubule. (From A. C. Guyton, *Function of the Human Body*, Philadelphia, W. B. Saunders, 1969)

sodium. As the filtrate flows through the loop, it becomes very dilute and is hypotonic by the time it enters the collecting tubule. The epithelium of the collecting duct alters its permeability to water in response to the posterior pituitary antidiuretic hormone (ADH).

When ADH is released, most of the water is reabsorbed from the urine in the collecting tubules and the urine is concentrated. The release of ADH is effected by special neural osmoreceptors located in the supraoptic nuclei near the hypothalamus in the brain. When extracellular fluid is too concentrated these neurons stimulate the release of ADH from the posterior pituitary. In the presence of dilute extracellular fluid ADH is not released and a dilute urine is produced, decreasing extracellular fluid volume.

summary of renal function

The total blood flow into the nephrons of both kidneys is estimated to be about 1,200 ml. per minute. Of this total amount, about 650 ml. is plasma. Approximately one fifth of the plasma filters through the glomerular membranes into the Bowman's capsules, forming 125 ml. glomerular filtrate per minute. This filtrate is essentially plasma minus proteins. The pH of glomerular filtrate is equal to that of plasma, or 7.4. As the glomerular filtrate passes through the proximal tubules, nearly 80 percent of the water and electrolytes, all of the glucose, proteins and most of the amino acids are reabsorbed. The glomerular filtrate passes on through remaining tubules where water and electrolytes are reabsorbed, depending upon the need of body fluids and the effectiveness of the regulatory mechanism responsible for maintaining their normal levels. The pH of the forming urine may rise or fall, depending upon the relative amount of acidic and basic ions which are reabsorbed by the tubule walls. The osmotic pressure of the tubular fluid will depend upon the amounts of electrolytes and water that are reabsorbed. Because of those factors, urine pH may vary from 4.5 to 8.2 and osmotic pressure may vary from one fourth that of plasma to approximately 4 times plasma pressure. The amount of urine delivered to the renal pelvis is usually about $1/125$ the amount of glomerular filtrate produced or about 1 ml. per minute. This 1 ml. of urine will contain nearly one half of the urea contained in the original 125 ml. of glomerular filtrate, all of the creatinine, and large proportions of uric acid, phosphate, potassium, sulfates, nitrates, and phenols. It should be pointed out that even though all glucose and proteins, nearly all amino acids, and large amounts of water and sodium in the original glomerular filtrate are reabsorbed, a very large proportion of the waste products are never reabsorbed and are found in the urine in highly concentrated form.

ALLEN C. ALFREY, M.D.
DONALD E. BUTKUS, M.D.

16

renal failure: pathophysiology and management

pathophysiology of renal failure

The adverse effect of reduced renal perfusion on renal function, as a consequence of various shock states, has been recognized for over a hundred years. However, it was during and following World War II that most of the knowledge in regard to understanding the pathogenesis, physiology, and management of renal ischemia was obtained. Since about 1950 evidence has been accumulated to suggest that early diagnosis of renal failure in association with aggressive treatment of the shock state can reverse functional abnormalities and prevent acute tubular necrosis.

Because of the large amount of renal blood flow required to maintain normal renal function, changes in urinary composition occur early in the shock state when renal perfusion is decreased. Normally the kidneys receive 20 to 25 percent of the cardiac output (approximately 1,200 ml. per minute). Almost 90 percent of the blood flow to the kidney is concerned with cortical distribution and, in turn, glomerular filtration. The kidney has an intrinsic ability to regulate blood flow (autoregulation) so that the glomerular filtration rate is kept constant over a blood pressure range of 80 to 180 mm. Hg. This is accomplished by variations in the tone of pre- and postglomerular arterioles.

However, when renal blood flow is severely compromised as a result of either reduction in effective blood volume, fall in cardiac output, or decrease in blood pressure below 80 mm. Hg, characteristic changes occur in renal function. Thus the capacity for complete autoregulation is exceeded. The glomerular filtration rate falls. The amount of tubular fluid is reduced and the fluid travels through the tubule more slowly. This results in increased sodium and water reabsorption. Because of the reduced renal circulation the solutes reabsorbed from the tubular fluid are removed more slowly than normal from the interstitium of the renal medulla. This results in increased medullary tonicity, which in turn further augments water reabsorption from the tubular fluid. Therefore, the urinary changes are typical in the shock state. The urinary volume is reduced to less than 400 ml. per day (17 ml. per hour), urinary specific gravity is increased, and urinary sodium concentration is low (usually less than 5 mEq. per liter).

In addition, substances such as creatinine and urea which are normally filtered but poorly reabsorbed from the renal tubule are present in high concentration in the urine as a result of the increased water reabsorption. Because of the characteristic changes associated with renal underperfusion, measurement of urinary volume and specific gravity is a simple method of determining the effect of shock management on renal perfusion. An increase in systemic blood pressure does not necessarily imply improvement in renal perfusion. This may be especially evident when drugs such as norepinephrine (Levophed) are used to correct the hypotension associated with states of volume depletion. These drugs may be associated with further reduction in renal blood flow as a consequence of constriction of renal arteries. This is manifested by a further fall in urinary volume and rise in specific gravity. In turn, if the shock state is more appropriately and specifically treated by replacing volume, improving cardiac output, correcting arrhythmias, or by giving isoproterenol (Isuprel), the improved renal perfusion will be manifested as an increased urinary volume and a fall in specific gravity of the urine.

management of acute reversible renal failure

Primary management of renal function impairment is directed at the adequate and specific management of the shock state. The three most common causes for reduced renal perfusion are decreased cardiac output, altered peripheral vascular resistance, and hypovolemia.

decreased cardiac output

Factors such as cardiac arrhythmias, acute myocardial infarction, and acute pericardial tamponade, all of which decrease cardiac output, may be associated with a reduction in renal blood flow. The reversibility of the renal failure is thus dependent on the ability to improve cardiac function. The specific management has been discussed in earlier chapters.

With the above conditions cardiac output is usually acutely and severely compromised. However, when cardiac output is impaired to a lesser extent over a more chronic period of time, features of congestive heart failure occur. Again there is reduced renal perfusion, although to a lesser extent. The major feature of this state, from the renal aspect, is avid sodium reabsorption, which results in increased extracellular fluid volume, elevation of central venous pressure and edema.

Several mechanisms are responsible for the increased tubular reabsorption of sodium. First, there is a greater reduction in renal blood flow than in glomerular filtration, bringing into play the mechanisms discussed earlier. Second, it has been suggested that blood flow to the superficial cortex is reduced while blood flow to the inner cortical area is increased. It is also thought that the nephrons in the inner cortical region reabsorb a greater percentage of the filtered sodium than the nephrons in the outer cortex of the kidney. Other factors include increased proximal and distal tubule sodium reabsorption. The mechanisms responsible for the increased proximal tubule sodium reabsorption are poorly understood; however, aldosterone is largely responsible for the increased distal tubule sodium reabsorption. It can be seen that numerous mechanisms are responsible for the increased tubular reabsorption of sodium in congestive heart failure.

Therapy is largely directed at increasing urinary sodium excretion. At times this can be accomplished by improving cardiac output which in turn increases renal perfusion. This is not always possible, however. Diuretics are frequently used to increase sodium excretion. These agents directly inhibit sodium reabsorption in the renal tubule. The potency of a diuretic is primarily determined by the site in the renal tubule where sodium reabsorption is blocked. The two most potent diuretics presently available are furosemide (Lasix) and ethacrynic acid (Edecrin). These agents block sodium reabsorption in the ascending limb of the loop of Henle and in the distal tubule. It is still unclear whether they have an effect in the proximal tubule as well. The thiazide diuretics have their major site of action in the distal tubule and are therefore somewhat less potent than the above agents. Another diuretic commonly used is spironolactone (Aldactone) which increases urinary sodium by blocking the renal tubular effect of aldosterone.

altered peripheral vascular resistance

Renal perfusion is compromised in these states as a result of increased size of the intravascular compartment and redistribution of blood volume. This may be a consequence of gram-negative septicemia, certain drug overdoses, anaphylactic reactions, and electrolyte disturbances such as acidosis. Management is primarily directed at treating the basic disturbance with appropriate specific therapy plus fluid, electrolyte, and colloid replacement. The controversy in regard to the use of steroids and various pressor agents in gram-negative sepsis is beyond the scope of this discussion.

hypovolemia

Restoration of extracellular fluid and blood volume is of major importance in the management of any shock state. Evidence for extracellular volume depletion is usually obtained from the history and physical examination. Historically the patient may give evidence of external sodium and water loss as a result of vomiting, diarrhea, excessive sweating, or surgical procedures. Blood volume may also be compromised as a result of fluid redistribution as seen both with burns and with inflammatory processes in the abdomen, such as pancreatitis or peritonitis. The physical findings associated with extracellular volume depletion are sunken eyes, dry mouth, loss of skin turgor and tachycardia. Postural hypotension may also be noted. Therapy is directed at sodium and water replacement. Response to treatment can be judged by changes in urinary volume, specific gravity, central venous pressure and the above physical findings.

maintenance of urinary flow

At times in spite of adequate treatment of the shock state, urinary volume remains low. This may be a result of either continuing functional impairment in the postshock period or parenchymal renal damage suffered as a consequence of the shock state. Not only is it necessary to differentiate these two states from each other, but a number of authors also feel that prolonged oliguria, if allowed to persist, may eventually lead to acute tubular necrosis. Mannitol and furosemide have been used in this setting for both diagnosis and maintenance of urinary function.

Mannitol is the reduced form of the six-carbon sugar mannose. It is distributed in the extracellular fluid and is essentially not metabolized. It is freely filtered at the glomerulus and not reabsorbed by the tubule. Because of its small molecular size (180) it exerts a significant osmotic effect and in turn increases urinary flow. Mannitol is usually infused rather rapidly. The more rapid the infusion the higher the blood level and in turn the filtered load. Urine flow is dependent on the amount of mannitol filtered, and if the infusion is too slow, changes in urinary flow rate will be delayed and less apparent.

The usual test is 12.5 gm. given intravenously as a 25 percent solution over 3 to 5 minutes. If urine flow increases to greater than 40 ml. per hour, the patient is felt to have reversible renal failure and his urine volume is then maintained at 100 ml. per hour with additional mannitol.

More recently furosemide and ethacrynic acid have largely replaced mannitol in the diagnosis of reversible renal failure. A number of patients who fail to develop a diuresis following mannitol will have an acceptable increase in urinary volume following furosemide or ethacrynic acid. Furosemide in dosages of 200 to 1,000 mg. is given intravenously. The peak diuresis usually occurs within 2 hours of its administration. If furosemide is effective in increasing urinary volume, it is then repeated at 4- to 6-hour intervals to maintain the urinary flow rate. In patients failing to respond to furosemide a diagnosis of acute tubular necrosis is seriously entertained. In patients who respond to furosemide and mannitol it is important to realize that sodium and water depletion will occur if losses are not replaced. Usually urine volume is replaced by half-strength normal saline. In addition potassium replacement is frequently required.

acute tubular necrosis

Although approximately 30 percent of the cases of acute tubular necrosis occur without a specific etiology being found, some of the more common causes for the development of this syndrome include shock, nephrotoxic agents and acute renal failure associated with myoglobinuria and hemoglobinuria.

There is little doubt that the severity and duration of traumatic shock play major roles in predisposing to the development of acute tubular necrosis. Over 40 percent of a large number of combat casualties in World War II developed acute tubular necrosis. In contrast, acute tubular necrosis was uncommon in Vietnam casualties. This reduced incidence has been attributed to early air evacuation and rapid treatment of shock.

A large number of chemicals and drugs have been found to be nephrotoxic. In the hospital patient probably the most common group of nephrotoxic agents are the antibiotics. These include gentamycin, cephaloridine, colistin, kanamycin, and polymyxin. Because of the frequency with which acute tubular necrosis occurs in patients receiving these agents, renal function should be routinely evaluated before and during treatment with these drugs.

A third major category of acute tubular necrosis is that associated with abnormal release of body pigments (myoglobin and hemoglobin). Characteristically the urine is dark in color and positive for hemoglobin. Patients with states associated with intravascular hemolysis such as transfusion reactions, malaria, and arsine intoxication, may develop acute tubular necrosis. In addition, acute renal failure commonly occurs in patients with myoglobinuria of a variety of etiologies.

Numerous investigations have been carried out to define the mechanisms by which nephrotoxic agents and shock induce acute tubular necrosis and oliguria, but to date these have not been clearly defined. Renal blood flow has been found to be reduced to approximately one third of normal in acute tubular necrosis, whereas the glomerular filtration rate is almost completely suppressed. This is in contrast to other states in which a similar reduction in renal blood flow is accompanied by much better maintenance of glomerular filtration and renal function.

Numerous animal studies have suggested that intratubular obstruction from casts and cellular debris may be involved in the suppression of glomerular filtration. If this obstruction is relieved, renal function returns. Other studies have suggested that there is disruption of the tubule epithelium with excessive back flow of the filtrate out of the tubule lumen, thus explaining the lack of urine formation in the face of continuing, although reduced, renal blood flow.

Hollenberg and his colleagues have put forth evidence that cortical blood flow is severely compromised in acute tubular necrosis resulting from ischemia as well as nephrotoxic agents.[1] The mechanism responsible for the decreased superficial cortical blood flow in the kidney with acute tubular necrosis has not been defined. However, the recent demonstration of converting enzyme being present in the kidney suggests that renin-angiotensin may play a role in this phenomenon.

Classically patients have oliguria in association with acute tubular necrosis; however this is not invariably so. A group of patients present with acute nonoliguric (partially reversible) renal failure. This state is especially common in patients receiving nephrotoxic antibiotics. If antibiotics are discontinued before renal function is markedly reduced, the patient frequently sustains moderate functional impairment for 7 to 10 days with gradual return to normal. In general, patients with nonoliguric acute renal failure have few symptoms and the disease is much less serious than the oliguric form of acute tubular necrosis.

The more classical or oliguric form of acute tubular necrosis begins with an acute precipitating event immediately followed by oliguria (urine volume less than 400 ml. per day). The mean duration of oliguria is around 12 days although it may last only 2 to 3 days or as long as 30 days. This is accompanied by a usual rise in BUN of 25 to 30 mg. per 100 ml. per day and creatinine of 1.5 to 2 mg. per 100 ml. per day. The most common complication in this period is overhydration with resulting cardiac failure, pulmonary edema, and death. In addition the patient may develop acidosis, hyperkalemia, and symptoms of uremia.

The oliguric phase is followed by gradual return of renal function as manifested by a stepwise increase in urine volume (the diuretic stage). The degree of diuresis is primarily determined by the state of hydration at the time the patient enters the diuretic stage. If the patient is markedly overloaded, urinary volume may eventually exceed 4 to 5 liters per day. This may result in marked sodium wasting, with death resulting from electrolyte depletion. Because of the slow return of renal function during the diuretic phase the degree of azotemia may increase during the early part of the diuretic period and the patient will have similar complications as noted in the oliguric phase. A period of several months is required for full recovery of renal function after the end of the diuretic period.

differentiating acute tubular necrosis from decreased renal perfusion

During the immediate postshock period the differentiation between continuing decreased renal perfusion and acute tubular necrosis has to be made. The routine urine analysis is usually of little help in differentiating these two states in that the changes are nonspecific. In both conditions there may be mild proteinuria in association with a moderate number of red blood cells, white blood cells, and granular casts. The major features of the two states are shown in Table 16-1.

The urinary changes present in patients with acute tubular necrosis are

table 16-1
use of lab values in differentiating acute tubular necrosis from decreased renal perfusion

TEST	ACUTE TUBULAR NECROSIS	REDUCED RENAL BLOOD FLOW
Urine		
Volume	Less than 400 ml./24 hr.	Less than 400 ml./24 hr.
Sodium	Between 40 and 100 mEq./L.	Less than 5 mEq./L.
Specific gravity	1.010	Usually greater than 1.020
Osmolality	250–350 mOsm/L.	Usually greater than 500 mOsm/L.
Urea	200–300 mg./100 ml.	Usually greater than 600 mg./100 ml.
Creatinine	Less than 60 mg./100 ml.	Usually greater than 150 mg./100 ml.
Blood		
BUN:Cr	10:1	Usually greater than 20:1
Response to		
Mannitol	None	None or flow increases to greater than 40 ml./hr.
Furosemide	None	Flow increases to greater than 40 ml./hr.

largely a consequence of loss of tubule function. Hypertension is uncommon in patients with acute tubular necrosis and when present suggests fluid and sodium excess.

When the patient presents to the hospital with oliguric renal failure, other causes of acute renal insufficiency must be considered such as lupus glomerulonephritis, periarteritis, rapidly progressive glomerulonephritis, post-streptococcal glomerulonephritis. In addition, the possibility of chronic parenchymal renal disease exists.

Rarely does the patient with acute tubular necrosis have total anuria. This is an important point in helping to differentiate acute tubular necrosis from obstructive uropathy. However, retrograde urography is frequently necessary to exclude obstruction.

management

Since acute tubular necrosis continues to carry a high mortality rate, the major objective is prevention of this complication. The feasibility of preventing the development of acute tubular necrosis in patients with major traumatic injuries by rapid replacement of blood loss and correction of fluid and electrolyte disturbances was clearly demonstrated in the Vietnam war. Similarly, patients receiving potentially nephrotoxic agents should have serial determinations to evaluate renal function during the course of the administration of these agents. This can most easily be done by measuring serum creatinine levels on an every-other-day schedule. If the serum creatinine begins to rise, the drug should be discontinued. In the majority of patients, functional deterioration stabilizes and the patient recovers without the development of severe impairment of renal function.

There is still considerable debate with regard to the effectiveness of mannitol and furosemide in the prevention of acute renal failure. In fact, some evidence has been accumulated which suggests that furosemide may actually increase the toxicity of certain nephrotoxic agents. Until this controversy is resolved it would seem desirable to use these agents sparingly in patients with nonoliguric acute tubular necrosis, especially when it is a consequence of drug intoxication.

After development of acute tubular necrosis, the primary consideration is maintenance of fluid and electrolyte balance. During the oliguric phase urinary volume is usually less than 300 ml. per day. Insensible losses average 800 to 1,000 ml. per day and are virtually free of electrolytes. In general, fluid replacement should be approximately 500 ml. per day. Additional water will be obtained from the water present in foods plus the water of oxidation from metabolism. Because of the utilization of body proteins and fats, the patient ideally should lose around 1 pound a day in order to maintain water balance. The danger of fluid overload with resulting congestive heart failure and pulmonary edema exists throughout the oliguric period. In contrast, during the diuretic phase of acute tubular necrosis there may be extensive sodium wasting in association with the increased urinary volumes. It is thus necessary to keep accurate intake and output records as well as daily weights during both phases. This is especially important when there are other avenues of fluid and electrolyte losses such as with vomiting, diarrhea, nasogastric suction, and drainages from fistulas. In general, losses occurring as a result of the above should be replaced in full.

Outside of adequate fluid and electrolyte replacement, intake is directed at supplying the patient with calories in the form of carbohydrates and fats to decrease the rate of breakdown of body protein. Since 1 gram of urea is formed from every 6 grams of protein metabolized, protein intake is usually restricted in order to prevent the BUN from rising at too fast a rate.

Certain drugs should be avoided or dosage reduced in any patient with markedly impaired renal function. Because of the possibility of magnesium intoxication, antacids containing magnesium should be avoided. Because of the reduced renal function, digitalis excretion may be reduced. Dosage should be altered to avoid excessively high blood levels. In addition, certain antibiotics should be given in much smaller dosages than usually employed (Table 16-2).

Before administering a drug to a patient with renal failure, it is wise to review the following questions:

1. Does the drug depend on the kidney for secretion?

table 16-2
recommended dosage for antibiotics

GROUP	ANTIBIOTIC	RECOMMENDED DOSE	
		SERUM CREATININE 4–10 mg. percent	SERUM CREATININE 10 mg. percent
1. Marked reduction in dosage	Tetracycline Oxytetracycline Kanamycin Streptomycin Colistimethate Polymyxin	Loading dose followed by standard doses at intervals of 1 to 2 days.	Loading dose followed by standard doses at intervals of 3 to 4 days.
2. Modest reduction in dosage	Penicillin G Lincomycin Cephalothin	Loading dose followed by: Standard doses at 4- to 5-hr. intervals. Standard doses at 6-hr. intervals. Standard doses at 12-hr. intervals.	Loading dose followed by: Standard doses at 8- to 10-hr. intervals. Standard doses at 12-hr. intervals. Standard doses at 24-hr. intervals.
3. No reduction in dosage	Chloramphenicol Erythromycin Methicillin Oxacillin Novobiocin	Same as in the normal.	Same as in the normal.

From W. B. Schwartz and J. P. Kassirer, *American Journal of Medicine,* Vol. 44 (1968), p. 796.

2. Does an excess blood level affect the kidney?
3. Does the drug add chemically to the pool of urea nitrogen?
4. Does the effect of the drug alter electrolyte imbalance?
5. Is the patient more susceptible to the drug because of kidney disease?
For additional information about the modification of drug dosages in uremia, see R. J. Anderson, J. G. Gambertoglio, and R. W. Schrier, *Clinical Use of Drugs in Renal Failure* (Springfield, Illinois: Charles C Thomas, 1976).

acidosis

Metabolic acidosis of moderate severity is usually present in patients with renal failure. This results from the inability of the kidneys to excrete fixed acids (e.g., H_2PO_4) produced from normal metabolic processes. The acidosis can usually be easily controlled by giving the patient 30 to 60 mEq. of sodium bicarbonate daily.

hyperkalemia

Hyperkalemia commonly occurs in patients with acute tubular necrosis. This is a consequence of both the reduced ability of the kidneys to excrete potassium and the release of intracellular potassium because of acidosis. The acidosis results in movement of the hydrogen ion into the cell, thus displacing potassium into the extracellular fluid. This maintains electrical neutrality but increases the hyperkalemic state. Hyperkalemia is manifested clinically by cardiac and neuromuscular changes. Both cardiac conduction disturbances and acute flaccid quadriplegia are life-threatening complications. These hyperkalemic changes are rapidly reversed by giving intravenous calcium gluconate which has a direct antagonist effect on the action of potassium. Reduction of the serum potassium can be accomplished by treating the acidosis with intravenous sodium bicarbonate. In addition, glucose and insulin are frequently used as an additional method of shifting extracellular potassium to intracellular pools. Hyperkalemia is usually preventable by avoiding potassium supplements, giving chronic therapy for acidosis and using sodium polystyrene sulfonate resin (Kayexalate) when serum potassium is even slightly elevated.

During the oliguric phase sodium retention may occur. However, with the onset of the diuretic period urinary volume and sodium excretion may markedly increase. Urinary volume is largely determined by the state of hydration at the onset of the diuretic period. Since urinary sodium concentration is relatively fixed, sodium losses are largely determined by urinary volume. Therefore, if the patient is markedly overhydrated at the onset of the diuretic phase, sodium losses may be severe. Clinically sodium depletion is characterized by either extracellular volume depletion as manifested by tachycardia and postural hypotension or water intoxication when sodium losses exceed water losses. This latter syndrome is characterized by markedly reduced serum sodium concentrations in association with personality changes, convulsions, coma, and death if allowed to progress untreated. With acute water intoxication, treatment is directed at raising the serum sodium concentration. This can usually be accomplished by giving hypertonic (3 to 5 percent) sodium chloride intravenously. Table 16-3 lists common fluid and electrolyte imbalances.

In addition to the above specific electrolyte disturbances, the patient may develop symptoms associated with any uremic state. Early the patient has nausea, anorexia, and vomiting. Later this progresses to stupor, convulsions, and coma. In addition, the patient may develop bleeding abnormalities, uremic pneumonitis, pericarditis, pleuritis, etc. Dialysis is indicated prior to the development of clinical symptoms of uremia. With the availability of hemodialysis or peritoneal dialysis in most hospitals, there is little reason for the clinical features of uremia to occur in patients with acute tubular necrosis. Most patients having oliguria for more than 4 to 5 days will require dialysis sometime during the course of their acute tubular necrosis. There is little doubt that dialysis has improved survival in patients with acute tubular

table 16-3
common fluid and electrolyte imbalances

ELECTROLYTE DISTURBANCE	MAJOR SYMPTOMS	MAJOR PHYSICAL FINDINGS	ETIOLOGY
Increased sodium and water	Dyspnea	Edema, anasarca, rales, increased jugular venous pressure	Congestive failure, renal disease, liver disease
Decreased sodium and water	Thirst Weakness	Tachycardia, postural hypotension, sunken eyes, dry mouth, decreased skin turgor	Excessive sweating, vomiting, diarrhea, Addison's disease, renal disease, diuretics without replacement
Decreased sodium and normal water	Headaches Psychological disorder	Hyperreflexia, pathological reflexes, convulsions, coma	Water without sodium replacement in above states; excess ADH
Normal sodium and decreased water	Thirst	Often no findings or those found in decreased sodium and water	Lack of water intake, diabetes insipidus, excessive sweating, fever
Hyperkalemia	Weakness	Paralysis, ECG changes: spiked T waves	Renal disease, excess potassium replacement
Hypokalemia	Weakness	Paralysis, paralytic ileus, hypoventilation, ECG changes: T waves and prominent U waves	Diuretics, renal disease, diarrhea, vomiting, excess laxatives
Acidosis	Weakness	Kussmaul respiration	Renal disease, diabetic acidosis, certain intoxications
Hypermagnesemia	Weakness	Muscle weakness, hypoventilation, hypotension, flushing	Antacids with renal disease

necrosis. During World War II, when dialysis was not available, the mortality rate was 90 percent in battle casualties developing renal failure. The mortality rate was reduced to 50 percent with hemodialysis in casualties with renal failure during the Korean war.

Prognosis is largely determined by the primary event that led to the development of acute tubular necrosis. Medical causes of acute tubular necrosis such as transfusion reactions, myoglobinuria, nephrotoxic agents, and simple volume depletion are accompanied by a mortality rate of around 25 percent, whereas cases resulting from trauma and severe surgical complications have a mortality rate of 70 to 80 percent. Death usually results as a complication of poor wound healing and sepsis. In view of the continuing high mortality rate associated with acute tubular necrosis, every effort should be directed toward the prevention of this complication when the patient is seen early during the course of his shock state.

REFERENCE

1. N. K. Hollenberg, D. F. Adams, D. E. Oken, H. L. Abrams, and J. P. Merrill, "Acute Renal Failure Due to Nephrotoxins," *New England Journal of Medicine*, Vol. 282 (1970), p. 1329.

selected tests used to monitor renal function

The patient whose condition is serious enough to warrant observation in the critical care unit will frequently manifest abnormalities of renal function, either as the result of impaired ability to excrete nitrogenous waste products or because of an inability to handle water loads efficiently, or both. It is therefore mandatory that certain aspects of renal function be monitored, on an intermittent or a continuing basis, in order that these complications can be detected early and appropriate therapy instituted. In most circumstances the parameters followed will include the urine output, the urine solute concentration (frequently in relation to the plasma solute concentration), and some parameter of the kidneys' ability to excrete nitrogenous waste products.

creatinine and creatinine clearance

The most commonly used tests of renal function are the serum creatinine and the blood urea nitrogen (BUN), but the most accurate test readily available is the creatinine clearance.

Creatinine is formed as a by-product of normal muscle metabolism and is excreted in the urine primarily as the result of glomerular filtration, with a small percentage secreted into the urine by the kidney tubules. It is therefore a useful indicator of the glomerular filtration rate. The amount of creatinine excreted in the urine of any given individual is related to his muscle mass and will remain quite constant unless muscle wasting occurs. The actual creatinine clearance is calculated by the formula:

$$\text{Clearance creatinine} = \frac{UV}{P}$$

where U is the urine creatinine concentration, V the urine volume, and P the plasma creatinine concentration. The most important technical aspect of this test is the accuracy of the urine collection, as it is important to know the exact time it took to form the sample and the exact amount of creatinine present. The expression UV tells how much creatinine appears in the urine during the period of collection, and this can be readily converted to mg. per minute which is the standard reference point. Dividing this by the plasma creatinine concentration (which has to be converted from mg. per 100 ml. to mg. per ml.) tells the minimum number of milliliters of plasma which must have been filtered by the glomeruli in order to produce the measured amount of creatinine in the urine. The final result is expressed in ml. per min. and the normal range varies between 80 and 120 ml. per minute, depending on the individual's size and age. The results should be corrected to a standard body size of 1.73 square meters, which can be derived from standard tables if the patient's height and weight are known.

If the kidneys are damaged by some disease process, the creatinine clearance will decrease and the serum creatinine concentration will rise. The urine creatinine excretion will initially decrease until the blood level rises to a point at which the amount of creatinine appearing in the urine is again equal to the amount being produced by the body. For example, a normal individual with a serum creatinine concentration of 1.0 mg. percent and a creatinine excretion of 1.0 mg. per minute has a creatinine clearance of 100 ml. per minute. If the individual develops renal disease with 50 percent loss of renal function, his serum creatinine will rise to 2.0 mg. percent and he will continue to excrete 1.0 mg. of creatinine in his urine per minute. In many situations where the patient has rapidly changing renal function and oliguria, as in acute tubular necrosis, the creatinine clearance becomes less reliable until the situation becomes more stable. It is therefore useful to follow the serum creatinine concentration as an indicator of the rate and direction of change until stability occurs.

blood urea nitrogen

The blood urea nitrogen (BUN) has also been used for many years as an indicator of kidney function, but, unlike the serum creatinine, its level tends to be influenced by a great many factors. Urea, as mentioned in an earlier section, has a clearance less than that of creatinine due largely to the fact that some urea diffuses out of the tubule back into the bloodstream. This is particularly true at low urine flow rates where more sodium and water, and consequently more urea, are being reabsorbed. Therefore, in states of relative or absolute volume depletion, the BUN will tend to rise out of proportion to any change in renal function. In addition, the amount of urea produced per day, unlike creatinine, is quite variable, especially in seriously ill patients. Increased urea production can result from increased protein intake (tube feedings and some forms of hyperalimentation) or increased tissue breakdown as with crush injuries, febrile illnesses, steroid or tetracycline administration, and reabsorption of blood from the intestine in a patient with intestinal hemorrhage. All of these may result in an increased urea production and an increased BUN even though renal function might be normal, and would also contribute to the rate of rise in BUN in an individual with renal failure. The opposite is true for patients with decreased protein intake or liver disease (both of which reduce urea production) and for patients with large urine volumes secondary to excessive fluid intake. The BUN is therefore less useful as a guide to changes in renal function than is the serum creatinine. The BUN is still of significant value, however, especially when looked at in comparison with the serum creatinine concentration. Normally these are present in a ratio of 10:1 (urea: creatinine). Discrepancies in this ratio might point toward a potentially correctable situation as noted in Table 16-4.

table 16-4
factors affecting serum urea: creatinine ratio

A. Decreased Urea:Creatinine ($<10:1$)
 1. Liver disease
 2. Protein restriction
 3. Excessive fluid intake
B. Increased Urea:Creatinine ($>10:1$)
 1. Volume depletion
 2. Decreased "effective" blood volume
 3. Catabolic states
 4. Excessive protein intake

urinary concentration and dilution

As noted earlier, the kidney possesses a considerable capacity to reabsorb filtered water. In individuals with normal renal function the final concentration of the urine is dependent upon the state of hydration. A patient who is well hydrated will excrete a very dilute urine, and a patient who is dehydrated will excrete a very concentrated urine, as the kidneys attempt to either eliminate or conserve water. The factor which governs the amount of water excreted, and, therefore, the urine concentration, is the amount of antidiuretic hormone (ADH) secreted by the pituitary gland. Urinary concentration may be measured by tests for specific gravity and/or osmolality.

Specific Gravity The specific gravity of the urine is the time-honored test of the kidneys' ability to concentrate and dilute the urine. The specific gravity measures the buoyancy of a solution compared to water and depends upon the number of particles in solution as well as their size and weight. Two methods have been used to obtain this measurement in clinical practice, the *hydrometer* and the *refractometer* (or TS meter, as it is frequently called). The hydrometer has been in clinical use for many years and is the less preferred of the two methods because (1) it requires a much larger volume of urine, (2) results are less reproducible, and (3) it requires a greater amount of time. The refractometer is highly reproducible and requires only a drop of urine for the measurement. In addition, this instrument can be used to measure the total solids of plasma (thus the name TS meter), which is a good indicator of the plasma protein concentration and a useful indicator of the state of a patient's fluid balance, especially when serial determinations are made. The refractometer, because of the above advantages, should replace the hydrometer for specific gravity determinations and should be used in the critical care unit.

The normal kidney has the capacity to dilute the urine to a specific gravity of 1.001 and to concentrate the urine to at least 1.022 (higher values are not unusual). Normally the individual's water balance will determine whether the urine is concentrated or dilute, a dilute urine being an indicator of water excess and a concentrated urine an indicator of water deficit. In many renal diseases the ability of the kidneys to form a concentrated urine is lost and the specific gravity becomes "fixed" at 1.010, a finding which might be seen in acute tubular necrosis and acute nephritis.

As with many simple laboratory tests there are limitations in the accuracy of the specific gravity determination. The specific gravity is not always the most accurate indicator of the ability of the kidneys to concentrate the urine because the concentrating ability is a reflection of the concentration of particles in the urine. In addition to the concentration of particles, the specific gravity is also in part dependent upon the size and weight of the particles in solution. Therefore, a falsely high specific gravity determination will be found when high-molecular-weight substances such as protein, glucose, mannitol, and radiographic contrast material are present in the urine. A greater degree of accuracy can be obtained with urine osmolality determinations.

Osmolality The *osmolality* of a solution is an expression of the total number (concentration) of particles in solution and is independent of the size, molecular weight, or electrical charge of the molecules. All substances in solution contribute to the osmolality to a certain degree. For example, a mol (gram molecular weight) of sodium chloride dissociates incompletely into Na^+ and Cl^- ions and produces 1.86 osmols when dissolved in a kilogram of solvent (such as plasma). A mol of nonionic solute (such as glucose or urea) produces only 1 osmol when dissolved in a kilogram of solvent. The total concentration of particles in a solution is the osmolality and is reported in units of osmols per kg. of solvent. In clinical situations, because we are dealing with much smaller concentrations, the osmolality is reported in milliosmols (thousandth of an osmol, abbreviated mOsm) per kilogram of solvent (plasma or serum).

The osmolality is determined in the laboratory by measuring the freezing point of the solution, the freezing point being directly related to the number of particles in solution. The normal serum osmolality is made up primarily of sodium and its accompanying anions, with urea and glucose contributing about 5 mOsm each. Therefore, knowing the serum sodium, urea and glucose concentrations, we can calculate the osmolality of plasma by the formula

$$\text{Osmolality} = 2 \, \text{Na} + \frac{\text{BUN}}{2.6} + \frac{\text{glucose}}{18}$$

The calculated osmolality will normally be within 10 mOsm of the measured osmolality, which normally averages 290 ± 5 mOsm per kg. The plasma osmolality in normal individuals is quite constant from day to day.

Because water permeates freely between the blood, interstitial fluid and tissues, a change in the osmolality of one body compartment will produce a shift in body fluids so that the osmolality of the plasma is always the same as that of the other body compartments, except in the most rapidly changing conditions, where a slight lag may occur.

The significance of the plasma osmolality lies in the fact that it is the main regulator of the release of antidiuretic hormone (ADH). When sufficient water is not being being taken in, the osmolality will rise, stimulating the release of ADH which signals the kidneys to conserve water and produce a more concentrated urine. When excessive amounts of water are ingested the osmolality decreases, ADH release is inhibited and the urine becomes more dilute. Under maximum ADH stimulation the kidneys can concentrate the urine to approximately 1,200 mOsm per kg., and with maximum ADH suppression (water load) the kidneys can dilute the urine to approximately 50 mOsm per kg. Thus there is no single normal urine osmolality but rather a range in which predicted values might be expected, depending upon the clinical setting. Also, unlike the plasma, the urine osmolality is less dependent on the urine sodium concentration, and other substances such as urea play a more important role. In renal disease one of the first renal functions to be lost is the ability to concentrate urine. As a reflection of this, the urine osmolality becomes fixed within 50 mOsm of the simultaneously determined serum osmolality. Therefore the osmolality is a useful parameter of renal function.

The serum and urine osmolality are of use in combination in a number of other circumstances. In the patient with diabetes insipidus, which results from neurological disease or injury, the urine volume would be increased with a low urine osmolality (50 to 100 mOsm) and the serum osmolality would be increased (310 mOsm or greater) unless the fluid loss had been replaced. On the other hand, the patient with carcinoma of the lung, porphyria, or CNS disease might have an excess production of ADH, or an ADH-like material, and have the opposite picture, with a low serum osmolality and a disproportionately high urine osmolality.

As already indicated, the serum osmolality may be increased or decreased in various states. A decrease in the serum osmolality can occur only when the serum sodium is decreased. An increase in the serum osmolality can occur whenever the serum sodium, urea, or glucose is elevated or when there are abnormal compounds present in the blood, such as drugs, poisons or metabolic waste products which are not usually measured, such as lactic acid. Symptoms due to increased osmolality usually occur when the osmolality is greater than 350 mOsm, and coma occurs when the osmolality is in the 400 range or above (see p. 337).

The usual close correlation between the measured and calculated osmolality has been mentioned. In certain circumstances the measured serum osmolality might be significantly higher than the calculated osmolality when substances of an unusual nature are present in the blood. Many drugs and toxins such as aspirin and alcohol raise the serum osmolality. In a comatose patient a discrepancy between the measured and calculated serum osmolalities might lead to the appropriate drug screen to provide the correct diagnosis. In patients with heart failure, hepatic disease, or shock, a discrepancy between the measured and calculated osmolalities, due to unknown metabolites of 40 or more mOsm, has been correlated with a mortality of 95 percent or greater.

serum sodium concentration

The serum sodium concentration is generally maintained in a narrow range (135 to 145 mEq. per liter) and is dependent upon the body's state of fluid balance as governed by the release of ADH and water intake. In a number of disease states, the serum sodium concentration may be reduced (hyponatremia) because of an inability of the kidneys to excrete free water. This is due to either a persistent release of ADH in response to a decrease in the total or effective intravascular volume* or to some inappropriate stimulation of ADH release (not due to volume or osmotic stimuli). Hyponatremia may be associated with an increased total body sodium and edema, a decreased total body sodium and hypovolemia, or a normal or slightly increased total body sodium and increased blood volume, depending upon the clinical disorder which gives rise to the hyponatremia (Table 16-5).

In patients with edema due to cirrhosis, congestive heart failure or the

table 16-5
hyponatremia

ACCOMPANIED BY	CAUSED BY
Increased total body sodium and edema	Congestive heart failure Decompensated cirrhosis Nephrotic syndrome
Decreased total body sodium and hypovolemia	Diuretics Renal salt wasting Adrenal insufficiency Hemorrhage
Normal total body sodium and hypervolemia	Syndrome of inappropriate ADH release which may accompany: CNS and pulmonary disease, tumors, porphyria, drugs, psychiatric disorders, myxedema

*A significant decrease in blood volume can override the normal osmotic stimulus to ADH release.

nephrotic syndrome, hyponatremia occurs frequently and may be enhanced by the use of diuretics. In these conditions, although there is an overall increase in body sodium and water, ADH release is stimulated because the *effective* blood volume is decreased. As a result the kidneys tend to reabsorb a greater percentage of filtered fluid, which causes further fluid retention and hyponatremia, especially if the patient has unlimited access to water. Treatment with thiazide diuretics, furosemide, or ethacrynic acid can seriously compound the hyponatremia because these drugs may further decrease the effective blood volume and because they decrease sodium transport in the ascending limb of Henle which is necessary for the kidneys' ability to excrete free water and maximally dilute the urine.

Patients with volume depletion from sodium or blood loss may also develop hyponatremia when the volume depletion is great enough to stimulate ADH release. In this circumstance, body sodium and blood volume are reduced and edema is not present. Diuretic administration, renal salt wasting, adrenal insufficiency, and hemorrhage are examples of this type of condition. Because of the decreased blood volume which accompanies these states, ADH release occurs and stimulates water reabsorption in an attempt to restore intravascular volume. If the patient ingests water without salt, or if hypotonic fluids are administered, hyponatremia will result. In this setting restoration of the blood volume takes precedence over the body's need to maintain its osmotic composition.

Hyponatremia may also occur in a number of conditions which are not associated with a decrease in either effective or absolute blood volume but in which either persistent release of ADH from the pituitary or ectopic production of ADH occurs. This unregulated production of ADH results in what is referred to as the syndrome of inappropriate ADH release (SIADH); this may occur with cerebral disease such as stroke, infection, or trauma; with pulmonary disease such as pneumonia, tuberculosis, or tumor; with systemic disorders such as porphyria and systemic lupus erythematosus; with certain drugs such as morphine and anesthetics; and with psychiatric disorders such as schizophrenia. When hyponatremia is due to the SIADH, blood volume is slightly increased due to water retention but edema does not occur. The BUN is generally low normal because of dilution, and the urine is abnormally concentrated in relation to the degree of hypo-osmolality because of the persistent ADH effect. The urine sodium concentration is frequently high despite the hyponatremia, probably because the mild volume expansion stimulates the kidneys to excrete sodium. The mechanism responsible for the persistent sodium excretion is unknown, but it may be the result of a humoral factor (also called *third factor*) released in response to volume expansion or of altered physical factors which govern tubular sodium reabsorption.

Hyponatremia is important because it can produce a wide range of neurological symptoms, including death. The severity of symptoms depends on the degree of hyponatremia and on the rate at which it has developed. Generally symptoms do not occur until the serum sodium is below 120 mEq. per liter. Table 16-6 depicts the symptoms to be expected in several ranges of

table 16-6
signs and symptoms related to hyponatremia

RANGE OF SERUM Na (mEq./L.)			
140–120	120–110	110–100	100–95
Generally none	Headache Apathy Lethargy Weakness Disorientation	Confusion Hostility Lethargy or violence Nausea and vomiting	Delirium Convulsions Coma Hypothermia Areflexia Cheyne-Stokes respiration Death

hyponatremia, but remember that for each level of sodium concentration, the severity of symptoms encountered will depend upon how rapidly the sodium concentration was lowered.

Treatment of hyponatremia depends upon the level of serum sodium, the patient's symptoms, and the cause. In most cases of mild hyponatremia associated with congestive heart failure or SIADH, fluid restriction to approximately 1,000 cc. per day is the only treatment necessary. In cases associated with true volume depletion, normal saline will usually correct the volume deficit and restore the sodium concentration to normal. For the most severe degrees of hyponatremia, with potentially life-threatening symptoms, hypertonic (3 percent) sodium chloride intravenously may be necessary. If fluid overload is also a problem, water restriction and intravenous furosemide or ethacrynic acid, both of which cause water loss in excess of sodium, may be the therapy of choice. For patients with chronic hyponatremia due to SIADH, demeclocycline, which blocks the ADH effect, may be the preferred treatment.

Hypernatremia results from primary water deficits in such situations as restricted intake, intestinal losses, and excessive insensible loss, or from nephrogenic or pituitary diabetes insipidus. Hypernatremia due to primary water loss results in a concentrated urine, whereas hypernatremia due to either form of diabetes insipidus is associated with a dilute urine. Symptoms of hypernatremia are generally the same as those of hyperosmolality and result from CNS dehydration. Mental confusion, stupor, seizures, coma and death may occur, in addition to other signs of dehydration such as fatigue, muscle weakness and cramps, and anorexia. The serum osmolality is generally above 350 mOsm per liter before significant symptoms are noted. This corresponds to a serum sodium of 165 to 170 mEq. per liter. Treatment consists of administration of free water (without salt), and vasopressin (Pitressin) in those cases due to pituitary diabetes insipidus.

The knowledgeable use and interpretation of the laboratory determinations described in the preceding paragraphs are of major importance in the assessment of the renal complications of the seriously ill patient. Their value lies in the prevention as well as the diagnosis of these complications. They are not cited to the exclusion of the usual parameters of close and accurate fluid and electrolyte balance, which are equally important to the understanding of the renal status of the patient.

BIBLIOGRAPHY

Baum, N., C. C. Dechoso, and C. E. Carlton, "Blood Urea Nitrogen and Serum Creatinine," *Urology,* Vol. 5 (1975), pp. 583–588.

Harrington, J. T., and J. J. Cohen, "Clinical Disorders of Urine Concentration and Dilution," *Archives of Internal Medicine,* Vol. 131 (1973), pp. 810–825.

Schrier, R. W., and T. Berl, "Hyponatremia and Related Disorders," *The Kidney,* Vol. 7 (1974), pp. 1–5.

ANNE T. BOBAL, R.N., B.S.

management modalities and assessment skills for the nurse: renal system

monitoring fluid balance

Body fluid equilibrium is based on intake and output—the amount of fluid taken in and the volume excreted. Water is lost through the kidneys, gastrointestinal tract, skin and lungs and is replaced by water from fluids and solid foods (which are 60 to 90 percent water), and from the oxidation of food and body tissues. Under normal circumstances and in the presence of adequate renal function, the losses equal the intake and the net balance is zero. Table 17-1 summarizes water gains and losses.

A review of the variables that interfere with normal fluid balance may assist the nurse in evaluating fluid problems in the clinical setting. Fluid imbalances may be the result of inadequate intake, excessive losses without adequate replacement, and impaired renal function.

inadequate intake

Inadequate fluid intake in the conscious patient may be the result of anorexia, apathy, lethargy, and difficulty in swallowing. Weak and feeble patients and infants are especially vulnerable simply because they cannot make their need for water known. In central nervous system disturbances the sense of thirst

table 17-1
ways in which water and
electrolytes balance each other in health

GAINS	RANGE IN ML.	LOSSES	RANGE IN ML.
Water from fluids	500–1,700	Water vapor loss through lungs and skin	850–1,200
Water from solid food	800–1,000	Water loss through urine	600–1,600
Water from oxidation of food and body tissues	200–300	Water loss through feces	50–200
Total	1,500–3,000	Total	1,500–3,000

The chief sources of fluid gain in health are...
- water present in liquids,
- water present in solid food, and
- water derived from oxidation.

These gains equal the losses caused by...
- water lost via insensible perspiration,
- water lost through urine, and
- water lost through feces.

Travenol Laboratories, Inc.

may be impaired, while in unconscious states the patient is entirely dependent on nursing personnel for fluid administration.

excessive losses

Circumstances which increase losses include the following:
1. Fever and increased respiratory rate. A patient with a temperature of 104°F (40°C) and a respiratory rate of 30 to 40 per minute can lose as much as 2,500 ml. in a 24-hour period.
2. Environment—hot and dry climates.
3. Activity—increased metabolic rate.
4. Hyperventilation.
5. Tracheostomy.
6. Increased gastrointestinal losses due to vomiting, diarrhea, gastric suction, fistulas, and ileostomies.
7. Burns—fluid loss through the skin may amount to 1,000 to 2,000 ml. per day.

8. Perspiration—with mild sweating a patient may lose up to 500 ml. per day, with profuse sweating up to 1,000 ml. per day.
9. Diuretic phase of acute tubular necrosis (see Chapter 16).

decreased renal function

The kidneys play an essential role in regulating water and electrolyte balance. Providing renal function is normal, a minimum of 400 ml. of fluid must be excreted as urine to prevent the accumulation of metabolic wastes. However, this minimum urinary volume is markedly influenced by the osmotic load excreted. In certain states such as hyperalimentation the increased urea production will necessitate a larger urinary volume. This also occurs in uncontrolled diabetes where marked glycosuria requires increased excretion.

nursing assessment

The nurse's role in the evaluation, correction, and maintenance of fluid balance includes accurate recording of intake-output, weight, and vital signs. The most sensitive indices of changes in body water content are serial weights and intake-output patterns, while trends in vital signs provide important supporting data. Assessment of fluid imbalance is based on observation and recognition of pertinent symptoms, and nursing action involves replacement or restriction of fluids.

intake and output

An accurate intake-output record will provide valuable data in evaluating and treating fluid imbalances. It is important that all nursing personnel, the patient, and the patient's visitors are involved and instructed. Circumstances will dictate how exact the record should be and what data will be included. For example, in an uncomplicated postsurgical situation, fluid replacement may be projected on estimated and actual losses for a 24-hour period. All measureable intake and output are recorded and totaled at the end of every shift. However, in the presence of excessive losses and/or deteriorating cardiac and renal function more detailed recording of every source of fluid intake and output is necessary. Calculations are often done on a q 1- to 4-hour basis. Intake includes not only pure liquids such as water and juices, but also those foods which are high in water content such as oranges, grapefruit, and those which become liquid at room temperature such as gelatin and ice cream. Ice chips and cubes must also be measured. It is useful to keep a list of fluid equivalents for fruits, ice cubes, and other sources of fluids. In severe electrolyte and fluid imbalances the time and type of fluid intake and the time and amount of each voiding should be recorded. This becomes important as it may be useful baseline data during tests for renal function.

A record of losses should also include emeses, stools, and drainages. When dressings are saturated with drainage, they should be weighed before and after changing. Other data such as temperature, pulse, respiratory rate and degree of perspiration should be available for estimating insensible losses.

weight

Rapid daily gains and losses in weight are usually related to changes in fluid volume. Because of the difficulties in obtaining accurate figures for intake and output records, serial weights are often more reliable. In addition, weight changes will usually pick up imbalances before symptoms are apparent. As with intake and output records the weighing procedure should be consistent. The patient should be weighed on the same scale with the same attire, preferably in the morning before breakfast and after voiding. Variations in the procedure should be noted and made known to the physician. A kilogram scale provides for greater accuracy since drug, fluid, and diet calculations utilize the metric system and conversion from pounds to kilograms may lead to discrepancies.

Normally, a patient with a balanced nutritional intake will maintain his weight. A patient whose protein intake is limited or who is catabolic will lose about a pound a day. A weight gain of more than 1 pound per day suggests fluid retention. A generally accepted guide is that a pint of fluid is reflected in one-half kilogram of weight gained.

assessment of hypovolemia and hypervolemia

The diagnosis of extracellular volume depletion or overload is seldom made on the basis of one parameter. The first clue to the nurse may be the patient's general appearance, after which more specific observations are noted. Symptoms will vary with the degree of imbalance, some symptoms being seen early in imbalance states and others not being evident until severe imbalances are reached. Table 17-2 lists the physical assessment and symptoms of fluid imbalance, and can be used as a guide for nursing assessment.

Other guidelines used to evaluate fluid states are hematocrit, central venous pressure, urine specific gravity, osmolality, and chest x-rays. CVP readings and specific gravity have been discussed in Chapters 10 and 16. In fluid overload, a chest x-ray may show the following changes: prominent vascular markings, increased heart size, pleural effusion, infiltrates, or frank pulmonary congestion. The hematocrit may be elevated in depletion states and decreased in overload, but other factors must be considered. For example, the hematocrit with hypovolemia may be low when significant blood loss has taken place. All data should be evaluated in the light of other influences. Trends are usually more significant than isolated values. For example, when the nurse notes a decrease in urine output, a systematic assessment should follow in order to determine why this is happening and what nursing interventions are most appropriate. Any system of assessment will work when it is consistent and thorough. After a review of the intake and output records for both the current and the previous day and an assessment of the symptoms and parameters just discussed, a decision to increase or decrease fluid intake can be made. In the absence of symptoms of fluid retention, when intra-

table 17-2
physical assessment and symptoms of imbalance

ASSESSMENT OF	HYPOVOLEMIA	HYPERVOLEMIA
Skin and subcutaneous tissues	Dry, loss of elasticity	Warm, moist, pitting edema over bony prominences, wrinkled skin from pressure of clothing
Face	Sunken eyes (late symptom)	Periorbital edema
Tongue	Dry, coated (early symptom), fissured (late symptom)	Moist
Saliva	Thick, scanty	Excessive, frothy
Thirst	Present	May not be significant
Temperature	May be elevated	May not be significant
Pulse	Rapid, weak, thready	Rapid
Respirations	Rapid, shallow	Rapid dyspnea, moist rales
Blood Pressure	Low, orthostatic hypotension, small pulse pressure	Normal to high
Weight	Loss	Gain

venous fluids are behind schedule and intake is inadequate for the patient's condition, missed fluids should be given. The patient's fluid status, especially his urine output, should be watched closely for the next few hours to evaluate whether or not the increase in fluid intake corrected the patient's fluid balance. If, however, urine output is zero or diminished in the presence of adequate fluid intake, no further fluids are given and the physician is called immediately. If a patient presents any of the symptoms of fluid overload discussed earlier, all fluid intake is restricted and the physician is notified immediately.

As stated previously, fluid replacement may be calculated for any given period of time, depending on the severity of the situation. For example, a

24-hour calculation of intake for a patient who is oliguric with normal insensible losses could be:

Previous 24-hour urine output	100 cc.
Insensible loss replacement	500 cc.
Total 24-hour fluid allowance	600 cc.

While the physician will specify the total amount and kind of fluid replacement, the details of distribution are often decided by the nurse. Priority is given to requirements for administration of drugs, both intravenous and oral. Distribution of the remaining fluid is then made according to patient preference. The nurse guides the patient in his selection to help him avoid using up the entire day's allowance early in the day. Because sodium and potassium may be restricted in the patient with renal failure, fluids such as ginger ale, 7-Up, and Kool Aid, which are low in sodium and potassium, are given.

hemodialysis

principles of operation

Dialysis refers to the diffusion of dissolved particles from one fluid compartment to another across a semipermeable membrane. In hemodialysis, the blood is one fluid compartment and the dialysate is the other. The semipermeable membrane is a thin, porous cellophane. The pore size of the membrane permits the passage of low-molecular-weight substances such as urea, creatinine, and uric acid to diffuse through the pores of the membrane. Water molecules are also very small and move freely through the membrane. Most plasma proteins, bacteria, and blood cells are too large to pass through the pores of the membrane. The difference in the concentration of the substances in the two compartments is called the *concentration gradient.* The blood, which contains waste products such as urea and creatinine, flows into the dialyzer or artificial kidney where it comes into contact with the dialysate containing no urea and creatinine. A maximum gradient is established so that movement of these substances is from the blood to the dialysate. Repeated passages of the blood through the dialyzer over a period of time (6 to 10 hours) reduces the level of these waste products to a near normal state. Hemodialysis is indicated in acute and chronic renal failure, drug and chemical intoxications, severe fluid and electrolyte imbalances, and hepatorenal syndrome.

The functions of the artificial kidney system are summarized as follows:
1. Removes the by-products of protein metabolism such as urea, creatinine, and uric acid.
2. Removes excess water (ultrafiltration) by changing osmotic pressure. This is done by adding a high concentration of dextrose to the dialy-

sate, or effecting a pressure differential between the blood and fluid compartments by mechanical means.
3. Maintains or restores the body buffer system.
4. Maintains or restores the level of electrolytes in the body.

major components of the artificial kidney system

A. The Dialyzer or Artificial Kidney This apparatus supports the cellophane compartments. Dialyzers vary in size, physical structure and efficiency. The efficiency of a dialyzer refers to its ability to remove water (ultrafiltration) and waste products (clearance). There are advantages and disadvantages to each dialyzer that must be considered in dialyzer selection. Whether the dialyzer will be used primarily for acute or chronic dialysis is one consideration. A highly efficient, shorter-run dialyzer may be more appropriate for use in drug intoxications or in acutely ill patients where a long dialysis is undesirable. Since some dialyzers have a greater propensity for clotting, a dialyzer requiring larger doses of heparin may be contraindicated for a patient with active or potential bleeding problems. Fluid overload may dictate using a dialyzer with maximum ultrafiltration capability. Rapid fluid and electrolyte changes characteristic of an efficient dialyzer are often avoided in the chronic patient. A low-blood volume dialyzer is advantageous in dialyzing children and small adults. Economy may dictate the selection of a shorter-run dialyzer to prevent higher personnel costs. Sometimes the final selection depends solely on the training and philosophy of personnel in charge of the hemodialysis unit.

B. Dialysate or Dialyzing Solution The dialysate or "bath" is a solution composed of water and the major electrolytes of normal serum. It is made in a clean system with filtered tap water and chemicals. It is not a sterile system, but since bacteria are too large to pass through the membrane, contamination from this source is not a major problem. Dialysate concentrates are usually provided by commercial manufacturers. A "standard" bath is generally used in chronic units but variations may be made to meet specific patient needs.

C. Dialysate Delivery System A single delivery unit provides dialysate for one patient; the multiple delivery system may supply up to twenty patient units. In either system, an automatic proportioning device along with metering and monitoring devices assures precise control of the water-concentrate ratio. The single delivery unit is usually used in acute dialyses. It is a mobile unit and dialysate requirements are easily tailored to meet individual patient needs.

D. Accessory Equipment This includes a blood pump, infusion pumps for heparin and protamine delivery, and monitoring devices to detect unsafe temperatures, dialysate concentration, pressure changes, air and blood leaks.

E. The Human Component Expertise in the use of highly technical equipment is accomplished through theoretical and practical training in the clinical setting. The operation and monitoring of dialysis equipment will differ, however. Reference to the manufacturer's instruction manuals will give the nurse guidelines for the safe operation of equipment. Although the technical aspects of hemodialysis may at first seem overwhelming, they can be learned fairly rapidly. A more critical aspect, one that takes long to achieve, is the understanding and knowledge that the nurse will utilize in her care of patients during dialysis. Because hemodialysis is a dynamic changing process, alterations in blood chemistries and fluid balance can occur. The nurse's observation skills, assessment of symptoms, and appropriate actions can make the difference between a smooth dialysis with a minimum of problems and one fraught with a series of crises for the patient and the nurse.

predialysis assessment

The degree and complexity of problems arising during hemodialysis will vary from patient to patient and will depend on many factors. Important variables are the patient's diagnosis, stage of illness, age, other medical problems, fluid and electrolyte balance, and emotional state.

An essential first step in the hemodialysis procedure is a review of the patient's history, the clinical records, laboratory reports, and finally the nurse's observation of the patient. After reviewing the data, and in consultation with the physician, the dialysis nurse will establish objectives for the dialysis treatment. The objectives will vary from one dialysis to the next in the acute renal failure patient whose condition may change rapidly. For example, fluid removal may take precedence over correcting an electrolyte imbalance or vice versa. Bleeding problems will determine the type of heparinization that will be used.

The patient's emotional state should be included in this initial evaluation. Anxiety and apprehension, especially during a first dialysis, may contribute to change in blood pressure, restlessness, and gastrointestinal upsets. The security provided by the presence of a nurse during the first dialysis is probably more desirable than giving the patient a drug that might precipitate changes in vital signs.

risk factors: prevention, assessment, and nursing intervention

FLUID IMBALANCES

Evaluation of fluid balance is desirable prior to dialysis so that corrective measures may be initiated early in the procedure. Parameters such as blood pressure, pulse, weight, intake and output, and the presence of certain symptoms will assist the nurse in estimating fluid overload or depletion.

The term "dry" or "ideal" weight is used to express the weight at which a patient's blood pressure is in a normal range for him and he is free of the symptoms of fluid imbalance. The figure is not an absolute one, but it gives the nurse a guideline for fluid removal or replacement. It requires frequent review and revision, especially in the newly dialyzed patient in whom frequent changes in weight are taking place due to fluid removal or accumulation and to tissue gains or losses.

HYPERVOLEMIA

The presence of some or all of the following may suggest fluid overload: blood-pressure elevation, increased pulse and respiratory rate, dyspnea, moist rales, cough, edema, excessive weight gain since last dialysis, and a history or record of excessive fluid intake in the absence of adequate losses.

A chest x-ray to assess heart size and/or pulmonary congestion may confirm the diagnosis of fluid overload, but may not be essential in the presence of overt symptoms. Increase in abdominal girth will suggest accumulation of fluid in the abdominal cavity. If ascites is present, measuring the abdominal girth will provide another useful tool in estimating correction of the problem.

Treatment of fluid overload during dialysis is directed toward the removal of the excess water. Care must be taken to avoid too rapid volume depletion during dialysis. Excessive fluid removal may lead to hypotension, and little is gained if intravenous fluids are given to correct the problem. Thus it is better to reduce the volume overload over a period of two or three dialyses, unless pulmonary congestion is life threatening. An analysis of the causes of the fluid overload is necessary to prevent reoccurrences. The intake and output record may provide a clue. For example, the patient may have been given excessive IV fluids in a "keep open" IV or fluids used as a vehicle for IV medications may not have been calculated in the intake. The patient may not have adhered to his fluid restriction or may have had a decrease in his fluid losses. For example, gastric suction may have been discontinued. Often, after the institution of chronic dialysis, urinary output decreases. If the patient continues his normal fluid intake he will become fluid-overloaded. In the chronic hemodialysis patient, fluid overload may be related to the intake of high sodium foods. Moderate restriction is necessary for all patients to prevent extracellular fluid overload. Change in weight provides an indication of water load; an acceptable weight gain is 0.5 kg. for each 24 hours between dialyses.

HYPOVOLEMIA

Assessment of hypovolemia is also made on the evaluation of trends in vital signs and symptoms. Clues to hypovolemia include falling blood pressure, increasing pulse and respiration rates, loss of skin turgor, dry mouth, a falling CVP, and a decreasing urine output. A history of excessive fluid loss through profuse perspiration, vomiting, diarrhea, and gastric suctioning with resulting weight loss will further substantiate the diagnosis. Treatment is directed toward the replacement of previous losses and the prevention of further losses during dialysis.

It is usual practice to phlebotomize the patient at the onset of dialysis. The patient's blood is pumped through the dialyzer, displacing the priming normal saline solution. In the hypovolemic patient the nurse can connect the venous return blood line immediately and infuse the normal saline into the patient. This 200 ml. of solution might be sufficient to restore balance or at least prevent further hypotension. Ultrafiltration will be avoided in the hypovolemic patient and he may even require additional fluids. Normal saline is the solution used most frequently to replace volume depletion during dialysis because small volumes usually produce the desired effect. Replacement in increments of 50 ml. are suggested, with frequent monitoring of blood pressure. Blood-volume expanders such as albumin are sometimes used in patients with a low serum protein. The treatment is expensive when the underlying cause of the hypoproteinemia is not corrected and repeated infusions become necessary.

HYPOTENSION

Hypotension during dialysis may be caused by preexisting hypovolemia, excessive ultrafiltration, loss of blood into the dialyzer, and antihypertensive drug therapy. Hypotension at the beginning of dialysis may occur in patients with a small blood volume such as children and small adults. Using a small-volume dialyzer or starting dialysis at a slower blood flow rate may avoid or minimize problems.

Hypotension later in dialysis is usually due to excessive ultrafiltration. This may be confirmed by weighing the patient and estimating fluid loss. Keeping the patient in a horizontal position, reducing the blood-flow rate, and discontinuing ultrafiltration may return the blood pressure to normal. If hypotension persists, saline or other plasma expanders may be administered. IV fluids should be kept to a minimum and discontinued as soon as the patient is normotensive. Salty liquids or foods may be given, but their effect is slower than intravenous administration. If hypotension persists in spite of adequate fluid replacement, other medical causes for hypotension should be considered.

Blood loss due to technical problems such as membrane leaks and line separations may lead to hypotension. The use of blood leak detectors and other monitoring devices has reduced the risk of excessive blood loss due to these causes, but they do occur. If separation of blood lines occurs, clamping the arterial blood line and stopping the blood pump immediately will minimize further blood loss. In a membrane leak the dialysis is discontinued and the dialyzer replaced. Although small leaks may seal over, they may progress to gross leaks and dialysate may cross the membrane into the blood compartment. In this situation, the blood may be returned to the patient, but he should be observed for pyrogenic reactions. If the patient's hematocrit is low, the risk of blood loss may be greater than the possibility of dialysate contamination. Some units have standing policies to cover this contingency; however, decisions may be made according to individual circumstances.

The use of antihypertensive drugs in the dialysis patient may precipitate hypotension during dialysis. To avoid this, it is standard practice in many units to omit antihypertensive drugs 4 to 6 hours before dialysis. Fluids and sodium restrictions are more desirable controls for hypertension. Sedatives and tranquilizers may also cause hypotension and should be avoided if possible.

HYPERTENSION

The most frequent causes of hypertension during dialysis are fluid overload, disequilibrium syndrome, and anxiety.

Hypertension during dialysis is usually caused by sodium and water excesses. This can be confirmed by comparing the patient's present weight to his ideal or dry weight. If fluid overload is the cause of hypertension, ultrafiltration will usually bring about a reduction in the blood pressure.

Some patients who may be normotensive before dialysis become hypertensive during dialysis. The rise may occur either gradually or abruptly. The cause is not well understood, but may be the result of increased cardiac output as fluid overload is corrected.

Hypertension is a common finding in dialysis disequilibrium syndrome and will usually respond to correction of that condition. If the diastolic blood pressure is over 120 or the patient has symptoms, small doses of hydralazine (Apresoline) may be given intravenously into the venous blood line. An initial dose of 10 mg. may bring about a favorable response. Hydralazine is preferred to methyldopa (Aldomet) because its effect is more rapid. Blood pressure is monitored at frequent intervals following the administration of antihypertensive drugs.

Anxiety, fear, and apprehension, especially during the first dialysis, may cause transient and erratic hypertension. Sedatives may be necessary, but confidence in the staff and a smooth, problem-free dialysis will help reduce anxiety during subsequent treatments.

DIALYSIS DISEQUILIBRIUM SYNDROME

Dialysis disequilibrium syndrome is manifested by a group of symptoms suggestive of cerebral dysfunction. Symptoms range in severity from mild nausea, vomiting, headache, and hypertension to agitation, twitching, mental confusion, and convulsions. It is thought that rapid efficient dialysis results in shifts in water, pH, and osmolality between cerebrospinal fluid and blood, causing the symptoms.

Disequilibrium syndrome in the acutely uremic patient may be avoided by dialyzing the patient slowly for short periods daily for two or three treatments. Phenytoin (Dilantin) is sometimes used prior to and during dialysis in the new patient to reduce the risk of CNS symptoms.

Restlessness, confusion, twitching, nausea, and vomiting may suggest early disequilibrium. Reduction of the blood flow rate and administration of sedatives may prevent more severe symptoms, but it may be necessary to discontinue dialysis if symptoms persist or worsen.

ELECTROLYTE IMBALANCE

With the trend toward early and adequate dialysis the severe extremes of electrolyte imbalances are not seen with the same frequency as before the widespread use of hemodialysis. Critical electrolyte changes and their management have been discussed in Chapter 16.

Maintenance and restoration of electrolyte balance in the dialysis patient are accomplished primarily with dialysis and to a lesser degree with dietary controls. With the exception of potassium, very few changes in the standard concentration of electrolytes in the dialysate are necessary.

Laboratory tests to evaluate electrolyte status are done before and after each dialysis in acute renal failure. The nurse's role includes knowledge of normal values, recognition of symptoms of imbalance, and evaluation of probable causes. In many institutions nursing intervention also includes taking the necessary corrective measures as defined by the policies of the critical care unit. For example, a patient complains of extreme muscle weakness. The nurse notes excessive amounts of gastric drainage during the previous 24-hour period. The situation suggests hypokalemia and the nurse orders a stat serum K^+ level. If the result is low, the nurse increases the potassium level in the dialysate from the standard 2.0 mEq. per liter to 3.5 mEq. per liter. She also monitors the patient for possible cardiac arrhythmias during the procedure.

The electrolytes of main concern in dialysis, which are normally corrected during the procedure, are sodium, potassium, bicarbonate, calcium, phosphorus, and magnesium.

A. Serum Sodium   Serum sodium concentration normally varies between 135 mEq. per liter and 145 mEq. per liter and is a reflection of water volume. A low serum sodium usually indicates water intake in excess of sodium and is characterized by an increase in body weight. A high serum sodium usually indicates water loss in excess of sodium and is reflected in weight loss. Serum sodium extremes do not, as a rule, become a problem unless the values fall below 120 or rise above 160 mEq. per liter. The rate of change is probably more important than the absolute value (see p. 337).

Although serum sodium extremes are not usually seen in the adequately dialyzed patient, nevertheless thirst may indicate sodium excess. The patient who is thirsty because of excessive sodium intake will drink excessive amounts of water, which can lead to hypertension and fluid overload. Evaluation of sodium intake should be made in the patient who gains excessive amounts of fluid between dialyses. Again, the recommended weight gain is approximately 1 pound for each day between dialysis. Shifts in sodium and water during hemodialysis may lead to muscle cramping. This can be alleviated by reducing the flow rate and ultrafiltration.

B. Potassium   Both hypo- and hyperkalemia occur in renal failure. Normal serum concentration is between 3.5 and 5.0 mEq. per liter. Levels below 3.0 and above 7.0 mEq. per liter may lead to generalized muscle weakness and cardiac arrhythmias (see Chapter 10). Extremes in the serum potassium level are seen more frequently in the acute patient and may result from either the disease or the therapy. Crushing injuries with extensive tissue destruction, blood transfusions, potassium-containing drugs, and acidosis all contribute to hyperkalemia. Vomiting, diarrhea, and gastric suction may lead to hypokalemia. Rapid correction of serum potassium in either direction should be avoided. Patients on digitalis are of special concern because a low serum potassium potentiates the effects of digitalis. Therefore, rapid lowering of the potassium level during dialysis can lead to hypokalemia, to increased effects of digitalis, and possibly to serious and sometimes fatal arrhythmias (see Chapter 10). The potassium level in the bath is kept at 3 to 3.5 mEq. per liter, whichever is more appropriate for the individual patient. Patients with overt or potential problems should be monitored for cardiac function during dialysis.

C. Bicarbonate   Bicarbonate protects the body from excessive acid loads. Normal concentration varies between 25 and 30 mEq. per liter. In uremia, the bicarbonate is depleted because it has been used to buffer the acidosis resulting from the inability of the kidneys to excrete acids. Acidosis in the uremic patient who has not been started on dialysis is corrected by giving sodium bicarbonate. During dialysis, acidosis is corrected by adding acetate to the dialysate. Acetate diffuses into the blood where it is metabolized to form bicarbonate.

D. Calcium   Normal serum calcium levels range between 8 and 10.3 mg. percent although this will vary among laboratories. Disturbances in calcium metabolism which result in hypocalcemia occur in renal failure and are thought to involve impaired absorption of dietary calcium and resistance to the action of vitamin D. The dialysate calcium is kept at 3 mEq. per liter to prevent the loss of calcium from the blood to the dialysate. Dialysis, however, does not seem to correct the bone problems which occur in the chronic patient as a result of calcium-phosphorus imbalances (see Chapter 18).

E. Phosphorus   In chronic renal failure antacids are used to bind phosphorus in the intestinal tract and prevent its absorption. The lowered serum phosphorus reduces the risk of soft-tissue calcifications. Antacids are usually given during or after meals; however, because of the medication's unpleasant taste and consistency, patients often omit taking antacids. A high serum phosphorus is an indication to the nurse that the patient is not adhering to the prescribed dose. Some patients save their meager amounts of fluids to wash away the unpleasant taste. Rinsing the mouth with water or a mouth-wash may also help.

F. Magnesium   The normal plasma level of magnesium is 1.5 to 1.7 mEq. per liter. Magnesium accumulates in the serum, bone, and muscle in the presence of renal failure. It is thought to be involved, along with calcium and phosphorus, in the bone problems accompanying chronic renal failure. Although magnesium is removed by the artificial kidney, high levels remain in the bone. It is also difficult to reduce magnesium intake in the diet and provide palatable and nutritious meals. The regular use of magnesium-containing drugs should be avoided. This applies particularly to antacids which are taken regularly by patients on chronic dialysis. Acceptable nonmagnesium antacids include aluminum hydroxide gel (Amphojel), dihydroxyaluminum amino-acetate (Robalate), and basic aluminum carbonate gel (Basaljel).

INFECTION

The uremic patient has a lowered resistance to infection, which is thought to be due to a decreased immunological response. Therefore, all possible foci of infection should be eliminated. Indwelling urinary catheters and intra-caths should be removed as soon as possible, or their use should be avoided altogether. Strict aseptic technique is essential in catheterizations, veni-punctures, wound dressings, and tracheal suctioning.

Pulmonary infections are a leading cause of death in the acute uremic patient. Contributing factors include depression of the cough reflex and respiratory effort due to central nervous system disturbances, increased viscosity of pulmonary secretions due to dehydration and mouth breathing, especially in the unresponsive patient, and pulmonary congestion due to fluid overload. Fluid in the lungs not only acts as a medium for growing bacteria but also impedes respiratory excursion. Nursing techniques which prevent or minimize pulmonary complications cannot be overlooked during the hemodialysis procedure. They include frequent turning, deep breathing and coughing, early ambulation, adequate humidification, hydration, tracheal aspiration, use of intermittent positive pressure machines, and oxygen therapy. Oral hygiene is important because bleeding from the oral mucous membrane and the accumulation of dry secretions promote growth of bacteria in the mouth which can lead to a pneumonia.

BLEEDING AND HEPARINIZATION

Bleeding during dialysis may be due to an underlying medical condition such an ulcer or gastritis, or may be the result of excessive anticoagulation. Blood in the extracorporeal system, such as the dialyzer and blood lines, clots rapidly unless some method of anticoagulation is used. Heparin is the drug of choice because it is simple to administer, increases clotting time rapidly, is easily monitored, and may be reversed with protamine.

Specific heparinization procedures vary, but the primary goal in any method is to prevent clotting in the dialyzer with the least amount of heparin. Two methods are commonly used: intermittent and constant infusion. In both cases an initial priming dose of heparin is given, followed by smaller doses either at intervals or at a constant rate by an infusion pump. The resulting effect is *systemic heparinization,* in which the clotting times of the patient and the dialyzer are essentially the same.

Absolute guidelines are difficult to give as methods and dialyzer requirements vary. The normal clotting time of 6 to 10 minutes may be increased to the range of 30 to 60 minutes. The effect of heparin is monitored by the modified Lee White method, which measures the length of time it takes for 1 cc. of blood to form a solid clot in a clean standard Lee White tube, tipped at 1-minute intervals. More recently, activated partial thromboplastin time and activated coagulation time methods have come into use. These have the advantage of providing results in seconds but require more sophisticated laboratory equipment.

Systemic heparinization usually presents no risk to the patient unless he has overt bleeding such as GI bleeding, epistaxis, or hemoptysis, is 3 to 7 days postsurgery, or has uremic pericarditis. In these situations, *regional heparinization* is employed. In this technique the patient's clotting time is kept normal while that of the dialyzer is increased. This is accomplished by infusing heparin at a constant rate into the dialyzer and simultaneously neutralizing its effects with protamine sulfate before the blood returns to the patient. As with systemic heparinization there is no standard heparin-protamine ratio.

Frequent monitoring of the clotting times is the best way to achieve effective regional heparinization. Because of the rebound phenomenon which may cause bleeding problems following regional heparinization, some dialysis units have switched to low-dose heparinization. In this method, a dialyzer having low heparin requirements is used with minimal heparin dosage. Although some clotting may take place in the dialyzer, this small blood loss is preferable to the risk of profound bleeding.

Bleeding problems occasionally occur because of accidental heparin overdose. This may be caused by infusion pump malfunction or carelessness in setting the delivery rate. Because of the hazards, the importance of careful, frequent monitoring of heparin delivery cannot be overemphasized.

PROBLEMS WITH EQUIPMENT

One of the major objectives of a dialysis unit is the prevention of complications resulting from the treatment itself. Hemodialysis involves the use of highly technical equipment. The efficiency of the dialysis, as well as the patient's comfort and safety, is compromised if both the patient and the equipment are not adequately monitored. Mechanical monitors provide a margin of safety, but should not replace the observations and actions of the nurse.

Monitoring devices are designed to monitor many parameters, the most important of which are flow, concentration, and temperature of the dialysate, and flow and leakage of blood. The design and operation of dialysis equipment and monitoring devices vary greatly; however, they have a common purpose.

A. Dialysate Flow   Inadequate dialysate flow will not harm the patient, but it will compromise dialysis efficiency. Flow is maintained at the rate recommended for each particular dialyzer. The nurse usually checks the flow at least every hour and makes adjustments as necessary.

B. Dialysate Concentrate   Sudden or rapid changes in dialysate concentrate may result in red blood cell hemolysis and cerebral disturbances. Mild symptoms include nausea, vomiting, and headache. In severe cases, convulsions, coma, and death may ensue. If several patients in a unit develop similar symptoms simultaneously, dialysate concentrate imbalance should be thought of immediately. If a patient is accidentally dialyzed against water, the first symptom may be sudden severe pain in the returning vein. Because of hemolysis, blood will immediately turn dark brown to black. Dialysis is discontinued at once.

In a single delivery, proportioning system, monitoring devices are built into the system and the concentrate is monitored continuously. If the concentrate exceeds the predetermined limits, dialysate automatically bypasses the dialyzer until the problem is corrected. The problem may have been caused by an interruption in the water or concentrate delivery. Inflow lines should be checked for kinking and the concentrate container checked for quantity.

In a central delivery system the electrolyte concentration is also checked continuously by a meter which measures the electrical conductivity of the solution. If the solution exceeds the limits, the transfer valve between the mix tank and the supply tank is automatically closed so that no solution in unsafe concentrations is delivered to the supply tank. The solution is discarded and another batch is mixed and rechecked. A system of visual and audible alarms alerts dialysis personnel to problems.

In a batch system, the bath may be checked in a number of ways. The test for chloride ion is commonly used. It is done before dialysis commences and any time the bath is changed.

C. Temperature Most dialysate delivery systems use a heating element to maintain dialysate temperature at optimal levels (98 to 101°F or 36.7 to 38.3°C). Some systems include alarms; others require visual observation of the temperature gauge. Cool temperatures may cause chilling and vessel spasm. Sometimes chilling in the patient is the first indication of a drop in dialysate temperature. High temperatures (over 101°F or 38.3°C) may produce fever and discomfort in the patient, while extremely high temperatures (of 110°F or 43.3°C) will cause hemolysis. Corrections should be made as soon as the temperature reaches 101°F (38.3°C).

D. Blood Flow Monitoring adequate blood flow rate throughout dialysis is essential to dialysis efficiency. Factors that influence blood flow rate are blood pressure, shunt and fistula function, and the extracorporeal circuit. A manometer connected to the drip chamber is used to measure the pressure in the blood lines. Changes in blood line pressures are transmitted to the drip chamber and register on the manometer as high- or low-pressure alarms. A high-pressure alarm indicates a problem in the venous blood line, vessel spasm, or a clotted vein. Vessel spasm is seen in new shunts or with chilling, and a heating pad over the shunt may help to relax the vessel. If a clot is suspected, the vein is irrigated with a heparinized saline solution. A low-pressure alarm reflects an obstruction to blood flow from the patient. Arterial spasm, clotting, displacement of a fistula needle, and a drop in blood pressure are possible causes. Correction is again directed to the cause.

E. Blood Leaks A blood leak detector is invaluable when outflow dialysate is not visible, as in a single-pass delivery system. One type of blood leak detector is a color-sensitive photocell which picks up color variations in the outflow dialysate. Any foreign material such as blood will be detected and an alarm set off. Since false alarms are sometimes set off by air bubbles, the nurse will check the dialysate visually for a gross leak and with a hemostix for smaller leaks. Dialysis is usually discontinued immediately with a gross leak. Whether or not the blood is returned to the patient is either a matter of unit policy or an individual determination. If the patient is severely anemic, the risk of losing the blood in the dialyzer may outweigh the risk of a reaction to dialysate contaminated blood. Sometimes minor leaks, in which there is no visible blood in the dialysate and only a small hemostix reaction, seal over and dialysis is continued.

F. Air Embolism The risk of air embolism is one of the most serious patient safety problems in the hemodialysis unit. Air can enter the patient's circulation through defective blood tubing, faulty blood line connections, vented intravenous fluid containers or accidental displacement of the arterial needle. The use of air leak detectors and plastic fluid containers has minimized air embolus risks but the prevention of potential problems by strict attention to technical details and visual monitoring cannot be overemphasized.

access to circulation

Successful repeated hemodialysis depends on access to the patient's circulation. Methods commonly used are the arteriovenous shunt, the arteriovenous fistula, the bovine graft, and the femoral vein catheter.

ARTERIOVENOUS SHUNT

The A-V shunt consists of two soft plastic (Silastic) cannulas, one of which is inserted into an artery and the other into a vein. Between dialyses, the cannulas are joined by a hard, plastic (Teflon) connector and blood flows freely between the two vessels. At the time of dialysis the two cannulas are separated and attached to the blood tubing of the dialyzer. Cannulation is a surgical procedure performed in the operating room under local anesthesia. The cannula is usually inserted in the forearm of the nondominant arm, although circumstances may dictate placement in other extremities. Presurgical care should include avoiding venipunctures, intravenous administrations, tourniquets, and blood-pressure cuffs in the affected limb. Nursing care is directed at maintenance of good function and prevention of clotting and infection beginning in the immediate postsurgical period. General recommendations for promoting shunt life are:

1. *Limiting activity in the postoperative period.* Shunt functioning can be promoted by elevating the affected extremity for two to three days to reduce swelling and discomfort, and avoiding weight bearing in a leg shunt for at least a week.
2. *Cleanliness.* The shunt site should be kept clean and dry. Good aseptic technique is essential in dressing changes and handling of the shunt. Daily dressing changes are not recommended unless infection with drainage is present. Cleansing at the time of dialysis is usually sufficient and should be done from the exit sites outward. Separate gauze and applicators are used for each exit to prevent cross-contamination. Picking at crusts should be avoided.
3. *Proper alignment.* Misalignment may occur if the cannulas are twisted during either the hookup procedure or the reconnection at the end of dialysis. Distortions should be corrected immediately as tension at the exits may lead to small tears in the epithelium which in turn contribute to clotting and infection. An outer dressing such as Kling, which conforms to the contours of the extremity, is recommended because it prevents the shunt and other dressings from slipping around with normal motions.
4. *Gentleness.* Careful, gentle handling of shunt parts is important in extending shunt life. Therefore, jerking and pulling on the cannulas during dialysis procedures should be avoided.

5. *Frequent observation.* Early detection and attention to symptoms may lead to the prevention of more serious problems. Clotting and infection are the two major complications.

6. *Preventing clotting.* A clue to good blood flow through the shunt is a sound or burst heard with a stethoscope. The sound has been likened to the sound of rushing water. Sometimes the bruit is so strong it can be palpated with the fingers. This is called a thrill. If the bruit is faint or absent, the dressing is removed in order to observe the shunt. The color of the blood should be uniformly red and the shunt warm to the touch. If the shunt if clotted, the blood is quite dark and the red cells and serum may have already separated. Declotting may or may not be successful, depending on the length of time that has elapsed between clotting and detection. The routine declotting procedure consists of evacuating the clots by irrigating each cannula with a weak heparinized saline solution. Aseptic technique is again emphasized. Once flow has been reestablished, the shunt is reconnected and observed closely. It has been the experience of dialysis personnel that once clotting occurs, it will recur unless the cause has been determined and corrective measures taken. A history of trauma, obstruction to flow caused by sleeping with a limb bent or legs crossed, hypotention, and infections is often found. The patient, however, may have an intrinsic clotting problem which may indicate the use of an anticoagulant such as sodium warfarin (Coumadin). This will necessitate the usual observations and precautions taken with anticoagulation therapy. The patient will also need a readjustment in heparin dosage during dialysis.

7. *Preventing infection.* The shunt is routinely inspected at the time of dialysis. It is also inspected when the patient develops any unusual symptoms, such as pain or bleeding at exits, between dialysis. Any of the signs of inflammation, such as redness, swelling, tenderness, and drainage, is cause for concern and requires prompt attention. Cultures are routinely done by the nurse if drainage is noted. Each exit site is cultured separately. Some physicians will treat the infection without cultures, assuming that most shunts are infected with *Staphylococcus aureus.* However, *Pseudomonas* and *Escherichia coli* are sometimes cultured out. Aside from the possibility of further shunt surgery, the most serious complication of a shunt infection is septicemia. To forestall this possibility, some physicians choose to remove an extremely infected shunt immediately. Whether this is done or not, the patient should be observed closely especially during the hemodialysis procedure when contamination of the bloodstream from an infected shunt is a strong possibility. The development of chills, fever, and hypotension in a patient with an infected shunt should be regarded as a serious sign. Blood cultures should be drawn immediately and the physician notified promptly.

A complication that occurs rarely but one which requires immediate nursing intervention is accidental separation of the cannulas or displacement of the arterial cannula. The appearance of large amounts of bright red blood on the shunt dressing constitutes an emergency and should be investigated without hesitation. If the cannulas have become separated, they should be clamped immediately and then reconnected. For this reason it is essential that shunt clamps be attached to each person who has an A-V shunt. If the arterial cannula has slipped out of the vessel, direct pressure is applied over the artery until medical assistance is available.

ARTERIOVENOUS FISTULA

The arteriovenous fistula technique was developed in response to the frequent complications encountered with the arteriovenous shunt.

In this procedure the surgeon anastomoses an artery and a vein, creating a fistula or artificial opening between them. Arterial blood flowing into the venous system results in marked dilatation of the veins which are then easily punctured with a large bore 14-gauge needle. Two venipunctures are made at the time of dialysis, one for a blood source and one for a return. The arterial needle is inserted toward the fistula to obtain the best blood flow, but the tip should not be placed closer than 1 to 1½ inches from the fistula. A traumatic puncture might lead to damage and closure of the fistula. The venous needle is directed away from the fistula in the direction of normal venous flow. It may be placed in either the same vessel, another vein in the same arm, or even in another extremity. If both needles are inserted into the same vessel, the tips should be at least 8 to 10 cm. apart to avoid mixing of the blood which would result in inadequate dialysis. If it is necessary to place the needles close to each other, a tourniquet is applied between the two needles.

Care of the arteriovenous fistula is less complicated than with the arteriovenous shunt. Normal showering or bathing with soap provides adequate skin cleansing. Traumatic venipunctures or repetition in the same site should be avoided as these lead to excessive bleeding, hematoma and scar formation. Excessive manipulation and adjustment of the needles should also be avoided for the same reasons. Postdialysis care includes adequate pressure on the puncture sites after the needles are removed.

BOVINE GRAFT

The bovine graft was developed in response to a need for blood access in those patients with inadequate blood vessels of their own. A bovine graft is a segment of selected bovine carotid artery which is processed and sterilized for human use. The section is anastomosed between an artery and a vein. After a suitable healing period, the vessel is used in the same manner as an arteriovenous fistula. The procedures for preventing complications are the same as those for arteriovenous fistula.

FEMORAL CATHETERS

Femoral catheters (also called Shaldon catheters) are used for hemodialysis when other means of access to the bloodstream are not available. This method is used primarily in acute dialysis, but may also be used for chronic dialysis patients because of shunt or fistula failure. It should be considered a temporary measure. The procedure involves inserting one or two Teflon catheters into the femoral vein. If an arm vein can be used for blood return, only one catheter is used. When two catheters are needed, the lower one is used for the blood supply, the higher one for the return. Femoral catheterization trays are standard equipment in dialysis units and in critical care units which perform acute dialysis.

The femoral catheters must be secured to the leg to prevent accidental slipping, and observed frequently for bleeding during hemodialysis. The catheters are usually removed after dialysis, but may be left in place if the patient is scheduled for another dialysis within 24 hours. Leaving femoral catheters in place over 24 hours may lead to infection. Catheters left in place are irrigated periodically with a weak heparinized saline solution to prevent clotting. The usual dilution is 1,000 units of heparin to 30 cc. of normal saline, and 4 to 5 cc. are instilled into the catheter q 2 to 4 hours. If the catheters are removed at the end of dialysis, pressure is applied to the puncture sites until complete clotting occurs. The site is checked for several hours thereafter to detect any renewal of bleeding.

peritoneal dialysis

Peritoneal dialysis accomplishes the same functions and operates on the same principles of diffusion and osmosis as hemodialysis. In this instance, however, the peritoneum is the semipermeable membrane.

Peritoneal dialysis is an effective alternate treatment when hemodialysis is not available or when access to the bloodstream is not possible. It is sometimes utilized as an initial treatment for renal failure while the patient is being evaluated for a hemodialysis program. The advantages of peritoneal dialysis over hemodialysis include use of less complicated technical equipment, less need for highly skilled personnel, availability of supplies and equipment, and minimizing of adverse symptoms of the more efficient hemodialysis. This may be important in patients who cannot tolerate rapid hemodynamic changes.

On the other hand, peritoneal dialysis requires more time to adequately remove metabolic wastes and to restore electrolyte and fluid balance. In addition, repeated treatments may lead to peritonitis, while long periods of immobility may lead to such complications as pulmonary congestion and venous stasis. Because fluid is introduced into the peritoneal cavity, peritoneal dialysis is contraindicated in existing peritonitis, recent or extensive abdominal surgery, the presence of abdominal adhesions, and impending kidney transplantation.

materials used in peritoneal dialysis

1. Solutions. As in hemodialyses, peritoneal dialysis solutions contain "ideal" concentrations of electrolytes, but lack urea, creatinine, and

other substances which are to be removed. Unlike dialysate used in hemodialyses, solutions must be sterile. Solutions vary in dextrose concentrations. A 1.5 percent dextrose solution is usually used for drug intoxications and acute renal failure if excessive fluid removal is not necessary. A 7 percent dextrose solution is used with patients who are severely fluid-overloaded. Since this concentration of dextrose may lead to excessive fluid removal with hypotension, it is sometimes used only for several exchanges. If hyperkalemia is not a problem, 4 mEq. of potassium chloride is added to each liter.

2. Dialysis administration set.
3. Peritoneal dialysis catheter set. The set usually includes the catheter, a connecting tube for connecting the catheter to the administration set, and a metal stylet. The stylet is used for dislodging fibrin clots which may form and collect in the catheter.
4. Trocar set. Commercially prepared materials have the advantage of being prepackaged and sterile.
5. Ancillary drugs:
   a. Local anesthetic solution—2 percent lidocaine (Xylocaine)
   b. Aqueous heparin—1,000 units per cc.
   c. Potassium chloride.
   d. Broad-spectrum antibiotics.

preliminary procedures

1. The bladder should be emptied just prior to the procedure to avoid accidental puncture with the trocar.
2. The abdomen is shaved, prepped, and draped as for a surgical procedure.
3. The dialyzing fluid is warmed to body temperature or slightly warmer.
4. Baseline vital signs, such as temperature, pulse, respirations and weight, are recorded. If possible, an in-bed scale is ideal as the patient's weight can be monitored frequently. Moving a lethargic or disoriented patient to a scale may create problems such as catheter displacement.
5. Specific orders regarding fluid removal, replacement and drug administration should be written by the physician prior to the procedure.

procedure

Under sterile conditions, a small midline incision is made just below the umbilicus. A trocar is inserted through the incision into the peritoneal cavity. The obturator is removed and the catheter secured. The dialysis solution flows into the abdominal cavity by gravity as rapidly as possible (5 to 10 minutes). If it flows in too slowly, the catheter may need repositioning. When the solution is infused, the tubing is clamped and the solution remains in the abdominal cavity for 30 to 45 minutes. Then the solution bottles are placed on the floor and the fluid is drained out of the peritoneal cavity by gravity. If the system is patent and the catheter well placed, the fluid will drain in a steady forceful stream. Drainage should take no more than 10 minutes. This cycle is repeated continuously for the prescribed number of hours which varies from 12 to 36 hours, depending on the purpose of the treatment, the patient's condition, and the proper functioning of the system.

automated peritoneal dialysis systems

In the past few years automated peritoneal dialysate systems have been developed. These are comparable to hemodialysis systems in that they mix water and dialysate in proper dilution, have built-in monitors and a system of automatic timing devices which cycle the infusion and removal of peritoneal fluid. Automated peritoneal delivery systems are more appropriately used for chronic peritoneal dialysis utilizing a permanent, indwelling peritoneal catheter. Less sophisticated devices which minimize the necessity for manual bottle exchanges are more appropriate for the unit which may do an occasional peritoneal dialysis.

essential features of nursing care

1. Maintenance of accurate intake and output records to assess volume depletion or overload.
2. Frequent monitoring of the patient's vital signs, weight, and general condition.
3. Correction of technical difficulties before they result in physiological problems.
4. Prevention of the complications of immobility.
5. Provision of an environment which will assist the patient in accepting a long and potentially tiring treatment.

complications of peritoneal dialysis and nursing intervention

TECHNICAL COMPLICATIONS

1. Incomplete recovery of fluid with each exchange. The fluid removed should at least equal or exceed that of the amount inserted. If less fluid is removed or drains very slowly, the catheter tip may be buried in the omentum or clogged with fibrin. Turning the patient from side to side, elevating the head of the bed, and gently massaging the abdomen may facilitate drainage. If clots are suspected, introducing the stylet into the catheter may reopen it. Adding heparin to the solution may prevent the formation of fibrinous clots in the catheter. The specific dose is ordered by the physician but will be in a range of 500 to 1,000 units per liter.
2. Leakage or bleeding. Superficial leaking and bleeding may occur with the first exchange. These may be controlled by a purse-string suture. Since persistent leakage around the incision site will act as a medium for bacterial contamination, the problem should be solved early. Blood-tinged drainage due to the trauma of insertion may be noted in the first few passes. Gross bleeding at any time is an indication of a more serious problem and should be investigated immediately.

PHYSIOLOGICAL COMPLICATIONS

1. Hypotension may occur if excessive fluid is removed. Vital signs are monitored frequently, especially if a hypertonic solution is used. A progressive drop in blood pressure and weight should alert the nurse to potential problems.
2. Hypertension and fluid overload may occur if all the fluid is not removed in each cycle. The exact amount in the bottles should be noted. Some manufacturers add 1,050 ml. to a 1,000-ml. bottle; over a period of hours this can make a considerable difference. The patient is observed for signs of respiratory distress which may indicate pulmonary congestion. In the absence of other symptoms of fluid overload, hypertension may be the result of anxiety and apprehension. Reassuring the patient and promptly correcting problems are preferable to the administration of sedatives and tranquilizers.

PAIN

Mild abdominal discomfort may be experienced at any time during the procedure and is probably related to the constant distention or chemical irritation of the peritoneum. If a mild analgesic doesn't provide relief, inserting 5 cc. of 2 percent lidocaine (Xylocaine) directly into the catheter may help. The patient may be less uncomfortable if nourishment is given in small amounts, when the fluid is draining out rather than when the abdominal cavity is distended.

Severe pain may indicate more serious problems of infection or paralytic ileus. Infection is not likely in the first 24 hours. Aseptic technique and the use of prophylactic antibiotics minimize the risk of infection. Periodic cultures of the outflowing fluid will assist in the early detection of pathogenic organisms.

PULMONARY COMPLICATIONS

Immobility may lead to hypostatic pneumonia, especially in the debilitated or elderly patient. Deep breathing, turning, and coughing should be encouraged during the procedure. Leg exercises and the use of elastic stockings may prevent the development of venous thrombi and emboli.

Further nursing measures are directed at making the patient as comfortable as possible during the lengthy procedure. Diversions such as having visitors, reading, or watching TV should be encouraged.

BIBLIOGRAPHY

Abbott Laboratories, *Fluid and Electrolytes* (North Chicago, Ill., 1970).
Black, D. A. K., *Essentials of Fluid Balance* (Oxford: Blackwell Scientific Publications, 1964).
Gilmore, Joseph P., *Renal Physiology* (Baltimore: Williams & Wilkins, 1972).

Goldberg, Emmanuel, *A Primer of Water Electrolyte and Acid-Base Syndromes* (Philadelphia: Lea & Febiger, 1970).

Gutch, C. F., and Martha H. Stoner, *Review of Hemodialysis for Nurses and Dialysis Personnel*, second edition (St. Louis: C. V. Mosby, 1975).

Light, Jimmy A., "A Review of Vascular Access Management," *Dialysis and Transplantation*, Vol. 4, No. 1 (December–January 1975), pp. 20–31.

Merrill, John P., and Constantine Hampers, *Uremia—Progress in Pathophysiology and Treatment* (New York: Grune & Stratton, 1971).

Pendras, Jerry P., and Gerald W. Stenson, *The Hemodialysis Manual* (Seattle, Wash.: Seattle Artificial Kidney Center and University of Washington, 1969).

Schemmel, Rachael, "Fluid Intake and Renal Failure," *Dialysis and Transplantation*, Vol. 4, No. 5 (August–September 1975), pp. 50–54.

Shoemaker, William C., and William F. Walker, *Fluid Electrolyte Therapy in Acute Illness* (Chicago: Year Book Medical Publishers, 1970).

Soffer, Rae-Ann, "The Nurse and Hemodialysis," *Nursing Care* (October 1973), pp. 14–18.

KAREN CHOATE ROBBINS, R.N., B.S.N.
ANN MARIE POWERS, R.N., B.S.N.

18

renal transplantation

Transplantation research began in the early 1900s, although it was not until the early 1950s that transplantation became a realistic and therapeutic approach for chronic renal failure in humans. Originally, kidneys were grafted into the thigh using the femoral vessels for vascularization. Experience with this procedure was limited to a very few patients. Since this site was obviously not practical for long-term graft survival, surgeons began grafting kidneys into the iliac fossa in the mid 1950s, the site still used today. Since that time, many centers in the country are performing renal transplants as definitive therapy for *endstage renal disease* (ESRD).* As more centers evolved, so too have a multitude of approaches and philosophies, with the major differences revolving around the immunosuppressive therapy. This chapter does not encompass all possible management approaches, but will, however, discuss the major points of transplantation and care which are common to all centers and are well documented in the literature. It will provide the critical care nurse with sufficient information that she may competently care for the transplant recipient.

endstage renal disease

Renal failure is rarely an "all or none" phenomenon, but instead is a gradual loss of function involving either part or all of the nephrons, depending on the basic disease process. When a patient has minimal renal damage, the

---

*The acceptable federal terminology for chronic renal failure is endstage renal disease. As of July 1, 1973, patients with endstage renal disease became eligible for Medicare coverage regardless of age. As a result, no one is denied replacement therapy due to lack of funds.

table 18-1
effects of endstage renal disease treated by dialysis or well-functioning renal graft

EFFECT ON	WITH DIALYSIS	WITH WELL-FUNCTIONING TRANSPLANT
Renal filtration	Only during dialysis	24 hours/day
Nutrition	Na, K, protein and fluid restrictions	Possible Na restriction for up to 1 year after transplant
Erythropoietic system	Anemia, fatigue	Normal red blood cells and hematocrit
Skeletal system	Renal osteodystrophy	No further bone resorption
	Hyperparathyroidism	Possible hyperparathyroidism
		Avascular necrosis
Nervous system	Peripheral, gastrointestinal and genitourinary neuropathy	Neuropathy will not progress, and may improve
Sexuality	Decreased libido	Improved libido
	Frequent impotence	Impotence may persist
Liver	Increased risk of hepatitis from recurrent extracorporeal circulation and transfusion	10% incidence of hepatitis due to azathioprine therapy
Cardiovascular system	Risk of shunt infection, clotting, exsanguination and frequent site changes	No need for vascular access
	Accelerated atherosclerosis	Decrease in atherosclerotic process
	Ventricular hypertrophy, heart failure	Ventricular size sometimes returns to normal
	Uremic pericarditis	
	Cardiac tamponade	
Muscular system	Decreased muscle mass due to dietary limits	Myopathy which improves when steroid dosage decreases and patient's activity increases
	Decreased exercise tolerance	

EFFECT ON	WITH DIALYSIS	WITH WELL-FUNCTIONING TRANSPLANT
Lungs	Risk of pulmonary edema, congestive heart failure	Pulmonary infections secondary to immunosuppressive therapy
Dependence	Dependent on machine to support life	Dependent on medications
Mortality	10% for first and second years, 36% for third year and increasing	20% for first year, then decreases

body may compensate for certain lost functions and the patient will have few symptoms. If the process is acute and reversible, the effects of long-term failure (e.g., anemia, osteodystrophy) will not be seen. For many patients, however, the process is a long and exhausting one which affects all body systems. It is not until irreversible damage to the majority of nephrons (approximately 2 million) occurs and the glomerular filtration rate decreases to 10 cc. per minute that a patient is considered to have ESRD (see Chapters 15 and 16).

transplant or dialysis: the patient's dilemma

Once a patient has reached endstage renal disease, he has three options: no treatment and death, chronic dialysis (either peritoneal dialysis or hemodialysis), or transplantation.

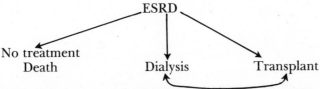

Although the option of no treatment and death is considered and occasionally chosen by the patient, the focus here will be on the treatment options of dialysis and transplant (called *replacement therapy*). Although dialysis and transplant are separate options, each of these therapies is an integral part of the other. Transplantation cannot be done without the support of dialysis, and, if the transplant fails, dialysis is resumed. Both ESRD and replacement therapy cause symptoms. Therefore, the patient needs to consider the effects of the disease as well as the risks of therapy. Table 18-1 outlines the effects of dialysis and transplantation on endstage renal disease.

Renal Filtration   In ESRD the GFR and urinary output are grossly diminished. Therefore hemodialysis must be done on a regular basis to provide the vital process of renal filtration. With a well-functioning renal graft, however, renal filtration is constant.

Nutrition   Diet is severely restricted in the majority of dialysis patients. These restrictions, which include protein, sodium, potassium and fluid, are necessary since the equivalent of renal filtration occurs for only a limited number of hours per week. When the diet is followed, it changes lifetime eating habits and poses severe limits on the patient's social activities. Gross abuse of the diet can result in malignant hypertension, congestive heart failure, pulmonary edema, hyperkalemia or, potentially, cardiac arrest. After transplantation, the only dietary restriction sometimes imposed upon the patient with good renal function is sodium. Rather than a fluid restriction, the patient is encouraged to drink at least 2 liters per day. Therefore, following successful transplant, the diet more closely approaches a normal one and is much more conducive to socialization.

Erythropoietic System   Anemia is common to all patients with ESRD. Because the kidney is no longer able to produce adequate amounts of erythropoietic stimulating factor, red blood cell production is low. This, along with shorter red blood cell survival in the uremic patient, causes hematocrits one half that of normal. This anemia is thought to cause the fatigue which is one of the most frustrating problems for the ESRD patient. Dietary restrictions limit iron and vitamin B_{12} intake, reducing the amount of iron that can be absorbed from the gut. The recent use of iron and androgen therapy has been of benefit to many patients, although normal hematocrits are rarely seen in spite of such therapy. Increased blood losses in the hemodialysis patient further contribute to low hematocrits. Ruptures and clotting of the dialyzer, residual blood in the dialyzer following termination of the dialysis, and routine laboratory tests constitute a blood loss in excess of 600 cc. per month per patient.[1]

In contrast, several months after the transplant, anemia is seldom a problem, and the patient will have a near normal, if not normal, hematocrit. Although the kidney was denervated when transplanted, this does not affect the erythropoiesis of the graft. While blood loss from laboratory tests is appreciable immediately following the transplant, it is markedly reduced following hospital discharge. The patient has a normal protein intake, an increased ability to absorb iron, and normal red blood cell survival time, all increasing the ability to maintain the hematocrit at a higher level.

Skeletal System   In the absence of renal function, the calcium/phosphorus ratio cannot be maintained. Phosphorus cannot be properly excreted and the patient must therefore take phosphorus binders in an attempt to maintain a near normal level. Because the kidney can no longer convert vitamin D, which is inactive, to I,25 dehydroxycholecalciferal, the form necessary for calcium absorption in the GI tract, calcium levels are low. The low calcium levels stimulate the production of parathyroid hormone in an effort to elevate the serum calcium to normal levels. When calcium levels remain low, the parathyroid hormone stimulates resorption of calcium stores from the bones and teeth. This causes a multitude of problems known as renal osteodystrophy which range from faulty bone formation in children to fractures, ruptured tendons, and vascular and soft tissue calcifications in adults. The persistent stimulation of parathyroid hormone often leads to secondary hyperparathyroidism which in turn may necessitate subtotal parathyroidectomy. These problems are somewhat lessened by the recent use of dihydrotachysterol, a synthetic form of vitamin D which increases calcium absorption from the GI tract. This is used along with either dietary or oral calcium supplementation. Following a transplant, calcium-phosphorus equilibration and vitamin D metabolism are again normal due to the presence of the functioning graft. Hyperparathyroidism is often reversed, although occasionally it continues, and is called tertiary hyperparathyroidism. While not a function of calcium-phosphorus metabolism, avascular necrosis is the most disabling complication of transplantation and is thought to be due to chronic steroid therapy. It occurs in about 10 percent of the transplant population but is rarely seen in the dialysis population. The femoral head is the part most commonly affected, and total hip replacement is sometimes necessary.

Nervous System Though the mechanism is poorly understood, neuropathies may develop in the presence of severe or chronic uremia. The neuropathies cause muscle weakness which sometime requires the use of braces, walkers or crutches for ambulation. Neuropathy should not increase in severity following transplantation, and, depending upon the severity of the neuropathy, there may be partial or total reversal following successful transplantation.

Sexuality Impotence is prevalent among the dialysis patient population. While women may be physically capable of engaging in sexual intercourse, libido is often markedly decreased, lowering their desire for sexual activity. Most male patients are impotent, perhaps because of their disease or because of antihypertensive medications. The etiology of this complication is probably physiological as well as psychological. Marriages and other comparable relationships can be adversely affected, and the long-term effects can be devastating. Some patients remain impotent following transplantation, although this is most frequently associated with antihypertensive medication and steroid therapy. The libido, which is decreased while the patient is on dialysis, seems to return to normal following transplant. Women usually cease to have menstrual periods while on dialysis, and following transplant will once again ovulate and menstruate. Therefore, some means of contraception should be used, as pregnancy can pose some potential problems for both the expectant woman and the child.

Liver Problems associated with the dialysis treatments alone are considerable. Hepatitis is an ever-present threat due to the frequent extracorporeal circulation. Hepatitis from multiple blood transfusions is diminished when fresh frozen red blood cells are used, since the hepatitis virus does not withstand freezing. Once over the initial postoperative period, transplant recipients rarely receive transfusions. However, noninfectious hepatitis associated with the use of the immunosuppressant azathioprine occurs occasionally among transplant recipients. This is usually resolved by discontinuing azathioprine and replacing it with cyclophosphamide.

Cardiovascular System Vascular access must be maintained in the hemodialysis patient, and loss of sites can sometimes pose life-threatening problems. Shunts, arteriovenous fistulas, bovine heterograft fistulas, Sparks-Mandrill grafts and polytetrofluroethylene (PTFE) grafts may be used in various combinations to gain permanent access to the circulation. Infections, clotting, high output cardiac failure, and exsanguination are persistent threats with any type of access. With each access failure, the number of potential sites is reduced until finally all possible sites are exhausted. Access problems account for a significant number of hospital admissions of hemodialysis patients. For the peritoneal dialysis patient, the surgically placed peritoneal catheter is left in place, but the potential for peritonitis is ever present. The transplant patient need not maintain a vascular access site; in fact, the greatest problem of access is simply to find blood vessels from which to draw blood for laboratory studies to monitor renal function.

Perhaps the most dramatic complication of ESRD is the rate of accelerated atherosclerosis. The etiology is not understood, but the greatest cause of mortality in long-term dialysis patients is cardiovascular accidents. Some of the most advanced atherosclerosis seen at postmortem examination has been in long-term dialysis patients. Because of protein restrictions, most calories are taken in the form of carbohydrates, which leads to an increased level of cholesterol. In addition, there is a hypertriglyceremia thought to be due to increased synthesis by the liver and decreased clearing by the kidney of lipoprotein and lipase. The apparent arrest of this rapid atherosclerosis is one of the greatest advantages of transplantation. Again, the return to a normal diet can decrease the dietary contributions to atherosclerotic changes.

Because the dialysis patient usually has little or no fluid output, an increased intake of sodium or fluid will cause hypervolemia which, because the vascular system has difficulty accommodating this fluid excess, can lead to congestive heart failure. Some patients lose as much as 15 pounds of fluid with a single dialysis treatment. Hypervolemia can occur in the transplant recipient when decreased urinary output occurs as the result of rejection episodes or acute tubular necrosis and is managed by either diuretic therapy or hemodialysis support.

The specific mechanism causing uremic pericarditis is unclear. Depending on the severity and chronicity of pericarditis, a pericardial window or a pericardectomy is sometime necessary to control this problem. If the patient has fluid overload, a pericardial rub may not be heard due to the fluid contair.d in the pericardial sac. What seems to be an appropriate therapy, dialyzing to remove excess fluid, can actually increase the patient's pain because the fluid is removed and the friction is increased. At this point a rub is very prominent. Conservative management of pericarditis varies greatly and may include anti-inflammatory agents.

A patient with uremic pericarditis may develop cardiac tamponade. The treatment for the ESRD patient is the same as for any other patient: an attempt to remove the blood from the pericardial sac before an arrest occurs. Cardiac tamponade is an ominous complication with high mortality.

Muscular System   A loss of muscle mass is not uncommon in the ESRD patient. Limited dietary intake and inability to exert oneself due to the fatigue associated with anemia are probably the major contributing factors. The transplant recipient will frequently experience myopathies due to steroid therapy. This loss in muscle mass can be recovered with exercise, particularly when the steroids are reduced. In an attempt to avoid severe myopathies, the transplant recipient is encouraged to walk, climb stairs and exercise as much as possible.

Lungs   Hypervolemia as the result of ESRD can cause congestive heart failure, pulmonary congestion, and pulmonary edema (see p. 368). After transplantation, the risk of congestive heart failure and pulmonary edema diminishes because fluid balance can be maintained by the functioning kidney graft. However, after transplant there is greater risk of pulmonary infection as the result of immunosuppressant therapy (see p. 380).

Dependence   Patients with ESRD need dialysis to live, and therefore are physiologically dependent upon a machine. The average hemodialysis patient spends approximately 15 hours per week attached to the machine, while a peritoneal dialysis patient spends even greater lengths of time attached to the machine. Because of the life-sustaining value of dialysis, as well as the time devoted to the procedure, patients have varying degrees of emotional dependence upon the treatment. Some patients keep their dependence in perspective by looking on dialysis as a necessary but not exclusive part of their lives and make an effort to keep the rest of their lives as fulfilling as possible. Others adapt to the dependency by having all their emotional energy revolve around the treatment and the personnel who provide care. Conversely, the transplant recipient is no longer dependent upon a machine, but rather on medication to support the function of the graft. Patients usually find dependence upon the medication far more acceptable than dependence upon a machine.

Mortality   The mortality rate associated with long-term maintenance dialysis is 10 percent for the first and second years, 25 percent for the third year and 40 percent by the fifth year.[2] While there are mechanical problems with the dialysis treatments, most of the deaths are cardiovascular in nature. Hyperkalemia, "the silent killer," may account for more deaths than is realized, particularly if the patient expires out of the hospital setting.

The mortality rate for those receiving organs from living related donors is 11.5 percent for the first year and 15.4 percent for the second year; for cadaver donors, the rate is 28 percent for the first year and 34 percent for the second year.[3] Most transplant deaths are related to infection.

Endstage renal disease is chronic and complex and presents a multitude of problems for the patient, his family and the health care team, whether the decision is continued dialysis or transplantation. Many patients will choose transplantation. One of the next steps, then, is tissue typing to find a suitable donor.

finding a donor for renal transplant

Just as red blood cells can be typed for both donor and recipient to prevent reaction between them, tissue can also be typed to prevent similar reactions when organs are transplanted. The tissue typing system, called HL-A, defines specific tissue antigens which each person possesses. Each person has four HL-A antigens, having inherited two from each parent. Since more than 30 HL-A antigens have been identified, there are more than 30,000 possible combinations of tissue types; it quickly becomes apparent that a donor from within the family provides greater potential for a compatible tissue match. Lymphocytes contain the tissue antigens, and are used to determine an individual's tissue type. It is also essential that the donor and recipient have compatible ABO blood types, although Rh factor compatibility is not necessary.

living related donors

As the name indicates, a living related donor is a donor from within the family. The possibility of an HL-A compatible donor from within the family should be explored for every potential recipient. The possible combinations include: a 4-antigen match, also called an "HL-A identical" match, which would have to be a sibling of the potential recipient; a 3-antigen match, which is uncommon since the antigens are usually inherited in pairs or haplotypes; and a 2-antigen match, which is the most frequently seen compatibility. The presence of four completely different antigens is considered a complete mismatch, and is not a desirable situation for a transplant to be performed, since no similarity exists between the tissues. Once a potential living related donor is identified, he has a thorough medical evaluation to determine that he is free of underlying disease, that he has two kidneys, and that donation could in no obvious way jeopardize his well-being. Once this evaluation is successfully completed, a living related transplant may be performed.

cadaver donors

Approximately one fourth of the people who are in need of a transplant have a suitable living donor, which means three fourths of all potential recipients must wait for a suitable cadaver donor. A potential cadaver kidney donor is a person who dies from a problem not involving the kidneys. Some illnesses which exclude a person from becoming a donor are malignancy (except primary brain tumors), long-standing diabetes mellitus, chronic hypertension, hepatitis, tuberculosis and sepsis. Patients with persistent hypotension resulting in oliguria or anuria are not reasonable donors. Age is not necessarily a limiting factor and donors have been less than one year old and more than sixty years old. Many donors are trauma victims, while others die from cerebral aneurysms and surgery.

The cadaver donor is tissue typed to identify his HL-A antigens. Once the ABO and HL-A types have been identified, potential recipients can be considered. A further test, called a crossmatch, is set up to screen the potential recipients for antibodies they might have against the donor. This crossmatch takes 6 to 8 hours to complete and involves mixing serum from the potential recipients with donor lymphocytes. A positive crossmatch means that the recipient has antibodies against the donor. This response can be thought of as *in vitro* rejection. Thus a *negative* crossmatch is necessary for recipient selection. Occasionally a crossmatch is negative when, in fact, the recipient has antibodies against the donor in insufficient titers to elicit a positive test. This crossmatch is also performed for a living related transplant and must also be negative. A number of other screening tests are being studied but are still research endeavors without clear-cut clinical application for predicting graft survival.

Criteria for Determining Death Historically, death was acknowledged when irreversible cardiac or respiratory arrest occurred. In the mid 1960s, however, the concept of *brain death* came into existence and is now medically accepted as an additional way in which death can be diagnosed. Only a minority of states, however, accept brain death as a legal definition of death. Brain death refers to the cessation of brain activity at both cortical and lower levels even though heart and respiratory functions can be maintained mechanically. The acknowledgment of brain death is important in obtaining kidneys from cadaver donors since the kidneys should be removed within 30 minutes after respiration and circulation cease. This time limit insures viable organs for transplant. As a result of technological advances which sustain life, and because both physicians and the public want to be protected against premature diagnosis of death, various groups have tried to refine criteria which indicate death. The most widely accepted criteria for defining death are referred to as the "Harvard Criteria."[4] All criteria must be met on two separate occasions, 24 hours apart, without any change in the findings, unless it is not possible to maintain respiratory and cardiac function. The criteria include:

1. Complete unresponsiveness: total unawareness to external stimuli, i.e., irreversible coma.
2. No spontaneous muscular movements including respiration. If the patient has been on a mechanical respirator, it can be turned off for 3 minutes to observe whether or not the patient breathes spontaneously. For this criterion to be valid, the patient must have a normal carbon dioxide tension and must breathe room air for at least 10 minutes before the test.
3. Absent reflexes, spontaneous or elicited.
4. A flat electroencephalogram for at least 10 and preferably 20 minutes is a confirmatory rather than an essential criterion. There are further procedural criteria for the way the test should be done. Electroencephalogram results are not valid when there is hypothermia or central nervous system depression from drugs.

The issue of determining death is included in this chapter because of the increasing numbers of patients awaiting organs for transplant. Because of the large number needed, the transplant team must seek out potential organs for donation and are therefore sometimes viewed by personnel as hoping for death and awaiting the bounty. Supplying the names of patients who have slim chances of surviving means that health care workers must acknowledge that a patient they care about may die in the near future whether or not his organs are donated for transplant. The transplant team member who needs the information usually recognizes the double-edged nature of the task and walks the tightrope of trying to obtain information without seeming either nonchalant or eager. Knowing that there are criteria adhered to in determining death should reassure health care providers that death will not be premature even though it is anticipated and plans are made for obtaining viable transplant organs.

The Nurse's Role When a patient meets the criteria and becomes a potential donor, it is necessary to maintain the blood pressure as near normal as possible to provide adequate perfusion of the organ. At that time there is probably also the need to support a family who may be troubled not only by the donor's impending death, but also by their decision to donate organs. On the one hand, keeping an organ viable may be frustrating, particularly when the vigilant monitoring and regulation of blood pressure are viewed as taking care away from other patients who will survive. On the other hand, these efforts can be viewed as giving two people a chance at a longer and better life. Visiting a transplant recipient, particularly one who has received a cadaver organ from a patient they cared for, has helped nurses realize that the organ donation and the help needed to keep it viable are indeed worthwhile.

care of the transplant recipient

The transplant recipient is usually cared for in a specially designated area throughout both acute and convalescent phases of recovery. This not only allows for highly proficient nursing care, but also eliminates patient transfer, decreases fragmentation of care and reduces exposure to infection for the newly immunosuppressed patient. In addition, the transplant recipient is usually not critically ill and so many times does not fit the criteria for admission to a critical care area. Nevertheless, there may be times when transplant patients will be cared for in a critical care area, especially during the acute postoperative phase or when complications occur.

postoperative phase of transplant recipient care

Immediately after surgery, the transplant recipient is cared for in a closely monitored area until his condition stabilizes. As the patient arrives in this recovery or intensive care area, the following assessment can be made:

1. Check the patient's level of consciousness and degree of pain.
2. Check the number of intravenous lines present, noting the site, type of solution and flow rate.

3. Observe the abdominal dressing for drainage, noting whether a Hemovac or drain is present.
4. Check for the presence of Foley and ureteral catheters and observe the patency and urinary drainage of each.
5. Locate the vascular access site and determine its patency by placing either fingers or a stethoscope directly over the access site and feeling or listening for a characteristically loud pulsating noise called a *bruit*.
6. Check the blood pressure, apical pulse, respirations, temperature and central venous pressure. Blood pressure should be taken on the extremity that does *not* have a functioning vascular access site, because even momentary interference with arterial blood flow may lead to access malfunction.
7. If a nasogastric tube is present, attach it to an appropriate drainage system.
8. Weigh the patient on a bed scale.

Answers to the following questions will provide additional baseline information.

1. Are the patient's own kidneys present in addition to the graft, and if so, how much urine do they produce daily? This information will help determine how much of the urine produced is from the transplanted kidney. If the chart does not provide answers, the patient and family can. In addition, flank scars usually indicate nephrectomy.
2. When was the last dialysis treatment?
3. What are the preoperative results of laboratory tests (serum electrolytes, urea nitrogen, creatinine, liver function, calcium, phosphorus, CBC with differential and platelet counts, urine electrolytes, specific gravity, creatinine clearance)?
4. How much and what kind of intravenous fluid has the patient received?
5. Did the patient receive a loading dose of immunosuppressive drugs preoperatively? What is the present dose schedule?
6. Was methylprednisolone (Solu-Medrol) given in the operating room, and what is the ongoing dose schedule?
7. Is the patient to receive antilymphocytic globulin? This drug information helps not only to clarify the regimen, but also to estimate the degree of immunosuppression.
8. What preoperative teaching has been done? Patients who have received some teaching tend to be less anxious and more cooperative, since they know what to expect. A cadaver donor recipient who receives a graft shortly after being placed on the waiting list might be poorly informed because preoperative teaching was not done. In this case, additional explanation is needed.
9. Which physician is to be called—how, where and when—for ongoing medical care? Clarifying and recording this information may enhance communication and efficiency, especially in case of emergency.

Many nursing responsibilities revolve around observing the function of the transplanted kidney, monitoring fluid and electrolyte balance, helping the patient avoid sources of infection, picking up early signs of complications and supporting the patient and family through recovery phases.

Monitoring Renal Graft Function   The transplanted kidney may function immediately after revascularization and produce large amounts of urine (200 to 1,000 cc. per hour), small amounts of urine (<20 cc. per hour), or no urine at all. The amount of urine produced is related to the length of time the donor kidney was ischemic. The ischemic time tends to be shorter in the living related transplant situation than in the cadaver transplant situation. Therefore, the living related donor kidney has less ischemic damage and tends to produce more urine in the initial recovery phase. However, the hourly production of large amounts of urine is called post-transplant diuresis and is thought to be the result of a proximal tubular defect. The proximal tubule is responsible for 80 percent reabsorption of water, electrolytes and glucose, and interference with its function allows more filtrate than normal to be excreted. This is a reversible state in which tubular reabsorptive functions are temporarily lost or greatly diminished because of an ischemic time period from clamping the renal artery in the donor to the end of the venous revascularization of the recipient.

The ischemic time is prolonged in the cadaver donor situation since it may take hours to find a suitable recipient after the donor has expired and the graft harvested. In this situation the graft is placed on an organ preservation machine or in a preservation solution until a suitable recipient is found. Acceptable time of preservation is under 50 hours. This preservation time, added to the extreme hypotensive period in cadaver donor patients, points out how long the ischemic period may be and why there is renal tissue damage and low output. Nevertheless, this damage is usually reversible. The graft, in this situation, may produce either a small quantity or no urine at all for up to four weeks after the transplant operation. This output phase is referred to as acute tubular necrosis.

The quantity of urine does not have to correlate with the quality of graft function. Renal function is assessed by periodic serum urea nitrogen and creatinine levels and by a renal scan, which is a radioisotope test used to determine renal perfusion, filtration and excretion. It is frequently done in the first 24 hours as a baseline and periodically in the postoperative phase depending upon the patient's recovery and the presence of complications.

When a change in urinary output occurs, such as a large volume one hour to a diminished amount the next, mechanical factors which interfere with urinary drainage should be suspected. Clotted, kinked or compressed tubing in the urinary drainage system may be the cause of the decreased output. When the catheter is occluded by a clot, the patient may complain of pain, feel an urgency to void, or have bloody leakage around the catheter. Milking is the preferred way to dislodge clots, since irrigation, even under aseptic conditions, increases the risk of infection.

Urinary leakage on the abdominal dressing and severe abdominal discomfort or distention may indicate retroperitoneal leakage from the ureteral anastomosis site. Decreased urinary output or severe abdominal pain in the presence of good renal function and adequate pain medication should be reported since technical and surgical complications account for a 10 percent loss of graft function.[5]

Two major types of graft anastomoses are performed. In the first type, the donor kidney is anastomosed at the ureteropelvic junction to the recipient ureter. A Foley catheter is commonly used with this anastomosis. In the second type, the donor ureter is implanted into the recipient's bladder and a Foley and/or ureteral catheter may be used to provide drainage. The urinary drainage from the ureteropelvic anastomosis tends to be bloody initially but turns pink in a few hours. The urinary drainage from the second type of anastomosis tends to be bloody for the first few days, and clotting is more problematic. The urine is bloody because the bladder is very vascular and tends to bleed after being sutured. With urine outflow, some clots are carried down the catheter while others occlude the lumen.

Maintaining Fluid and Electrolyte Balance   Maintaining fluid and electrolyte balance follows the same principles outlined in Chapter 17. Intake is provided intravenously while the patient is unable to take fluids by mouth. A standard maintenance solution of 1,200 cc. per 24 hours for an adult is based on insensible water losses, while replacement solution is calculated for each patient according to such things as urine output, gastric and wound drainage and CVP readings. When urinary output is high as in post-transplant diuresis replacement will be large, while in oliguric or anuric states, replacement will be small. The solutions used most often include 0.09 percent normal saline, 5 percent dextrose in water, 0.45 percent saline and 2.5 percent dextrose in water.

The slow maintenance intravenous solution may be infused through a CVP line, but large amounts of fluid, e.g. 500 cc., should not be infused directly into the heart. Replacement intravenous solution is generally infused through a peripheral site on the extremity which does *not* have a vascular access site. It is highly unlikely to have an infusion into a vein that has an access because if the renal graft does not function immediately, the patient will need to be dialyzed within the first few days. For this the patient will need a healthy access site.

Serum electrolytes are drawn shortly after the patient arrives in the unit. The frequency of these tests usually depends on graft function. If the patient has a large volume of output, laboratory tests may be done every four or six hours for the first 24 to 36 hours. If the patient is anuric but otherwise stable, tests for electrolytes are done daily except for potassium, which may be ordered more frequently. Excessive blood drawing should be kept to a minimum since the recipient is anemic in the initial recovery phase because of ESRD. The most frequent electrolyte disturbance in the acute postoperative phase is hyperkalemia. Most transplant recipients are dialyzed within 24 hours of surgery and therefore have a normal serum potassium in the operating room. If the graft functions and excretes a high volume of urine, it is also generally able to excrete the excessive serum potassium created by surgical tissue damage. If the patient is oliguric or anuric after surgery, serum potassium will increase to unacceptable levels and will need to be lowered initially by sodium polystyrene sulfonate (Kayexalate) enemas and then possibly by dialysis.

Preventing Infection Infection is a frequent complication and the most frequent cause of graft failure. The immunosuppressive drugs decrease the patient's defense system and prolong graft survival (see discussion below). The detrimental effect is that patients are more susceptible to organisms, even those normally found in the environment. Since most infections are endogenous, strict isolation technique has been abandoned in the postoperative phase. It not only creates psychological problems for the patient, but compliance by all team members is difficult to enforce. Nevertheless, visitors, nurses and other personnel who have upper respiratory or any other type of infection should not visit or give care to the patient.

Cleansing the catheter and perineal area around the urethral meatus with an antiseptic solution every eight hours will decrease urinary tract infections. Changing intravenous tubing daily as well as when it is contaminated will also decrease the risk of sepsis. Wet dressings should be changed often since they are excellent media for organism growth. Thorough handwashing before and after patient care is a simple and effective way to decrease organisms in the recipient's environment.

Because pulmonary infections are high on the list of transplant recipient complications, enhancing ventilation and promoting drainage of secretions is paramount. Observing the rate and character of respirations and listening to breath sounds will help determine how often the patient should turn, deep breathe, cough, walk, use blow bottles or tubes, or need postural drainage. Transplant patients can turn to the operative side; in fact, doing so promotes wound drainage and decreases the incidence of hematomas and lymphoceles.

complications of renal transplantation

immunity and the rejection phenomenon

The most frequently occurring noninfectious complication is graft rejection. To begin to understand these phenomena, one needs to understand antigen-antibody reaction. There are two basic types of acquired immunity — humoral and cellular — and both are involved in the rejection process.

Humoral immunity refers to the system responsible for antigen-antibody reactions. Antigens are large protein complexes which invade the body and elicit an antibody response. Antibodies are globulin molecules which are made in response to a specific antigen. Once formed, these antibodies are capable of attacking the antigen any time after the initial exposure.

Cellular immunity develops when lymphocytes become specifically sensitized against a foreign agent. Lymphocytes, which constitute about 1 percent of the total number of leukocytes, "bind antigen and then release a host of pharmacological factors called lymphokines which produce a specific inflammatory response that leads to the elimination of antigen."[6]

The transplanted kidney is a foreign antigen implanted in a recipient. Eventually, the recipient's body will recognize the kidney as a foreign antigen and mobilize its defense system to try to rid itself of this foreign substance. This process is called *rejection*. It is important to realize that all transplant recipients' defense immune systems eventually see the kidney as foreign and in some way respond to it. The only exceptions to this are recipients who are nonresponders. Such persons either do not respond to any foreign antigen stimulation or respond poorly to stimulation. The nonresponders, however, are few in number; therefore, what becomes important is observing how strongly the immune defensive system responds. Rejection can be broken down into four basic categories: hyperacute, accelerated, acute and chronic.

Hyperacute rejection can occur within minutes to hours following transplantation. This may occur either because of a major blood group incompatibility, or, more commonly, because preformed antibodies existed in titers too low to be detected in the tissue typing tests. There is no treatment for hyperacute rejection and it always results in loss of the graft.

Accelerated rejection is a slower form of hyperacute rejection, occurring within a few days to approximately one week following the transplant. This, again, is probably a function of preformed antibodies and does not respond to any form of therapy. It destroys the kidney, which must then be removed. Both hyperacute and accelerated rejection are results of humoral immunity.

Acute rejection occurs after the first postoperative week. It is the most frequently seen form of rejection and fortunately the type which responds best to therapy. During an acute rejection episode, the patient may experience any, all, or none of the following:
1. Decrease in urine output
2. Weight gain
3. Edema
4. A temperature of 100°F (37.8°C) or greater
5. Tenderness over the graft site with possible swelling of the kidney itself
6. General malaise
7. Increased blood pressure

Laboratory findings indicating an acute rejection episode include:
1. Increased serum creatinine
2. Decreased urine creatinine and creatinine clearance
3. Possible decrease in urine sodium
4. Increased BUN

Chronic rejection is a gradual deterioration of kidney function and is the result of repeated insults from acute rejection episodes. The symptoms are similar to those of acute rejection except that fever and graft enlargement may not occur. Chronic rejection results in scarring of renal tissue and infarction of renal vessels from the vasculitis accompanying acute rejection. Therefore in chronic rejection the inflammatory signs are absent. Laboratory findings are similar in both acute and chronic rejection. The rate of deterioration in chronic rejection can vary and the patient may have adequate renal function from a few months up to a year before replacement therapy is indicated. There is no effective therapy known to treat this type of rejection.

table 18-2
immunosuppressive drugs used in renal transplantation

DRUG	ADVERSE REACTIONS	DOSAGE	COMMENTS
Azathioprine (Imuran) (IV or PO)	Bone marrow suppression: leukopenia, thrombocytopenia, anemia, pancytopenia Rash Alopecia Liver damage, jaundice Increased susceptibility to infection Anorexia, nausea, vomiting and diarrhea from large doses	Regulated to keep WBCs 5,000 to 10,000. Drug usually stopped when WBCs 3,000 or less. Initial: 5-10 mg./kg. of body weight Maintenance: 2-3 mg./kg. of body weight During rejection: maximum of 3 mg./kg. of body weight	Lower doses are given when: 1. Renal function is poor since drug is excreted by kidney 2. Given concurrently with allopurinol which delays metabolism of azathioprine (allopurinol and azathioprine are synergistic)
Methylprednisolone (Solu-Medrol) (IV) Prednisone (PO)	Diabetogenic effect Increased susceptibility to infection Masks symptoms of infection Peptic ulcer, GI bleeding Delayed healing Increased sodium and water retention Increased appetite, weight gain Behavior and personality changes	Initial: 2-3 mg./kg. of body weight, tapered to an adequate oral maintenance dose During rejection: methylprednisolone may be given in IV boluses up to 1 gm./dose	Methylprednisolone is given only until the patient tolerates liquids Cardiac arrest can occur if IV bolus of 1 gm. is given rapidly An antacid is taken while patient is on steroids to reduce the risk of gastric irritation and ulceration

DRUG	ADVERSE REACTIONS	DOSAGE	COMMENTS
Methylprednisolone (Solu-Medrol) (IV) Prednisone (PO) *Continued*	Negative nitrogen balance Adrenal gland suppression Osteoporosis with long-term therapy Muscle weakness Easy bruising Skin atrophy, striae Glaucoma, cataracts Acne Hirsutism Cushing syndrome		Sodium restriction may be necessary when steroid dosage is high or when fluid retention increases
Antilymphocyte globulin (ALG) Antithymocyte globulin (ATG) (IV, IM, or deep SC)	Anaphylactic shock due to hypersensitivity to animal serum Fever (up to 105°F or 40.6°C) and chills Increased susceptibility to infections due to decreased lymphocytes IM or deep SC injection site may be swollen, red and painful with abscess formation Difficulty walking, if injection given in thigh	Dosage may vary	Skin test for hypersensitivity to animal serum before giving initial dose Lymphocytes and/or platelets decrease sharply with drug administration; therefore, draw bloodwork for lymphocyte count before infusion is started

immunosuppression

As the term implies, immunosuppression is the use of drug therapy to suppress the immune response in order to permit acceptance of transplanted organs, most often with a type of tissue at least partially different from that of the recipient. The difficulty of this therapy is in providing enough suppression to prevent rejection without rendering the recipient grossly susceptible to opportunistic infections. The drugs given to control the immune response are azathioprine (Imuran), methylprednisolone (Solu-Medrol), prednisone and antilymphocytic globulin. Major points about these drugs are summarized in Table 18-2 (pp. 378–379). The drug cyclophosphamide (Cytoxan) may be used in place of azathioprine if the latter drug causes hepatotoxicity.

Azathioprine, an antimetabolite, is the mainstay of immunosuppression. The patient's ability to consistently tolerate 2 to 3 mg. per kg. dosage is important for long-term graft survival. Azathioprine cannot be increased to treat rejection because of its bone marrow suppression effects and its cumulative effects in the presence of little or no renal function.

Methylprednisolone is the parenteral steroid used in the initial postoperative period until the patient is able to tolerate oral medications, at which time prednisone is started. Oral prednisone may be given in a variety of schedules and doses, and the philosophy varies from center to center, just as it does with the use of methylprednisolone in the treatment of rejection episodes. Treatment of rejection episodes may include intravenous injections of methylprednisolone in boluses up to 1 gram per dose. It is recommended that it be administered over 20 to 30 minutes. This is particularly important since several cardiac arrests have been reported following the administration of 1 gram of methylprednisolone, IV push.

Antilymphocyte or antithymocyte globulin is used in a number of centers in an effort to prevent rejection by providing the patient with antibodies against lymphocytes or thymocytes, which are the cells responsible for rejection. These antibodies are produced by injecting human lymph or thymus cells into an animal (horse, rabbit or goat) which then produces antibodies against these cells.

infection

One of the greatest crises for the recipient is sepsis, since it is still one of the greatest threats to recipient survival. The origin of sepsis may be the blood (septicemia) or a single organ, such as the liver, lungs, or pancreas; or the entire body, i.e., a disseminated infection may be involved. Pulmonary infections are probably the most frequent cause of death from an infection, and the patient requires mechanical respiratory support and good pulmonary toilet. The pathogens vary from the more commonly seen bacterial organisms to fungal, viral, or even protozoan organisms. The latter organisms are referred to as "opportunistic pathogens." These are organisms normally found in humans and in the environment and are generally considered harmless. However, the patient with a compromised immune system such as a transplant recipient is susceptible to infections from these organisms: thus the term "opportunistic," since the microorganisms take advantage of the decreased host defenses. Specific examples of these opportunistic infections include herpes simplex, herpes zoster, *Candida albicans*, Aspergillus, Cryptococcus, Nocardia, and cytomegalovirus (CMV). The presence of any of these infections should be monitored closely, as they could pose life-threatening crises.

If immunosuppressive therapy is reduced or discontinued in the presence of a life-threatening situation resulting from an opportunistic infection, the emphasis *must* be on the patient's life rather than on the graft. Therefore, rejection of the graft is permitted in an effort to save the patient's life. If the graft is totally rejected, the patient is supported with dialysis therapy, and, once the infectious process is resolved, the patient can then be considered for retransplantation.

Another problem which contributes to loss of renal function is the antibiotic therapy necessary to control the infection. Amphotericin B, a drug used to treat the fungal infections, is nephrotoxic in that it decreases renal perfusion. The use of mannitol in the amphotericin B solution can counteract the problem of decreased perfusion, because it increases renal perfusion. Because many antibiotics and antifungal agents are nephrotoxic, treatment of infections can pose difficult management problems.

cardiovascular complications

Although cardiovascular accidents can occur in the acute postoperative period, more frequently they occur a year after transplant, and are considered late complications of transplantation. Should the complications occur in the early postoperative period, graft survival and vascular problems are of concern. However, if they occur as late complications of transplantation, graft function has usually stabilized, and vascular complications are the major concern. Patients with a functioning graft may succumb to this type of complication. The Twelfth Transplant Registry Report lists myocardial infarction and cerebral hemorrhage as leading noninfectious causes of death. A greater percentage of patients receiving cadaver transplants succumb to these complications, with more than one half of the patients having a functioning graft at the time of the insult.

The cause of death from vascular problems occurring years after transplant is under investigation. Since the early 1970s, higher risk patients, such as those with diabetes, vasculitis, systemic lupus erythematosus, and those 50 to 70 years old, have had transplants. In fact, patients with cardiac disease treated by coronary bypass surgery have later received renal transplants. Perhaps these higher risks have contributed to an increase in death from vascular complications. In addition, it may be that the long-term complications are just beginning to surface, since patients are now reaching a point ten years or more post-transplant.

gastrointestinal complications

Gastrointestinal complications may pose serious and even life-threatening situations for the recipient. Massive gastrointestinal bleeding may occur as the result of steroid therapy, stress, and the decreased viability of tissues due to earlier protein restrictions. GI complications most often will occur in the acute postoperative phase, at the point when graft survival is still of major concern. Again, forfeiture of the graft may be necessary in an effort to save the patient's life. Other serious GI complications include acute pancreatitis, obstruction from bowel adhesions, and ulcerative colitis. Should the patient have an intestinal perforation, then not only is the GI complication a threat, but so is infection. It should therefore be stressed that a transplant recipient may have one or more of these complications simultaneously, increasing the complexity of both medical and nursing care. The following patient situations point out how interwoven complications may become and how necessary it is to observe for their subtle clues.

Patient Situation No. 1

A 54-year-old recipient of a cadaver kidney was admitted with a fever of 102°F (38.9°C) and lethargy. Diagnostic tests showed chronic rejection with azotemia and bowel obstruction. Laparotomy and a temporary colostomy were performed. The patient returned to hemodialysis three times per week. The abdominal incision became infected with *Escherichia coli,* while pulmonary atelectasis in the postoperative period progressed to infectious pneumonia. Within one week, the patient required intubation and ventilatory support. She was placed in a critical care area. She then developed secondary iatrogenic diabetes mellitus as another complication of steroid therapy. Within a few weeks, she died from disseminated intravascular coagulation and overwhelming, irreversible lung infection.

Patient Situation No. 2

A 50-year-old man was the recipient of a cadaver transplant. The patient was known to have renin-dependent hypertension and was receiving propranolol four times per day. Throughout the immediate post-transplant period, the patient complained of "gas pains." Due to this chronic complaint, an evaluation was undertaken but with negative findings. Approximately three weeks post-transplant, a duodenal ulcer perforated. Because of steroid therapy, the symptoms of perforation were masked to the extent that none of the classical signs of peritonitis were present. In addition, the myocardial effects of propranolol therapy prevented the patient's heart from responding to the sympathetic drive, and as a result his apical rate never varied from approximately 60, in spite of his perforation. About eight hours following the perforation, the patient's blood pressure began to drop, and bowel sounds were no longer heard. The diagnosis of perforation was made. Thus, the combination of drugs markedly masked the otherwise classical symptoms the patient might have demonstrated.

The need for nurses to be aware of drug actions such as those described above cannot be overemphasized. Constant and thorough evaluation is mandatory in caring for this very complex group of patients. Detailed information concerning the infectious complications, cardiovascular problems, and gastrointestinal complications of the transplant recipient is not within the scope of this chapter, and the reader is referred to the bibliography.

hypertension

Hypertension is a common but often transitory complication following renal transplantation. Many patients requiring chronic antihypertensive therapy are hypertensive before the transplant, and their hypertension is made worse by post-transplant steroid therapy. Various factors are responsible for post-transplant hypertension.

Transplant recipients are placed on steroids, usually prednisone and/or methylprednisolone. Although these are glucocorticoids, they are converted into mineralocorticoids, and cause sodium and water retention. While patients may be on a sodium-restricted diet, drug therapy is often necessary. Spironolactone, an aldosterone-blocking agent, is often useful in treating steroid-induced hypertension along with the diuretic, hydrochlorothiazide. Nurses must monitor for potential electrolyte imbalances (specifically, hyponatremia and hypokalemia) and instruct the patient and his family about the signs and symptoms of these imbalances and what to do should they occur. The effect of these drugs does not occur immediately, and therefore electrolyte imbalances are usually not seen until several days after the medications are started. At this time, a brisk diuresis may follow, increasing the potential for both hypovolemia and electrolyte imbalances. Because rapid fluid loss will result in weight loss, the patient's weight should be carefully recorded.

While steroid treatment is one mechanism which causes post-transplant hypertension, a second mechanism, renin-dependent hypertension, is seen rather frequently. Immediately following the transplant procedure, the recipient may have markedly elevated blood pressure. Due to the ischemic injury to the organ between time of removal and time of implantation, excessive amounts of renin may be released. Once adequate circulation has been established within the organ, this mechanism should "turn off," resulting in a return of the pressure to the preoperative level within a few days following the transplant. While renin itself is not a potent vasoconstrictor, its conversion to angiotensin I and angiotensin II causes vasoconstriction. The immediate postoperative period is not the only time in the progress of the transplant recipient's course that renin-dependent hypertension can occur.

Hypertension may be one of the first clinical manifestations of rejection. The basis of this hypertension is renin. Since rejection is an inflammatory response, vasculitis within the kidney impedes normal circulation and results in elevated renin levels. Renin levels are elevated in virtually all patients who have hypertension during an acute rejection episode. This phenomenon occurs in chronic rejection as well. Therefore, the nurse should pose the question of ensuing rejection when she first detects an elevated blood pressure.

Renal artery stenosis can also result in renin-dependent hypertension. The stenosis may cause a decrease in renal perfusion leading to increased renin production. When this occurs, an abdominal bruit may be auscultated lateral to the midline and medial to the kidney. The sudden appearance of a bruit or an increase in an abdominal bruit previously present is strongly suggestive of a renal artery stenosis. Surgical correction of the stenosis is almost always successful, and there is rarely loss of renal function as a result of the surgery. In fact, loss of renal function is more likely to occur when surgery is not performed.

Propranolol is often used to treat renin-dependent hypertension because it is thought to act as a renin inhibitor. Because this drug is a cardiac depressant, congestive heart failure may result from its prolonged use. The use of a diuretic may help to avoid this complication. However, the use of catecholamine-depleting agents such as reserpine is unwise since the patient is unable to respond to a sympathetic drive because of the beta adrenergic blocking effects of propranolol. Recent, but limited, use of an experimental drug, minoxidil, has been effective in treating renin-dependent hypertension which does not respond to therapy with propranolol. Hirsutism, the major obvious side effect of minoxidil, can be very distressing to the patient and may actually affect compliance with this therapeutic regimen.

Volume-dependent hypertension is another problem for the transplant recipient. During rejection episodes or periods of acute tubular necrosis, the patient may become fluid-overloaded due to inadequate fluid output from the kidney. If the patient does not respond to diuretic therapy, the use of dialysis may be indicated to further control the hypervolemic and hypertensive state until renal function recovers. The development of malignant hypertension precipitating hypertensive crisis is managed as with any other patient.

Problems associated with antihypertensive therapy are not unique to the transplant patient. Lethargy, impotence, and orthostatic hypotension are just some of the untoward effects of such therapy. However, once renal function has become stable, the patient's steroid dose has been reduced, and his urine output is satisfactory, the need for antihypertensive medications is markedly reduced.

a patient's view

How do patients who have experienced many complications view their decision to have a renal transplant? One patient received a cadaver transplant which chronically rejected after three and a half years, underwent bilateral total hip replacements for aseptic necrosis and had impaired vision due to cataracts. When asked if it had been worth it to him to be off dialysis and whether he would like to receive a new kidney graft, he responded without question or hesitation with an emphatic, "Absolutely!" People who have had successful renal transplantation, even in the face of complications, state unequivocally that they would not alter their decision to have received a renal graft. It is the success of such patients and their appreciation of new lives that makes transplantation a challenging and richly rewarding field.

REFERENCES

1. R. E. Lonecker et al., "Chronic Blood Loss in the Hemodialysis Patient," *Dialysis and Transplantation* (February–March 1975), pp. 32–37.
2. A. Lyndner and K. Curtis, "Morbidity and Mortality Associated with Long-Term Hemodialysis," *Hospital Practice*, Vol. 9 (November 1974), p. 147.
3. Advisory Committee of the Renal Transplant Registry, *The Twelfth Report of the Human Renal Transplant Registry*, p. 7.
4. A Report by the Task Force on Death and Dying of the Institute of Society, Ethics and the Life Sciences, "Refinements in Criteria for the Determination of Death: An Appraisal," *Journal of the American Medical Association*, Vol. 221 (1972), pp. 48–53.
5. Advisory Committee of the Renal Transplant Registry, *op. cit.*, p. 21.
6. John M. Dwyer, "Understanding Modern Immunology. I: The Development of the Human Immune System," *Connecticut Medicine* (March 1975), pp. 170–174.

BIBLIOGRAPHY

American Association of Nephrology Nurses and Technicians, *Standards of Clinical Practice. Section II: Transplantation.* Available from the American Association of Nephrology Nurses and Technicians, 2 Talcott Road, Suite 8, Park Ridge, Illinois, 60068.

Balk, Michael, et al., "Influence of Rejection Therapy on Fungal and Myocardial Infections in Renal Transplant Recipients," *The Lancet* (January 27, 1973), pp. 180–184.

Bennett, W. M., I. Singer, and C. J. Coggins, "A Guide to Drug Therapy in Renal Failure," *Journal of the American Medical Association*, Vol. 230 (1974), p. 1544.

Blount, Mary, and Anna Belle Kinney, "Chronic Steroid Therapy," *American Journal of Nursing* (December 1974), pp. 1626–1631.

Burton, John R., et al., "Aspergillosis in Four Renal Transplant Recipients—Diagnosis and Effective Treatment with Amphotericin B," *Annals of Internal Medicine*, Vol. 77 (1972), pp. 383–388.

Cosimi, A. Benedict, et al., "Experience with Large Dose Intravenous Antithymocyte Globulin in Primates and Man," *Surgery*, Vol. 68 (June 1970), pp. 54–61.

De Luca, Hector, "The Kidney as an Endocrine Organ for the Production of 1,25 Dihydroxy Vitamin D_3, a Calcium-Mobilzing Hormone," *New England Journal of Medicine* (August 16, 1973), pp. 359–365.

Friedman, Barry, and Kenneth Newmark, "Orthopedic Problems in Renal Patients," *Dialysis and Transplantation* (April-May 1975), pp. 71-72.

Harrington, Joan DeLong, and Etta Rae Brener, *Patient Care in Renal Failure* (Philadelphia: W. B. Saunders, 1976).

Kootstad, G., et al., "Spontaneous Rupture of Homografted Kidneys," *Archives of Surgery,* Vol. 108 (January 1974), pp. 107–112.

Lucas, Zoltan, et al., "Renal Allotransplantation in Humans. I: Systemic Immunosuppressive Therapy," *Archives of Surgery,* Vol. 100 (February 1970), pp. 113–124.

Mandell, Gerald Lee and Edward W. Hook, "Opportunistic Infections," *Hospital Medicine* (December 1968), pp. 40–48.

Medical Staff Conference, "Medical Management of Chronic Renal Disease," *California Medicine,* Vol. 3, No. 4 (April 1971), pp. 44–53.

Merrill, John, and Constantine Hampers, "Uremia, Part I," *New England Journal of Medicine* (April 23, 1970), pp. 953–961.

Misha, M. K., et al., "Major Colonic Diseases Complicating Renal Transplantation," *Surgery,* Vol. 73, No. 6 (June 1973), pp. 942–948.

Robbins, Karen C., "Hypertension in the Renal Transplant Recipient," *Journal of the American Association of Nephrology Nurses and Technicians,* Vol. 2, No. 4 (1975), pp. 171–177.

Sachs, Bonnie, *Renal Transplantation: A Nursing Perspective* (Flushing, New York: Medical Examination Publishing Company, 1977).

Salvatierra, Oscar, et al., "The Advantages of I-Orthoiodohippurate Scintophotography in the Management of Patients After Renal Transplantation," *Annals of Surgery,* Vol. 180, No. 3 (September 1974), pp. 336–342.

Schweizer, Robert, and Stanley Bartus, "Renal Transplantation as Definitive Therapy for Endstage Renal Disease," *Connecticut Medicine,* Vol. 40, No. 2 (February 1976) pp. 83–85.

Sheil, A. G. R., et al., "Anti-Lymphocyte Globulin in Patients with Renal Allografts from Cadaveric Donors," *The Lancet* (August 4, 1973), pp. 227–228.

Simmons, Richard L., et al., "Cytomegalovirus: Clinical Virological Correlations in Renal Transplant Recipients," *Annals of Surgery* (October 1974), 22. 623–634.

Streeten, David, "Corticosteroid Therapy II, Complications and Therapeutic Indications," *Journal of the American Medical Association,* Vol. 232 (June 9, 1975), pp. 1046–1049.

Toper, Michele A., "Kidney Transplantation Especially in Pediatric Patients," *Nursing Clinics of North America,* Vol. 10, No. 3 (September 1975), pp. 503–516.

Vineyard, Gordon, et al., "Evaluation of Corticosteroid Therapy for Acute Renal Allograft Rejection," *Surgery, Gynecology and Obstetrics,* Vol. 138 (February 1974), pp. 225–228.

Wolf, Zane R., "What Patients Awaiting Kidney Transplant Want to Know," *American Journal of Nursing* (January 1976), pp. 92–94.

MARGARET ANN BERRY, R.N., M.A., M.S.

normal structure and function of the nervous system

The basic organization of the nervous system is similar to other systems of the body. Its basic functional unit is the *neuron* consisting of a cell body and filament outgrowths, the *nerve fibers*. These fibers are responsible for the transmission of information from one part of the nervous system to the other. Neurons in the central nervous system process incoming peripheral information and then determine what information will be sent to various parts of the body to initiate specific activities. The nervous system consists of three major divisions which perform these functions: (1) the *sensory system*, (2) the *motor system*, and (3) the *integrative system*.

Figure 19-1 is a schematic illustration of the organization of the two larger divisions, the sensory and motor divisions.

The *sensory system* is the site of origination of most nervous system activities. That is, stimuli received and processed by this system, whether sight, sound, touch, or taste, cause a response somewhere else in the nervous system. The response may be an immediate motor response, or the information may be stored in the brain and then used to determine bodily reactions later. The sensory system, in general, transmits impulses from the body surface and deep structures into the spinal cord at all levels through the spinal nerves. From here the information is sent to the basal regions of the brain which include the medulla and the pons and to the higher brain centers, the thalamus and the cerebral cortex. These are the primary areas of the nervous

387

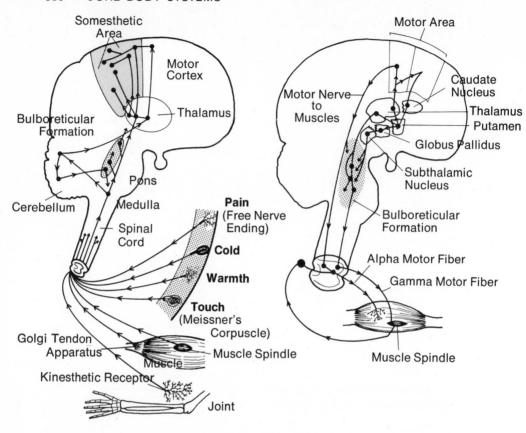

Fig. 19-1. General organization of the sensory (*left*) and motor (*right*) divisions of the nervous system. (From A. C. Guyton, *Function of the Human Body,* Philadelphia, W. B. Saunders, 1964, p. 260)

system for handling sensory input; essentially all other parts secondarily receive and process sensory input.

The *motor division* of the nervous system is responsible for control of bodily functions. This is mediated through the control of the contraction of skeletal muscle and of smooth muscle of internal organs, and by the secretions of the exocrine and endocrine glands. In this division the impulses arise in the motor area of the cerebral cortex, the basal regions of the brain, and the spinal cord. Those messages arising in the basilar areas of the brain and in the spinal cord are primarily automatic responses to sensory stimuli. The higher regions are concerned with voluntary, deliberate movements associated with thought processes of the cerebrum.

The *integrative system* is concerned with processing signals to determine accurate and appropriate motor responses. It is also believed to be involved in abstract thinking. Numerous areas in both the cord and the brain are concerned almost exclusively with integrative activities. Lying adjacent to sensory and motor areas, these centers determine the qualities and characteristics of sensory input. Is it painful? intense? weak? Having determined this, the areas then ascertain the appropriate motor responses and transport signals to the appropriate motor area. Another extremely important function of this division is one of storing information. This activity is readily recognized as memory.

As stated earlier, the basic functional unit of the nervous system is the *neuron,* and all information and activity whether sensory, motor and/or integrative is processed by it. The precise characteristic of individual neurons is determined by their specific function. Some are extremely large and may give rise to extremely long nerve fibers. Transmission velocities in the long fibers may be as high as 100 meters per second, while smaller neurons with very small fibers demonstrate velocities of 1 meter per second. Some neurons connect to many different neurons in a "network," and still others have few connections to other cells of the nervous system.

It has been estimated that there are twelve billion neurons in the central nervous system. Three fourths of these neurons are located in the cerebral cortex where information transmitted through the nervous system is processed. This processing, as indicated above, includes not only the determination of appropriate and effective responses, but also the storage of memory and the development of associative motor and thought patterns.

The pattern of information processing is basically as follows: (1) sensory information is received, (2) this information is transmitted to the central nervous area, and (3) a motor response is determined and carried to an end organ. Many times this pattern is strictly reflexive and simple in its neuronal involvement. These instantaneous and automatic motor responses to sensory input are called *reflex* responses and involve a *receptor,* a *transmitter,* and an *effector.* A sensation such as touch, cold, or heat is detected by the receptor and transmitted to the transmitter to the central nervous system. This may be a single neuron or several neurons in series. The effector is the end organ which receives the motor impulse, such as a skeletal muscle, internal organs such as the gut or heart, or an exocrine or endocrine gland.

Many reflexes such as the withdrawal of an arm or leg from a painful stimulus involve only the spinal cord, while other reflexes are much more complex and involve the integrative division. These more complex reflexes may involve information stored from earlier experiences; thus previous experience is associated with the current one. The more complex responses that involve many neurons and several areas of the nervous system are commonly called *higher functions* as opposed to the simple reflexes just described.

The above discussion has implied a basic hierarchical organization of the nervous system and indeed this is the case. There are three levels of organization: (1) the *spinal cord,* controlling many basic reflex responses: (2) the *basal regions of the brain,* controlling bodily functions such as equilibrium, eating, walking, and (3) the *cerebral cortex,* controlling voluntary, discrete motor activities and thought processes.

Even though many sensory activities are responded to and carried out at spinal levels, many sensations from the body *(somesthetic sensations)* are interpreted by the brain. The interpretation of these messages enables us to determine body position, and conditions of the immediate external environment as well as conditions of the internal environment. These are called *proprioceptive, exteroceptive,* and *visceral* sensations respectively.

As indicated above, proprioceptive sensations are those sensations which describe the physical position state of the body such as tension in muscle, flexion or extension of joints, tendon tension, and deep pressure in dependent parts like the feet while standing or the buttocks while seated. Exteroceptive sensations are those that monitor the conditions on the body surface. These include temperature and pain. Visceral sensations are like exteroceptive sensations except that they originate from within and monitor pain, pressure, and fullness from internal organs.

Figure 19-1 indicates the possible pathways for processing somesthetic sensations. The fibers ending in the spinal cord initiate the cord reflexes discussed previously. Brain-stem fibers initiate reflexes such as those that position the trunk and aid in upright posture. All of these are more complex than spinal reflexes but are still subconscious. As the sensations are transmitted to higher levels they terminate in the thalamus, where the *general* origin of the sensation and the modality (type) of the sensation are determined. However, the *discrete* localization and modality of the sensations are determined in the cerebral cortex where information from past experiences is involved in interpretation.

The sensory receptors for somesthetic sensations include both free nerve endings and specialized end organs. Free nerve endings are nothing more than small filamentous branches of the dendritic fibers. They detect crude sensations of touch, pain, heat, and cold. The precision is crude because there are many interconnections between the free endings of different neurons. However, they are the most profusely distributed and perform the general discriminatory functions, whereas the more specialized receptors discriminate between very slight differences in degrees of touch, heat, and cold. Structurally the special exteroceptive end organs for detection of cold, warmth, and light touch differ from each other and are quite specific in their function as seen in Fig. 19-1. The physiological basis for this specific function has not been determined but is presumed to be based upon some specific physical effect on the organ itself. There are three proprioceptive receptors. Joint kinesthetic receptors are found in the joint capsules and send messages concerning the angulation of a joint and the rate at which it is changing. Information from muscles concerning the degree of stretch is transmitted to the nervous system from the muscle spindle apparatus, while the Golgi tendon determines the overall tension applied to the tendons.

When a sensory effector is stimulated it responds with an increased frequency of firing. At first there is a burst of impulses; if the stimulus persists, the frequency of impulses transmitted begins to decrease. All sensory receptors show this phenomenon of *adaptation* to varying degrees and at different rates. Adaptation to light touch and pressure occurs in a few seconds, whereas pain and proprioceptive sensation adapt very little if at all, and at a very slow rate. The determination of the intensity of sensation is on a relative rather than an absolute basis and follows a logarithmic response. Therefore while the intensity of a sensation increases logarithmically, the frequency of response in the nerve ending increases linearly.

Although there are structurally different receptors for detecting each type of sensation, it is the area of the brain to which the information is transmitted that determines the *modality* or type of sensation the individual feels. The thalamus, hypothalamus, and somesthetic area of the cerebral cortex operate together to determine the various sensory qualities. As sensory input arrives at the central nervous system the different characteristics such as a pain element or a touch element are determined by the cooperative effort of the areas.

The sense of pain warrants special consideration, since it plays such an important protective role for the body. At the same time there is a wide variation in individual response to pain. Whenever there is tissue damage, pain receptors are stimulated and the sensation of pain is felt. This sensation is usually felt during the time that tissue is undergoing damage, and ceases when the damage ends. This condition is due to the release of chemicals and metabolites such as histamine and bradykinin from damaged cells. Typical damaging stimuli are trauma (cutting, crushing, tearing), ischemia, intense heat or cold and chemical irritation. Most people *perceive* the pain at the same degree of tissue damage. However, there is a wide variation in the extent to which individuals *react* to pain. Differences in reactivity to pain are due to the psychic makeup of the individual and not to differences in pain-receptor sensitivity.

The nervous system responds to sensory input through motor mechanisms which control bodily function and position. As demonstrated in Fig. 19-1, the motor division of the central nervous system is organized in a hierarchical manner like the sensory division. That is, a large number of reflexive motor functions are mediated through the spinal cord, while others operate through brain-stem centers and still others through cortical centers. The largest number of motor activities are controlled by the spinal cord and brain stem, and therefore operate primarily at subconscious reflexive levels.

Simple cord reflexes include the *axon reflexes* which provide increased blood flow to damaged tissues in the skin. Proprioceptor reflexes which are processed at the spinal cord include the *stretch reflex*, which helps maintain normal muscle tone, posture, and positioning of limbs with respect to the rest of the body. Another proprioceptive reflex mediated at the spinal level is the *tendon protective reflex*, which protects the tendon and muscle against excessive stretch. The *extensor thrust reflex* aids in the support of the body against gravity.

Also included in spinal reflexes is the *withdrawal,* pain, or flexor reflex. The purpose of this reflex is obvious. Operating in association with this reflex is the *crossed extensor reflex.* When one limb flexes in withdrawal from a painful stimulus the opposite limb extends, pushing the whole body away from the source of the painful stimulus. An important feature of all reflexes is reciprocal inhibition which occurs in the antagonist muscle of the one stimulated. For example, when a flexor reflex stimulates the biceps, it also inhibits its antagonist, the triceps, and provides for more efficient performance of motor activities in the upper arm.

Spinal cord activities also include reflex circuits which aid in the control of visceral functions of the body. Sensory input arises from visceral sensory receptors and is transmitted to the spinal cord, where reflex patterns appropriate to the sensory input are determined. The signals are then transmitted to autonomic motor neurons in the gray matter of the spinal cord which send impulses to the sympathetic nerves innervating visceral motor end organs. A most important autonomic reflex is the *peritoneal reflex.* Tissue damage in any portion of the peritoneum results in the response of this reflex, which slows or stops all motor activity in the nearby viscera. In the presence of transectional injuries at the brain stem, cord reflexes are also capable of modifying local blood flow in response to cold, pain, and heat. This vascular control by autonomic reflexes in the spinal cord operates as a backup mechanism for the usual brain-stem control patterns.

Also included in the autonomic reflexes of the spinal cord are those causing the emptying of the urinary bladder and the rectum. When the bowel or bladder becomes distended, sensory signals are transmitted to the autonomic internuncial neurons of the cord. Motor signals via the parasympathetic neurons excite the main portion of the bowel or bladder, at the same time inhibiting the internal sphincters of the urethra or anus, thus causing the organ to empty. Normally these reflexes are overridden by cortical centers until an appropriate time and place for evacuation arises.

The lower brain stem, composed of the medulla, the pons, and the mesencephalon, contains the areas which control blood pressure, respiration, and gastrointestinal regulation. The brain stem's motor functions also include maintaining bodily support against gravity and maintaining equilibrium. Located within the brain stem is the structural area in which these latter two integrative functions occur, the bulboreticular formation. This area receives information from a variety of sources which includes all areas of the peripheral sensory receptors via the spinal cord, the cerebellum, the inner-ear equilibrium apparatus, the motor cortex, and the basal ganglia. The bulboreticular area, then, is an integrative area for sensory information, motor information from the cerebral cortex, equilibrium information from the vestibular apparatus, and proprioceptive information from the cerebellum; it also controls many involuntary muscular activities.

Even though most of the essential motor functions are performed by the lower levels of the central nervous system, one of the distinguishing characteristics of human beings is their ability to perform intricate, complex voluntary muscular activity such as talking and writing.

These precise, complex functions are controlled by specific areas of the cerebral cortex. There are, however, many stereotyped movements which are much more complex than postural functions of the lower brain stem but less complex than the intricate functions of the cerebral cortex. These movements are controlled by the basal ganglia, which are large conglomerates of neurons that have connections with the cerebral cortex and the thalamus. Special dampening functions for smoothing out tremors and jerkiness inherent in raw muscular activity are controlled by the cerebellum.

Verbal communication is dependent upon the ability to interpret speech and to translate thought into speech. Ideas are usually communicated between individuals by either spoken or written word. With the spoken word the sensory input of information is through the primary auditory cortex. In auditory association areas the sounds are interpreted as words and the words as sentences. These sentences are then interpreted by the common integrative area of the cerebral cortex as thoughts. The common integrative area also develops thoughts to be communicated. Letters seen by the eyes are associated as words, thoughts and sentences in the visual association area and integrated into thought in this area also. Operating in conjunction with facial regions of the somesthetic sensory area, the common integrative area initiates a series of impulses, each representing a syllable or word, and transmits them to the secondary motor area controlling the larynx and mouth. The speech center, in addition to controlling motor activity of the larynx and mouth, sends impulses to the respiratory center of the secondary motor cortex to provide appropriate breath patterns for the speech process.

The major portion of this discussion has dealt with sensory, motor, and integrative activities of the spinal cord, brain stem, and cerebral cortex. These activities may be unconscious, subconscious, or voluntary. Only short references have been made to the autonomic or involuntary function with regard to bowel and bladder emptying, control of blood flow, peritoneal reflex, and the like. The function of the *autonomic nervous system* is far more diffuse than this however, in the control of internal functions of the body. This system is subdivided into *sympathetic* and *parasympathetic* sections on the basis of (1) the anatomical distribution of nerve fibers, (2) the antagonistic effects of the two divisions on the organs they innervate, and (3) the secretion of two different neural transmitters by the postganglionic fibers of the two divisions. Figure 19-2 shows the anatomy of the sympathetic and parasympathetic nervous systems.

As seen in Fig. 19-2, the sympathetic system is comprised of a chain of perivertebral ganglia receiving fibers from the thoracolumbar region of the spinal cord and distributing postganglionic fibers to the various organs innervated. The parasympathetic system, on the other hand, has rather long preganglionic fibers coming from the craniosacral area of the central nervous system which terminate in ganglia that are closely associated with the

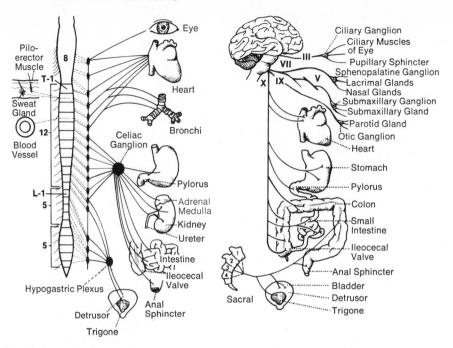

Fig. 19-2. Anatomy of the autonomic nervous system. (From A. C. Guyton, *Function of the Human Body*, Philadelphia, W. B. Saunders, 1964, pp. 333–334)

organ innervated. Short postganglionic fibers then innervate the tissues of the organs directly. A major difference between the two divisions of the autonomic nervous system is the neural transmitters secreted by the postganglionic fibers. Parasympathetic postganglionic nerve fibers secrete acetylcholine and thus are referred to as *cholinergic* fibers, whereas sympathetic postganglionic fibers are called *andrenergic* fibers, since they secrete noradrenalin (norepinephrine). The actions of these two antagonistic chemical transmitters are summarized in Table 19-1.

Impulses are transmitted continuously at a slow rate from both divisions at all times. This *tonic effect* of the individual divisions allows each to exert independently both positive and negative effects on a given organ—increasing the discharge frequency has a positive effect and decreasing the frequency a negative effect. For example, if sympathetic discharge to vasoconstrictor vessels was "on" or "off," this would result only in constriction of vessels during "on" periods. But since there is a normal resting frequency, increasing it causes more vasoconstriction and decreasing it results in less vasoconstriction or vasodilatation. This tonic effect persists throughout both the sympathetic and the parasympathetic divisions of the autonomic nervous system and is responsible for the high degree of effectiveness of the system in the regulation of visceral activities.

table 19-1
autonomic effects on various organs of the body

ORGAN	EFFECT OF SYMPATHETIC STIMULATION	EFFECT OF PARASYMPATHETIC STIMULATION
Eye: Pupil	Dilated	Contracted
Ciliary muscle	None	Excited
Gastrointestinal glands	Vasoconstriction	Stimulation of thin, copious secretion containing many enzymes
Sweat glands	Copious sweating (cholinergic)	None
Heart: Muscle	Increased activity	Decreased activity
Coronaries	Vasodilated	Constricted
Systemic blood vessels:		
Abdominal	Constricted	None
Muscle	Dilated (cholinergic)	None
Skin	Constricted or dilated (cholinergic)	None
Lungs: Bronchi	Dilated	Constricted
Blood vessels	Mildly constricted	None
Gut: Lumen	Decreased peristalsis and tone	Increased peristalsis and tone
Sphincters	Increased tone	Decreased tone
Liver	Glucose released	None
Kidney	Decreased output	None
Bladder: Body	Inhibited	Excited
Sphincter	Excited	Inhibited
Male sexual act	Ejaculation	Erection
Blood glucose	Increased	None
Basal metabolism	Increased up to 50%	None
Adrenal cortical secretion	Increased	None
Mental activity	Increased	None

From A. C. Guyton, *Function of the Human Body*, ed. 3, Philadelphia, W. B. Saunders, 1964, p. 335.

The function of the autonomic nervous system can also be regulated by stimulation of widespread areas of the bulboreticular formation of the medulla, pons, and mesencephalon. The hypothalamus also regulates many of the autonomic functions, and stimulation of certain areas of the cerebral cortex also causes both diffuse and discrete autonomic effects. Exact mechanisms for these interactions are not well known but seem to be those of integrative functions similar to that in motor and sensory integration.

ROBERT W. HENDEE, JR., M.D.
M. LYNN McCRACKEN, R.N., M.S.
MARILYNN J. WASHBURN, R.N., B.S.N.

20

pathophysiology of the central nervous system

Nurses in a critical care unit caring for individuals having acute nervous system injury or illness serve as the patient's first line of defense. In order to insure superior care a multitude of routine supportive acts must be performed in repetition. Concomitantly, the nurse must carry out frequent neurological and (in cases of multiple systems injuries) other evaluations with constant vigil for subtle changes in blood pressure, pulse rate and regularity, respiratory activity, sensorial status (level of consciousness), and motor and sensory function. Alterations when they occur may be the initial indication of impending deterioration, leading to rapid demise unless immediate action is taken to alleviate the underlying pathology. An example may be helpful.

Patient Situation

A nineteen-year-old right-handed female was seen in the emergency room following a vehicular-induced closed head injury. During the initial neuro-surgical evaluation her arousal mechanism was moderately depressed, but she responded purposefully and uniformly upon request. No focal or lateralizing signs were evident except for tendency for enlargement of the left pupil (pupillary inequality is termed *anisocoria*). One hour later following repair of facial lacerations and with stability of sensorial status, she was moved to the critical care unit for further observation. The patient's condition was discussed with the receiving nurse by the neuro-surgical resident.

Soon thereafter the nurse noted definite, persistent anisocoria, with diminished reaction to light of the dilating pupil and more difficulty in arousing the patient. Immediately the resident was called, and in the interim mannitol was prepared for intravenous administration. This was begun upon the physician's arrival as a deteriorating situation was apparent. The patient was transferred to the operating room, by which time her respiratory condition required external assistance, both pupils had dilated, and she was unresponsive to painful stimuli. Emergency trephinations revealed an acute subdural hematoma over one cerebral hemisphere and an epidural hematoma over the opposite hemisphere.

Fortunately the young woman recovered with minimal neurological damage. Her life was undoubtedly saved by the awareness and prompt action of the critical care nurse.

Opportunity for the nurse to discover other interesting and extremely important findings is ever present. Serosanguineous drainage from ears, nose, or scalp wound, even when it has been debrided and repaired but incompletely explored in the emergency unit, will represent cerebrospinal fluid (CSF) leak until proven otherwise. Progressive urinary output of abnormally high levels following injury or certain types of intracranial and facial surgery may represent diabetes insipidus. Neither of these conditions need cause concern about the immediate demise of the patient. If left unobserved too long, however, they may result in unnecessary intracranial infection or hypovolemia and severe electrolyte imbalance. These in turn will lead to new problems of care and worsened condition of the patient, possibly precluding complete recovery or ultimately leading to death.

Experience aids the nurse in sharpening her powers of observation to recognize the slight changes that may be the precursors of the full constellation of signs of increased intracranial pressure and/or brain herniation. The same holds for alterations in lower-extremity motor and sensory function after incomplete spinal cord injury. Experience also imparts confidence to the nurse, as does knowledge of the more common patterns of deterioration, in assisting her to determine whether additional observation is warranted or whether she should seek the physician's reevaluation immediately.

Physicians rendering quality care in the treatment of critically ill patients should always allocate time to discuss with the nurse, even briefly, the particulars of each new patient upon arrival in the critical care unit. At that time the nurse must establish *precise* baseline information to her own satisfaction and seek clarification if necessary.

In these days of vehicular abuse, exposure to dangerous equipment, and utilization of complex mechanical recreational devices, many of the patients in any large and active critical care unit are those with acute cranial and/or spinal injuries. Intracranial abscesses, aneurysms, arteriovenous malformations and tumors, and nontraumatic spinal cord lesions also continue to require neurosurgical care. This section will discuss some of the common problems that may arise in the general neurosurgical population.

neurosurgical problems

increased intracranial pressure

Elevated intracranial pressure may be acute, subacute, or chronic, depending on the duration, severity, and rapidity with which it develops. The magnitude of the effects is determined by the extent to which the intracranial structures adapt and the time allowed for the process. It then refers to a situation wherein the normal central nervous system contents are obliged to compete for space within the bony confines of the cranium. Additional limitations are imposed by the sensitivity of the brain in general to trauma and of the cranial nerves and vessels to stretch and compression. The fibrous partitions between parts of the brain (falx cerebri, tentorium cerebelli) also act as intrinsic barriers to displacement of the cranial contents, and may result in pressure against the nervous and vascular structures.

Competition with the normal intracranial contents may arise extrinsic to the brain—for example, from epidural or subdural hematomas, or tumors arising from the covering of the brain (meningiomas), all of which may exert pressure against any of the brain's surfaces. Intrinsically, hydrocephalus (due to tumors located in the posterior fossa or elsewhere, subarachnoid hemorrhage, or congential anomalies), intracerebral or intracerebellar hematomas (due, for example, to hemorrhage from aneurysms), malformations, and cerebral edema all may create abnormal intracranial pressure.

A focal or diffuse intracranial lesion of sufficient size, regardless of the etiology or whether extracerebral or intracerebral, imparts a mass effect, the result of which is an obligatory shift of the normal contents. If the pressure is acute and the mass significantly large, dramatically rapid adverse effects will be noted, as in the case of most epidural hematomas. These are usually due to temporal bone fracture and laceration of the middle meningeal artery, implying more rapid hemorrhage than that which is venous in origin, unless large venous structures such as the major venous sinuses are involved. Such structures are the origin of major venous bleeding which may lead to early tragedy.

The ultimate result, even in the case of long-standing, slowly evolving subdural hematomas, is some degree of impingement upon the superficial cerebral substance and secondary distortion of the cranial nerves, vessels, and brain stem.

Pressure of the medial aspect (uncus) of the medially displaced temporal lobe on the superior part of the third cranial (oculomotor) nerve results in progressive pupillary dilatation on the same side because of interference with the pupilloconstrictor fibers carried by that nerve. Occasionally the opposite oculomotor nerve will be compressed against its ipsilateral cerebral peduncle, with false lateralization of the abnormal (enlarged) pupil.

A sign of early increased intracranial pressure may be seen in injury to the sixth cranial (abducens) nerve, which is manifested by impaired abduction of the appropriate globe. The abducens nerve traverses the greatest distance between sites of origin and function and thereby has the greatest theoretical chance of injury by compression or stretch.

Compression of the cerebral hemispheres and/or distortion of or injury to the brain stem will result in alterations in arousal. In the latter structure the reticular activating system is involved. Interference with the cardiorespiratory centers will be evidenced by depression and perhaps irregularity of pulse rate and concomitant elevation of blood pressure, as well as abnormalities visible on the cardiac monitor suggestive of primary cardiac disease. In addition there will be abnormalities of respiratory depth, rate, and regularity. Pupillary abnormality, decreased spontaneous movement and weakness of the opposite limbs, and, where the dominant side of the brain is involved, speech dysfunction (dysphasia) will also be apparent. It should be noted, however, that lateralizing signs (hemiparesis, speech disorders, pupillary changes) may not be present initially; rather, headache, progressively severe nausea, emesis, and sensorial depression leading to obtundation will be the most striking symptoms and findings.

It is helpful for both nurse and physician to have concise understanding of the terminology used for the various pathological levels of consciousness:

Stuporous/very lethargic—sleepy or trancelike but can still be aroused to respond with volitional, well-defined and purposeful acts, whether the acts be socially acceptable or not.

Semicomatose—does not perform volitional acts upon request but does have individual, purposeful movements (defensive withdrawal) or motor activity that is categorized as:

  a. *decerebrate*—extension of lower extremities, extension and inward rotation of upper extremities.

  b. *decorticate*—extension of lower extremities, flexion and internal or external rotation of forearms.

  c. *opisthotonic*—extension of extremities, neck and trunk.

Coma—implies no spontaneous or induced response except that noted, for example, in the pulse and respiratory rate when nociceptive (painful) stimulation is utilized.

It is burdensome to rely on more categories than those listed above.

cerebral concussion and contusion

A cerebral concussion is the "transient stage in which consciousness is lost"[1] after a blow to the head. Implied or inherent therein is interruption of normal neural activity. The loss of consciousness is "usually reversible," according to Rowbotham.[2] Retrograde amnesia (loss of memory of events prior to the injury, usually recent rather than remote) occurs, varying in severity depending on the degree of injury. It is obvious that severe head injuries may be sustained without cerebral concussion by the strict definition —that is, without loss of consciousness, even briefly. Moreover, patients with injuries that consist purely of concussion should be expected to recover without any neurological sequelae. Individuals who remain unconscious for more than one hour must be suspected of having suffered more than a simple concussion. It is worth emphasizing that loss of consciousness is not mandatory for a diagnosis of severe head injury, at the same time recognizing that a certain percentage of patients with a clinical diagnosis of "simple" cerebral concussion will upon observation be found to have or develop significant injury.

This is well illustrated in the "classic" case of epidural hematoma, in which the patient is initially rendered unconscious, perhaps only for a minute or so, and appears to recover, refusing medical assistance. A short time afterward the patient becomes drowsy, eventually obtunded, and hemiparetic, and develops anisocoria. Unless neurosurgical intervention occurs, virtually all victims will die. This is the reason head-injury patients must be observed so closely in the critical care unit even though they may at the onset and, for the great percentage, later, appear quite normal.

Cerebral contusion per se is usually more serious and refers to injury resulting in bruising of the brain. This may be minimal or a widespread, massive, and fatal nerve tissue insult. Contusions in general carry a higher risk than concussions regarding permanent damage and significant lesions. Contusions may be accompanied by brain lacerations and hematomas and may lead to depressing problems of intractable, fatal cerebral edema. Individuals with focal and/or lateralizing neurological signs are evaluated by specific neurodiagnostic procedures (computerized axial tomography if available and time permits, or cerebral angiography) to differentiate brain contusion, a nonoperative problem, from traumatic space-occupying lesions which may be surgically remediable.

Treatment for contusion without accompanying surgical injury consists of excellent general supportive care and usually steroids to preclude or reduce concomitant cerebral edema.

cerebral edema

A fairly frequent and frustrating situation to deal with is that in which significant cerebral edema is present after head injury. Often no concomitant surgical lesion is present which, once removed, might alleviate pressure, and medical therapeutics may be to no avail. The result is that the patient succumbs.

Edema of the brain consists of swelling (excess fluid), which causes increased bulk in which the white matter is more vulnerable than the gray. It may be especially evident in the cerebral tissue surrounding tumors or abscesses, or following the removal of a tumor or hematoma from the surface of the brain when significant compression with accompanying vascular stasis has occurred. Cerebral edema may be associated not only with cerebral contusions related to impact forces, but may be present after thrombosis of cortical veins (in overwhelming sepsis or dehydration), hypoxia, water intoxication, vascular inflammation, exposure to cold, tin poisoning, and hormonal imbalance. This has been called "benign" intracranial hypertension or pseudotumor cerebri, wherein presence of a tumor is mimicked.

Therapy directed at relief of cerebral edema consists of both medical and surgical modalities. The latter includes a technique of decompression.[3] Among the former are adequate respiratory care (airway and ventilation) to preclude or reduce hypoxia which may lead to further edema if persistent, and cerebral dehydrating agents which are hyperosmolar in nature (urea, mannitol) and serve to attract fluids into the cerebral vascular space for transport to the kidneys, acting rapidly to create diuresis. However, these agents have the propensity to create a "rebound" phenomenon unless a longer-acting agent is utilized at the same time. It is speculated that 4 to 5 hours after administration of urea or mannitol, plasma osmotic pressure becomes lower than tissue osmotic pressure as a result of the induced diuresis. Consequently, fluid shifts to the interstitial compartment and cerebral edema can again become a problem. Steroids such as dexamethasone (Decadron), which act to reduce swelling by means as yet not clearly understood but perhaps related to a stabilizing effect on membrane permeability, have a slower onset of action but may reduce the "rebound" effect when used in conjunction with the cerebral dehydrating agents. Other methods include relative dehydration of the body in toto by restriction of replacement fluid and use of salt-containing fluids to maintain the patient on the low or dry side of fluid maintenance; hypothermia to decrease the metabolic needs of the injured cerebral tissue; elevation of the head when feasible to promote venous return from the brain to the heart; and cautious use, when deemed necessary, of intermittent positive pressure breathing techniques, which, although beneficial to pulmonary care, may increase intracranial pressure.

Experience proves that, in general, younger patients tend to show higher rates of recovery following cerebral contusions and edema than do individuals past the second or third decade.

The signs of cerebral edema are those of any space-occupying situation if the intracranial pressure is sufficiently elevated. Severe, intractable edema may be present from the onset or appear later (by hours or days), even acutely, despite the appearance of a relatively stable course and the use of the entire spectrum of preventive or therapeutic measures.

Because of the importance of observation unaffected by outside influences, sedatives and analgesics are rarely used during periods of neurological evaluation, even in the face of other injuries (for example, femoral or other long-bone fractures). Paraldehyde seems to be most efficacious in those with head injuries, however, only when the patient is severely confused and/or combative, threatening more harm to himself by his thrashing and inability to rest. Should the patient show more depression in sensorial status at any time, squeezing the trapezius or discreet use of a safety pin in the sole will assist in determining whether arousal is possible, as from an exhausted slumber which is known to occur when a patient is exposed to a critical care unit environment for several days. If the patient is severely ill to begin with, recognition of changes indicative of deterioration becomes more difficult postoperatively or after trauma, for there is less room for physiological change.

cerebrospinal fluid fistula

Fistulas that allow leakage of cerebrospinal fluid (CSF) are dangerous in that they may predispose to meningeal infection, cerebritis, and death. They frequently follow injuries causing basilar skull fractures and meningeal tear, or depressed skull fractures where the irregular bone edge interrupts the meningeal integrity. CSF leak may occur spontaneously without antecedent trauma in situations of chronic, progressive elevated intracranial pressure. Fracture at the base involving the posterior or middle cranial fossae may allow drainage of the bloody or serosanguineous fluid via the external auditory canal. Eventually the fluid becomes xanthochromic, then clear, and if infected, may be purulent. Drainage from the nares via the paranasal or frontal sinuses is seen in basilar or low frontal fractures in the frontal fossa. Patients who are sufficiently alert may complain of fluid trickling into the oropharynx when reclining or partially seated. Often discharge via the nares is noted by a spurt or flow of fluid when the patient sits or stands and leans forward.

A specimen of the discharge should be obtained in any case for evaluation by the physician. If the fluid does not contain blood or its disintegration products, a positive glucose test (qualitative) confirms the fluid as CSF.

It is possible to be more vigilant for CSF leaks if basilar skull fracture is identified on examination of the skull radiographs, if the patient has Battle's sign (ecchymosis, edema, and tenderness over the mastoid bone) or periorbital and/or nasal discoloration and edema. Suspicion should be raised promptly whenever dressings covering a scalp wound become stained with watery, usually serosanguineous, fluid. There may exist a previously undetected fracture with underlying meningeal laceration. Postoperative staining of a craniotomy dressing will indicate inadequate meningeal closure or elevated intracranial pressure decompressing itself by CSF leak via the meningeal suture line.

In any case, it is of utmost importance that prophylactic antibiotics be administered until the fistula heals spontaneously (with the assistance of lumbar punctures to lower the CSF pressure, if necessary) or correction of wounds or operative closure is carried out. It is usual to maintain as far as possible, with appropriate right- or left-sided dependent posturing, a head-up position to allow better drainage. This lowers the intracranial CSF "pressure head" and precludes pooling of CSF in, for example, the paranasal sinuses, whereby bacterial organisms then have a better chance to congregate for access via the fistula to the intracranial fluid. In the presence of CSF leak one should not try to clear the nose by blowing, as this allows forceful retrograde displacement of organisms into the fistula.

diabetes insipidus

Diabetes insipidus (DI) represents a pathological state wherein abnormally great quantities of dilute urine are excreted, at times up to 20 liters per day. The kidneys have lost ability to control the amount of fluid output because of absence or deficit in antidiuretic hormone (ADH), which is produced in the supraoptic and paraventricular nuclei of the hypothalamus. The hormone is eventually released by the neurohypophysis (posterior pituitary) and appears to act on the distal renal tubules to promote reabsorption of water. Approximately 85 percent of the hypothalamic nuclei involved in production of the hormone must be impaired before insufficient ADH is available.

The excessive urinary output is matched by excessive thirst in persons alert enough to recognize it, requiring increased fluid intake. This contrasts with the situation found in psychogenic polydipsia, where excess water is conumed resulting secondarily in excess output.

Individuals with depressed arousal and inability to regulate their own intake will eventually lose enough fluid to lead to hypovolemia and death unless replacement in proper amounts is supplied for them. Replacement of water and glucose alone without appropriate electrolytes will result in water intoxication and cerebral edema, since electrolytes accompany the water lost by the kidneys.

Control of water balance is more complicated than one may be led to believe based on the preceding information alone. The entire complex mechanism is not fully understood, but it incorporates not only ADH but osmoreceptors and baroreceptors and one additional hormone at least, namely aldosterone. In general, however, if the water available to the body is decreased, the secretion of ADH is increased leading to water retention. In states of excess body water, ADH secretion is normally diminished, allowing for loss of the excess fluid.

Diabetes insipidus is usually expected, transiently at least, but at times it occurs in florid and permanent fashion following open procedures for pituitary and parasellar lesions (craniopharyngioma), and in transsphenoidal approaches utilizing cryotherapy for pituitary ablation. It is hoped that newer transsphenoidal microsurgical techniques, where applicable, will preclude leaving a postoperative pituitary cripple and reduce the chances for diabetes insipidus.

DI may also be seen in other surgical procedures performed in the region of the hypothalamus, and in head injuries with basilar fractures involving the sphenoid bone, gunshot wounds of the head, hypothalamic tumors, hydrocephalus, maxillofacial injuries with displaced fractures, nasopharyngeal tumors invasive of the base of the skull, aneurysms encroaching upon the sellar or suprasellar space, and the like. Of course, some patients without traumatic lesions may have DI among other symptoms or as the sole presenting symptom.

In cases of DI it is essential that evaluation be carried out for concomitant anterior pituitary insufficiency. This is usually manifested initially as adrenal crisis with hypotension, generalized weakness, anorexia, depressed arousal, hypothermia, and psychotic symptoms.

Recognition of DI in the early postoperative period may be difficult if cerebral dehydrating agents have been used before and/or during surgery, for the diuresis created by them may continue for the first postoperative day or so. Utilization of steroids may also cause increased urinary output. If the patient is awake, however, he will complain of progressively severe thirst if DI is present. Urine output will increase and persist despite the amount of fluid intake (which is usually maintained below normal replacement levels after cranial neurosurgery), and urine specific gravity will fall or remain below about 1.007 to 1.008. Suspicion of the entity is confirmed by serum and urine electrolyte and osmolarity determinations (see Chapter 10).

The presence of persistent DI will result in exhaustion of the alert patient who is unable to rest for long because of the frequent need to micturate and replenish fluids, the replacement fluids consisting of iced juices and other electrolyte-containing liquids. In this case, vasopressin (Pitressin) will eventually be required, just as in severe, continuing DI in patients unable to voluntarily replace their losses.

It should be reemphasized that patients developing florid DI may lose enormous amounts of urine in a relatively short period of time, leading to hypovolemia, unless a diagnosis is surmised or established and treatment undertaken. When the diagnosis is secure it is most efficacious to allow the patient to satisfy his replacement needs by drinking according to his thirst. It is more difficult in those requiring intravenous therapy, but especially in the latter cases, meticulous quantitation of intake and output is mandatory.

It should also be noted that transient, manageable DI may occur and then undergo spontaneous total remission even after a florid initial course. The utilization of vasopressin, unless as a short-acting form, coincident with the spontaneous remission might lead to relative renal insufficiency and oliguria until effects of the extrinsic vasopressin are completed.

intracranial hemorrhage

Intracranial hemorrhage not related to trauma is encountered most frequently secondary to rupture of cerebral aneurysms. It may also occur from vascular malformation, rupture of weakened vessels under the strain of systemic hypertension, or occasionally in relation to cerebral neoplasms per se or leukemic infiltrates or aggregates. More common than generally recognized are hemorrhages during periods of anticoagulation therapy for previous myocardial infarction, because of vascular insufficiency, and as prophylaxis of pulmonary embolus in phlebitis of the lower extremities. Admittedly there is usually an antecedent minor head injury or episode of severe straining in anticoagulated patients. Massive, rapid hemorrhages also may occur in diffuse intravascular coagulopathy (DIC) whatever the basic cause. The hemorrhage may be confined to the spaces associated with the meningeal layers or involve the intracerebral substance.

In ruptured aneurysms, unless a space-occupying lesion is present necessitating emergency surgery, such as subdural and/or intracerebral hematoma, the patient is frequently too ill for immediate surgery because of severe spasm in the cerebral vessels. He generally does not become a candidate for direct attack on the aneurysm unless the neurological situation improves markedly and repeat arteriography confirms remission of vascular spasms. This holds true despite the knowledge that a significant percentage may be expected to have a recurrent hemorrhage that could prove fatal in the interval while awaiting sufficient improvement to allow surgery. Headache (frequently severe), nausea, emesis, stiff and tender neck, and photophobia are common complaints if the patient is adequately alert.

spinal cord injury

Trauma to the spinal cord is not uncommon in automobile, motorcycle, and mountain-climbing accidents. It also occurs from the use of trampolines and sky kites and seems increasingly frequent in skiers. Care of the patient with a complete or significant incomplete lesion involves psychological difficulties for both nurse and patient as soon as the permanency of the neurological deficit becomes apparent to the latter. *Immediate and complete* lesions hold little if any chance of recovery.

"Spinal shock" is the term used to denote complete loss of voluntary neurological integrity distal to the level of injury. It is the *fact* of cord sectioning, not the *act*, that produces spinal shock and implies paralysis of the muscles and anesthesia of the tissue below the lesion; i.e., sensation and voluntary motion are abolished and are never recovered. The stretch reflexes, although lost initially, do recover and eventually become overactive several weeks after the injury. The mass-reflex response usually appears several months later with exaggerated withdrawal reflexes and spread of the reflex activity to the visceral autonomic outflow. Thus by merely stroking the sole of the foot a patient may be stimulated to perspire, withdraw extremities, and empty bladder and bowel. The mass reflex activity may be spontaneous at times.

Return of spinal reflexes is noted in the initial one to three weeks, beginning with withdrawal upon stimulation of the sole. Later in the period, anal and genital reflexes and the presence of a Babinski sign are noted. Progressively vigorous and brisk withdrawal is elicited and the zone of positive elicitation becomes larger.

Autonomic reflexes remain suppressed following injury longer than somatic reflexes. Thus the patient's skin is completely dry during the first four to eight weeks, but perspiration later may be severely intense.

Injury to the spinal cord above the cervical levels of 3 and 4 is usually not compatible with survival due to interruption of the innervation to the diaphragmatic muscles which supply respiratory function when the intercostal musculature is lost by lower cervical injuries. Higher cervical trauma may also contribute to edema, more cephalad, involving important medullary centers.

Because of the initial loss of sympathetic outflow, patients are often hypotensive as a result of loss of vascular tonus below the injury. For the same reason hypothermia may be profound because of loss of heat through the dilated vessels.

Patients with cervical injury often seem to be unstable from the standpoint of regulation of blood pressure and maintenance of respiratory activity when initially turned on their frames, especially in rotating from supine to prone position. It is necessary to be prepared to render immediate respiratory assistance and to return the patient to the supine position if significant cardiac and blood pressure irregularities occur.

syndrome of inappropriate secretion of antidiuretic hormone (SIADH)

This phenomenon was initially described by Schwartz et al.[4] and further defined by Bartter.[5] The features are hyponatremia and hypotonicity of the plasma in conjunction with excretion of urine which is hypertonic to plasma and which contains appreciable amounts of sodium. In addition there is absence of hypokalemia and edema, normal cardiac, renal and adrenal function, and normal or expanded plasma and extracellular fluid volumes (i.e., no evidence of dehydration or hypovolemia). The presence of low serum blood urea nitrogen and uric acid levels assists in confirming the diagnosis.

The secretion of antidiuretic hormone (vasopressin) is "inappropriate" in that it continues despite the decreased osmolality of the plasma.

According to Bartter some neoplastic conditions (carcinoma of the lung, duodenum or pancreas, or thymomas) may produce a chemical substance which is similar or identical to the arginine vasopressin produced in the hypothalamopituitary system but which is independent of normal physiological controls. Thus, an aberrant secretion is the factor in these cases.

In other conditions such as hemorrhage, trauma, central nervous system infection or disease, or pulmonary disease, or in the postoperative period, abnormal secretion of ADH endogenously is the etiology. Utilization of medications such as vincristine, chlorpropamide, hydrochlorothiazide, and carbomazepine (Tegretol) may also result in the syndrome.

The symptomatology of SIADH is basically that of water retention at one end of the spectrum proceeding to water intoxication at the other end. In this regard, the author has seen definite symptoms that subsequently cleared with the usual therapy even with a serum sodium reduced no more than the range of 120 to 125.

Bartter states that water retention (and concomitant dilution of the serum sodium concentration) occurring slowly or when not severe causes headache, asthenia, somnolence, lethargy, and confusion. More rapidly occurring dilution, or water intoxication per se, is associated with anorexia, nausea and emesis, proceeding to delirium, fits, aberrant respirations, hypothermia, and coma. Prior to coma the stretch reflexes may become absent, the presence of Babinski's sign is noted, and pseudobulbar palsy may occur.

Diagnosis can be established by readily available laboratory procedures although radioimmunoassay of plasma ADH might be the most confirmatory method. The serum sodium concentration and serum osmolality are the best routine indices.

Treatment consists of restriction of fluid intake (even limited to perhaps 500 cc. per day maximum in severe cases) and where applicable the treatment of underlying disorders (e.g., administration of cortisone in Addison's disease), or the discontinuation of carbomazepine or other causative medications. Administration of salt (sodium chloride solutions) is usually of only transient benefit but may be considered where water intoxication is severe in order to attempt to acutely increase serum osmolality.

REFERENCES

1. Joseph P. Evans, *Acute Head Injury* (Springfield, Ill.: Charles C Thomas, 1963), p. 89.
2. G. F. Rowbotham, *Acute Injuries of the Head* (New York: Longman, 1964), p. 27.
3. R. N. Kjellberg and A. Priesto, "Bifrontal Decompressive Craniotomy for Massive Cerebral Edema," *Journal of Neurosurgery*, Vol. 34 (April 1971), pp. 488-493.
4. W. B. Schwartz, W. Bennett, S. Curelop, and F. C. Bartter, "A Syndrome of Renal Sodium Loss and Hyponatremia Probably Resulting from Inappropriate Secretion of Antidiuretic Hormone," *American Journal of Medicine*, Vol. 23 (1957), pp. 529-542.
5. F. C. Bartter, "The Syndrome of Inappropriate Secretion of Antidiuretic Hormone," *Disease-A-Month*, Year Book Medical Publishers (November 1973).

thrombus, embolus, hypotension, spasm

The thrombus-caused CVA usually occurs while the patient is quiet and inactive. Atherosclerosis is frequently the cause and the patient fits into the atherosclerotic risk profile. This patient often has had transient ischemic attacks (small strokes). Some of these premonitory symptoms consist of falls or dropping attacks for no reason, blurring of vision or transient monocular blindness, transient paresthesia, ataxia, dysphasia, nerve palsies, disorientation, vertigo or light-headedness, or behavior change noted by family and friends (Table 20-1). (Incidentally, if the nurse or some other person had been

table 20-1
symptoms occurring during transient ischemic attacks (TIAs)

CAROTID OCCLUSION	VERTEBRAL-BASILAR OCCLUSION
1. Aphasia	1. Vertigo or dizziness
2. General or focal seizure	2. Hearing loss or tinnitus
3. Contralateral weakness or numbness	3. Visual graying or loss
4. Ipsilateral migraine-type headache	4. Diplopia
5. Transient blurring of vision or blindness in ipsilateral eye	5. Dysarthria
6. Homonymous visual field loss	6. Dysphagia
	7. Hemiparesis
	8. Occipital headache
	9. Homonymous visual field loss

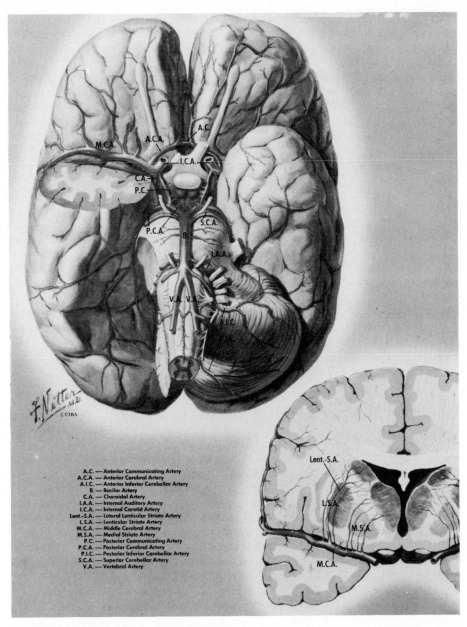

A.C. — Anterior Communicating Artery
A.C.A. — Anterior Cerebral Artery
A.I.C. — Anterior Inferior Cerebellar Artery
B. — Basilar Artery
C.A. — Choroidal Artery
I.A.A. — Internal Auditory Artery
I.C.A. — Internal Carotid Artery
Lent.-S.A. — Lateral Lenticular Striate Artery
L.S.A. — Lenticular Striate Artery
M.C.A. — Middle Cerebral Artery
M.S.A. — Medial Striate Artery
P.C. — Posterior Communicating Artery
P.C.A. — Posterior Cerebral Artery
P.I.C. — Posterior Inferior Cerebellar Artery
S.C.A. — Superior Cerebellar Artery
V.A. — Vertebral Artery

Fig. 20-1. Blood supply of the brain. [© Copyright 1953, 1972 CIBA Pharmaceutical Company, Division of CIBA-GEIGY Corporation. Reproduced, with permission, from THE CIBA COLLECTION OF MEDICAL ILLUSTRATIONS by Frank H. Netter, M.D. All rights reserved.]

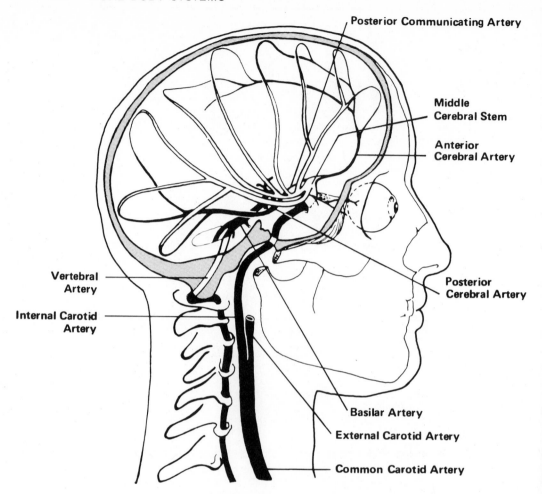

Fig. 20-2. Blood supply of the brain.

sensitive to these warning signs and directed the patient to appropriate medical care, this CVA might have been prevented.) The embolus-caused CVA is usually related to primary heart disease (chronic atrial fibrillation, rheumatic valve disease, or the mural thrombus of a myocardial infarction). Hypotension from acute blood loss, myocardial infarction, hypotensive drugs, or cardiac arrhythmias are other causes of CVAs. The thrombus, embolus, or hypotensive-caused CVA will cause similar symptoms as will those related to arterial spasm. Symptoms vary depending on the site of interference with the blood supply to the brain (Figs. 20-1 and 20-2).

hemorrhage

Hemorrhage, while probably less frequent than the above causes of CVA, is more likely to occur on exertion. Hypertension and atherosclerosis are often involved. The patient may have severe headache, nausea and vomiting, more severe motor deficit, and frequently may be comatose. If there is blood in the spinal fluid, he will have signs of meningeal irritation (nuchal rigidity, positive Kernig's sign, photophobia).

Recognition of the above patterns will assist the nurse in collecting data for the physician who will make the diagnosis. The point is not for the nurse to make the diagnosis, but in planning appropriate nursing care, the nurse needs adequate data. The patient with intracranial hemorrhage will be treated so as to avoid any rebleeding. The Valsalva maneuver is avoided as is anything that might elevate the blood pressure. CVAs due to other causes will initially be treated with more aggressive patient activity toward rehabilitation.

The hemiplegia of the stroke patient is the result of an upper motor neuron lesion. It follows the general rule that upper motor neuron lesions yield spastic paralysis, while lower motor neuron lesions yield flaccid paralysis (Fig. 20-3).

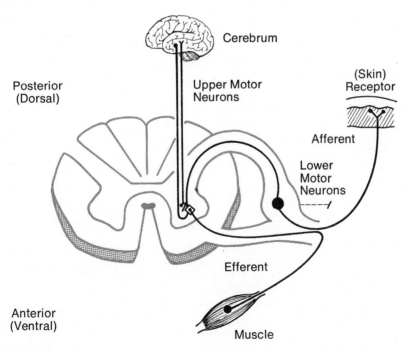

Fig. 20-3. Upper motor neurons vs. lower motor neurons (spinal reflex arc). (Courtesy of Sylvia Meeks.)

The spinal reflex arc (lower motor neurons) when interrupted yields a flaccid paralysis. When the efferent nerve in the arc is interrupted, this also prevents stimulation or inhibition from the upper motor neuron (arising in the intracranial central nervous system) for voluntary motor function. When the upper motor neuron is interrupted (as in stroke or traumatic brain damage) the spinal reflex arc remains intact. Thus whenever the afferent nerve is stimulated in the arc, the corresponding efferent function occurs.

Accordingly, stroke patients develop spasticity because of the interruption of the upper motor neuron influence. The pyramidal and extrapyramidal systems are also both involved in the control of resultant tonus.

The nurse must recognize that while occasional upper motor neuron lesions may yield a permanent flaccid paralysis, this is relatively rare. The initial flaccid paralysis is caused by a state of "shock" or depressed reflex function that occurs with sudden nerve damage. Soon spasticity will appear. Exercise will maintain joint range of motion as well as "fatigue out" some muscle spasms. It must be brought to the patient's attention that exercises will maintain muscle tone and joint function and reduce disability, should significant function return. The nurse must also inform the patient that frozen, flexed joints, particularly in the upper extremity (1) are painful, (2) reduce social acceptance when one is unable to wash the axilla, (3) inhibit one's dressing, (4) do not allow for the assistive functions that even a paralyzed limb has to offer, such as stabilizing objects while the other hand works on them. Exercise in controlling spasticity is very important to the patient's maximum rehabilitation.

A stroke patient's motor deficit (hemiplegia or hemiparesis) is on the opposite side to the brain damage when the middle cerebral artery is affected because the pyramidal tracts (the voluntary motor nerves) cross at the level of the medulla.

seizures

The convulsive state is the mode of expression of the nervous system to overwhelming stimuli resulting in sudden, transient alterations of brain function. Paroxysmal, excessive neural discharge may result from acute cerebral anoxia, hypoglycemia, other metabolic disturbances, overhydration, cerebral vascular accident, intracranial infection, and brain tumor. Most commonly, the abnormal discharge is due to the presence of an organic lesion, with the irritable focus being in the partially damaged tissue adjacent to the brain tumor, vascular malformation or lesion, or brain abscess. The type of injury and the severity of damage to the brain are significant considerations when one is predicting the occurrence of seizure activity following cranial trauma. Various figures of incidence are reported. The average prediction is that one person out of four with severe open head injury will experience seizure activity in the first year. The seizures will often cease spontaneously or with medication.

classification of seizures

The variety of physical and psychological characteristics of convulsive activity has led to the establishment of a general classification of seizures. It should be noted that there is no single convulsive type, but certain similar characteristics facilitate the formation of basic categories. The common factor in all seizure types is the occurrence of dysrhythmic electrical disturbances of characteristic form and voltage found on the electroencephalogram. The EEG is the most effective tool available for diagnostic appraisal of seizure activity. Seizure activity is classified using the characteristic configuration and spacing of spikes and waves shown on the EEG tracing (Fig. 20-4).

Grand Mal   Often the most alarming in terms of physical manifestation, this type of seizure is frequently preceded by an "aura" in the conscious patient. About half of the patients experience this personalized warning which may be a temporary visual, olfactory, or auditory sensation such as a flash of lights, a particular smell, or a feeling of impending distress. With abrupt onset, the person may cry out before entering a phase of tonic contraction, lasting about 60 seconds and during which respirations cease and cyanosis occurs. The activity then becomes clonic in nature as the muscles of the face and extremities display jerky movements; breathing is resumed, although irregular and stertorous. Bowel and bladder incontinence may occur, teeth are clenched, and physical injury is often sustained before the person relaxes. He may remain unconscious for several minutes, awakening in a confused, drowsy state often followed by sleep. Todd's palsy, which is temporary paresis or paralysis of the extremities following the clonic phase, may or may not occur. Often the person has no recollection of the event upon awaking.

Petit Mal   This type of activity rarely occurs in adults, and is common in childhood. Unlike the grand mal type, petit mal seizures have no aura and are much shorter in duration (5 to 30 seconds). Transient clouding of consciousness (a blank stare) is often the only symptom. Eye blinking and minor movements of the head may be noted, but major physical manifestations are not present. This type of seizure may occur several times in a day and frequently goes unnoticed.

Psychomotor (Temporal Lobe)   Occurring more commonly in adults than in children, these episodes are at times confused with psychic equivalents of temporal lobe origin such as deja vu (an abnormal feeling of having lived through a new situation before) and hysteria, due to the sometimes bizarre physical activity. Of longer duration than the petit mal, an attack often begins with an inappropriate gesture, followed by a repetitive, seemingly purposeful activity which often does not fit the situation. Automatic behavior may consist of lip-smacking, hand-wringing, or disrobing. Postseizure amnesia follows.

Focal   This seizure results from focal irritation of a part of the motor cortex and may remain localized in the appropriate peripheral area. The Jacksonian seizure often begins in the hand or foot and progresses in "march"-type fashion through the other muscle groups to generalized motor activity

EEG CLASSIFICATIONS

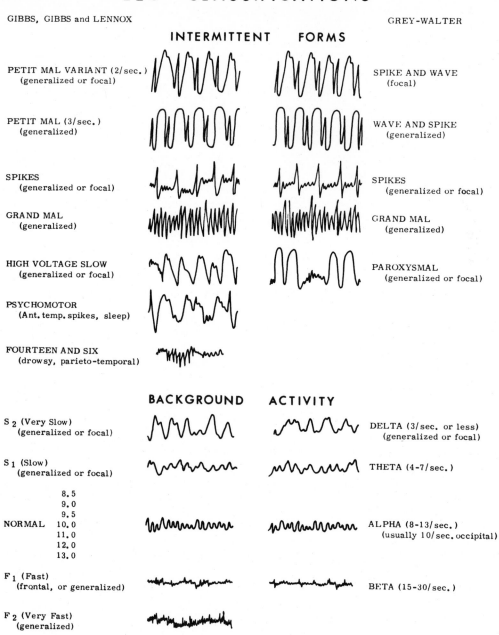

GIBBS, GIBBS and LENNOX   GREY-WALTER

INTERMITTENT FORMS

PETIT MAL VARIANT (2/sec.)
(generalized or focal)
                                        SPIKE AND WAVE
                                        (focal)

PETIT MAL (3/sec.)
(generalized)
                                        WAVE AND SPIKE
                                        (generalized)

SPIKES
(generalized or focal)
                                        SPIKES
                                        (generalized or focal)

GRAND MAL
(generalized)
                                        GRAND MAL
                                        (generalized)

HIGH VOLTAGE SLOW
(generalized or focal)
                                        PAROXYSMAL
                                        (generalized or focal)

PSYCHOMOTOR
(Ant. temp. spikes, sleep)

FOURTEEN AND SIX
(drowsy, parieto-temporal)

BACKGROUND ACTIVITY

S_2 (Very Slow)
(generalized or focal)
                                        DELTA (3/sec. or less)
                                        (generalized or focal)

S_1 (Slow)
(generalized or focal)
                                        THETA (4-7/sec.)

          8.5
          9.0
          9.5
NORMAL   10.0
          11.0
          12.0
          13.0
                                        ALPHA (8-13/sec.)
                                        (usually 10/sec. occipital)

F_1 (Fast)
(frontal, or generalized)
                                        BETA (15-30/sec.)

F_2 (Very Fast)
(generalized)

Fig. 20-4. EEG classifications. (From C. M. MacBryde and R. S. Blacklow, *Signs and Symptoms*, ed. 5, Philadelphia, J. B. Lippincott, 1970, p. 684)

414

which may continue to progress to a grand mal episode. Consciousness may be retained in focal seizures, and posticteric weakness in the affected muscle groups follows for a time.

Status Epilepticus   This refers to a succession of epileptic attacks, either grand mal or petit mal, in which the postseizure phase of one episode overlaps with the discharge of the next, with the patient never fully regaining consciousness. Sustained grand mal activity is an emergency situation with potential lethal outcome, requiring immediate intervention. Intravenous barbiturates or diazepam is usually administered, with appropriate measures for airway establishment and physical protection. General anesthesia may be required for control if other measures are unsuccessful.

nursing responsibility

A grand mal seizure seldom goes unnoticed, and can be a frightening scene when first witnessed. The nurse in the critical care unit must know the measures to institute to protect the patient from injury. Accurate observation is essential. Of primary important is remaining with the patient and staying calm. Loosen restrictive clothing and be sure there is something soft beneath the patient's head. Remember that the cyanotic state is unpreventable and transient. Position the patient on his side, if possible, to facilitate drainage of mucus and saliva. Do not attempt to open clenched teeth, even with a padded tongue blade. Teeth clenching occurs almost immediately and it is too late to prevent biting of the tongue if it was between the teeth at the onset of the attack. Observations to be made include: the seizure pattern and the duration of each phase, the types of movement and the body parts involved, bowel or bladder incontinence, pupil size and eye movement, loss of consciousness, and patient behavior following the episode, e.g., falling asleep, inability to speak, temporary paralysis.

The term "seizure" has a frightening connotation to patient and family alike. Often the patient has no awareness or understanding of his behavior. Accurate observations by the nurse and discussion with the patient following such an event will assist in appropriate assessment and management.

MARILYNN J. WASHBURN, R.N., B.S.N.
CARY LOU MARTINSON, R.N., B.S.N.
CAROLE K. JOHNSON, M.A.T., C.C.C.-SP.
CYNTHIA JOHNSON, M.A., C.C.C.-SP.
MARGARET KERSENBROCK, R.N., B.S.N.
MARILYNN MITCHELL, R.N., B.S.N.
CAROLYN M. HUDAK, R.N., M.S.

21 21

management modalities: nervous system

care of the brain-injured patient
individual response to brain injury

Neurological damage does not occur without effecting some change in a person's behavior response. His personality and entire characteristic behavior pattern will undergo some changes, either temporary or permanent, depending upon the locus and severity of the injury. Lesions of the temporal, parietal, and occipital lobes, which comprise the posterior cerebrum, will affect the quality of reception and interpretation of sensory input from the environment. More specifically, each of the principal lobes of the brain can be associated with a particular function. The occipital lobe at the posterior of the skull is crucial for visual perception, while the temporal lobe is associated with auditory reception and interpretation. Visual-spatial perception involving the nonauditory and nonvisual functions of touch, space and movement are attributed to the parietal lobe. The frontal lobe in the anterior cerebrum plays a major role in integrating emotion with social behavior, mediating personality. Coordination, balance and rhythm are functions of the cerebellum.

Types of maladaptive behavior have been conveniently labeled and can be attributed to injury of various lobes of the brain. One of the most frequently used labels is "frontal lobe syndrome," describing that behavior which is a consequence of injury to the frontal lobe. The frontal lobe is essential to the planning and carrying out of goals, coordinating the "self-concept" with external social forces, and organizing volitional activity. "Frontal" patients will

417

display a flat affect and an apathetic response to any situation, and will have difficulty in displaying appropriate social behavior. Their "I don't care" attitude may lead to unfounded judgments of "lazy," "worthless," and "indifferent." Involvement in group activities of short duration is useful therapy in this situation.

Following severe brain trauma, the patient may exhibit an inability to control his emotions. Frequently, he may cry continually, or burst into inappropriate paroxysms of laughter. Often the content of his dialogue will not fit the emotion displayed. Such affective lability is due to an impairment of the "fine tuning" ability to control emotional response. Interruption of inappropriate emotional responses helps the patient to gain control and conserve energy.

Prompt feedback following inappropriate behavior may be helpful; angry comments will only perpetuate the behavior. Behavior modification techniques may be successful in some instances if the staff approach is very consistent. For example, if a patient uses abusive language when talking with another person, the staff may modify this behavior by consistently ignoring it or terminating the conversation once the patient becomes abusive. The situation should be discussed with the patient first, and then dealt with in a consistent fashion.

States of confusion are also common following brain injury. Due to sustained memory impairment, the patient may not be able to state correctly where he is now, but may accurately describe an event in his past. He may regress in time, consistently answering neuro exam questions with the same incorrect responses, e.g., "It's 1951, Truman is the president," etc. The ability to retain new learning, such as his doctor's name or what he had for breakfast, is impaired, leading to a significant effect on behavior.

Even more difficult to cope with than confusion is the hostile, combative phase common in cases of severe head injury. The patient who displays loud, physically aggressive and verbally abusive behavior is a serious management problem in the critical care unit. This phase is often temporary, lasting days or weeks. Prevention of physical injury, as well as unlimited patience, is of prime importance during this time.

Tranquilizing agents are contraindicated due to their effect on the central nervous system of masking or altering changes which may be symptomatic. Paraldehyde is probably the drug of choice when there is no alternative. It has been found to be most effective when administered on a scheduled basis as opposed to prn usage. Restraints are suggested only as a last resort to prevent physical harm to patient or staff. Soft restraints of wrists and ankles should be released when the nurse is with the patient, to allow for unrestricted muscle movement. The Michelle Craig bed was designed to provide a padded, soft environment in which the patient can move about without risk of physical injury (Fig. 21-1).

In evaluating patient response and behavior change, it is important to have some idea of what the patient was like prior to injury. Emotional outbursts or consistent behavior responses may be part of the patient's premorbid personality and not a direct consequence of the injury. The patient's family or

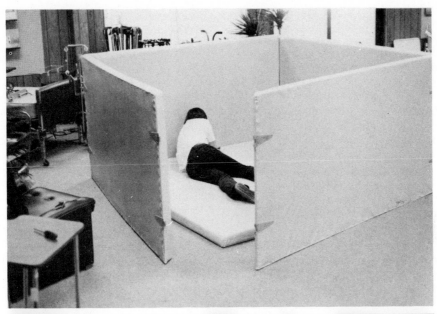

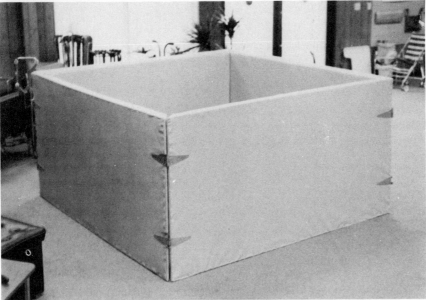

Fig. 21-1. The Michelle Craig Bed provides a protective environment for the restless brain-injured patient. (Available from Wheelchairs, Inc., 3500 South Corona Street, Englewood, Colorado.)

significant others provide a vital link to understanding the patient's behavior prior to injury.

Sensory reception is often significantly impaired following neurological injury. Compounding this impairment is the environment of the critical care unit, devoid of stimuli having any meaning to the patient. Incapable of verbal response, the comatose patient should be assumed to receive sensory input, and staff and visitors alike should direct conversation *to* him, not *about* him.

Sensory deprivation can be diminished by supplying short, frequent periods of sensory input that is meaningful to the patient. A favorite radio program, tape recording, or thirty minutes of music from the patient's favorite radio station provide more meaningful stimulation than constant radio accompaniment, which becomes as meaningless as the continual bleep of the cardiac monitor. Brief explanations of nursing actions, such as, "I'm going to take your blood pressure now," provide verbal stimuli and aid in orienting the patient. A calendar with the days marked off and a clock also reinforce orientation.

Essential to any treatment of the brain-injured patient is the establishment of routine. In addition to the memory impairment and confusion brought on by injury, most brain-injured patients have an impaired ability to transfer learning from one situation to another. The consistency of a schedule of daily activities strengthens learning and memory by repetition, and alleviates anxiety. The nurse in the critical care unit can do much to establish a schedule specific to the patient. Using information obtained from relatives, a daily routine of activities can be established which incorporates the patient's pre-injury preferences and habits. Mobilizing the patient in a wheelchair and dressing him in his own clothes, even while comatose, are effective means of stimulation, appropriate even in the critical care unit. Early mobilization and passive range of motion are essential for prevention of contractures and other complications which will impede rehabilitation.

BIBLIOGRAPHY

Carini, E., and G. Owens, *Neurological and Neurosurgical Nursing,* ed. 6 (St. Louis: C. V. Mosby, 1974).

Carozza, V., "The Nature of Epilepsy," *Nursing Clinics of North America,* Vol. 5 (March 1970), pp. 18–22.

Chusid, J., *Correlative Neuroanatomy and Functional Neurology,* ed. 16 (Los Altos: Lange Medical Publications, 1976).

Fowler, R. S. Jr., and W. E. Fordyce, "Adapting Care for the Brain-Damaged Patient," *American Journal of Nursing,* Vol. 72, Nos. 10 and 11 (October-November, 1972), pp. 1832–1835, 2056–2059.

Gardner, H., *The Shattered Mind* (New York: Alfred A. Knopf, 1975).

MacBryde, C. M., and R. S. Blacklow, *Signs and Symptoms,* ed. 5 (Philadelphia, J. B. Lippincott, 1970).

Merritt, H. H., "The Treatment of Convulsive Disorders," *Medical Clinics of North America,* Vol. 56, No. 6 (November 1972), pp. 1225–1231.

Norsworthy, E., "Nursing Rehabilitation After Severe Head Trauma," *American Journal of Nursing,* Vol. 74 (July 1974), pp. 1246–1250.

respiratory function

Respiratory distress is a common component of brain injury. With decreased levels of consciousness an airway must be maintained. An endotracheal tube can be used for days, but to prevent complications a tracheostomy should be considered. Since the neurophysiology of respiration is so complex, the neurological insult could produce problems at any of a number of levels. The highest level of respiratory control is found in the brain-stem structures of the pneumotaxic center, the nucleus solitarius, and the medulla oblongata. These brain-stem centers can be injured by increased intracranial pressure and hypoxia, as well as direct trauma or interruption of blood supply. When the brain-stem centers are affected the patient becomes dependent on an external source of control and thus becomes ventilator dependent.

Different respiratory patterns can be identified when there is an intracranial dysfunction (Fig. 21-2). Cheyne-Stokes breathing is periodic breathing with the depth of each breath increasing to a peak and then decreasing to a state of apnea. The hyperpneic phase usually lasts longer than the apneic phase. Cheyne-Stokes respiration usually indicates bilateral lesions located deep in the cerebral hemispheres. With traumatic brain injury, the onset of Cheyne-Stokes breathing might be due to herniation of the cerebral hemi-

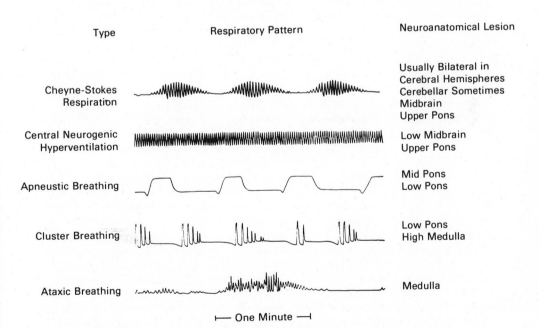

Type	Respiratory Pattern	Neuroanatomical Lesion
Cheyne-Stokes Respiration		Usually Bilateral in Cerebral Hemispheres Cerebellar Sometimes Midbrain Upper Pons
Central Neurogenic Hyperventilation		Low Midbrain Upper Pons
Apneustic Breathing		Mid Pons Low Pons
Cluster Breathing		Low Pons High Medulla
Ataxic Breathing		Medulla

⊢— One Minute —⊣

Fig. 21-2. Abnormal respiratory patterns associated with coma. (From R. R. M. Gifford and M. R. Plaut, "Abnormal Respiratory Patterns in the Comatose Patient Caused by Intracranial Dysfunction," *Journal of Neurosurgical Nursing*, Vol. 7, No. 1, July 1975, p. 58)

spheres through the tentorium, indicating a deteriorating neurological condition. This herniation can also cause compression of the midbrain, and central neurogenic hyperventilation will be observed. This hyperventilation is sustained, regular, rapid and fairly deep. It is usually caused by a lesion of the low midbrain or upper pons.

Apneustic breathing indicates respiration with a pause at full inspiration and full expiration. The etiology of this pattern is usually occlusion of the basilar artery causing infarction of the lateral portions of the brain stem. Cluster breathing may be seen when the lesion is high in the medulla or low in the pons. This pattern of respiration is seen as gasping breaths with irregular pauses.

The real centers of inspiration and expiration are located in the medulla oblongata. Any rapidly expanding intracranial lesion, such as cerebellar hemorrhage, can compress the medulla and ataxic breathing will result. This is totally irregular breathing with both deep and shallow breaths associated with irregular pauses. When this pattern of respiration occurs, a ventilator should be made available to the patient as there is no predicting respiratory rhythm or continuation of respiration.

Interference with some cranial nerves can also influence respiration. The brain-stem centers receive information from chemoreceptors in the carotid artery and aorta and from stretch receptors in the lungs by way of the glossopharyngeal (IX) and the vagus (X) nerves. Outgoing information from the brain stem then travels by way of the phrenic nerve, which leaves the spinal cord with the third cervical nerve and activates the diaphragm. The intercostal muscles which expand the chest wall are activated by the intracostal nerves of the thoracic spinal cord. Even if the brain-stem centers, the cranial nerves, and the thoracic nerves are all intact, the patient may still develop respiratory problems if pulmonary hygiene is inadequate.

The majority of brain-injured patients will have perfectly normal respiratory rates and adequate oxygen exchange, but still may not tolerate closing of an open tracheostomy because of the inability to handle their secretions. Pulmonary hygiene then becomes the responsibility of the nurse.

It is important to observe the patient for spontaneous coughing. Also note if he takes occasional deep breaths (sighs). Coughs and sighs are essential to keep the lungs fully expanded and to prevent pooling of secretions which lead to infection. Preventing atelectasis and pneumonia is the goal in the immobile patient with a decreased level of consciousness. This can be accomplished by frequently stimulating the cough reflex and suctioning secretions via either the nasopharyngeal route or an open tracheostomy. Turning the patient frequently not only helps prevent skin sores, but also mobilizes secretions and decreases pooling in the dependent lobes. Actually, any movement of an inactive patient helps the pulmonary status. By getting a brain-injured patient up in a chair or on a tilt table or even doing range of motion, you are stimulating the patient to do some deep breathing.Without nursing stimulation and vigilant suctioning, respiratory complications can easily be fatal to a brain-injured patient.

urinary control

In the acute brain-injured patient, fluid management is essential and a Foley catheter is necessary to accurately measure urinary output. Too often the Foley catheter is forgotten as a source of irritation as well as potential infection. Even though a brain-injured patient has lost voluntary control of his bladder, the reflexes for normal voiding may be intact. For the male patient, an indwelling catheter can be removed and an external (condom-type) collector used. Care must be taken to monitor the patient's voiding to insure that the bladder does not become overdistended or that a high residual volume is not left in the bladder. When a Foley catheter is removed, a straight catheter should be used to measure the postvoid residual volume. If the volume is below 100 cc. for at least three residual checks, the patient may remain catheter free. Residuals above 100 cc. indicate the presence of constant static urine, which increases the possibility of bladder infection.

Of course, if the patient does not void within a reasonable period of time as indicated by fluid intake, a catheter should be used to prevent distention. Unfortunately, external collectors are not available for female patients, but success can be obtained by transferring the patient to the toilet on a regular schedule when she is at least partially responding to the environment, and her condition permits. Environmental cues such as sitting on a toilet and being in a bathroom might be adequate to stimulate the patient to void even though she is unable to communicate needs.

Many brain-injured patients with motor control involvement develop very spastic bladders and have painful bladder spasms. To the brain-injured patient with decreased ability to understand his situation and to communicate his difficulties, an uncomfortable Foley catheter and painful bladder spasms are a source of great irritation. As a result, the patient may become more agitated and preoccupied with discomfort and less able to focus on more important environmental stimuli. Therefore, removing the Foley catheter can aid in reorientation of a brain-injured patient, as well as decrease the complication of bladder infection.

bowel control

Many complications can be avoided if a good bowel program is started in the critical care unit. Straining to evacuate stool can increase intracranial pressure and produce a decreased level of consciousness. Thus, it is important to give adequate stool softeners and to facilitate evacuation on a regular basis. The actual mechanism of emptying the bowel is basically a reflex activity at the spinal cord level. With brain injury, the voluntary control of stimulating or inhibiting the reflex is impaired. The reflex may be artificially stimulated by a gloved, lubricated finger touching the external rectal sphincter, or by enemas or suppositories.

All of these methods enable the nurse to control evacuation. Establishing a regular routine for daily bowel movements prevents constipation and impaction, accidental bowel movements or continuous small stools, and avoids embarrassment for the patient and visiting family members.

bed positioning

With damage at the brain-stem level, there is a release of tonic reflexes which result in the assumption of abnormal postures. Abnormal muscle tone is reinforced by these reflexes and, in time, can create complications such as increased spasticity, scoliosis, contractures, and hip subluxation. It is easier to "mold" a patient's posture and muscle tone early postinjury. Proper positioning helps to inhibit abnormal tone and allows for easier handling by the physical and occupational therapists and nurses who are helping the patient maintain full range of motion.

Most common in the brain-injured patient is opisthotonic posturing. This is a forward arching of the back and hyperextention of the head with all extremities rigid and straight or hyperextended. This posturing is exaggerated when the patient is supine. Trunk rotation and flexion of the lower extremities will help break up this posturing (Fig. 21-3). If the patient is left flat on his back with legs out straight, you will see an increase in extensor

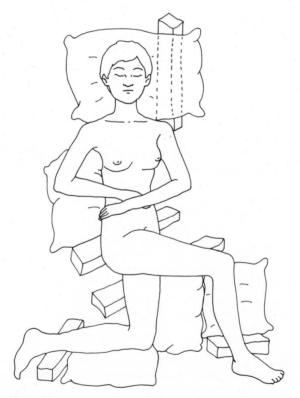

Fig. 21-3. Bed positioning for reflex inhibition in brain-injured patients. This position uses trunk rotation and lower-extremity flexion to relax abnormal muscle tone.

muscle tone. Turn the hips to side lying and flex the knees, and you will see the tone relax.

Head positioning is important because of an asymmetrical tonic neck reflex. This reflex is demonstrated when the extremities on the same side to which the head is turned extend, and the opposite extremities flex. Therefore, to do range of motion on a tightly drawn up arm, try turning the head to that side and see if the muscle tone decreases. Each brain-injured patient will have different reflexive posturing and the nurse must evaluate what positions can be accomplished. The goal of effective positioning is to break up reflexive patterns and decrease abnormal muscle tone.

Passive range of motion is used to stretch muscles and to maintain joint mobility. With the immobile patient, the nurse should move each joint through its normal range of motion on a regular basis. This activity is accomplished easily during a bath. When tightness does occur, splinting may help regain lost range of motion. An easy and effective way to splint an extremity is with pillow splinting. Put one or two pillows along the outstretched arm and secure them tightly with an Ace bandage. The pillow splint can be left in place for approximately an hour at a time if skin pressure points are not a problem. With proper use of pillow splints, range of motion in the elbow joint can be increased and maintained. With a tight hand grip, either voluntary or involuntary, a cone can be used to decrease the development of hand contractures. Pressure on the insertion of a muscle inhibits muscle contraction; thus, the use of a hand cone as opposed to a soft wash cloth can actually cause relaxation of the hand and maintain normal functioning.

With loss of sensory and motor function, the brain-injured patient is left vulnerable to skin breakdown, and bed positioning becomes an important concern from this aspect. There is one simple rule to follow to prevent pressure sores: prevent pressure. With current technology, there are numerous tools to help achieve this goal, such as alternating pressure air mattresses, water mattresses, Stryker-gel pads and sheepskins. But the fact remains that

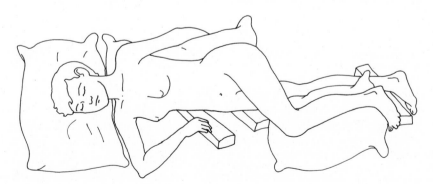

Fig. 21-4. Side lying position. Pads are used above and below the trochanter and lateral malleolus to relieve pressure.

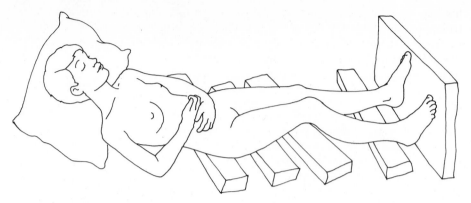

Fig. 21-5. Supine position. Pads are used above and below the sacrum and above the heels to relieve pressure. A pad above the knees prevents hyperextension of the knees and relieves pressure on the popliteal space.

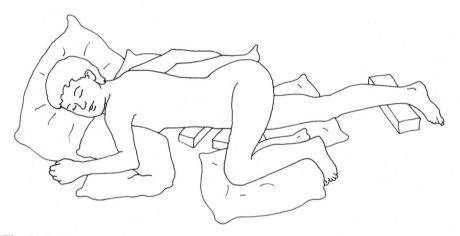

Fig. 21-6. Coma position. Shoulders are turned almost prone for better drainage of the oral and nasal passages.

an immobile patient who is not turned regularly can develop pressure sores in time, no matter what mattress is used. Each patient must be evaluated individually as to his skin tolerance (how fast his skin turns red without being turned). However, two hours is an average skin pressure tolerance time for an acutely ill patient.

Another technique helpful in preventing pressure problems is to pad above and below prominent bony processes. For example, when the patient is on his side, put a rectangular foam pad or small pillow above and below the hip trochanter and above the lateral malleolus of the ankle. Also pad between bony pressure points such as the knees (Fig. 21-4). The nurse should place her hand under the bony processes to confirm that pressure has been relieved. When the patient is on his back, place a pad above and below the sacrum and above the heels (Fig. 21-5). Circular pads called "doughnuts" may actually impair circulation by causing circular pressure around the protected area. Use of rectangular pads allows for collateral circulation, while still relieving pressure.

During initial coma, the patient may be very flaccid, and the "coma position" is recommended to facilitate handling of oral secretions or vomitus to prevent aspiration (Fig. 21-6).

BIBLIOGRAPHY

Chusid, J., *Correlative Neuroanatomy and Functional Neurology,* ed. 16 (Los Altos: Lange Medical Publications, 1976), p. 33.

Farber, S. D., *Sensorimotor Evaluation and Treatment Procedures for Allied Health Personnel* (Indiana University Foundation, 1974), p. 42.

Gifford, R. R. M., and M. R. Plaut, "Abnormal Respiratory Patterns in the Comatose Patient Caused by Intracranial Dysfunction," *Journal of Neurosurgical Nursing,* Vol. 7, No. 1 (July 1975), pp. 57, 61.

Netter, F. H., *Nervous System,* Volume I (New York: The Ciba Collection of Medical Illustrations, 1962), p. 61.

Plum, F., and J. B. Posner, *The Diagnosis of Stupor and Coma,* ed. 2 (Philadelphia: F. A. Davis), 1972.

communication disorders

Because the brain contains the centers for all thought processes, the patient who has sustained brain injury from any cause is likely to demonstrate some kind of communication disorder. Areas which may be affected include language, memory, visual perception, problem solving, concentration and thought organization. The site of injury and etiology determine the kind of problems the patient will evidence.

Language and speech are centered in the left cerebral hemisphere in most people. Therefore, as a general rule, the patient who has sustained injury to the left temporal-parietal area, particularly from CVA, will demonstrate decreased abilities to understand or produce language. This acquired loss of the ability to use language is termed aphasia. Language encompasses all aspects of the learned symbols used to communicate—writing, reading, numbers and the spoken word. An aphasic patient may have difficulty understanding or producing any form of language, although he attempts to make his needs known. He may be unable to think of words he wants to say. He may say inappropriate words or jargon words. What he hears or reads may be meaningless. He may not be able to write the word he wants to write.

The word "aphasia" is often misused to describe patients who do not follow commands or who do not talk. It is accurate to say that the comatose patient shows a decreased ability to process and respond to his environment. However, it is not possible to assess the language abilities of a patient who demonstrates limited response to his surroundings. As his level of awareness increases, he may or may not exhibit language problems.

In communicating with an aphasic patient, it is helpful to use both words and gestures. Pointing to what you are talking about gives the patient extra information about what you are saying. Encourage him to use gestures also.

The phrase "Show me" may reduce frustration for both the patient and the staff. Try to speak slowly and in simple terms without talking down to the patient. Give him time to process what you are saying and to formulate his response. Speak in a normal tone of voice. Aphasics are not deaf but merely have difficulty understanding the meaning of what they hear. Use short sentences; the patient may forget the first part of a long sentence by the time you finish saying it. Avoid useless chatter which may confuse him. Try to ask questions which require a Yes or No response. Evaluation by a speech pathologist may help determine the patient's best means of communicating.

Dysarthria (slurred speech caused by muscle weakness), paralysis, and incoordination may also be present in the right hemiplegic. Encourage the patient to speak slowly and to overemphasize the articulatory movements of the tongue.

Apraxia is another problem often seen with left hemisphere damage. It means the patient knows what he wants to say or do, but is unable to perform at a volitional level. This inability to perform an act cannot be accounted for by muscle weakness, decreased sensation or lack of understanding. Often the patient can do things at an automatic level. For example, he may be able to say the word "coffee" when you provide him with the lead-in phrase "I'd like a cup of _____." Yet he cannot repeat the word after you or name the object. Apraxia may be seen in any voluntary movement such as pointing, swallowing, brushing teeth or speaking.

If apraxia is apparent, try to avoid giving the patient a command to follow. Instead of saying "Take a drink of water," simply hand him the glass and let him perform the act automatically.

The right cerebral hemisphere is the center of visual-spatial functions. A patient who has sustained right hemisphere damage, usually resulting in left hemiplegia, is likely to speak clearly and in complete sentences, but evidence problems in visual perception and spatial planning. These difficulties sometimes go undiagnosed because the patient is highly verbal and appears to be functioning normally. However, the patient tends to ignore or deny the affected side of the body and things placed on the left side. He has great difficulty orienting his body in space and will easily become lost on the unit if he is mobile. Often he will make excuses for these deficits rather than acknowledge their existence.

It is usually necessary to retrain the patient to be consciously aware of his left side in everyday activities. He must be reminded to look on the left side of his plate for additional food during meals, to look to the left when his wheelchair is caught and will not move, or to look on his left when he hears a voice but does not see a visitor. It is helpful to keep things that the patient may need on his good side, and to position him so that he can see approaching visitors and staff. Generally this patient requires much supervision initially because he tends to deny his problems and will attempt acts of which he is incapable.

Homonymous hemianopia is a visual field deficit which often occurs following a CVA. Since neural pathways for vision cross at the optic chiasm, lesions occurring in the occipital area (visual cortex) produce blindness in half of both eyes on the opposite side of the lesion (see Fig. 22-2 in Chapter 22).

Visual field deficits can often be observed when the patient is engaged in functional activities such as eating or taking care of personal hygiene. Notice also whether he responds to approaching visitors on both sides of the bed or runs into objects while wheeling a chair. Turning his head slightly so that he can utilize the intact side of both eyes may help the patient see better and learn to scan visually. Place objects on his good side and position the bed so he can see approaching visitors or staff.

Patients who sustain brain injury from trauma are likely to exhibit different kinds of communication problems. Language and visual perception skills may be intact but the patient may have difficulty with memory, thought organization, concentration, and relating past experience to present situations. Coma or decreased level of response may persist for several weeks or months. Patient responses may be limited in nature (reflex movements, increased gross body movement, opening eyes) and may be noted only when stimulation is present. When left alone, the patient may remain quiet and still. As level of awareness increases, he may begin to respond to discomfort by pulling at his nasogastric or tracheostomy tube or by becoming restless or agitated. Although he is apparently unresponsive to environmental stimulation, he does respond to his own internal agitation and stimulation, often in a nonpurposeful manner.

With increased awareness, the patient begins to respond to things around him, although he has difficulty maintaining selected attention for any length of time. Short-term memory is extremely impaired, although long-term memory may be intact. The patient may begin to wander with the intention of going home. Agitation may persist but is more goal-directed and aimed at external stimuli. The patient may be able to tolerate irritations (catheter, nasogastric tube, etc.) once they have been explained to him.

As the patient's ability to concentrate increases, improvements in short-term memory and learning will be evident. He will begin to show carry-over for old learning tasks (dressing, hygiene, etc.); new learning tasks show little carry-over. He may have difficulty organizing his thoughts to perform an activity. Since a great deal of retraining is based on language and reasoning, the speech pathologist can often provide guidance in improving the patient's functional abilities.

reestablishment of oral intake

NORMAL SWALLOWING FUNCTION

Knowledge of normal swallowing function is essential before initiating an oral intake program with a brain-injured patient. Swallowing is primarily a reflexive action and is usually described in three stages. In the oral stage, the tongue controls a bolus of food or liquid by pressing it against the soft palate and forming a seal around it. There is a respiratory pause on inspiration as the larynx moves up and forward to close and protect the airway. The seal around the bolus is broken as the soft palate elevates and closes the nasopharynx to prevent nasal regurgitation. The oral stage may include some volitional tongue movements, but is primarily a reflexive action. In the pharyngeal stage, with the soft palate elevated and the airway occluded, the tongue propels the bolus back against the posterior pharyngeal wall with anterior to posterior rippling motions. The muscles of the pharynx then contract sequentially to move the bolus down through the pharynx. The cricopharyngeal sphincter relaxes and opens in the esophageal stage as the bolus of food enters the esophagus. Peristaltic waves carry the bolus down the esophagus and into the stomach.

The swallowing reflex can be initiated by sensory stimulation of three cranial nerves. The glossopharyngeal nerve (IX) innervates the posterior tongue, the mucosa of the oropharynx, the soft palate, and the tonsillar area. The vagus nerve (X) provides sensory innervation to the mucosa of the larynx above the level of the vocal cords, the epiglottis, portions of the pharynx, and the esophagus. The trigeminal nerve (V) provides sensory innervation to the mucosa of the palate, the uvula, and the tonsillar area. Sensory stimulation to initiate a swallow is conveyed to the cranial nuclei in the medulla of the brain stem which coordinates the simultaneous inhibition of respiration and the motor act of swallowing.

Over twenty different muscle pairs are involved in the swallowing process, and they are innervated by six cranial nerves and the motor neurons of the first three cervical levels of the spinal cord. The cranial nerves involved include the hypoglossal (XII) for tongue movements; the vagus (X) for movement of the larynx, pharynx, and esophagus; the glossopharyngeal (IX) for pharyngeal muscle contractions and elevation of the soft palate; the facial (VII) for portions of the laryngeal action; and the trigeminal (V) to activate the tensor muscle of the soft palate. Swallowing is the most complex "all-or-none" reflex[1] that results in an integrated, synchronized pattern which is individually constant and occurs below the level of consciousness.[2]

FACTORS TO CONSIDER BEFORE INITIATION OF ORAL INTAKE

The patient's medical condition should be stable before oral intake is initiated. Conditions which contraindicate oral intake include fever (which may mask signs of aspiration pneumonia), the necessity of frequent suctioning, respiratory insufficiency, or other acute medical problems. Aspiration pneumonia can seriously complicate the patient's condition, especially in the presence of other medical problems.

The level of consciousness should at least allow for generalized responses to noxious stimulation, such as grimaces, restlessness, or pushing away. The patient's eyes should be open, but maintenance of eye contact or eye tracking is not necessary.

Swallowing ability should be evaluated and determined to be adequate without danger of aspiration. The most effective evaluation technique is cinefluorography (barium swallow) with the patient in an upright position. Anteroposterior and lateral views of the passage of barium in the swallowing sequence can easily reveal swallowing dysfunctions, such as poor tongue control, difficulty in initiation of the swallow, nasopharyngeal regurgitation, pharyngeal retention, inadequate relaxation of the cricopharyngeal area, or aspiration into the larynx.[3,4] If cinefluorography demonstrates significant aspiration, an oral intake program is contraindicated.

Swallowing function is evaluated by subjective observation as well, and in some settings this may be the only method available. Many patients can be made to swallow with tactile stimulation around the mouth or larynx, or simply observed when swallowing saliva. The action of the tongue, the upward movement of the larynx, and the respiratory pattern are observed for rate, duration, and sequence, and compared to normal function. Some patients also demonstrate primitive oral reflexes with stimulation of the oral area. These are the same reflexes that a newborn has, and are usually controlled by higher brain centers by the age of 1 year. The patient's brain injury has removed the inhibitory control mechanisms of the higher brain centers, and, consequently, the primitive brain-stem reflexes are released. The most easily observed primitive oral reflexes are a suckling pattern (a repetitive forward, up, and backward movement of the tongue usually followed by a swallow), chewing (rhythmical chewing motions without jaw closure), and biting (jaw closure and holding when the area between the teeth or the gums is stimulated).

Another major consideration before the beginning of oral intake is the patient's respiratory status. Respiratory function should be adequate with a small Jackson trach tube (size 4 or below), a Kistner button, or a normal airway. If the patient's respiratory function is such that a cuffed trach tube or a Jackson, size 5 or larger, is required, the oral intake program should be postponed, since a large tracheostomy gives the patient an artificial airway which alters the normal coordination of respiration and swallowing. The tracheostomy tube can limit up and forward movement of the larynx, as the tube itself anchors the trachea to the muscles and skin of the neck. Regurgitation and aspiration into the larynx may result from compression of the cervical esophagus by the tracheostomy tube.[5] The larger trach tubes with inflated cuffs cause even more compression of the esophagus; food or secretions may overflow and rest above the inflated cuff, and pressures from the swallow itself force liquids and even semisolids around the cuff into the trachea.[6] Consequently, larger tracheostomy tubes are a negative factor in attempting to reestablish safe swallowing function. The normal nasal-oral airway should be established by plugging the smaller Jackson trach tubes, using a Kistner button, or removing the tracheostomy, before a patient is started on an oral intake program.

The final consideration is evaluation of cough strength. The patient should demonstrate a cough reflex adequate for protection of the airway. A weak cough will not clear the airway in the event of aspiration, and thus the patient should not be started on oral intake.

The patient is ready to initiate an oral intake program if the above five factors are met: medical condition is stable; at least generalized responses to noxious stimuli are present; swallowing function is present; respiratory function is adequate; and the cough reflex is strong. Most severely brain-injured patients require at least a few weeks to elapse postinjury before all these requirements are met.

TECHNIQUES FOR ORAL INTAKE

If the patient has a nasogastric tube, it should be removed at least a few hours before food is introduced orally. The nasogastric tube can cause nasal and pharyngeal irritation, esophagitis, and laryngeal edema. The irritation and inflammation produce excessive secretions which are difficult to remove and interfere with the swallowing process. The presence of a foreign object passing through the nasal, oral, pharyngeal, and esophageal areas only interferes with swallowing efficiency.

The patient is best positioned in bed or in a chair from 45 to 90 degrees upright, with the neck slightly flexed. Care should be taken not to extend the neck, as this makes upward movement of the larynx (to protect the airway from aspiration) more difficult. The ideal environment is free from distracting noises and movements for more effective concentration on the swallowing process.

Often the physician will order clear liquids for the initial oral trial. Thin liquids are easily affected by gravity, and they flow through the mouth and pharynx quickly, before the patient is able to initiate a swallow. Consequently, solids with a clear liquid base, such as gelatin or popcicles, are a better choice as they can more easily be controlled in the mouth. Food should be chosen to provide maximum stimulation in temperature, taste, color, and texture when possible. Bland tastes and lukewarm temperatures (such as tepid tap water) provide minimal stimulation to the patient and should be avoided in the initial stages, especially for patients with a reduced level of awareness. Milk products and sweets should be avoided as well, as these cause excess mucus production.

Pureed foods are introduced if the patient demonstrates adequate control of the clear solids. The diet expands as the patient gains swallowing efficiency and control. From pureed foods, the patient progresses to foods that require minimal chewing, such as finely chopped meat, fruit, and vegetables. As chewing ability and tongue control improve, foods are chopped in larger pieces until the patient is able to tolerate a regular diet. Foods the patient did not enjoy prior to injury are to be avoided. Close contact should be maintained with the dietary department to provide nutritious and attractive meals within the patient's swallowing ability. The dietitian can also be helpful in recommending various protein or caloric supplements if indicated.

Techniques used during an oral intake session depend on the patient's individual swallowing pattern, but some general suggestions apply to most patients. It is important to verbalize the entire process to the patient, even if understanding is questionable. The food or liquid should be described as to taste, smell, and appearance. The swallowing process is emphasized with comments such as "Move your tongue," "Push that food back," "Hold your breath," and "Swallow." The food is introduced as far posteriorly in the mouth as possible with firm pressure from the spoon. Metal spoons should always be used, as plastic spoons can easily break and shatter, especially if the patient has a biting reflex.

In hemiplegic patients with unilateral sensory and/or motor impairment of the face, food and liquid should be placed in the mouth on the intact side. Also, swallowing efficiency can be improved if the patient's head is tilted slightly to the intact side so gravity will direct the food or liquid to the area of normal sensory and motor function. "Pocketing" of food in the impaired side of the mouth is characteristic of hemiplegic patients, and they need to be reminded to clear food from the mouth on both sides. Following a meal, it is important to carefully check the oral cavity and clear any residual food that may have lodged in the impaired side.

The amount per swallow is initially small, approximately 5 cc. or less. Patients with poor tongue control lose food in the sides of the mouth, and large amounts are not completely evacuated after the first swallow. The food remaining in the oral cavity can easily slide down the pharynx after the swallow is completed and cause choking. Many patients have greater difficulty with liquids than with solids; consequently, liquids should initially be given carefully in small amounts.

If the introduction of food or liquid into the mouth fails to set off the reflexive swallow, additional stimulation is provided. Firm upward pressure on the floor of the mouth, light upward stroking of the larynx, or light tactile stimulation around the mouth may provide the stimulation necessary to trigger the swallowing reflex.

Staff members who feed the severely brain-injured patient must be carefully observant of the patient's swallowing behaviors. The staff member provides external control of the swallowing process with the introduction of food into the mouth, the amount per swallow, and the stimulation of the swallowing reflex. Too much food given too fast greatly increases the likelihood of aspiration.

Goals are established for the total amount of fluid and caloric intake needed in 24 hours. All care givers participating in the oral intake program should use a consistent feeding technique and accurately record the amount of fluid and caloric intake. Supplemental methods of intake are used when the patient is unable to maintain adequate nutrition orally. These supplemental methods may include intravenous feeding or gastrostomy. Reinsertion of the nasogastric tube should be avoided, if possible, due to the irritation of the swallowing mechanism and interference with the swallowing process. In cases of significant swallowing dysfunction with slow improvement in swallowing ability, a gastrostomy is ideal as the patient can continue on a consistent feeding program and adequate nutrition can be maintained.

Careful monitoring of oral intake to maintain adequate nutrition is essential, especially in the initial stages. Periodic serum electrolytes and nitrogen balance checks are indicated. Weight should be charted on a regular basis.

WHEN TO DISCONTINUE ORAL INTAKE

Oral intake should be discontinued if the patient shows evidence of aspiration pneumonia. A sudden spike in temperature, a chest x-ray showing right lower lobe infiltration, or increased right lower lobe sounds after feeding are all indicative of aspiration.

Aspiration pneumonia is most frequently found in the right lower lobe of the lung due to the effect of gravity and the relatively straight downward course of the right bronchus as compared to the more acute angle of the left bronchus. The oral intake program should also be discontinued if the patient develops other complications which require priority treatment, or if the tracheostomy tube is increased above a Jackson size 4 or changed to a cuffed trach tube. Any significant decrease in the patient's level of consciousness may indicate neurological complications, and the oral intake program should again be terminated.

REFERENCES

1. R. W. Doty, "Influence of Stimulus Pattern on Reflex Deglutition," *American Journal of Physiology*, Vol. 166 (1951), pp. 142-158.
2. C. H. Best and N. B. Taylor, *The Physiological Basis of Medical Practice* (Baltimore: Williams & Wilkins, 1950), pp. 561-563.
3. M. W. Donner and M. L. Silbiger, "Cinefluorographic Analysis of Pharnygeal Swallowing in Neuromuscular Disorders," *American Journal of the Medical Sciences* (May 1966), pp. 134-150.
4. A. Silverstein and D. Faegenburg, "Cineradiography of Swallowing," *Archives of Neurology*, Vol. 12 (January 1965), pp. 67-71.
5. P. C. Bonanno, "Swallowing Dysfunction After Tracheostomy," *Annals of Surgery*, Vol. 174, No. 1 (July 1971), pp. 29-33.
6. N. B. Pinkus, "The Dangers of Oral Feeding in the Presence of Cuffed Tracheostomy Tubes," *Medical Journal of Australia* (June 1973), pp. 1238-1240.

care of the patient with spinal cord injury

The care of cord-injured patients has improved since the advent of special care units. With alertness, close observation, and good judgment on the part of the critical care nurse, many of the complications of cord injury no longer occur, or at least are recognized early, so appropriate treatment is initiated.

Traumatic spinal cord injury is one of the most devastating of all traumatic injuries. Nursing care must be directed toward the concomitant physical, emotional, and social problems. Realistic goal setting will be determined by the level and extent of the injury.

Basic evaluation of the patient with possible traumatic spinal cord injury should be carried out immediately upon his arrival at the hospital. This initial evaluation will be the baseline with which all future observations are compared.

It is important to establish whether the patient lost consciousness, how his injury occurred, and whether he has numbness, pain, burning paresthesias, involuntary spasms, or weakness of the trunk or extremities. Whether he was incontinent of urine or stool is also important.

The patient is said to have an areflexic paraplegia or tetraplegia if there was an immediate complete loss of motor power, sensation, and deep reflexes. If this total paralysis has existed for more than 24 hours, the prognosis for significant recovery is not at all promising. If, however, there is some retention of sensation or motor power, the lesion is considered incomplete and the prognosis is better.

In examining the patient, localizing the level of the lesion is important. Keep in mind that in early childhood there is a disparity in the growth rate of the spinal cord and the spine, with the bony spine growing more quickly. Thus, by adulthood the cord segments lie at a higher level than do their correspondingly designated vertebrae.

There is a rule of thumb for remembering the relationship between the spine and the level of the cord in adults. The rule is to add 2 to the number of the spinous process; the sum is the number of the underlying spinal segment. This applies from the spinous process of C_2 to that of T_{10}. For example, spinous process C_5 overlies spinal segment C_7. T_{11}, T_{12}, and L_1 spinous processes overlie eleven spinal segments (L_1 through L_5 and S_1 through S_5 and the first coccygeal segment).

The extent of motor and sensory loss will greatly depend upon the location of the spinal cord lesion. With a C_1–C_4 lesion, the trapezius, sternomastoid, and platysma muscles remain functional. Intercostal muscles and the diaphragm are paralyzed and there is no voluntary movement below the spinal transection. The segmental innervation of the phrenic nerve may be sufficient to maintain respiration. As spinal shock resolves, the muscles become spastic. There is a marked paralytic vasodilation of the face, a blockage of the nasal passages, and an increase in the respiratory rate. The patient generally has difficulty talking and swallowing, is unable to cough, and may be irrational secondary to hypoxia. Sensory loss for levels C_1 through C_3 includes the occipital region, the ears, and some regions of the face.

When the C_5 segment of the cord is damaged, the function of the diaphragm is impaired secondary to post-traumatic edema in the acute phase. Intestinal paralysis compounds the respiratory distress. The upper extremities are outwardly rotated from impairment of the supra- and infraspinous muscles. The shoulders may be markedly elevated due to the uninhibited action of the levator scapulae and trapezius muscles. Following the acute phase, reflexes below the level of the lesion are exaggerated. Sensation is present in the neck and the triangular area of the anterior aspect of the upper arms.

In a C_6 segment lesion, respiratory distress may occur because of intestinal paralysis and ascending edema of the spinal cord. The shoulders are usually elevated, with arms abducted and forearms flexed. This is due to the uninhibited action of the deltoid, biceps and brachioradialis muscles. Functional recovery of the triceps is dependent upon correct positioning of the arms (forearm in extension, arm in adduction). Sensation remains over the lateral aspect of the arms and the dorsolateral aspect of the forearm.

Cord lesions at the level of C_7 allow the diaphragm and accessory muscles to compensate for the affected abdominal and intercostal muscles. The upper extremities assume the same position as in C_6 lesions. Finger flexion is usually exaggerated when the reflex action returns.

The abnormal position of the upper extremities is not present in C_8 lesions because the adductors and internal rotators are able to counteract the antagonists. The latissimus dorsi and trapezius muscles are strong enough to support a sitting position. Postural hypotension occurs when the patient is raised to the sitting position due to the loss of vasomotor control. This postural hypotension can be minimized by having the patient make a gradual change from the lying to the sitting position. The patient's fingers usually assume a claw position. Most patients are able to function at a level that includes writing, self-feeding, dressing, and some sports.

Lesions in the T_1–T_5 region may cause diaphramatic breathing. The inspiratory function of the lungs increases as the level of the thoracic lesion descends. Postural hypotension is usually present. A partial paralysis of the adductor pollicis, interosseous and lumbrical muscles of the hands is present, as is sensory loss for touch, pain and temperature.

Lesions at the T_6 level abolish all abdominal reflexes. From the level of T_6 down, individual segments are functioning, and at the level of T_{12}, all abdominal reflexes are present. There is spastic paralysis of the lower limbs. Patients with lesions at a thoracic level should be functionally independent.

The upper limits of sensory loss in thoracic lesions are as follows:

Level of Lesion	Upper Limit of Sensory Loss
T_2	Entire body to the inner side of the upper arm
T_3	Axilla
T_5	Nipple
T_6	Xyphoid process
T_7, T_8	Lower costal margin
T_{10}	Umbilicus
T_{12}	Groin

Bowel and bladder function may return with the reflex automatism.

The sensory loss involved in L_1 through L_5 lesions is as follows:

Level of Lesion	*Sensory Loss*
L$_1$	All areas of the lower limbs, extending to the groin and the back of the buttocks
L$_2$	Lower limbs excepting the upper third of the anterior aspect of the thigh
L$_3$	Lower limbs and saddle area
L$_4$	Same as in L$_3$ lesions, excepting the anterior aspect of the thigh
L$_5$	Outer aspects of the legs and ankles, and the posterior aspect of the lower limb and saddle area

Patients with these lesions should attain total independence.

With lesions involving S$_1$ through S$_5$, there may be some displacement of the foot. From S$_3$ through S$_5$, there is no paralysis of the leg muscles. The loss of sensation involves the saddle area, scrotum, glans penis, perineum, anal area, and the upper third of the posterior aspect of the thigh.

autonomic dysreflexia

Autonomic dysreflexia or hyperreflexia is a syndrome which sometimes occurs in patients with a spinal cord lesion at T$_5$ or above and constitutes a medical emergency. The syndrome presents quickly and can precipitate a seizure or cerebrovascular accident. Even death can occur if the cause is not relieved.

Impulses produced by tactile, painful, or thermal stimulation of the skin and visceral distention or contraction of the bladder or bowel are transmitted through the pelvic and presacral nerves to the spinal cord via the lateral spinothalamic tracts and the posterior columns. These impulses ascend to the cord lesion, where a sympathetic reflex is activated, and massive sympathetic nerve overactivity results below the level of the lesion. Stimulation of pressure receptors in the carotid sinus and the aorta occurs. The centers respond with vagal stimulation by way of the vasomotor center in the brain stem, and produce bradycardia. Impulses from the vasomotor center which would cause splanchnic pooling and allow a decrease in blood pressure are blocked at the cord lesion.

The clinical signs of hyperreflexia include bradycardia, sweating, rhinorrhea, pounding headache, and severe paroxysmal hypertension. Cutis ansernia (gooseflesh) and urticaria may be present. Hypertension and bradycardia usually persist until the cause of the autonomic crisis is removed.

When hyperreflexia is recognized, there are several things the alert nurse can quickly do. The head of the bed should be elevated and frequent checks of the blood pressure should be made. The patient's bladder drainage system should be checked. If it is clamped, the clamp should be removed. Kinks in the tubing should be looked for, and the collection bag checked to make sure it is not full. The catheter may slowly be irrigated with 30 cc. of irrigating solution to determine its patency. If the symptoms persist after these checks are made, the catheter should be changed to allow the bladder to empty. If the patient's blood pressure does not return to normal, the use of a ganglionic blocking agent, such as atropine sulfate, may be indicated.

The patient should also be examined for bowel impaction, for pressure areas, and for other inflammatory processes as possible causes of the hyper-reflexia.

complete vs. incomplete cord lesions

Once the level of the spinal cord lesion has been determined, there are other factors to consider. One of these is the extent of damage to the cord. The lesion may be complete or incomplete. Spinal cord *concussion* is one type of incomplete cord injury. Concussion generally implies a traumatic physio-logical interruption of spinal cord function which is usually transient, lasting hours to several weeks. The diagnosis of cord concussion is usually made when the patient presents with a neurological deficit following trauma, and there is no evidence of fracture, dislocation, or the presence of a foreign body in the spinal canal. The spinal fluid shows no evidence of subarachnoid block, and the myelogram is normal.

A spinal cord *contusion* often involves some degree of anatomical as well as physiological interruption of cord function. There is usually subpial ecchymosis and swelling secondary to cord compression. A contusion implies some permanent neurological deficit.

Laceration of the spinal cord implies a tear of the pia mater and the cord substance, and is associated with hemorrhage and edema. Lacerations may be small, but if severe fracture/dislocation has occurred, there may be ex-tensive damage with complete cord transection. Complete cord transection results in immediate and complete loss of all motor, sensory, autonomic and reflex responses.

Spinal shock is associated with complete transection and may last weeks or months. Spinal shock differs from traumatic shock in several ways. In tran-sections above the sympathetic outflow (T_5), there is an initial fall in blood pressure due to spinal shock. This hypotension is more pronounced in cervical lesions. The blood pressure returns to normal soon, but the reflex depression remains unchanged for a long period. In distal cord lesions, the blood pressure may remain normal, but spinal shock can be severe. Blood transfusions have no effect on this phenomenon.

The reduced peripheral resistance and consequent pooling of blood in spinal shock is due to the vasomotor paralysis which occurs in spinal injury above the level of T_6 and produces hypotension. In this instance, the hypo-tension is like that of neurogenic shock. The low blood pressure in uncompli-cated cord injury is accompanied by bradycardia due to reflex vagal activity. When other injuries are present, there may be hypovolemia and tachycardia. Cardiac arrest is a potential danger in spinal shock due to this vasomotor instability. There is also the potential for deep vein thrombosis in the spinal shock phase, but it is more apt to occur after reflex activity has returned.

Spinal shock with complete cord transection is eventually replaced by a purely reflex state in which hyperreflexia and hypertonicity are present.

Mass reflexes develop and can be initiated by such stimuli as having the patient take a deep breath, by stroking his foot, or by pricking the skin. These mass reflexes are often misunderstood by the family and patient. They tend to think the reflexes are a sign of returning cord function and may develop false hope unless the situation is explained to them. Eventually spasticity develops, and with it comes the potential for contractures in the limbs.

Incomplete lesions of the spinal cord may be associated with the same initial degree of spinal shock as seen with complete transection. Several syndromes may be identified in incomplete cord lesions which further aid in localizing the injury. The acute anterior cervical spinal cord syndrome is one in which the damage is concentrated in the anterior aspect of the cord. There is complete motor paralysis below the level of the lesion (corticospinal tracts), and loss of sensations of pain, temperature, and touch (spinothalamic tracts). Light touch sensation, proprioception, and position (posterior columns) are preserved.

In the acute central cervical cord syndrome, cord damage is centrally located. Damage is mainly confined to cervical tracts lying centrally which supply the arms. There is less damage to the lumbar and sacral segments which lie peripherally and supply the legs and bladder.

The Brown-Séquard syndrome occurs when the damage is located on one side of the spinal cord. There may be increased or decreased cutaneous sensation of pain, temperature, and touch at the level of the lesion. Below the level of the lesion on the same side, there is complete motor paralysis. On the opposite side below the level of the lesion, there is loss of sensations of pain, temperature, and touch, since the spinothalamic tracts cross after entering the cord. Functionally, the limb with the best motor power has the poorest sensation.

nursing care considerations

There are certain commonalities in caring for patients with spinal cord injuries, regardless of the level of injury or the extent of damage.

Respiratory Hypoventilation from inadequate respiratory movement may occur secondary to the spinal paralysis. Respiratory dysfunction may be further compounded by preexisting pulmonary disease or coexistent chest injuries. Alveolar ventilation may be directly affected by the pulmonary collapse and/or by consolidation from retained mucus, or aspiration of vomitus. Pulmonary edema may also result from incorrect management of intravenous fluids. Paralytic ileus and gastric dilatation may contribute to the respiratory compromise by increasing pressure on the diaphragm. Interference with the cough reflex and the fluid imbalance may also combine to obstruct the airways.

By means of the quad coughing technique, the patient may be able to effectively clear his lungs, despite weakness or loss of the respiratory muscles which produce the automatic cough reflex. This technique consists of compressing the sides of the patient's chest (if on his side or abdomen), or the diaphragm (if supine), when he begins to cough (Fig. 21-7). Often, position

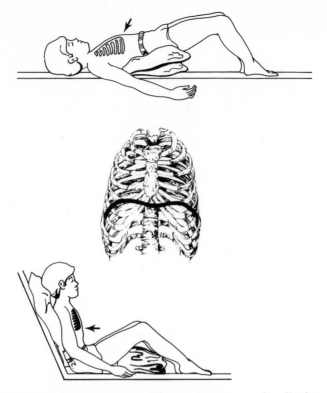

Fig. 21-7. Quad coughing technique. These positions are for diaphragmatic quad coughing only. (*Top*) To push the diaphragm, place one hand flat in the middle of the torso above the stomach and below the ribs. (*Middle*) Front view of the ribs; diaphragm indicated by heavy line. (*Bottom*) To compress the chest, place both hands flat and position on both sides of the chest. Do not move on top of the rib cage, as this could cause damage.

change and/or chest percussion will stimulate the patient to begin to cough. Compression of the chest should not be forceful, and should be done only during exhalation. The patient should be allowed to rest periodically during this procedure.

Metabolic The patient with a spinal cord injury demonstrates a surprisingly florid metabolic response to an injury that is usually associated with little tissue damage. If the injury is uncomplicated, the metabolic derangement reaches a peak within 48 to 72 hours postinjury. A return to normal may be anticipated between 10 and 14 days postinjury. When the spinal injury is complicated by other factors such as surgical intervention or other medical problems, the metabolic response is greater and more prolonged. This response is characterized by a marked retention of sodium and water, increased potassium excretion, breakdown of body protein, and an oliguric period followed by diuresis. A reduced glomerular filtration rate secondary to hypotension compounds the sodium and water retention. Starvation is also a factor in the metabolic disturbance since the majority of cord-injured patients are unable to tolerate oral food or fluid for at least a week following the injury.

Since it may be difficult to ascertain the patient's state of hydration on admission, monitoring of fluid intake and output is necessary to prevent pulmonary edema, tubular necrosis, electrolyte imbalance, and congestive heart failure. Additives to the intravenous fluid should include potassium chloride, occasional sodium bicarbonate, and amino acids. The intravenous caloric content should approximate 2,000 calories per 24 hours.

Gastrointestinal Cord-injured patients often have gastrointestinal difficulties. This complication is seen most frequently in the patient whose lesion is above the sympathetic outflow. The cessation of smooth muscle function lasts for about five to seven days. There is an accumulation of fluid in the stomach and intestines with vomiting and abdominal distention. Acute gastric dilatation frequently occurs in patients with high cord lesions, with or without paralytic ileus. Acute gastrointestinal hemorrhage may also occur secondary to a stress ulcer.

The combination of starvation and gastrointestinal and metabolic changes may precipitate ketosis, dehydration, and other electrolyte and acid-base imbalances. Because of the gastrointestinal complications, a nasogastric tube should be inserted and bowel sounds monitored. Oral fluids may be started at 25 to 50 cc. per hour after bowel sounds have returned. If there is no evidence of residual gastric aspirate, oral fluids may gradually be increased. Food intake may begin when the patient can tolerate 75 to 150 cc. of fluid per hour. A small amount of antacid medication should be instilled via the gastric tube whenever the pH of the gastric aspirate is below 3.

Bowel Program Smooth muscle peristalsis begins as soon as the ileus secondary to spinal shock resolves. Keep in mind that bowel impaction frequently occurs during the period of ileus. The impaction may precipitate autonomic dysreflexia as the reflex automatism returns. The defecation reflex remains intact with lesions above the sacral segments. The reflex is interrupted with lower motor neuron lesions but the autonomous bowel has an intrinsic contractile response. Bowel training is based on a fixed time pattern which takes the place of the cerebrally monitored urge. For the patient with an upper motor neuron lesion, the program takes advantage of the intact reflex by establishing the program at a convenient time for the patient. With a lower motor neuron lesion, continence is assured by regularly evacuating the bowel.

Peristalsis should be stimulated as soon as bowel sounds are present. This is safely done with stool softeners, mild laxatives, or suppositories. A suppository with a stimulant effect is preferred initially. Enemas, other than the oil retention type, should be avoided as the risk of intestinal perforation is high.

The actual bowel program is begun at the time of the initial bowel clean-out. The time of day should be established in relation to the patient's future social needs. A stool softener is used the night before the program is to begin. At the established time, a suppository is inserted for mechanical effect, or digital stimulation of the nerve endings in the rectum may be performed. These methods may be used separately or together to achieve an evacuated bowel. A spastic rectal sphincter will need to be held aside to allow for evacuation.

The usual goal of a bowel program is an every other day evacuation. Occasionally, a bowel pattern identical to that before injury can be reestablished.

Urinary   Acute tubular necrosis may occur during the first 48 hours postinjury as a result of hypotension. In the acute phase of injury, the urine output should be measured hourly. An indwelling catheter is necessary to accomplish this. The urine should be tested for specific gravity, blood, protein, bile, and sugar to help monitor electrolyte balance.

The long-range objective of bladder management, regardless of the level of the lesion, is to achieve a means whereby the bladder consistently empties, the urine is sterile, and the patient remains continent. The ultimate goal would be to have the patient catheter-free, with consistent low-residual urine checks, no urinary tract infection, and no evidence of damage to the upper urinary tract structures.

There are two ways to achieve bladder management. One is a pattern of clamping and draining the catheter. This method usually establishes a schedule for draining the bladder every four hours. The urine volume is measured each time. This pattern is an attempt to eventually establish a catheter-free status.

The other method of bladder management is intermittent catheterization, and it may be begun in the early recovery phase. The purpose of this program is to exercise the detrusor muscle, with the goal again being to have the patient catheter-free. The advantage of this program is that no irritant remains in the bladder.

The bladder is drained every four hours. As the patient gains strength, he can be taught methods to stimulate voiding. Gradually the number of catheterizations is decreased, as the residual amount of urine decreases to less than 100 cc. The patient's oral intake should be gauged to approach 500 cc. between catheterizations.

Each catheterization, for the intermittent catheterization program or for routine catheter changes, must be managed as a sterile surgical procedure. The catheter material has some effect on the condition of the urinary tract mucosa. Latex rubber indwelling catheters are more irritating to the mucosa than catheters made of, or coated by, inert substances. The drainage system must be sterile and it is advisable to change the system daily.

Perineal hygiene should consist of washing the perineal area and the outside of the catheter with soap and water two to three times daily. Particular attention should be given to the scrotum, the foreskin, the labial folds, and the groin area.

A balanced bladder is one in which the residual urine volume is consistently low. The amount of residual urine is not as important as the percentage of the voided volume it represents. The objective is to achieve a repeatable residual urine volume of 10 percent of the voided volume. Factors which hinder efforts to achieve a balanced bladder include bowel impactions, cystitis, bladder stones, pressure sores, systemic infections, and anxiety.

Skin Pressure is a common cause of structural damage to a muscle and its peripheral nerve supply. There is a definite time/pressure relationship in the development of pressure sores. Skin can tolerate minute pressure indefinitely, but great pressure for a short time is disruptive. Microscopic tissue changes secondary to local ischemia occur in less than 30 minutes. Pressure interferes with arteriolar and capillary blood flow. When the pressure is prolonged, there is definite superficial circulatory and tissue damage. The damage may be associated with congestion and induration of the area, or blistering and loss of superficial epidermal layers of the skin. As the pressure continues, the deeper skin layers are lost, leading to superficial necrosis and ulceration. Serous drainage from such an ulceration can constitute a continuous protein loss of as much as 50 grams per day. Prolonging the pressure results in deep penetrating necrosis of the skin, subcutaneous tissue, fascia, and muscle. The destruction may progress to gangrene of the underlying bony structure. Pressure necrosis can begin from within the tissue over a bony prominence where the body weight is greatest per square inch.

A turn schedule for the patient is obviously important. It should be carried out every two hours. The vital signs and skin condition should be checked before and after the position change. If the cord injury precludes a position change, the patient can be lifted and held for a period of three to five minutes every eight hours. Use of an alternating pressure mattress will assist in preventing skin problems, but does not preclude the need to turn.

Neurological Assessment It is most crucial in the acute phase of cord injury that frequent vital sign and neurological checks be made. The frequency of these checks can be reduced when there is evidence of vasomotor stability. Sharp and dull sensation must be evaluated above the level of the lesion because of the possibility of an ascending lesion. Patients with a high cord lesion need to be evaluated for possible head injury. This assessment includes level of consciousness, pupillary reaction, and response to questions relating to time and place.

Venous Thrombosis Deep vein thrombosis is a silent problem in cord-injured patients and carries with it the hazard of pulmonary embolism. The development of a thrombosis is influenced by stasis in the venous system, local trauma, continuous contact of the patient's calves and thighs with the bed, prolonged immobilization, and the patient's inability to sense pain. With the development of venous thrombosis, there is swelling of the involved limb, local redness, increased skin warmth, and a slight systemic temperature rise.

The routine turn schedule for skin prophylaxis also mobilizes the patient sufficiency to help prevent venous thrombosis. Elastic stockings or bandages properly applied also have prophylactic value. They should be removed for about 30 minutes once each eight-hour period.

Other preventive measures include determining the patient's leg circumference 20 cm. above and below the upper border of the patella upon admission to the hospital, and then twice daily at specified times. Passive range of motion to the lower extremities should be carried out at least twice a day. Anticoagulant therapy may also be considered.

Medications   Some medications are commonly used in patients with spinal cord injuries, and others are contraindicated. Cortisone (dexamethasone MSD) may be used initially for a short period to relieve the physiological stress phenomenon. Intravenous therapy (hyperalimentation) may be indicated during the spinal shock phase, or possibly for longer periods depending upon coexistent complications. The intravenous site of choice is the subclavian vein as there is less chance of thrombosis secondary to the vasomotor paralysis. For this reason, the veins of the lower extremities should never be used for intravenous administration.

Subcutaneous and intramuscular injections are not absorbed well because of the lack of muscle tone. Sterile abscesses may result, causing autonomic dysreflexia or increasing spasms. Injection sites are the deltoid area, the anterior thigh, and the abdominal area. These sites should be rotated and the volume injected should not exceed 1 cc. at any one site.

As a rule, sensation in cord-injured patients is limited. Intractable pain may be present after spinal shock and is due to nerve root damage. Abnormal sensation may occur at the level of the lesion in injuries causing diverse nerve root damage, such as with gunshot wounds or knife wounds. Narcotics are not favored because of the high probability of addiction. Attention to position and other comfort measures, along with the use of mild analgesics such as aspirin or propoxyphene hydrochloride, is a more acceptable approach.

Tranquilizers (ataractics) can be used to dull the environment during the initial stage following cord injury. As reflex automatism returns, relief of spasms has been achieved with diazepam.

Behavioral problems are not relieved by tranquilizers. The psychological stages of the recovery process must be resolved and this cannot be accomplished if the patient remains sedated.

Physical Therapy   A program of physical therapy and rehabilitation should be organized shortly after the patient's admission. Short- and long-range goals must be set jointly with the patient. Rehabilitation is often a very protracted program. The patient must be aware that results from the program will not be seen overnight. Thus it is important that the patient and his family be part of the rehabilitation conference when goals are discussed.

A myriad of problems can surround the patient with a spinal cord injury. Each person responds differently and adjusts to his injury in different ways. When his whole life style must be changed because of a spinal cord injury, the emotional and social problems, as well as the physical ones, can seem overwhelming. Patients need the support of family and significant others at this time. The critical care nurse assumes a major role in helping both patient and family to cope with the problems.

Rehabilitation of the cord-injured patient can be slow and tedious, and psychologically draining for the nurse, but it also offers great rewards in terms of the personal satisfaction that comes from meeting the challenge.

BIBLIOGRAPHY

Burke, D. C., "Resuscitation and Parenteral Nutrition in Patients with Acute Spinal Cord Injuries and Associated Injuries," lecture to the American Spinal Injury Association, Austin Hospital, Hidleberg.

Carini, E., and G. Owens, *Neurological and Neurosurgical Nursing*, ed. 6 (St. Louis: C. V. Mosby, 1974).

Cheshire, D. J. E., "The Complete and Centralized Treatment of Paraplegia," *International Journal of Paraplegia*, Vol. 6 (1968), pp. 59-73.

Crosby, E. E., et al., *Correlative Anatomy of the Nervous System* (New York: Macmillan, 1962).

Feiring, E. H., *Brock's Injuries of the Brain and Spinal Cord and Their Coverings*, ed. 5 (New York: Springer, 1974).

Ford, J. R., and B. Duckworth, *Physical Management for the Quadriplegic Patient* (Philadelphia: F. A. Davis, 1974).

Gardner, E., *Fundamentals of Neurology*, ed. 6 (Philadelphia: W. B. Saunders, 1975).

Guttman, L., *Spinal Cord Injuries: Comprehensive Management and Research* (London: Blackwell, 1973).

Haymaker, W., and B. Woodall, *Peripheral Nerve Injuries*, ed. 2 (Philadelphia: W. B. Saunders, 1953).

Kahn, E. A., et al., *Correlative Neurosurgery*, ed. 2 (Springfield, Ill.: Charles C Thomas, 1969).

hypothermia

The use of hypothermia (lowered body temperature) in clinical situations ranges from treating gastric hemorrhage to attempting to prevent irreversible cerebral damage. Decreased body temperature reduces cellular activity and consequently the oxygen requirement of tissues. Hypothermia is therefore induced in situations involving interrupted or reduced blood flow to vital areas to minimize tissue damage due to diminished oxygen delivery. This is the rationale for using hypothermia during open heart and neurosurgical procedures.

The presence of fever (hyperthemia) in any patient produces greater cellular oxygen requirements because of the increased rate of metabolism. Each degree of temperature elevation above normal increases metabolism approximately 7 percent. This fact becomes especially significant in the patient whose vital centers may already be compromised because of cerebral edema surgically induced or resulting from another form of insult such as hypoxia from cardiac arrest. It is to provide some margin of safety in these situations until injured tissue can recover that the body temperature is lowered or maintained at normothermic levels. Current emphasis is on preventing marked elevations in body temperature as opposed to markedly lowering the temperature. Physiological responses to cold remain the same, and there are occasions when actual hypothermia is desirable.

Since the critical care nurse is usually responsible for inducing the hypothermic state and monitoring the patient during this therapy, she must be aware of the physiological manifestations of the various phases of body cooling.

phases of hypothermia

1. COOLING PHASE

For the conscious patient, lowering body temperature is at best a most unpleasant experience. It goes without saying that adequate explanation and support for the patient and his family are integral parts of nursing care.

Although the method of inducing hypothermia will depend upon the situation and the equipment available, there are essentially two ways to proceed—surface cooling or the more direct method of bloodstream cooling. The latter is the method employed during open heart surgical procedures when the blood passes through the cooling coils in the cardiopulmonary bypass machine. Surface cooling with the use of blankets circulating a refrigerant is the method usually employed in critical care units. The cooling blanket may be placed directly against the patient, or more esthetically a sheet can cover the blanket and be tucked under the mattress to hold the blanket in place. (This should not negate turning the blanket with the patient to maintain skin contact with the cooling device.) The important point here is to avoid placing any degree of thickness between the patient and the blanket, as this will serve as an insulator and impede the cooling process.

When cooling is initiated, one blanket may be placed under the patient and another placed on top to hasten the cooling process. If a top blanket is used, care must be exercised in observing the patient's respiratory status, as the weight of the cooling blanket may limit chest excursion. Keeping the blanket in contact with areas of superficial blood flow such as the axilla and groin will also expedite cooling. In the event that a cooling device is not available, ice bags can be used to initiate the cooling process, utilizing these same principles.

The body's initial reaction to cold exposure is an attempt to conserve body heat and to increase heat production. Skin pallor that occurs is due to a vasoconstrictor response which limits superficial blood flow and thus loss of body heat. Intense activity in the form of shivering occurs to maintain body heat. The effects of these compensatory responses will be reflected in the vital signs, and it is important that the nurse understand these transient variations and consider them in evaluating the patient.

During the first 15 to 20 minutes of hypothermia induction, all vital signs increase. Pulse and blood pressure rise in response to the increased venous return produced by vasoconstriction. Respiratory rate increases to meet the added oxygen requirements of increased metabolic activity produced by shivering and to eliminate the additional carbon dioxide produced. If the patient hyperventilates with shivering, respiratory alkalosis can develop. The initial rise in temperature is a reflection of this increased cellular activity.

Since the patient requiring hypothermia usually has an existing cellular oxygenation problem, the increased oxygen consumption induced by shivering is undesirable. For this reason, chlorpromazine (Thorazine) may be given at the beginning of induction to reduce hypothalamic response. Hypoglycemia is a potential occurrence during vigorous shivering, as increased glucose is required for the increased metabolic activity.

After approximately 15 minutes the vasoconstrictor effect is broken by means of a negative feedback loop, and warm blood flow to the body surface is reestablished. This accounts for the reddened skin color following initial skin pallor. This same phenomenon can be demonstrated by holding an ice cube in the hand for a short period of time.

As superficial warm blood flow is reestablished, body heat is lost and body temperature begins to drop. The temperature can be monitored by a rectal probe taped in place which allows for frequent or continuous readings. Fecal material should be removed before the probe is inserted. Because blood cooled at the body surface continues to circulate through the body core, "downward drift" of the temperature usually continues for approximately 1 degree after the cooling blanket is turned off. In the obese patient, a greater degree of drift may be experienced. For this reason, the cooling device should be turned off before the desired hypothermic level is actually attained. Close temperature monitoring will be necessary to determine if the trend remains downward or whether an increase in temperature occurs, requiring use of the blanket again.

Skin care becomes particularly crucial due to the presence of cold and its circulatory effects. Position can be changed to eliminate pressure points, taking care to move the blanket with the patient so that body contact is maintained with the cooling device. Experience has indicated that the skin can be protected by applying a thin coating of lotion followed by talcum powder which does not appear to impede the cooling process. The application can be repeated in accordance with the skin care program, but the skin should be gently washed at least every eight hours to remove the accumulated coating.

2. HYPOTHERMIA

When the desired level of hypothermia is achieved, usually around 32°C (89.6°F), a number of other physiological changes become apparent. The vital signs at this stage are all diminished. The development of respiratory acidosis is a real possibility, since at deeper levels of hypothermia, ventilation falls off more rapidly than does reduced carbon dioxide production. Also, with increasing hypothermia the oxygen dissociation curve shifts to the left, and at lower tensions oxygen is not readily released by hemoglobin to the tissues. Because of the developing circulatory insufficiency and increased metabolic activity due to shivering, metabolic acidosis is also a possibility. Secretion of antidiuretic hormone is inhibited and an increase in urine output may be noted with a drop in the specific gravity. During hypothermia, water shifts from the intravascular spaces to the interstitial and intracellular spaces. This results from sodium moving into the cell in exchange for potassium and taking water with it. This fluid shift produces hemoconcentration, and nursing measures must be taken to prevent embolization. Such measures would include passive range of motion exercises and frequent change of position.

In hypothermic states, for every degree of temperature below normothermic levels, cerebral metabolism is decreased 6.7 percent. At 25°C (77°F) the brain volume is reduced 4.1 percent and extracellular space increases about 31.5 percent. The sensorium fades at 34 to 33°C (93 to 91.4°F). This becomes increasingly significant for the nurse working with the neurological patient who already has a depressed sensorium. She must then rely on other measures to evaluate changes in the patient's level of response. This may be accomplished by evaluating purposeful or nonpurposeful movements in response to painful stimuli and the degree of painful stimuli necessary to elicit a response.

As all cellular activity diminishes with hypothermia, cerebral activity decreases and hearing fades at approximately 34 to 33°C (93 to 91.4°F) due to reduced cochlear response. At 18 to 30°C (82 to 86°F) there is no corneal or gag reflex, and pulse irregularities may be noted due to myocardial irritability, which probably occurs as a result of potassium moving into the cell. Ventricular fibrillation is a common occurrence at this level, and consequently the patient is usually maintained at a hypothermic level around 32°C (89.6°F) to avoid cardiac problems.

Drugs tend to have a cumulative effect in the hypothermic patient. Decreased perfusion at the injection site and decreased enzyme activity result in slower chemical reactions. Therefore the intravenous route is preferred, and intramuscular or subcutaneous injections should be avoided. If a drug must be given hypodermically, it should be given deeply IM and vigilance maintained during the rewarming phase for accumulative effects.

Another potential occurrence in hypothermia is that of fat necrosis. This results from prolonged exposure to cold and decreased circulation which allows crystals to form in the fluid elements of the cells, leading to necrosis and cellular death. Nursing measures which can minimize this occurrence are turning the patient frequently, massaging the skin to increase circulation, and avoiding prolonged application of cold to any one area.

When the patient has reached the desired hypothermic level, vital signs will also level out at reduced values. Changes in vital signs must therefore be evaluated in light of the patient's hypothermic state. For example, if you are caring for a neurosurgical patient cooled to 32°C (89.6°F) and if his vital signs have decreased as you would normally expect, an increase in pulse, respirations, blood pressure to "normal levels" must be interpreted in view of the hypothermic state. Is an infectious process present? Are changes occurring in the patient's neurological status? Is intracranial pressure increasing?

If the patient is to be maintained at the hypothermic level for a prolonged period of time, this can be accomplished in a number of ways. The patient (after his temperature has risen several degrees) may need to be placed on the cooling blanket periodically and returned to the desired level. Nursing measures should be carried out gently, with a minimal degree of activity to the patient to prevent an increase in body heat, such as providing passive range of motion exercises. Bathing of the patient should be done with tepid or cool water to avoid increasing temperature in this manner. It cannot be overemphasized that prevention of pulmonary problems in the hypothermic patient is almost entirely dependent upon nursing care. Change of position allowing for postural drainage, measures to promote adequate ventilation, and suctioning to remove accumulated secretions are all extremely important in this patient.

3. REWARMING

Once it is determined that the patient no longer requires the hypothermic state, rewarming can be accomplished by a number of methods. These methods include surface rewarming, bloodstream rewarming, or rewarming naturally. Allowing the patient to rewarm naturally is the preferred method. The cooling device is removed. Blankets may be used to cover the patient but no artificial heat is used and the patient is allowed to warm at his own rate. As the patient approaches normothermic levels, it is to be anticipated that vital signs will return to precooling levels due to reversal of the physiological events. One of the hazards of artificially inducing rewarming is that of warming the skin and muscles before the heart. The heart remains in a cooled state and is unable to pump sufficient blood to meet the oxygen demands of the superficial areas. Further warming increases the dilatation of peripheral vessels and blood pools, resulting in decreased circulating volume, decreased venous return, and therefore decreased cardiac output. This sequence of events can be avoided if the heart is warmed first, as in the bloodstream method or by allowing the body to rewarm naturally. Other complications which may occur during the rewarming process are hyperpyrexia, shock (for reasons just cited), and acidosis. The acidosis occurs as a result of the increase in metabolic activity in those areas already warmed and an insufficient circulation to meet the metabolic requirements of this increased activity. Oliguria may also result, probably due to antidiuretic hormone secretion. During this rewarming phase the patient must be monitored closely for indications necessitating recooling. Using the patient's normothermic status as a baseline, these indications would include a fading sensorium, greater increase in pulse and respirations than would normally be expected with the warming process, and a drop in the blood pressure. Another important facet to be monitored is the cumulative effect of drugs given previously.

The necessity for interpreting clinical changes in the patient on the basis of the physiological changes brought about through cooling and then rewarming cannot be overemphasized. The nurse must anticipate changes and findings based on the patient's pathology and other variables present which would alter those findings. When those findings that she is anticipating do not occur, and when there is a deviation from the anticipated, the critical care nurse must be prepared to ask the question *Why?* and go about systematically determining why the anticipated change is not present. Only when she is able to do this can she render optimum nursing care.

CORINNE A. CLOUGHEN, R.N.
RAE NADINE SMITH, R.N., M.S.

22

assessment skills for the nurse: nervous system

neurological nursing assessment of head-injured and stroke patients

Nursing care of the neurological patient must be approached with the attitude that the patient can resume a useful life and be an asset to society. Nursing assessment must be done completely and systematically to establish a baseline of function and to identify when change has occurred. Understanding the physiology involved in change allows for proper nursing judgments on the appropriate intervention. Certainly a proportion of head-injured and stroke patients die or function at less than their potential, not because of pathophysiology, but as a result of nurse-allowed or nurse-induced disability. Assessment will be discussed so that disability is abolished as far as possible and not induced (or allowed to occur). The objectives for neurological crisis care are (1) to maintain and support life, (2) to prevent complications and further neurological deficit, and (3) to help the patient to accept and adjust to his limitations.

The first things the nurse should notice upon admission are the patient's general appearance, age, sex, general health and symmetry of appearance. Check for any bruising, lacerations, and involuntary movement. While examining the patient, ascertain any complaints he may have (e.g., headache, pain, seizure, dizziness, visual problems, loss of balance). Ascertain the time of occurrence and duration of the symptoms which the patient mentions. This may help you and the physician in pinpointing specific areas of dysfunction which may deserve special attention when neurological checks are made.

A medical history is important in order to pick up evidence of vascular disease, diabetes, renal disease, anemia, cancer and other metabolic dysfunctions that can complicate the neurological picture. The patient's mental and emotional status as well as general intelligence should be noted. These aspects of the assessment may be delayed if the patient is in need of immediate medical attention.

There should be a standard neurological check sheet that is utilized by the nursing staff to note any changes in the patient's condition. It should include vital signs, level of consciousness, extremity movement, and comments relative to the patient's condition. The terms used in describing the levels of consciousness should be clearly defined and utilized by all care givers (e.g., stuporous to one person may mean lethargic to another).

level of consciousness

Level of consciousness is the most reliable index for determining neurological status. Since numerous terms exist for describing levels of consciousness, and these may not have the same meaning for everyone, it is better to describe the patient's actions and state of awareness. Does he arouse to verbal stimuli? Is he oriented to time, place, person, and recent events? Are his actions and responses appropriate? Is he confused? Can he answer simple questions and follow simple commands? If the patient does not respond to verbal stimuli, does he respond to noxious stimulation by purposeful withdrawal or primitive reflexes, or is there no response to painful stimuli? Note what stimulus is used to issue a response, beginning with light touch and progressing to deep pain. Progressive restlessness and agitation should not be interpreted as an improvement in the level of consciousness, as it may be an indication of increased intracranial pressure. Sedation should therefore be avoided in cases of agitation.

vital signs

Classical signs of increased intracranial pressure include an elevated systolic pressure in conjunction with a widening pulse pressure, slow bounding pulse and respiratory irregularities.

Following any emergency treatment which may be indicated, such as maintenance of the airway for adequate ventilation, vital signs should be taken immediately and followed frequently. Any indication of shock should alert one to search for signs of thoracic and intra-abdominal injuries. It must be remembered that vital signs are only signs and are not infallible in determining the patient's neurological status (Fig. 22-1).

Hypoventilation following cerebral trauma can lead to respiratory acidosis. As the blood CO_2 increases and blood O_2 decreases, cerebral hypoxia and edema can result in secondary brain trauma. Hyperventilation following cerebral trauma produces respiratory alkalosis with increased blood O_2 and

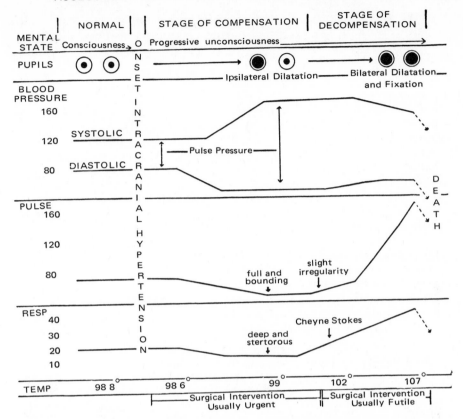

Fig. 22-1. Chart showing changes in mental state, pupils, blood pressure, pulse rate, respiratory rate, and temperature before and after the onset of fatal increase of intracranial pressure.

decreased blood CO_2 levels. This causes vasoconstriction of cerebral vessels, decreases oxygen consumption and results in cerebral hypoxia.

Since temperature elevation increases cellular metabolism, measures should be implemented to maintain temperature in the normal range, or hypothermia may be induced if indicated.

pupillary changes

In conjunction with checking the level of consciousness and vital signs, pupils must be checked frequently. Pupils are best checked in a darkened room for size, shape, equality and reaction to light. Light directed into one eye should constrict the pupil in both eyes (consensual pupillary reflex). Anisocoria (unequal pupils) may be normal in a small percentage of the population or may be an indication of neural dysfunction. Ipsilateral dilation (dilation of the pupil on the same side as the injury) can be an indication of increasing intra-cranial pressure. Severe central or bilateral pressure may cause dilation and fixation of both pupils. Bilaterally constricted pupils may be due to damage to the pons and midbrain which paralyzes the sympathetic fibers to the oculomotor nerve.

extremity movement and strength

Extremity movement and strength should also be evaluated frequently. The upper extremities can be checked by having the patient push away from and pull against your resistance. Grasp is not a reliable index for testing upper extremity strength since a weak grasp may be indicative of peripheral neuropathy alone. If weakness is noted, have the patient hold his arms straight out with eyes closed and observe for any drift of an extremity. The lower extremities are checked by having the patient raise his legs against your resistance. Weakness noted in any of these tests indicates damage to the pyramidal tracts or within the pyramidal system which controls voluntary movement.

Size, tone and muscle strength should be tested throughout the major muscle groups of the body. Careful observation for a resting or intentional tremor should be included at this time.

Superficial and deep reflexes are tested on symmetrical sides of the body and compared in relation to the strength of contraction elicited. Pathological

table 22-1
tests for reflex status

| | DEEP REFLEXES | | |
REFLEX	SITE OF STIMULUS	NORMAL RESPONSE	PERTINENT CENTRAL NERVOUS SYSTEM SEGMENT
Biceps	Biceps tendon	Contraction of biceps	Cervical 5 & 6
Brachioradialis	Styloid process of radius	Flexion of the elbow and pronation of the forearm	Cervical 5 & 6
Triceps	Triceps tendon above the olecranon	Extension of the elbow	Cervical 6, 7 & 8
Patellar	Patellar tendon	Extension of the leg at the knee	Lumbar 2, 3 & 4
Achilles	Achilles tendon	Plantar flexion of the foot	Sacral 1 & 2

SUPERFICIAL REFLEXES

REFLEX	NORMAL RESPONSE	PERTINENT CENTRAL NERVOUS SYSTEM SEGMENT
Upper abdominal	Umbilicus moves up and toward area being stroked	Thoracic 7, 8 & 9
Lower abdominal	Umbilicus moves down	Thoracic 11 & 12
Cremasteric	Scrotum elevates	Thoracic 12 & lumbar 1
Plantar	Flexion of the toes	Sacral 1 & 2
Gluteal	Skin tenses at gluteal area	Lumbar 4 through sacral 3

PATHOLOGICAL REFLEXES

REFLEX	HOW ELICITED	RESPONSE
Babinski	Stroke lateral aspect of sole of foot	In pyramidal tract disease, an extension or dorsiflexion of the big toe occurs—in addition to fanning of the toes
Chaddock	Stroke lateral aspect of foot beneath the lateral malleolus	Same type of response
Oppenheim	Stroke the anteromedial tibial surface	Same type of response
Gordon	Squeeze the calf muscles firmly	Same type of response

R. N. DeJong and A. L. Sahs et al., *Essentials of the Neurological Examination*, Philadelphia, Smith Kline Corporation, 1976, pp. 39–47.

reflexes should be noted, including the presence of a Babinski sign (dorsiflexion of the big toe and fanning of the toes when the sole of the foot is stroked). This indicates pyramidal tract disease in a person over two to three years of age. (See Table 22-1.)

cranial nerves

I. Olfactory Contains sensory fibers for the sense of smell. This test is usually deferred unless the patient complains of an inability to smell. The nerve is tested by placing aromatic substances near the patient's nose while his eyes are closed, for identification. Each nostril is checked separately. Loss of smell may be caused by a fracture of the cribriform plate or in the ethmoid area.

II. Optic Gross visual acuity is checked by having the patient read ordinary newsprint. The patient's preinjury need for glasses should be noted. Visual field testing should be done by having the patient look straight ahead with one eye covered. The examiner will move her finger from the periphery of each quadrant of vision toward the patient's center of vision. The patient should indicate when he sees the examiner's finger. This is done for both eyes and the results compared with the examiner's visual fields, which are assumed to be normal. Damage to the retina will produce a blind spot. An optic nerve lesion will produce partial or complete blindness on the same side. Damage to the optic chiasm results in bitemporal hemianopsia, blindness in both lateral visual fields. Pressure on the optic tract can cause homonymous hemianopsia, half blindness on the opposite side of the lesion in both eyes. A lesion in the parietal or temporal lobe may produce contralateral blindness in the upper or lower quadrant of vision respectively in both eyes (this is known as quadrant deficit). Damage in the occipital lobe may cause homonymous hemianopsia with central vision sparing (Fig. 22-2).

An opthalmoscopic examination should be done, with close observation of the optic disk, the vessels, and the periphery of the retina.

III. Oculomotor IV. Trochlear VI. Abducens These cranial nerves are checked together since they all innervate extraocular muscles. The parasympathetic fibers of the oculomotor nerve are responsible for lens accommodation through control of the ciliary muscle and regulation of the iris and pupillary change. The motor fibers of the oculomotor nerve innervate the muscles that elevate the eyelid as well as move the eyes up, down, and medially, including the superior rectus, inferior oblique, inferior rectus and medial rectus muscles. The trochlear nerve innervates the superior oblique muscle to move the eyes down and out. The lateral rectus muscle moves the eyes laterally and is innervated by the abducens nerve. Diplopia, nystagmus, conjugate deviation, and ptosis may indicate dysfunction of these cranial nerves. These nerves are tested by having the patient follow the examiner's finger with his eyes as it is moved in all directions of gaze (Fig. 22-3).

V. Trigeminal The trigeminal nerve has three divisions: ophthalmic, maxillary and mandibular. The sensory portion of this nerve controls sensation to the face and cornea. The motor portion controls the muscles of mastication. This nerve is partially tested by checking the corneal reflex; if it is intact, the patient will blink when the cornea is stroked with a wisp of cotton. Facial sensation can be tested by comparing light touch, temperature and pinprick on symmetrical sides of the face. The ability to chew or clench the jaw should also be observed.

VII. Facial The sensory portion of this nerve is concerned with taste on the anterior two thirds of the tongue. The motor portion controls muscles of facial expression. With a central (supranuclear) lesion, there is muscle paraly-

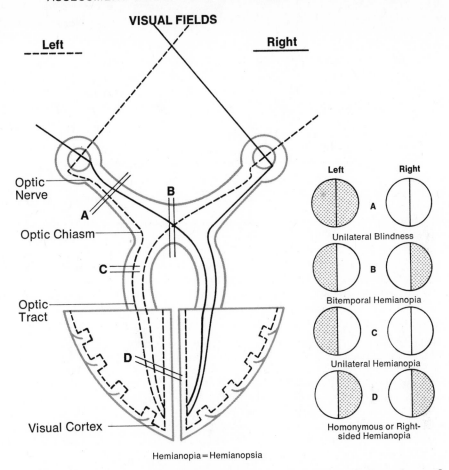

Hemianopia = Hemianopsia

Fig. 22-2. Neural pathways for vision. One can see that some of the pathways for vision cross. By creating a lesion in the occipital area (visual cortex) as in a CVA, one creates a half-blind state in both eyes on the opposite side as the brain damage. This is called *homonymous hemianopsia* (or hemianopia) (Lesion D). Note that the visual field defect is on the same side as a stroke patient's motor deficit. (Adapted from W. B. Youman, *Fundamentals of Human Physiology,* ed. 2, Chicago, Year Book Medical Publishers, 1962, p. 198)

sis of the lower half of the face on the side opposite the lesion. The muscles about the eyes and forehead are not affected. In a peripheral (nuclear or infranuclear) lesion, there is complete paralysis of facial muscles on the same side as the lesion. The most common type of peripheral facial paralysis is Bell's palsy, which consists of ipsilateral facial paralysis. There is drooping of

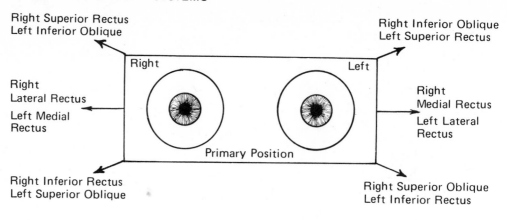

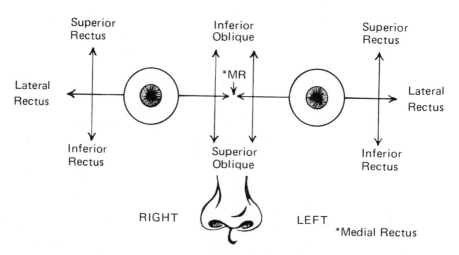

Fig. 22-3. (*Top*) Muscles used in conjugate ocular movements in the six cardinal directions of gaze. (*Bottom*) Diagram of eye muscle action. (From Joseph G. Chusid, *Correlative Neuroanatomy and Functional Neurology,* ed. 16, Los Altos, Lange Medical Publications, 1976, p. 90)

the upper lid with the lower lid slightly everted, and facial lines on the same side are obliterated with the mouth drawn toward the normal side. Artificial tears as well as taping the eye closed may be indicated to prevent corneal abrasion and irritation.

VIII. Acoustic This nerve is divided into the cochlear and vestibular branches which control hearing and equilibrium respectively. The vestibular nerve is not routinely evaluated but can be checked by doing a caloric test, usually performed on the pathological side first. The test consists of irrigating the ear canal with ice water until the patient complains of nausea or dizziness or until nystagmus is noted, which usually takes 20 to 30 seconds. If no reaction occurs within three minutes, the test is discontinued.

The cochlear nerve is tested by air and bone conduction. A vibrating tuning fork is placed on the mastoid process; after the patient can no longer hear the fork he should be able to hear it for a few seconds longer when it is placed in front of his ear (Rinne's test). The patient may complain of tinnitus or decreased hearing if this nerve is damaged.

IX. Glossopharyngeal X. Vagus   These cranial nerves are usually tested together. The glossopharyngeal nerve supplies sensory fibers to the posterior third of the tongue as well as the uvula and soft palate. The vagus innervates the larynx, pharynx, and soft palate, as well as conveys autonomic responses to the heart, stomach, lungs and small intestines. Autonomic vagal functions are not usually tested since they are checked on the general physical exam. These nerves can be tested by eliciting a gag reflex, observing the uvula for symmetrical movement when the patient says "ah," or observing midline elevation of the uvula when both sides are stroked. Inability to cough forcefully, difficulty swallowing, and hoarseness may be signs of dysfunction.

XI. Spinal Accessory   This nerve controls the trapezius and sternocleidomastoid muscles. It is tested by having the patient shrug his shoulders against resistance.

XII. Hypoglossal   This nerve controls tongue movement. It can be checked by having the patient protrude his tongue. Check for deviation from midline, tremor and atrophy. If deviation is noted secondary to damage of the nerve, it will be to the side of the lesion.

higher intellectual function tests

Intellectual performance should be evaluated within the context of the patient's educational and socioeconomic background. The quality of language production can be ascertained by the patient's ability to speak, read, write and comprehend. Deficiency in any of these language functions is known as aphasia. Depending on the type of aphasia noted, different areas of damage in the brain can be located.

Abstract reasoning is often evaluated by having the patient explain simple proverbs and slogans, such as, "A rolling stone gathers no moss." Keep in mind that many "normal" people have difficulty with this exercise. Subtraction of serial 7's from 100 is a test of calculation and attention span.

The inability to recognize objects by sight, touch or sound is termed agnosia. The ability to recognize and identify objects by touch is called stereognosis, and is a function of the parietal lobe. Identification of an object by the sense of sight is a function of the parieto-occipital junction. The temporal lobe is responsible for identification of objects by sound. Each of these senses should be tested separately. For example, a patient may not be able to identify a whistle by its sound, but may recognize it immediately if he holds it or looks at it.

sensory tests

The primary forms of sensation are evaluated first. These include light touch, superficial pain, temperature, and vibration. With the patient's eyes closed, multiple areas of the body are tested, including the hands, forearms, upper arms, trunk, thighs, lower legs and feet.

Note the patient's ability to perceive the sensation; compare distal areas to proximal areas and compare right and left sides at corresponding areas. Note if sensory change involves one entire side of the body. Abnormal results may indicate damage somewhere along the pathways of the receptors in the skin, muscles, joints and tendons, spinothalamic tracts, or sensory area of the cortex.

Cortical forms of sensation should also be tested. Disturbances of these forms, when the primary forms of sensation are intact, indicate damage to the parietal lobe. Cortical forms of sensation include:

1. Graphesthesia—the ability to recognize numbers or letters traced lightly on the skin. Bilateral sides are compared.
2. Point localization—the ability to locate a spot on the body touched by the examiner.
3. Two-point discrimination—tested by using two sharp objects and determining the smallest area in which two points can be perceived.
4. Extinction phenomenon—the inability to recognize that two areas have been touched when the examiner simultaneously touches two identical areas on opposite sides of the body.
5. Texture discrimination—the ability to recognize materials such as cotton, burlap and wool by feeling them.

All tests are done with the patient's eyes closed.

cerebellar function tests

The cerebellum controls balance and coordination and there are many tests of function. Some of the more common ones follow:

1. Romberg test—done by having the patient stand with his feet together, first with his eyes open, then with eyes closed. Observe for sway or direction of falling and be prepared to catch the patient if necessary.
2. Tandem walking—done by having the patient walk heel to toe.
3. Finger to nose test—done by having the patient touch his finger to the examiner's finger, then touch his own nose. Overshooting or past pointing the mark is called dysmetria. Both sides are tested individually.
4. Heel to shin test—done by having the patient run the heel of one foot down the shin of the other leg. This is done on both sides.
5. Rapidly alternating movements (RAM)—checked on each side by having the patient touch each finger on one hand to his thumb in rapid succession, or by performing rapid pronation and supination of his hand on his leg. Observe for accuracy and smoothness of action in these tests. Ataxia and tremor are common manifestations of cerebellar dysfunction. Inability to perform rapid alternating movements is termed adiadokokinesia.

other observations

1. Battle's sign, bruising over the mastoid area, is suggestive of basal skull fracture.
2. Raccoon's eyes or periorbital edema is suggestive of fronto-basilar fracture.
3. Rhinorrhea, drainage of cerebral spinal fluid via the nose, is suggestive of fracture of the cribriform plate with herniation of a fragment of the dura and arachnoid through the fracture.
4. Otorrhea, drainage of cerebral spinal fluid from the ear, is usually associated with fracture of the petrous portion of the temporal bone.
5. Decorticate posturing occurs when the cortex of the brain is nonfunctioning (supratentorial damage). The arms are abducted and in rigid flexion, with the hands internally rotated and fingers flexed. The legs are in rigid extension.
6. Decerebrate rigidity indicates damage to the midbrain. Full extension of the arms and legs occurs, with internal rotation at the shoulder, flexed fingers and internally rotated toes.
7. Meningeal irritation can be detected by the presence of nuchal rigidity in conjunction with pyrexia, headache and photophobia. A positive Kernig's sign, pain in the neck when the thigh is flexed on the abdomen and the leg extended at the knee, may also be present.

Throughout the neurological assessment, the examiner should note the patient's behavior for appropriateness, emotional status, cooperativeness, attention span and memory.

Following the neurological exam, the nurse should record her findings, with particular emphasis on the abnormalities. Frequent reevaluation is necessary to ascertain change in the patient's condition.

Nursing care is directed toward returning the patient to maximum functioning, preventing complications and further neurological deficits, and helping the patient adjust to his limitations. Rehabilitation begins as soon as the patient enters the hospital. Adequate assessment of the neurological patient can not only prevent unnecessary complications and disability, but is the first ingredient for optimum rehabilitation.

BIBLIOGRAPHY

Chusid, J. G., *Correlative Neuroanatomy and Functional Neurology*, ed. 16 (Los Altos, Calif.: Lange Medical Publications, 1976).

DeJong, R. N., and A. L. Sahs, *Essentials of the Neurological Examination* (Philadelphia: Smith Kline Corporation, rev. 1976).

Jackson, F. E., "The Pathophysiology of Head Injuries," *Clinical Symposia*, Vol. 18, No. 3 (July-December 1966).

_____, "The Treatment of Head Injuries," *Clinical Symposia*, Vol. 19, No. 1 (January-March 1967).

Parsons, L. C., "Respiratory Changes in Head Injury," *American Journal of Nursing* (November 1971), pp. 2187–2191.

Perlo, V. P., "Answers to Questions of the Physical Examination in Central Nervous System Disease," *Hospital Rounds* (May 1971), pp. 129–150.

Ranschoff, J., and A. Fleisher, "Head Injuries," *Journal of the American Medical Association*, Vol. 234, No. 8 (November 24, 1975), pp. 861–864.

invasive neurological assessment techniques

Harvey Cushing, with his use of blood pressure measurement, is said to be the first neurosurgeon to introduce a form of instrument monitoring. We have progressed from this early intermittent and limited pressure monitoring into advanced techniques for continual pressure measurement. In 1952, Dr. Ryder opened the door to contemporary management of the neurosurgical patient with his work on intracranial pressure (ICP) measurement. Today, invasive techniques are frequently utilized to accurately and continuously assess the blood pressure, pulmonary artery pressure and intracranial pressure of the neurological patient. Correlating invasive measurements with noninvasive clinical assessment frequently reduces the amount of time required to accurately diagnose the problem, increases the amount of time available for treatment, and provides continual feedback on the patient's response to selected treatments.

indications for measurement

BLOOD PRESSURE

Direct or invasive blood pressure measurements of critically ill patients provide a variety of advantages over indirect or noninvasive techniques. These include: (1) accuracy (indirect or cuff pressures are particularly inaccurate during hypotensive episodes because of decreased cardiac output and increased vascular resistance), (2) ability to monitor the arterial mean pressure, (3) provision of a continual reading with an alarm system, (4) access for blood sampling, and (5) more efficient use of nursing time. Neurological conditions in which accurate and continual blood pressures are important include:

1. *Vascular lesions.* It is well established that an elevation of blood pressure is a cause of aneurysm rerupture. Aneurysms and subarachnoid hemorrhages are frequently treated by induced hypotension. Just as blood pressure is continuously monitored on a patient in shock being treated with vasopressors to increase pressure, it should likewise be monitored on the patient being treated with hypotensive agents to reduce pressure. In this situation, both hypertension and severe hypotension must be avoided.

2. *Strokes.* Mean arterial pressure must be maintained at a level above 60 to 70 mm. Hg to prevent the loss of autoregulation mechanisms in areas of focal cerebral ischemia.

3. *Increased intracranial pressure.* Both hypoxia and hypercarbia contribute

to alterations of intracranial pressure. An increased P_{CO_2} results in cerebral vasodilation, thereby increasing blood volume and intracranial pressure. Serial blood gases are necessary if P_{CO_2} is to be regulated by a method such as controlled hyperventilation. The majority of patients with severe head injuries develop hyperventilation with respiratory alkalosis. Early changes in respiratory patterns are usually too subtle for bedside detection. Serial blood gases obtained via an indwelling arterial cannula provide a safer, more efficient technique of blood sampling and certainly one more comfortable for the patient than repeated arterial punctures. The continual monitoring of the pressure between blood gas samplings protects the patient from the risks of bleedback and clotting of the cannula.

In patients with increased intracranial pressure or the potential to develop it, direct mean blood pressure measurement is compared with the mean intracranial pressure to determine the cerebral perfusion pressure (mean arterial blood pressure minus mean intracranial pressure). A normal cerebral perfusion pressure is at least 50 mm. Hg.

4. *Spinal cord injury.* During a laminectomy, increased blood pressure is often considered a warning sign of pressure on the spinal cord. Clinically, acute cervical cord injuries are often associated with hypotension. In this situation, blood pressure monitoring is often accompanied by blood volume monitoring, such as pulmonary artery and central venous pressure monitoring. During the hypotensive stage, patients with acute spinal cord injury have a low CVP. As sympathectomized muscles gradually regain tone, the blood-containing space contracts. If the patient has been receiving vigorous fluid replacement to correct his low blood pressure and low CVP, pulmonary edema may result. Increased fluid volume causes increased venous pressure on the left side of the heart which frequently is not manifested in CVP readings taken on the right side of the heart.

PULMONARY ARTERY PRESSURE

Pulmonary artery pressure measures pressure from the left side of the heart and gives an accurate determination of fluid volume as affected by IV fluid replacement or diuresis.

Examples of conditions in which accurate blood volume monitoring is indicated include:

1. *Cord injury.* Pulmonary edema usually develops within 11 to 24 hours after cord injury. Death from pulmonary edema is not uncommon in acute quadriplegia.
2. *Head injury.* Pulmonary edema often develops rapidly after head injury.
3. *Multiple trauma.* The blood volume picture is further complicated in the trauma patient who presents with acute cervical spinal cord injury with associated injury, particularly of the chest. It is often difficult to determine if the patient is hypotensive secondary to the sympathectomy effect or to the blood loss.

INTRACRANIAL PRESSURE

Intracranial pressure measurement usually provides an indication of changes in intracranial pressure dynamics before such changes are clinically evident, thereby prompting the initiation of measures to reduce increased intracranial pressure. The classical syndrome of increased intracranial pressure, which includes increased pulse pressure, decreased pulse, and decreased respirations with pupillary changes, usually occurs only in association with posterior fossa lesions and seldom with the more commonly observed supratentorial mass lesions, such as subdural hematoma. When these classical Kocher-Cushing signs do accompany a supratentorial lesion, they are associated with a sudden pressure increase and usually herald a state of decompensation. Brain damage is usually irreversible at this point and death is imminent.

Between the onset of increased intracranial pressure and herniation is a stage where a wide variety of treatments are available to reduce intracranial pressure. Measures such as hypothermia, the drainage of cerebral spinal fluid, hyperventilation and the use of corticosteroids and hypertonic solutions have proven valuable adjuncts to surgery. Since these techniques are usually most effective before the patient becomes clinically symptomatic, the need for pressure-reducing measures is best determined by direct pressure measurement.

Normal intracranial pressure ranges between 0 and 10 mm. Hg, with an upper limit of 15 mm. Hg. In acute situations, patients frequently become symptomatic at pressures around 20 to 25 mm. Hg. The patient's tolerance of changes in intracranial pressure varies with the acuteness of its onset. Patients with a slower buildup of intracranial pressure, such as occurs with certain brain tumors, are more tolerant of elevations in the ICP than patients with rapid development of pressure changes as seen in acute subdural hematoma.

The Monro-Kellie hypothesis states that the volume of the intracranium is equal to the volume of the brain, plus the volume of the blood, plus the volume of the cerebrospinal fluid (CSF). Any alterations in the volume of any of these components of the cranial vault, as well as the addition of a lesion, will lead to an increase in intracranial pressure.

Conditions which may be indications for intracranial pressure measurements are:

1. *Increased volume of brain.* Changes in the volume of the brain can occur secondary to ischemic changes, such as those which follow a stroke. Extensive manipulation of the brain during surgery or the trauma of closed head injury may lead to diffuse, generalized cerebral edema. Metastatic tumors can cause massive edema. Increased ICP is now recognized as a significant component of the Reye-Johnson syndrome.

2. *Increased volume of blood.* AV malformations and aneurysms are common causes of bleeding within the intracranial vault. Hemorrhagic strokes may cause massive bleeding. Subdural and epidural hematomas are seen frequently in critical care areas. Cerebral vasodilation following increases in Pco_2 may cause a significant increase in the volume of blood within the cranial vault.

3. *Increased volume of cerebrospinal fluid.* An increase in CSF production or a decrease in CSF absorption would change the volume of the CSF within the cranial vault. Patients with congenital hydrocephalus are often monitored following shunt revisions. More frequently seen in the critical care area are patients with decreased reabsorption of CSF, such as occurs with subarachnoid hemorrhage.

4. *Lesions.* Brain abscesses and brain tumors increase ICP.

Any of these conditions may result in an increase in intracranial pressure. As the ICP increases, cerebral blood flow decreases, leading to tissue hypoxia, a decrease in pH, an increase in P_{CO_2}, cerebral vasodilation, and edema, thus leading to further pressure increases. This malignant cycle continues until herniation occurs. The three major types of cerebral herniation are:

1. Herniation of the cingulate gyrus under the falx
2. Herniation of the uncus of the temporal lobe beneath the free edge of the tentorium
3. Downward displacement of the midbrain through the tentorial notch. With an open head injury, transcalvarial herniation may result.

techniques of measurement

Determination of these pressures requires the use of a transducer. A transducer can be defined as a device used to change varying pressures into proportionately varying signals which can be displayed on an oscilloscope, meter, and/or recorder (Fig. 22–4). The first report of the use of a transducer for

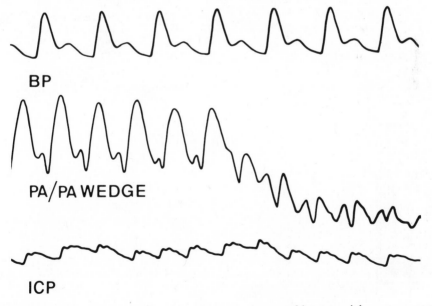

BP

PA/PA WEDGE

ICP

Fig. 22-4. Blood pressure, pulmonary artery pressure, and intracranial pressure waveforms.

human blood pressure measurement was in 1947. Various transducers are currently available for clinical application (see pp. 189–190).

BLOOD PRESSURE MEASUREMENT

The basic system for blood pressure measurement consists of a transducer which is connected via a tubing system directly to the patient's artery, usually the radial, brachial, or femoral. Pressure from the artery is transmitted to the transducer by a column of fluid and converted to a pressure tracing which can be read on a monitor (Fig. 22–5). To avoid clotting of the arterial cannula, a mildly heparinized flush solution, such as 5 percent dextrose and water, normal saline, or lactated Ringer's, is administered at a continual rate of 3 to 6 cc. per hour. To prevent bleeding back, the flush solution is maintained at a pressure higher than the patient's systolic arterial pressure. The complication of sepsis is avoided by maintaining a sterile system between the transducer and the patient. With a system such as this, Gardner's study reported the risk to be 0.2 percent with a total of 4,500 direct arterial lines in over 12,000 intensive care patient days. Other hospitals have published similar statistics.[1]

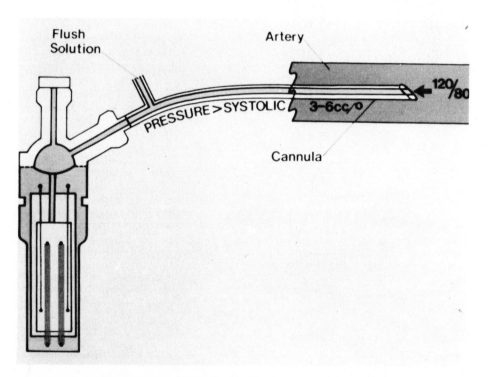

Fig. 22-5. Basic principle of blood pressure measurement.

The system provides a continual reading with an alarm system as the pressure from the artery is transmitted by the fluid column to the diaphragm of the transducer. In this particular example, the strain gauge wires are activated, converting the pulsating physiological pressure into an electrical signal that is displayed on a monitor.

PULMONARY ARTERY PRESSURE MEASUREMENT

To determine pulmonary artery (PA) and wedge pressures, a balloon-tipped catheter is inserted at the bedside (see p. 188). The catheter is inserted percutaneously or via venous cutdown into the antecubital, jugular, subclavian or femoral vein. It is then advanced through the vein into the right atrium, to the right ventricle and into the pulmonary artery. The progress of the catheter through the right side of the heart is followed by distinctive waveform changes on the oscilloscope or recorder (Fig. 22–6). With the balloon inflated, the catheter wedges into a distal branch of the pulmonary artery. This wedge (PAW) pressure reflects the pressure of the left side of the heart. Wedge pressures are taken intermittently; with the balloon deflated, continuous PA pressures are obtained. The basic system for setting up and maintaining the PA catheter is the same as that described for blood pressure measurement, using a continual IV flush rate of 3 cc. per hour.

INTRACRANIAL PRESSURE MEASUREMENT

There are basically three techniques for measuring intracranial pressure: (1) intraventricular, (2) subarachnoid (subdural), and (3) epidural.

Intraventricular Technique   The intraventricular technique of ICP measurement was first reported in 1952 and consists of placing a catheter into the lateral ventricle. A twist drill hole is placed lateral to the midline at the level of the coronal suture, usually on the nondominant side. A catheter is placed through the cerebrum into the anterior horn of the lateral ventricle. On occasion, the occipital horn is used. Connected to the ventricular catheter via stopcock and/or pressure tubing is a pressure transducer (Fig. 22–7). Saline or Ringer's lactate solution is used to provide the fluid column between the CSF and diaphragm of the transducer. Fifteen mm. Hg is considered the upper limit of normal ICP, with some patients having excursions to 100 mm. Hg.

Advantages
1. Direct measuring of pressure from the CSF.
2. Access for CSF drainage or sampling.
3. Access for determining volume-pressure responses.

Disadvantages
1. Risk of infection (Sundbärg et al. documented a clinically apparent CNS infection rate of 1.1 percent).[2]
2. Difficulty in locating the lateral ventricle following midline shifting of the ventricle, or collapse of the ventricle as a normal compensatory mechanism for increases in pressure.

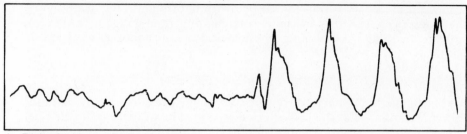

A. Right Atrium to Right Ventricle

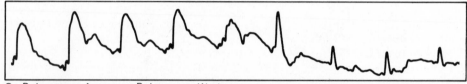

B. Right Ventricle to Pulmonary Artery

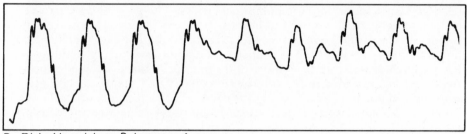

C. Pulmonary Artery to Pulmonary Wedge

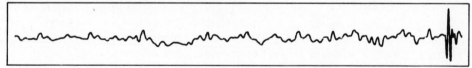

D. Pulmonary Wedge Pressure

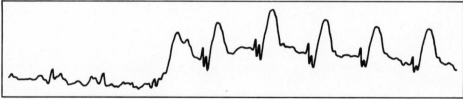

E. Wedge to Pulmonary Artery

Fig. 22-6. Waveforms produced by progression of catheter through right heart to pulmonary wedge position.

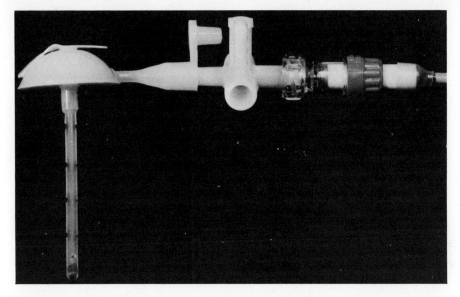

Fig. 22-7. Intraventricular cannula with subminiature transducer.

Subarachnoid Technique The measurement of ICP via a subarachnoid screw was first reported in 1973. The screw device is inserted via a twist drill hole and extends into the subdural or subarachnoid space. Although the cerebrum is not penetrated, pressures, as with the intraventricular technique, are measured directly from the CSF. A transducer filled with saline or Ringer's lactate solution may be fastened directly to the screw or connected via pressure tubing (Fig. 22-8). Volume-pressure responses have been determined using this technique.

Advantages
1. Direct pressure measurement from CSF.
2. Does not require penetration of cerebrum to locate ventricle.
3. Access for determining volume-pressure responses.
4. Access for CSF drainage and sampling.

Disadvantages
1. Risk of infection comparable to intraventricular technique.
2. Requires closed skull.

Epidural Technique This technique involves placing an epidural device such as a balloon with radioisotopes, a radio transmitter or a fiberoptic transducer between the skull and the dura. Some researchers feel that dural compression and surface tension, as well as thickening of the dura during prolonged monitoring, tend to cause inaccuracies in the pressure readings. Although subarachnoid and intraventricular pressures correlate well with each

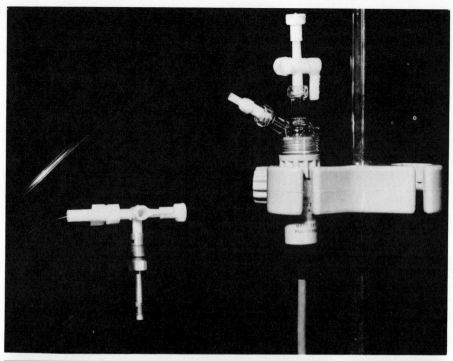

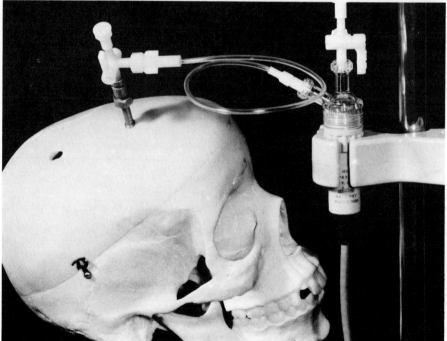

Fig. 22-8. (*Top*) Subarachnoid screw with standard transducer. (*Bottom*) Measurement of ICP via subarachnoid technique.

other, there have been inconsistent correlations between direct CSF pressure and the various epidural techniques.

Advantage
   1. Less invasive.

Disadvantages
   1. Questionable reflection of CSF pressure.
   2. No route for CSF drainage and sampling.
   3. Volume-pressure responses not feasible.

volume pressure response

The brain can accommodate or compensate for minimal changes in volume by partial collapse of the cisterns, ventricles and vascular systems. During this compensatory period, the intracranial pressure remains fairly constant. When these compensatory mechanisms have been fully utilized, pressure increases rapidly until the blood supply to the medulla is cut off. The status of these compensatory mechanisms can be evaluated by ICP monitoring. A technique utilized by Miller incorporates the injection of small amounts of fluid via an intraventricular catheter.[3] If the ICP increases less than 2 mm. Hg with a 1-ml. injection given over an interval of one second, the patient is not undergoing compensatory changes. A response of at least 3 mm. Hg per ml. per second is considered a sign of altered compensation or compliance. In selected cases, ventricular fluid is withdrawn.

pressure waveforms

Pressure waveforms of varying shape are displayed on the monitor. Hemodynamic and respiratory oscillations can be observed in the intracranial pressure traces. At times, the waveforms closely resemble arterial pressure waveforms, and other times resemble CVP waveforms.

Certain patients exhibit a phenomenon known as plateau waves. Plateau waves, as defined by Lundberg, are spontaneous rapid increases of pressure to 50 to 100 mm. Hg, usually occurring in patients with existing elevations of intracranial pressure.[4] They last approximately 5 to 20 minutes and are usually accompanied by a temporary increase in neurological deficits. Patients who sustain ICPs greater than 50 mm. Hg for periods longer than 20 minutes usually have a poor prognosis. Although the mechanisms of plateau waves or A waves are not clear, they have been correlated with certain clinical conditions. A report by Nornes correlates an increased frequency of plateau waves in the patient with an aneurysm who has a tendency to rebleed.[5] Although B and C waves have been described, these do not have the clinical significance of the A wave or plateau wave.

clinical implications

Clinical evaluation alone is not a reliable means of detecting changes in BP, PA pressure, ICP and the patient's response to treatment. The classical Kocher-Cushing syndrome is usually not a warning, but rather, a symptom of brain death. Recognizable clinical signs and symptoms of increased ICP usually occur after the patient has passed the optimal time for treatment, and sometimes not at all. By correlating clinical evaluations with invasive neurological assessments via direct BP, PA pressure and ICP measurements, patients can be diagnosed and treated in a more rational fashion. Increased ICP is now recognized as one of the mechanisms of death in Reye-Johnson syndrome. An autopsy study on patients with head injuries revealed transtentorial herniation as a cause of death in 34 percent of the automobile accident victims. Fifty percent of all deaths related to motorcycle accidents are secondary to head injuries.

In units where cerebral perfusion pressures are monitored, routine nursing measures such as suctioning and positioning have been found to have significant effects on this pressure. Interruptions in osmotherapy and ventilator support have resulted in dramatic alterations in the relationship between the BP and ICP. Invasive neurological assessment, providing continual feedback on parameters such as BP, PA pressure and ICP, has proven effective in determining diagnosis and the effectiveness of the therapeutic regimen.

REFERENCES

1. R. M. Gardner et al., "Percutaneous Indwelling Radial Artery Catheters for Monitoring Cardiovascular Function; Prospective Study of the Risk of Thrombosis and Infection," *New England Journal of Medicine*, Vol. 290 (1974), pp. 1227–1231.
2. G. Sundbärg et al., "Complications Due to Prolonged Ventricular Fluid Pressure Recording in Clinical Practice," *Intracranial Pressure*, M. Brock and H. Dietz, eds. (New York: Springer-Verlag, 1973).
3. J. D. Miller, "Volume and Pressure in the Craniospinal Axis," *Clinical Neurosurgery, Proceedings of the Congress of Neurological Surgeons*, Vol. 22 (Baltimore: Williams & Wilkins, 1975), ch. 7.
4. N. Lundberg, "Continuous Recording and Control of Ventricular Fluid Pressure in Neurosurgical Practice," *Acta Psychiatrica Scandinavica*, Vol. 36, Suppl. 149 (1960), pp. 1–193.
5. H. Nornes, "Monitoring of Patients with Intracranial Aneurysms," *Clinical Neurosurgery, Proceedings of the Congress of Neurological Surgeons*, Vol. 22 (Baltimore: Williams & Wilkins, 1975), ch. 18.

BIBLIOGRAPHY

Jorgenson, P., and J. Riishede, "Comparative Clinical Studies of Epidural and Ventricular Pressure," *Intracranial Pressure*, M. Brock and H. Dietz, eds. (New York: Springer-Verlag, 1972), pp. 41–45.

Langfitt, T. W., "Clinical Methods for Monitoring Intracranial Pressure and Measuring Cerebral Blood Flow," *Clinical Neurosurgery, Proceedings of the Congress of Neurological Surgeons*, Vol. 22 (Baltimore: Williams & Wilkins, 1975), ch. 17.

Mickell, J. J., et al., "Intracranial Pressure Monitoring in Reye-Johnson Syndrome," *Critical Care Medicine*, Vol. 4, No. 1 (January–February 1976), pp. 1–7.

Miller, J., and P. Leech, "Effects of Mannitol and Steroid Therapy in Intracranial Volume-Pressure Relationship in Patients," *Journal of Neurosurgery*, Vol. 42 (1975), p. 274.

Schroeder, J. S., and E. K. Daily, "Intra-Arterial Pressure Monitoring," *Techniques in Bedside Hemodynamic Monitoring* (St. Louis: C. V. Mosby, 1976), ch. 6.

Tindall, G. T., et al., "Monitoring of Patients with Head Injuries," *Clinical Neurosurgery, Proceedings of the Congress of Neurological Surgeons*, Vol. 22 (Baltimore: Williams & Wilkins, 1975), ch. 19.

Vries, J. K., et al., "A Subarachnoid Screw for Monitoring Intracranial Pressure," *Journal of Neurosurgery*, Vol. 39 (1973), pp. 416–419.

specific crisis situations

JOHN H. ALTSHULER, M.D.

disseminated intravascular coagulation syndrome

Disseminated intravascular coagulation syndrome has the singular distinction of being the oldest universally accepted hypercoagulable clinical state known. The many faces of this syndrome have led to synonyms so that it is known as consumption coagulopathy, diffuse intravascular clotting, and the defibrination syndrome. In most "clotting circles" however, the syndrome has become honorably dubbed "DIC" and will be referred to by this nickname throughout this chapter.

Unfortunately, DIC cannot be understood without a working knowledge of the clotting mechanism both *in vitro* and *in vivo* (as they differ). Lest the reader be discouraged by the thought of this task, let me assure her that the mystery of clotting will be sequentially and simply outlined in the pages that follow.

the blood coagulation mechanism

a. in vitro mechanism

If blood removed from a patient could remain unaltered in a syringe, it would not clot. However, upon exposure of blood to any surface outside of a blood vessel lining, (e.g., a syringe) changes in clotting factors start immediately. These changes are irreversible and cannot be stopped without the addition of inhibitory chemicals to blood. The changes that occur bear the relationship of enzyme (organic catalyst) to substrate (specific substance upon which an enzyme acts). The initiation of change referred to above is as yet unknown, although evidence suggests that exposure of blood to a foreign surface causes molecular alteration in one clotting factor. The unaltered clotting

477

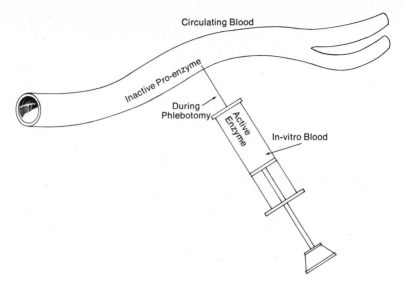

Fig. 23-1. *In vitro* clotting mechanism.

factor, known as a proenzyme, is thus converted to an altered state—an active enzyme (Fig. 23-1). One molecule of enzyme acts upon a specific substrate which is also a proenzyme clotting factor. The single active enzyme molecule is capable of converting not one but perhaps thousands of specific substrate molecules into other active enzymes. This is but a single event in what is to become an entire series of enzyme-substrate reactions. Hence a chain reaction is born whereby activation of a single proenzyme molecule may lead to activation of the entire clotting mechanism. The chain reaction involves at least nine well-defined clotting factors with 34 others reported as being involved in disputed points along the way. During the *in vitro* clotting process, at one place the reaction is known to be self-perpetuating so that a vicious cycle of clot activation ensues causing clot formation to accelerate rapidly. The cascade of events may be paralleled with a waterfall as represented in Fig. 23-2.

Understanding the basic concepts of clotting far outweighs knowledge of technical factors involved. However, some of these factors must be known. The first factor to be activated in clotting is inactive XII. The active enzymatic form of XII is annotated XIIa. The enzyme XIIa acts upon the next clotting proenzyme factor—inactive factor XI—converting it to the active enzyme XIa, and so on. Diagrammatically the clotting sequence may be represented as in Fig. 23-3.

Note that the activation of factor X requires factor VIII, and activation of factor prothrombin requires factor V. Furthermore, a fatty (lipid) substance derived from platelets (platelet cofactor −3) must be present at the site of activity of both factors VIII and V. The self-perpetuating effect in the mechanism takes place by creating the vicious cycle of activation of factor X through the effect of thrombin on factor VIII. Thrombin is a very potent enzyme converting fibrinogen to fibrin clot. The initial fibrin clot is further stabilized by yet another clotting factor (XIII).

As in most biological orders, a system antagonistic to the clotting mechanism exists—the fibrinolytic system. Again, a series of proenzymes, when activated, is converted to enzymes which are capable of dissolving blood clots. The dissolving or lytic enzyme is called *plasmin* and is derived from the proenzyme *plasminogen* normally present in whole blood. Unlike the coagulation mechanism, the fibrinolytic system is not activated by withdrawal of blood from the body. Nonetheless the state of the fibrinolytic system may be determined *in vitro* by assaying plasmin levels.

b. in vivo mechanism

In the normal state, the coagulation mechanism is inactive. Due to normal wear and tear of blood vessel linings, holes occur through which blood leaks out. The hole, however, is promptly plugged by the adherence of platelets

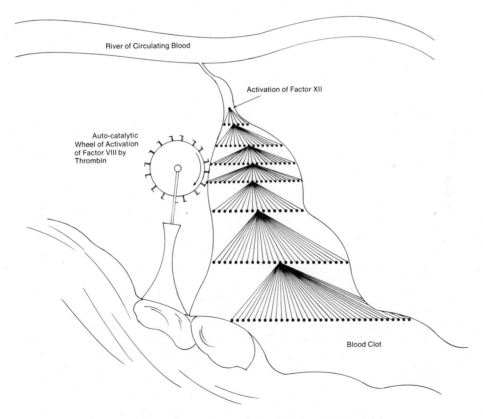

Fig. 23-2. Waterfall sequence of blood clotting.

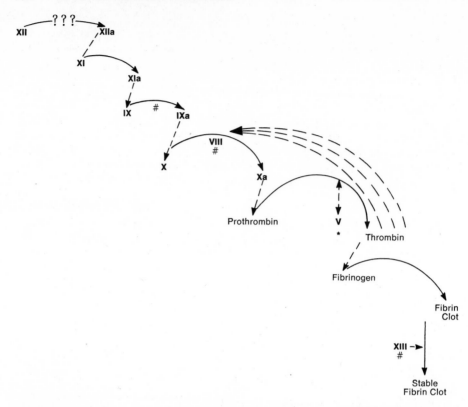

Fig. 23-3. Clotting sequence. [#—calcium ion required; *—calcium and fat (lipid) substance derived from platelets—both required.]

to the hole, thus preventing blood leakage outside of the vessel. The seepage of tissue juice into the rent in the vessel wall attracts platelets and causes the latter to adhere to the hole, effectively plugging up the leak. This phenomenon is further enhanced by the platelets' own ability to release a chemical (adenosine diphosphate—or ADP). Because platelet plugging may interfere with normal smooth flow (laminar flow) of blood through the vessel, eddy currents are set up which tend to activate the intrinsic clotting mechanism. Such activation would cause clots to form on top of the platelet plug, releasing thrombin in the process of clotting, further attracting platelets to the clot site, and causing additional clot to form at the local site of vessel leak. Total vessel occlusion by clot would occur if it were not for the fibrinolytic system which keeps a delicate balance between clot formation and clot lysis (Fig. 23-4).

A well-controlled balance between clotting and lysis is established in humans. Diagramatically, a seesaw plank depicts coagulation control (Fig. 23-5). On one side of the plank are the clotting factors (CF) and on the other side are the fibrinolytic factors (FF). Note that the plank may oscillate in a normal range. It is important to remember that the range of fluctuation may increase to a point where laboratory tests are abnormal but clinical evidence of pathological bleeding or clotting is not seen. Obviously, when this warning fluctu-

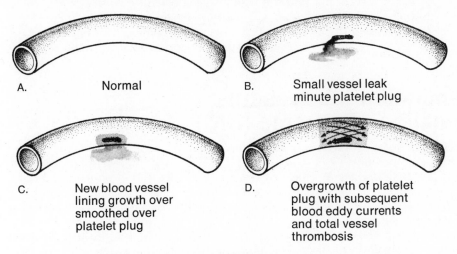

A.   Normal

B.   Small vessel leak minute platelet plug

C.   New blood vessel lining growth over smoothed over platelet plug

D.   Overgrowth of platelet plug with subsequent blood eddy currents and total vessel thrombosis

Fig. 23-4. Sequence of thrombus formation in blood vessels.

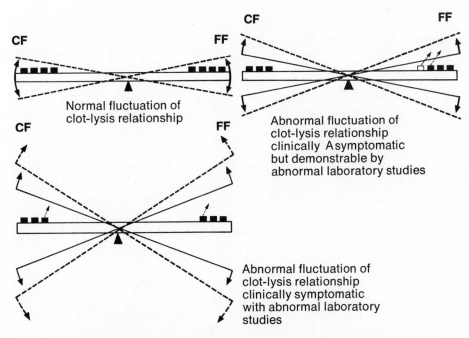

Normal fluctuation of clot-lysis relationship

Abnormal fluctuation of clot-lysis relationship clinically Asymptomatic but demonstrable by abnormal laboratory studies

Abnormal fluctuation of clot-lysis relationship clinically symptomatic with abnormal laboratory studies

Fig. 23-5. Normal and abnormal fluctuations in clot-lysis relationships.

ation range is exceeded, the patient will demonstrate overt clinical evidence of thrombosis or hemorrhage.

The balance may be upset by:

1. Decreasing clotting factors as in classic hemophilia where clotting factor VIII is low and the patient has a bleeding tendency.
2. Increasing fibrinolytic factors causing excessive bleeding.
3. Decreasing fibrinolytic factors causing pathological thromboses.
4. Increasing clotting factors causing hypercoagulability (still debated).

disseminated intravascular coagulation syndrome (DIC)

DIC is a syndrome of transient coagulation causing transformation of fibrinogen to fibrin clot, often associated with acute hemorrhage. The syndrome is secondary to a host of diseases and diversity of etiological factors. Paradoxically, DIC is a bleeding disorder resulting from an increased tendency to clot. Although the causes are varied, the syndrome itself has many common factors regardless of etiology. Almost uniformly, patients have arterial hypotension often associated with shock resulting in arterial vasoconstriction and capillary dilatation. Blood is then shunted to the venous side, bypassing dilated capillaries due to the opening of arteriovenous shunts (Fig. 23-6). The dilated capillaries now contain stagnant blood which accumulates metabolic by-products (pyruvic and lactic acid) rendering the blood acidotic. Further, the precipitating factors in DIC frequently cause release of procoagulant substances into the bloodstream (e.g., free hemoglobin, bacterial toxins, thrombosis-promoting placental tissue, amniotic fluid, cancer tissue fragments). We thus have three concomitant procoagulating effects in capillary blood: (1) acidosis—a potent coagulation activator, (2) blood stagnation, and (3) presence of coagulation-promoting substances in blood.

A special event in DIC may be the activation of clotting factors in cardiopulmonary bypass due to contact of blood with the extracorporeal apparatus. The result of DIC to this point is the accumulation of clot in the body's capillaries, the length of which exceeds 100,000 miles in the average adult. Thus the amount of blood clot sequestration in capillaries in acute DIC is enormous. Because of the rapidity of the process, clotting factors are effectively used up in the capillary clotting process at a rate exceeding factor replenishment. Circulating blood hence becomes depleted of clotting factors. With such depletion, the patient can no longer maintain normal hemostasis; therefore bleeding follows. Hemorrhage starts from needle and incisional sites and from the respiratory, genitourinary and gastrointestinal tracts. Blood cells now become suspended in serum rather than plasma—serum being the liquid portion of blood minus the clotting factors used up in clotting. Not all clotting factors are used up in clotting, although the platelet blood cell is totally removed in clotting. Table 23-1 shows the difference between serum and plasma.

ARTERIOLE - CAPILLARY - VENULE RELATIONSHIP IN NORMAL AND DIC

NORMAL

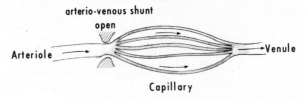

Capillary perfusion is normal, blood flow is rapid.

DIC

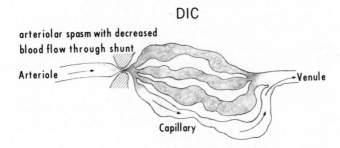

Capillary perfusion is impaired, blood flow is slow,
intracapillary thrombosis occurs with blood stagnation and acidosis.
Cells nourished by capillaries die of ischemia due to blood clotting.

Fig. 23-6. Effect of A-V shunting in DIC.

table 23-1
distribution of clotting factors in serum and plasma

CLOTTING FACTORS	PLASMA	SERUM
XII	†	†
XI	†	†
IX	†	†
VIII	†	0
X	†	†
V	†	0
Prothrombin	†	0
Fibrinogen	†	0
XIII	†	†
(Platelets)	(†)	(0)

† present; 0 absent; ( ) cellular component of blood.

Stress has a significant role in DIC as the former activates the fibrinolytic system. As stress is a primary cause of increased fibrinolysis, the DIC patient bleeds not only as the result of consumption of clotting factors but to some degree because of increased fibrinolysis. This effect not only brings about lysis of clots already formed but also causes production of certain degraded products of fibrin which further add to the bleeding diathesis. As may be recalled from the previous discussion, the clotting process elaborates thrombin, the most potent of all coagulation enzymes. In DIC, abundant intravascular thrombin is produced, rapidly converting fibrinogen to fibrin clot. When in the course of DIC fibrinogen is entirely used up, circulating thrombin persists in the intravascular space, just waiting for its substrate fibrinogen to arrive, converting it to clot. This arrival occurs either by additional body production of fibrinogen or by transfusion of blood, plasma, or fibrinogen, all of which serve to perpetuate the syndrome and worsen clinical hemorrhage. Although the body has naturally occurring antithrombins which inhibit thrombin activity, in DIC antithrombins are practically absent. The most important, *antithrombin (III)*, is not even present.

A summary diagram of the vicious cycle of DIC is given in Fig. 23-7.

Now that the pathogenesis of DIC is understood, let us discuss how the laboratory can aid clinicians in diagnosing DIC. Below is a list of the clotting factor and cell abnormalities found in DIC.

1. Clotting factor depleted plasma, hence the following clotting factors are reduced:
   a. Fibrinogen
   b. Factor VIII
   c. Factor V
   d. Prothrombin
2. Platelets markedly reduced (thrombocytopenia)
3. Absence of antithrombins
4. Abnormally high blood thrombin levels
5. Abnormally increased fibrinolytic activity
6. Abnormally increased fibrin degradation products

In classic DIC, the tests given in Table 23-2 are abnormal.

Recent investigation (unpublished data) suggests that clot tension strength is altered in DIC from a normal of 30 to 10–15 dyne per cm. These data are of prognostic importance because clot tension in patients recovering from DIC returns toward normal before conventional laboratory tests show normalization.

treatment of DIC

The backbone of therapy consists of removing the cause of DIC. If your kitchen is flooded by a broken pipe, adjacent flooding will not be averted by mopping alone. One must turn off the water supply to the broken pipe. If the cause of DIC cannot be removed (as in intravascular dissemination of cancer) therapy of the syndrome may control but not cure it.

Control of DIC is brought about by stopping the vicious cycle of thrombosis-hemorrhage as shown in Fig. 23-7. Heparin does this in three ways. First, it is antithrombin in activity and will neutralize free circulating thrombin. Second, heparin prevents propagation of thrombi that have formed in capillaries—in which capacity, heparin is functioning as an anticoagulant. Third, heparin has an inhibitory effect on the activation of blood clotting *in vivo*, principally due to its effect on factor IX.

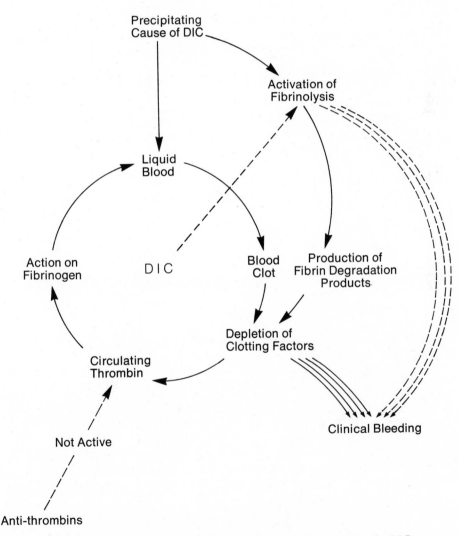

Fig. 23-7. Self-perpetuating cycle of clotting and hemorrhage in DIC.

table 23-2
laboratory findings in classic DIC

TEST	DIRECTION OF ABNORMAL VALUES	RATIONALE
Prothrombin time	Prolonged	Factor V and prothrombin are measured.
Partial thromboplastin time (PTT)	Prolonged	Factors V and VIII are measured and to a lesser degree—fibrinogen.
Platelet count	Low	Thrombocytopenia present.
Fibrinogen level	Low	Patient with DIC has reduced fibrinogen.
Euglobulin lysis time (ELT)	Shortened	ELT measures fibrinolytic activity.
Antithrombin III level	Low	Antithrombin III is absent in patient with DIC.
Thrombin time	Prolonged	Fibrinogen is indirectly measured by thrombin time.
Fibrin degradation products	Elevated	These products are increased in DIC.

In DIC, heparin should be given only *intravenously* for four reasons:

1. Dosage regulation is far easier via IV rather than subcutaneous administration because the absorption rate from tissue is affected by amount given, depth of injection, temperature of the patient and cardiovascular status.
2. Local hematoma formation when given subcutaneously may severely alter absorption of the drug.
3. The dose in severe, acute cases may be too large for proper blood levels to be obtained by any route except intravenously.
4. The time lag for therapeutic effect of subcutaneous heparin is too great compared to the immediate effect of the drug IV.

The amount of heparin to be given for acute DIC is not established. Most adults are given between 10,000 and 20,000 units (100 to 200 mg.) every two to four hours. Ideally, the stat dose of heparin is 2 to 2.5 mg. per kilo body weight with follow-up doses which keep the circulating level between 0.5 and 1 mg. per kilo body weight. The dosage may be determined by calculating the disappearance rate of heparin in the patient and giving a calculated dose every two hours to maintain the patient in the therapeutic range. The dosage of heparin required to treat DIC must be tempered by the clinical status of the patient, as heparin is eliminated from the body by renal excretion (in both an altered and unaltered state) and by heparinase activity in the liver. Patients with renal failure, inadequate liver perfusion, or both will thus have an abnormally prolonged heparin half-life, requiring far less heparin to control DIC. The author has experienced such cases in which a heparin dose of 1 mg. (100 units) every two hours was sufficient to control acute DIC.

The author's experience suggests that continuous drip of heparin does not work well in keeping the patient properly heparinized. Of course, once the primary precipitating cause of DIC has been removed and clinical and laboratory evidence suggests that the patient is on the way to recovery, heparin should be discontinued. In early acute DIC, a single large dose of heparin will arrest the DIC process if the primary factors have been eliminated.

Recent unpublished observations suggest that low doses of heparin in the range of 5 to 10 mg. (500 to 1,000 units) every two hours are enough to inhibit thrombin in the patient with active DIC. This inhibitory activity will break the cycle of clotting and hemorrhage.

The role of acidosis in this syndrome is sufficiently great to add another treatment goal in this disorder—the prevention of acidosis. Frequently patients in shock with DIC are acidotic, and correction of this acid-base imbalance should be part and parcel of the treatment of DIC bleeders.

Some authorities have recommended the use of epsilon amino caproic acid (eACA) (trade name, Amicar) in acute DIC. The rationale is to take advantage of the potent antifibrinolytic effect of eACA, hence reduce the fibrinolytic component of bleeding in acute DIC. Let us not forget that eACA is a double-edged sword. It inhibits not only pathological but also normal fibrinolysis, hence inhibiting a protective mechanism in the clot-lysis balance. Remember that DIC is after all a hypercoagulable state and eACA may render a patient even more hypercoagulable by destroying the lytic side of the balance. Certainly if one desires to control the pathological element of fibrinolysis, eACA must not be given unless the patient is adequately heparinized, and then only with great caution.

Thus far we have discussed the acute bleeding episodes of DIC. However, this syndrome occurs in both a subacute and a chronic phase. In the subacute stage bleeding may not be clinically obvious; however, at this stage the patient is in great danger of becoming an overt bleeder (acute DIC). Treatment of the subacute stage is important only to prevent the acute stage from occurring. The chronic form of DIC is usually unassociated with hemorrhage or abnormal clotting tests. The *only clue* may be a sudden *drop in hematocrit* in the absence of any demonstrable blood loss. It is assumed that hemoglobin is sequestered as clot in capillaries. Due to the slow replacement of red cell mass in circulating blood, the only manifestation of chronic DIC is a drop in circulating blood hemoglobin. Blood volume is kept normal with rapid plasma replacement. The typical chronic DIC patient is the one with a sudden episode of coronary shock with hemoglobin loss as a single occurrence.

"All that glitters is not gold." Likewise, all that bleeds is not DIC. All too often every bleeding crisis is diagnosed as DIC. There are numerous bleeding situations that mimic DIC and they should not be forgotten. To name a few— acute fibrinolytic activation, clotting factor depletion secondary to massive hemorrhage, and acquired clotting factor inhibitors. Unfortunately, routine laboratory data do not differentiate these syndromes with ease. Because treatment of the different bleeding disorders varies, correct diagnosis is essential if the patient's life is to be prolonged. Incorrect diagnosis, hence improper treatment, will hasten death.

summary

1. DIC is secondary to primary disease or symptom-sign complex.
2. DIC is a serious bleeding disorder resulting from a hypercoagulable state.
3. Massive capillary thrombosis leads to platelet and clotting factor depletion and hence to hemorrhage.
4. Simultaneous events in DIC include:
   a. Arterial hypotension
   b. Opening arteriovenous shunts
   c. Capillary blood stagnation
   d. Acidosis
   e. Capillary thrombosis.
5. Stress associated with DIC increases fibrinolytic activity.
6. Treatment of DIC requires a twofold approach:
   a. Removal of etiological factor(s) causing DIC
   b. Heparin use as outlined above.

HELEN C. BUSBY, R.N.

24

burns

Burns! A stark word! Grimly blunt in description of its process. It implies not only loss of the skin's integrity, but the vulnerability of all body functions. Burns—a challenge for every nurse to integrate her knowledge of the interrelatedness of all body systems and to provide the therapeutic interventions, supportive care, and maintenance care necessary for the person to cope with this precarious disequilibrium.

the skin

The burns discussed in this chapter are burns of the skin. Therefore, understanding the anatomy, physiology and function of the skin is vital to guiding the nurse's observations for determining the effects of burns on the internal body processes.

Sometimes it is hard to remember that the skin is the largest organ of the body, with three major layers, indispensable to life (Fig. 24-1). The epidermis is the thin outer layer which is constantly exposed to our external environment. It is composed of stratified epithelial cells that are continuously replacing themselves. Keratin, an insoluble protein, toughens and waterproofs this tissue, while chromatophores, the pigment cells, are present in varying numbers and give the color to our skin. Areas of localized concentrations, such as the nipples, present darker color.

The dermis is a layer of connective tissue fibers that lies immediately below the epidermis. This layer is richly supplied with blood and lymph vessels; nerve endings with sensory receptors for touch, temperature, pressure and pain; sweat glands which secrete a thin watery solution which helps regulate body temperature; sebaceous glands which secrete an oily substance (sebum)

489

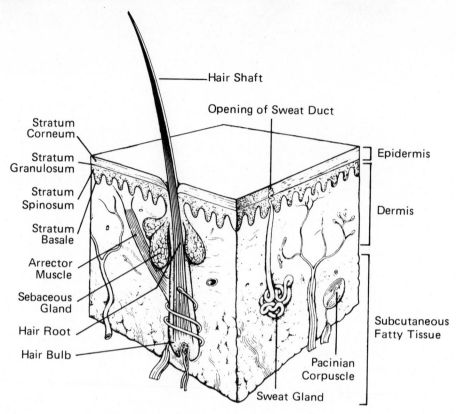

Fig. 24-1. A three-dimensional view of the skin.

for lubrication; and hair follicles with their arrector pili muscles that aid in temperature regulation. In the breasts, the mammary glands are specialized modifications of the sweat and sebaceous glands.

The subcutaneous layer is a layer of adipose tissue, a loose connective tissue filled with fat cells that protect the muscles and nerves and give the body shape and form.

These three layers of the skin perform multiple functions for the body. First, skin serves as the front-line protector against bacteria, parasites and other organisms, as well as preventing toxic materials and harmful environmental radiation from entering the body. The surface of the skin maintains a pH of 4 to 6.8 through the secretions of the sweat and sebaceous glands and the breakdown products from dead surface cells. This pH retards the growth of bacteria and fungi on the epidermis. The same properties that keep out invaders also keep in body fluids, thus preventing dehydration and fluid imbalance.

The skin is a principle contributor to the maintenance of a cor body temperature, commonly 98.6°F. The heat produced by the metabolic processes within the body must be controlled or the resulting increase in the cor temperature would cause irreparable cell damage. The blood vessels in the skin react to stimuli received from the hypothalamus. When the vessels dilate, more blood is allowed to flow through the skin, and heat is lost from the body by radiation, conduction or convection. If the blood vessels constrict, heat is conserved within the body as less blood passes through the upper layers of the skin where it would normally be cooled.

Signals from the hypothalamus also cause "sweating," which will lower the cor temperature by the expenditure of heat necessary to evaporate the fluid from the body surface and by the fact that the surface of the skin, where this transaction occurs, will be cooled.

The skin is also an excretory organ. Sweat glands continually secrete without our awareness (insensible perspiration). The sweat solution contains water, sodium chloride and some waste products of metabolism, such as ammonia. The body's water balance and acid-base balance are therefore assisted by the skin. In contrast, absorption can occur through the skin. Any substance that will dissolve the keratin will pass through the skin into the body. Thus, the paste Nitro-Bid, used for the relief of angina, is an effective treatment.

A constant barrage of stimuli from the environment is received by the skin. The sensory receptors located in the skin relay their reactions to these stimuli to the brain and we adapt ourselves accordingly. For example, we will withdraw from something that causes pain, but a gentle massage may cause a feeling of relaxation.

Last, but not least, the skin gives us our cosmetic makeup which plays a large role in our identity.

the burn and its severity

A burn injury to the skin will result in decreased or complete loss of function of the skin, depending upon the depth of the burn. However, the amount of bodily harm caused by a burn injury is not solely dependent on the depth of the burn. The severity of a burn depends on five factors: (1) the size of the burn injury, (2) the depth of the burn, (3) the part of the body involved, (4) the age of the patient, and (5) the patient's past medical history. Since treatment is directly related to the severity of the burn, all five factors must be evaluated.

The size of the burn injury is estimated as percentage of total body area. The following two basic methods utilize "shading in" the burned areas on anterior and posterior drawings of the body. From these outlines, the percentage of body area involved can be easily calculated. The first is Berkow's method (Fig. 24-2) which involves "shading in" the body area burned and then calculating the percentage according to a table based on the age of the patient. This method considers the changes in proportion of body areas (head

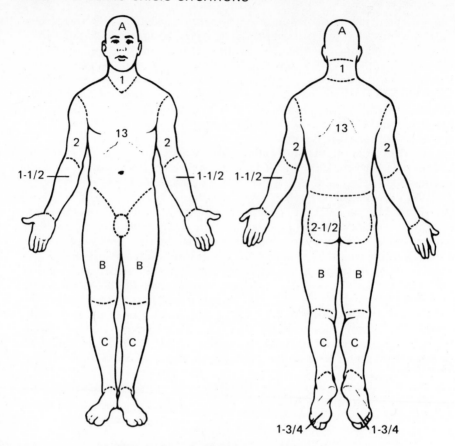

Relative Percentage of Areas Affected by Growth

	Age in years					
	0	1	5	10	15	Adult
A—1/2 of head	9-1/2	8-1/2	6-1/2	5-1/2	4-1/2	3-1/2
B—1/2 of one thigh	2-3/4	3-1/4	4	4-1/4	4-1/2	4-3/4
C—1/2 of one leg	2-1/2	2-1/2	2-3/4	3	3-1/4	3-1/2

Fig. 24-2. Berkow's method for determining percentage of body area with burn injury.

and lower extremities) that occur with growth. The proportion of the upper extremities to the trunk remains the same throughout life, and therefore these parts are given fixed values. All other areas will have a different value according to the age of the patient.

The "rule of nines" is the second method for determining the size of the

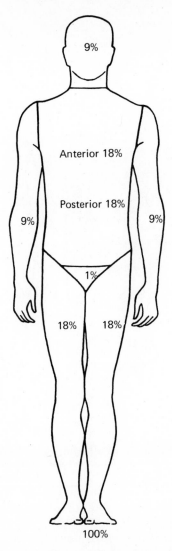

9%

Anterior 18%

Posterior 18%

9%   9%

1%

18%   18%

100%

Fig. 24-3. The "Rule of Nines" method for determining percentage of body area with burn injury.

burn area (Fig. 24-3). In this method the body is divided into areas equal to multiples or divisions of 9 percent. For example, the anterior arm is $4\frac{1}{2}$ percent and the posterior arm is $4\frac{1}{4}$ percent; therefore, the entire arm is 9 percent. The perineum is given a value of 1 percent. The total body areas add up to 100 percent.

The depth of the burn is not always visually apparent. It is only with time and the healing process that one can be exact as to the depth of the injury.

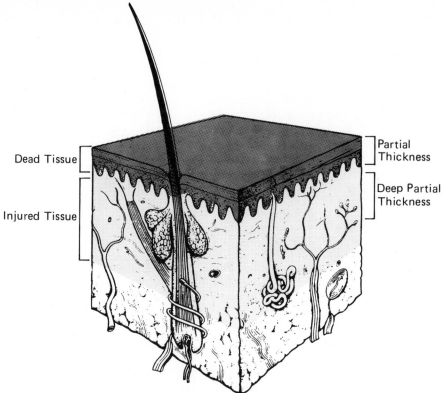

Fig. 24-4. Partial thickness burn.

Immediately after the injury occurs, one can estimate the depth by certain signs and symptoms. A partial thickness burn involves the epidermis and dermis layers of the skin (Fig. 24-4). The skin will have reddened areas that will blanch with finger pressure and refill readily. This degree of burn will heal by itself, if no further damage occurs, for sufficient epithelial cells are left intact to provide new epidermis.

A deep partial thickness burn (also shown in Fig. 24-4) destroys the epidermis and dermis and the deep dermis. It will have blisters that will increase in size during the first few hours post-burn. Full thickness burns destroy the epidermis, dermis, and possibly the muscle, tendon and bone. It is characterized by a leathery surface that may range in color from white to red to black. No blanching will occur. Small blisters may be present but will not increase in size. There will be no pain sensation as the nerve fibers of the dermis will have been destroyed.

Full thickness burns (Fig. 24-5) involve all layers of the skin and extend into the subcutaneous tissues. Regeneration of the skin is not possible and grafts must be provided to obtain normal skin function.

The part of the body involved is also important in evaluating the severity of the burn. A burn of the head, neck or chest may also involve injury to the pulmonary tree. Burns of the perineum are difficult to manage due to the high incidence of infection in this area.

The severity of the burn is very dependent on the age of the patient. It is a known fact that patients under two and those over 60 have a higher mortality rate than other age groups with burns of similar severity. The patient under two years of age is more susceptible to infection due to poor antibody response, while the patient over 60 has degenerative processes that may be aggravated by the bodily stress imposed by the burn. For example, the patient with arteriosclerosis may develop a myocardial infarction.

The fifth factor to be considered in evaluating the severity of a burn injury is the past medical history. If the patient has an illness prior to the burn (for example, diabetes or renal failure), this illness may become acute during the burn process.

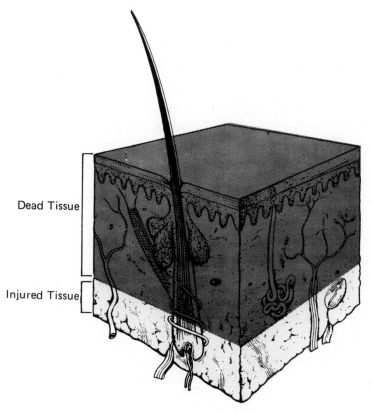

Fig. 24-5. Full thickness burn.

resultant systemic changes

A severe burn involves many systemic changes. The first to be considered must be the "fluid shift"—intravascular fluid leaking into the interstitial spaces. The severity of this phenomenon is directly related to the depth of the burn and the percentage of body surface involved. Since the depth of the burn is not easily determined at the time of admission, all burn patients must be closely observed for symptoms of hypovolemic shock. The shift of plasma and fluids into the interstitial spaces begins immediately at the time of the burn injury and is well underway within the first hour. Usually, this fluid leak continues up to 48 hours postburn.

The blood vessels in the burn area are traumatized and destroyed. This trauma increases capillary permeability due to the release of chemicals (as histamine) from injured cells and allows water and electrolytes to flow out into the interstitial spaces, thus causing edema in the burn site. This loss of fluid from the plasma results in an increase in protein concentration of the remaining circulating plasma. The high protein concentration within the blood vessels then causes fluid to be drawn out of the interstitial spaces in *un*burned areas into the vascular tree in order to maintain circulating blood volume. If fluid is not administered to compensate for this circulation loss, the interstitial spaces will become depleted and shock will occur. It is important to remember that this fluid loss is from the circulatory volume and not from the body per se, for it remains as increased interstitial fluid (edema) in the heat-damaged tissues.

Soon after the burn, protein will also start to leak through the injured capillary membranes. This leakage is not as rapid as that of water and electrolytes, for the protein molecule is larger. The albumin molecule is smaller than the globulin molecule, allowing for more albumin to leak into the interstitial space. Loss of protein from the circulating volume also contributes to hypovolemic shock if left untreated. Burn patients frequently have an altered A/G ratio, indicating this.

Electrolyte concentrations are altered within the body fluids not only from the leaking process but also from direct injury to the burned cells. Potassium is lost from intracellular fluid (K^+ concentration is higher within the cell than outside the cell) to interstitial fluid, and the hemolysis of red blood cells in the area of a severe burn releases free potassium. Potassium changes are more important after the first 48 hours rather than in the immediate postburn stage.

Serum sodium chloride leaks from the plasma into the interstitial fluid and is trapped in the edema at the burn site. If the burn wound has a large amount of exudate, hyponatremia will result as sodium (largest concentration of extracellular ions) is lost when the extracellular fluid is lost.

A calcium deficit may occur in extensively burned patients which may be due to calcium being trapped in the edema fluid of the damaged tissue and by extensive thermal injury to subcutaneous fat (saponification).

Insensible water loss is increased following a severe burn injury. The skin, which is our protector against loss of water and heat, is now impaired or destroyed. The amount of water and heat loss is related to the size of the full thickness burn. Fever and infection increase the metabolic process, thereby also increasing fluid loss. Vomiting, which often accompanies a severe burn, will also cause further water and electrolyte depletion.

The loss of fluid from the intravascular space results in a thickened sluggish flow of the remaining circulating blood. The effects reach to all body parts. The reduction of the circulating volume may decrease cardiac output. Low cardiac output results in poor tissue perfusion. Poor tissue perfusion results in metabolic acidosis and stasis of blood. This slowed circulation allows bacteria and cellular material in the blood vessels to precipitate to the lower part of the vessel, especially in the capillaries, resulting in intravascular coagulation. Other contributors to coagulation problems are the release of thromboplastin by the injury itself, the release of fibrinogen from injured platelets, an antigen-antibody reaction to the burned tissue, and bed rest. If thrombi occur, they may cause ischemia of the affected part and lead to necrosis. Since this is a widespread occurrence, any organ of the body—liver, heart, lung, brain, kidney—may be involved and organ failure can occur. This increased coagulation process may also develop into DIC (see Chapter 23).

One can readily see the importance of fluid therapy in the severely burned patient. Any patient with burns on over 20 percent of his body area should have a large intravenous catheter inserted as soon as possible postburn. If less than 20 percent of total body area is involved, fluid replacement is based on need, which is ascertained by close and knowledgeable observation of the patient.

At the end of 48 hours postburn, the capillaries have healed sufficiently to stop the loss of intravascular fluid. The increased interstitial fluid at the burn site will now begin reverse diffusion and be reabsorbed into the vascular system. At this point the parenteral intake is decreased to avoid fluid overload.

Another problem in a severe burn is hemolysis of red blood cells. The red cells are thermally destroyed as they pass through the burn area at the time of injury. The hemoglobin pigment is released in the bloodstream. Free hemoglobin pigment is filtered out of the circulation by the kidneys. If this free hemoglobin is not flushed through the kidneys, it will accumulate in the tubules and acute tubular necrosis will occur (see Chapter 16).

Red blood cells will be lost not only by hemolysis but also by (1) bleeding at the burn site, (2) thrombosis in the capillaries of the burn site, (3) hemolysis associated with septicemia, (4) delayed hemolysis of partially damaged red cells at the time of the injury (shorter survival time), and (5) bleeding due to debridement of wounds. The anemia that occurs from any or all of these causes is treated by replacing red blood cells as indicated by the patient's blood counts.

The gastrointestinal tract may also be affected. Gastric dilatation and paralytic ileus may occur in the first 24 hours postburn due to splenic constriction as a result of hypovolemia or to the stress on the body as a result of the injury itself. After the first few days, invasive wound sepsis is probably the cause of this phenomenon.

Curling's ulcer, the appearance of multiple ulcers in the stomach and duodenum of burn patients, may develop at any time during the course of recovery. Its etiology has not been established.

care of the person with burns

The first treatment of any burn injury is to STOP THE BURNING. The depth and severity of the burn is closely related to the causative agent and the length of time the skin is exposed. If flames are present, have the victim lie flat (to prevent inhalation of flame and smoke) and smother the flames with whatever means is available. Remove hot clothing immediately and cool the burned area with a cold liquid. Chemical agents should be neutralized or irrigated with copious amounts of water.

Once the burning is stopped, treatment is directed to any lifesaving measures that may be immediately necessary. The burn may be the most obvious injury, but the treatment of respiratory distress, hemorrhage, and/or shock takes precedence.

Every critical care nurse should be familiar with the clinical features of shock. Regardless of etiology, the shock syndrome results in a marked reduction of blood flow through the tissues. This leads to cellular hypoxia, which if not corrected leads to tissue death. The hypotension, reduced blood flow and hypoxia stimulate compensatory mechanisms in the body. Stimulation of the aortic and carotid pressor receptors increases pulse rate and selective vasoconstriction. (These pressure receptors will maintain normal blood pressure until approximately 20 percent of the blood volume has been lost.) The adrenal glands release epinephrine, which augments these responses. Respirations increase in rate and depth in order to promote venous return and cardiac filling. Changes in circulatory hydrostatic and osmotic pressures, due to the decreased volume, pull fluids from the interstitial spaces into the blood vessels. As has been explained, in a severe burn it is necessary to replace this fluid to prevent the shock process from continuing.

Due to increased activity of the sympathetic nervous system, adrenalin secretions are increased and the patient becomes restless and anxious. Decreased blood flow to the kidneys is reflected by a decreased urine output. Metabolic acidosis results from the accumulation of waste products of cellular metabolism brought about by inadequacy of the circulation.

The fundamental aims in the treatment of the shock state are to (1) improve circulation in order to perfuse body tissues and (2) correct the specific cause. The etiology of burn shock is known and fluid replacement will correlate to the fluid that is being lost. Several formulas (Table 24-1) have been devised to serve as a guide to fluid replacement in the burn patient. All of them replace saline and colloids, and include an electrolyte-free solution (D5W) to

table 24-1
sample formula for fluid replacement in an adult burn patient (Brooke formula)

FIRST 24 HOURS

1. Colloids solution	0.5 ml./kg./% of burn
2. Crystalloids solution	1.5 ml./kg./% of burn
3. Electrolyte-free solution	According to age and size of patient

SECOND 24 HOURS

One half of the amount of colloid and crystalloid solutions. Same amount of the electrolyte-free solution.

cover insensible fluid loss. Lactated Ringer's solution may be used to supply sodium and to help correct metabolic acidosis. Isotonic saline may be used to replace the large amount of lost sodium. Concentrated albumin may be given to replace the protein that leaks out. The amount of fluid infused must be determined for each individual patient. Fluid replacement is best gauged on the basis of the hourly urine output, the pulse rate, the blood pressure and the central venous pressure readings (see Chapter 10).

Once the patient is out of all life-threatening situations, wound care is instituted. The medical care of the burn wound is directed at maintaining healthy tissue and assisting the body to maintain skin function in the areas of deep partial and full thickness burns. By keeping the wound clean of exudate and crusts, we inhibit the growth of bacteria and allow the body to heal itself by epithelialization. If the body is unable to heal itself, then good wound care provides a clean bed of granulation tissue for grafting of skin.

Infection is one of the greatest and most devastating dangers to the burn patient. With the loss of its anatomical barrier, the body is open to invasion by pathogenic organisms. These organisms will survive and multiply in a wound that is not kept clean. Since the burn patient's resistance to infection is impaired, this localized wound infection may then spread throughout the body. Septicemia and pneumonia are the two leading causes of death in the burn patient.

The wound may be cared for by several methods.

Open or Exposed Wound In this method the wound is left exposed for the purpose of easy inspection and minimal bacterial growth (the theory is that bacterial growth will be diminished in the absence of moist warm dressings). The patient with this type of wound care is usually placed in reverse isolation to decrease the risk of acquired infections. The wound is kept free of exudate and crusts by frequent cleansings done either at the bedside, in a shower, or in a whirlpool bath. Any crusts (dried exudate) of a partial thickness burn are gently debrided away. Full thickness burns do not begin to loosen the eschar (thick leathery scab) until bacterial action causes collagen fibers to disintegrate. This loosened eschar should then be removed with each cleansing treatment. All debridement is done in a gentle manner, as vigorous scrubbing or pulling off of the scab may convert a partial thickness wound to a full thickness injury.

Semiopen Wound   This type of wound care consists of covering the injured areas with a topical antimicrobial agent. A thin layer of dressing may be used to help keep the medication in contact with the wound. Cleansing and debridement are still performed at prescribed intervals. The wound is thoroughly cleansed of all medication with each treatment and debridement, followed by a fresh application of the cream, ointment or liquid. The nurse must be knowledgeable of the medication used (as with any medication she administers) to recognize if the desired outcome is being achieved and/or the patient has adverse reactions.

Closed Wound (Occlusive)   This method of wound care consists of covering the wound with many layers of dressings which are not disturbed for several days. The dressings usually begin with a layer of fine mesh gauze immediately next to the wound. This allows the growth of new epithelium while allowing the exudate to drain away. An antimicrobial or lubricating agent may be incorporated into this layer. The next layer is a large amount of fluffy material that will absorb the exudate and hold it away from the surface of the wound. The outer layer is an elastic wrap to hold everything in place without causing constriction. This type of dressing will generally be used postgraft to stabilize and protect the new graft.

Wet Dressings   The wound is cared for by covering it with dressings saturated with a specific solution, such as normal saline or silver nitrate $\frac{1}{2}$ percent. For this method to be effective, the dressings must be kept *wet*. A dry covering reduces evaporation, making the patient more comfortable. A thin layer of gauze over the wound will help with debridement as it is removed with each dressing change. Dressing changes not only accomplish debridement, but allow for wound inspection. Maceration may occur with this treatment.

Biological Dressings   When the body must be assisted to form granulation tissue, a graft is placed over the burned area. These grafts may provide temporary coverage as heterografts (Bovine skin) or homografts (cadaver skin). Autografts, obtained from the patient's own body, are permanent placements.

The type of treatment prescribed will be determined by the extent and depth of the injury, associated injuries, the age of the patient and the cooperation of the patient.

A properly applied dressing will aid the body in conserving heat and water, minimize contractures, and make the patient more comfortable. Range of motion exercises should be performed with each dressing change to prevent loss of function. When body parts are positioned, the functional position should always be assumed. The body must not be allowed to chill during wound care, as chilling requires large expenditures of energy, which the burn patient cannot afford. Two burned areas should never touch for this will result in "webbing." Debridement times should be limited to 20-minute intervals so as not to overtax the patient. Burn wound care must be consistent!

An impatient nurse who is not willing to give the time necessary for effective wound care and healing is doing an injustice to the patient.

The nursing care of a severely burned patient requires a nurse who is knowledgeable in all aspects of critical care nursing. As complications may occur in any body system, she must be alert to any changes in the patient that may herald a crisis. However, above and beyond her technical knowledge, she must be able to deal with the tremendous psychological stress of any severe burn injury. She must be able to cope with her own attitudes, and therefore reactions, about caring for the victim of such a violent insult. She must be able to support a positive attitude in both the patient and his family. A firm considerate approach will help the patient accept the physical and emotional stress that must be endured. It has been pointed out that in many instances, the most that can be done is to help the patient endure his pain.

The care of a person with burns truly requires that we look beyond the scars and disfiguration to that part of the person that is more than the sum total of his parts.

BIBLIOGRAPHY

Feller, I., and C. Archambeault, *Nursing the Burned Patient* (Ann Arbor: Institute for Burn Medicine, 1974).

Jacoby, F. G., *Nursing Care of the Patient with Burns* (St. Louis: C. V. Mosby, 1972).

McClintic, J. R., *Basic Anatomy and Physiology of the Human Body* (New York: John Wiley & Sons, 1975).

Monafo, W. W. and C. Pappalardo, *The Treatment of Burns: Principles and Practice* (St. Louis: Warren Green, II, 1971).

Shepro, D., et al., *Human Anatomy and Physiology* (New York: Holt, Rinehart & Winston, 1974).

HELEN C. BUSBY, R.N.

25

hepatic failure:
ammonia intoxication

Liver function is essential to life. Fortunately, the liver has an exceptional functional ability and regenerative capacity. Liver disease may be acute or chronic and dysfunction may be reversible or irreversible, depending on the amount of tissue involved and the nature of the insult.

anatomy

The liver is the largest glandular organ in the human body. This two-lobed (right and left lobes) organ lies just below the diaphragm with its greatest portion located to the right side of the body. Its superior (rounded) surface fits into the curve of the diaphragm and is in contact with the anterior wall of the abdominal cavity. The inferior surface is molded over the stomach, the duodenum, the pancreas, the hepatic flexure of the colon, the right kidney and the right adrenal gland.

The functional unit of the liver is called a lobule. In the tissues surrounding each lobule are found the terminal branches of the portal vein, the hepatic artery and the bile ducts (Fig. 25-1).

The portal vein is formed behind the head of the pancreas by the union of the superior mesenteric and the splenic veins. At its entrance to the liver, the portal vein divides into two trunks which supply both lobes of the liver. The branches of the portal vein then disperse throughout the tissue of the liver and become the interlobular veins as they encircle each lobule. The blood sinusoids then pass toward the center of each lobule where they unite and

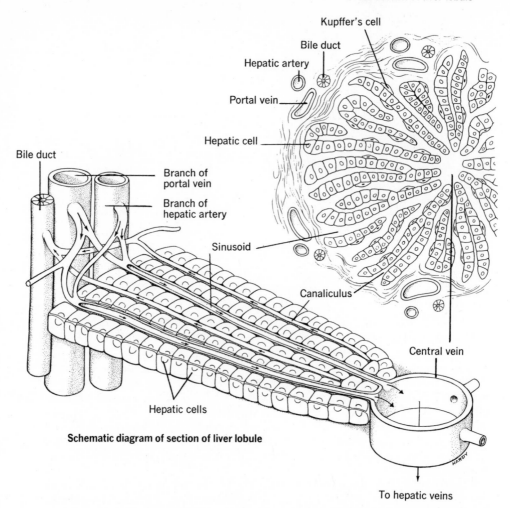

Cross section of liver lobule

Kupffer's cell

Bile duct

Hepatic artery

Portal vein

Hepatic cell

Sinusoid

Canaliculus

Central vein

Bile duct

Branch of portal vein

Branch of hepatic artery

Hepatic cells

Schematic diagram of section of liver lobule

To hepatic veins

Fig. 25-1. Liver lobule and sinusoids. (From E. E. Chaffee and E. M. Greisheimer, *Basic Physiology and Anatomy,* ed. 3; Philadelphia, J. B. Lippincott, 1974, p. 397)

form the central veins, which in turn form the sublobular veins, which then become the hepatic veins. The two hepatic veins drain into the inferior vena cava.

The hepatic artery supplies the liver with nutrients. This artery, along with the left gastric and splenic arteries, is the terminal branch of the celiac artery. The branches of the hepatic artery within the lobule of the liver form capil-

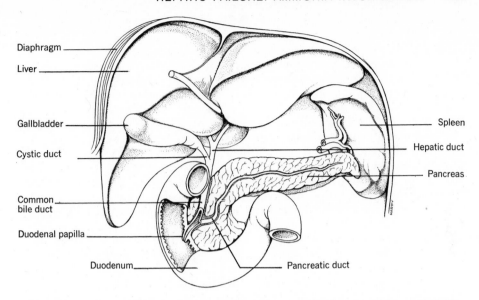

Diaphragm
Liver
Gallbladder
Cystic duct
Common bile duct
Duodenal papilla
Duodenum
Spleen
Hepatic duct
Pancreas
Pancreatic duct

Fig. 25-2. Liver and biliary system. (From E. E. Chaffee and E. M. Greisheimer, *Basic Physiology and Anatomy*, ed. 3, Philadelphia, J. B. Lippincott, 1974, p. 398)

laries which communicate with the sinusoids from the interlobular veins.

The bile ducts, which carry the bile secreted by the liver cells to the duodenum to aid in the digestion of fats, originate within the liver cells. They anastomose to each other and then pass to the periphery of the lobule where they form the primary bile ducts. These bile ducts from both lobes of the liver then unite to form the hepatic duct. The hepatic duct becomes the common bile duct after its connection with the cystic duct (Fig. 25-2). The cystic duct and the gallbladder are just an enlargement in the biliary system in which excess bile secretion may be stored. The gallbladder concentrates bile and then empties its contents, via the common bile duct, into the duodenum during digestion.

The common bile duct and the main duct from the pancreas usually unite just before the duct pierces the wall of the duodenum. There is often a dilation of the tube after this junction (the ampulla of Vater). The opening of the common bile duct in the duodenum is about 8 to 10 cm. from the pylorus.

physiology

The blood capillaries within the liver are situated to run along one or several sides of each parenchymal cell. Through these capillaries, by way of the portal vein, flows practically all the blood from the stomach, intestines, pancreas and spleen. This blood carries all the products of carbohydrate and protein digestion. Digested carbohydrate (glucose) is stored in the liver as glycogen and released into the bloodstream as glucose according to the body requirements. The parenchymal cells of the liver change the amino acids, derived from protein metabolism, into new proteins as fibrinogen, prothrombin, and plasma albumin. A certain amount of protein is stored in the liver to be released as required.

In liver cells, the poisonous nitrogenous by-products of protein digestion and metabolism are converted into nontoxic substances. For example, ammonia bodies are returned to the blood as urea, which is cleared from the bloodstream by the kidneys and excreted in the urine. Liver cells play a key role in the metabolism of fatty acids, producing glucose and ketone bodies. They also prepare, store and supply the body with vitamin B_{12}, which is necessary for the normal development of the immature red blood cells in the bone marrow. These cells also manufacture and store other vitamins, such as A, D, and many components of the B complex group. The liver stores certain metals, such as iron and copper, and excretes, modifies or absorbs certain drugs.

Another type of cell in the liver is the phagocytic cell (Kupffer cell) which engulfs particulate matter in the blood, such as defective or old red blood cells, and chemically splits the hemoglobin of these cells into an iron-containing fraction which is conserved for the formation of more hemoglobin. The remainder is converted into bile.

Bile formed by the liver is diverted into the gallbladder where a large proportion of its water is absorbed. The final solution of bile is five to ten times more concentrated than that originally secreted by the liver. Bile is used as an aid in the enzymatic intestinal digestion of fats by causing them to break up into small globules that are more easily attacked by the fat-splitting enzymes. It also serves as a vehicle for removal of substances that the liver cells clear from the blood as bilirubin and urobilinogen. Bilirubin is a by-product of the phagocytosis of hemoglobin (worn-out or defective erythrocytes). Attached to albumin, bilirubin circulates in the plasma until it comes in contact with a liver cell which absorbs it; separates it from its albumin; conjugates (joins) it with glucuronic acid; and secretes it into a bile canal from where it makes its way, via the common bile duct, into the duodenum. While in transit through the intestines, this bilirubin glucuronide becomes converted into urobilinogen by intestinal bacteria. Most of this urobilinogen makes its exit from the body in the feces. Some urobilinogen is reabsorbed into the bloodstream and some of this is excreted by the kidneys in the urine. The remainder is reconverted by the liver cells back into bilirubin and secreted in bile.

pathophysiology

Anything that affects the flow of blood through the liver, the metabolic action of the cells within the liver, or the flow of bile through the biliary tree will produce liver disease. If there is diffuse disease with parenchymal damage, dysfunction is marked.

Liver disease due to circulatory impairment is primarily caused by the shunting of portal blood around the liver. This can result from a venous obstruction within the liver itself or from hepatic congestion due to a high systemic venous pressure, as in right-sided heart failure. Disease of the liver parenchyma itself is caused by infectious agents (such as viral hepatitis), anoxia of the cells, metabolic disorders, toxins, drugs, and nutritional deficiencies (such as malnutrition in alcoholism). A less common cause of liver failure is associated with infection and or obstruction of the bile channels, either inside the liver or in the bile ducts outside the liver. Infection can spread from the gallbladder, through the hepatic duct to the small bile ducts in the liver substance. Extrahepatic obstruction may be caused by plugging of the bile duct by a gallstone, a tumor, an inflammatory process, or by an enlarged gland pressing on it. Intrahepatic obstruction is caused by pressure on the channels from inflammatory swelling of the liver substance, or by inflammatory exudate within the ducts themselves.

Disease of any one of these systems of the liver, if sufficiently extensive or prolonged, generally involves the others, and the end result is cirrhosis (excessive formation of connective tissue with shrinkage of the organ) with obstruction of bile channels and of portal blood flow. The liver has remarkable powers of recovery, and over 70 percent of the parenchyma may be damaged before function tests are abnormal.

Parenchymal liver cell function can be evaluated with serum protein studies. Enzyme tests indicate liver cell damage. Excretory function is tested by the dye clearance tests. Bilirubin tests are done to measure excretion or retention of bile (Table 25-1).

Obstructed portal blood flow results in an abnormally high venous pressure in the gastrointestinal tract. This increase of the collateral venous drainage leads to edema of the tract. Fluid will accumulate in the abdominal cavity (ascites), and varices will occur in the esophagus, rectum and abdominal wall. Abnormalities in the absorption of carbohydrate and protein digestion will be present.

When collateral channels develop as a result of portal bed block, the blood carrying the by-products of digestion bypasses the liver. Ammonia that is produced from the bacterial and enzymatic digestion of proteins bypasses the liver, where it would normally be converted into urea, and reaches high levels in the blood. As a result of this increased concentration of blood ammonia, the central nervous system is affected and, in an unknown manner, encephalopathy develops.

Any failure of the liver cells to detoxify ammonia will result in *ammonia intoxication* (hepatic coma). Blood ammonia will be increased if the intestines have a high nitrogenous load. Ammonia from this source will also be increased as a result of gastrointestinal bleeding, bacterial growth in the small intestine, the ingestion of ammonium salts (e.g., ammonium chloride, a diuretic) and a high protein diet.

table 25-1
liver function tests

TESTS	NORMAL VALUES	COMMENTS
1. *Protein Studies*		
Total (Serum)	*gm./100 ml.*	Albumin is a major part of total blood proteins. It is important in the maintenance of osmotic pressure between blood and tissue.
Albumin	6.5–8.0	
	4.0–5.5	
Globulins	2.0–3.0	Globulins are needed for the production of antibodies as well as helping maintain osmotic pressure.
Fibrinogen	0.2–0.4	Fibrinogen is necessary in the blood clotting process.
Electrophoresis	*Percent of 100% Total Protein*	Electrophoresis separates the various protein fractions by an electric current. In parenchymal liver cell disease, the amounts of serum proteins will be depressed or the ratio of the proteins to each other will be altered.
Albumin	53%	
Alpha globulins	14%	
Beta globulins	12%	
Gamma globulins	20%	
Prothrombin Time	12–15 sec.	Prothrombin is synthesized to thrombin (in the absence of vitamin K) by the liver. This test is a good index of prognosis, as a prolonged pro-time is indicative of severe functional loss.
2. *Enzyme Studies*		
SGOT	10–40 units	Transaminases are a catalyst in the breakdown of amino acids. SGPT is the specific enzyme released by damaged liver cells. LDH is present in large amounts in liver tissue.
SGPT	5–35 units	
LDH	165–300 units	

TESTS	NORMAL VALUES	COMMENTS
Alkaline phosphatase	2–5 Bodansky units	This enzyme hydrolyzes phosphate esters and is useful in differential diagnosis if jaundice is present. It is excreted through the biliary tract. If it is elevated, nucleotidase and leucine amino peptidase will determine if elevation is due to biliary obstruction.
3. *Bilirubin* Total	0.9–2.2 mg./100 ml. 0.8 mg%	This test measures the ability of the liver to conjugate and excrete bilirubin. If the conjugated bilirubin is low and the unconjugated high, it indicates a preliver block. If the conjugated bilirubin is high and the unconjugated normal or low, it indicates a postliver block.
Conjugated (direct)	0.05–1.4 mg./100 ml. 0.6 mg%	
Unconjugated (indirect)	0.4–0.8 mg./100 ml. 0.2 mg%	
4. *BSP* (Bromsulphalein dye clearance	95–100% excretion in 1 hour.	This test measures the ability of the liver to conjugate BSP and clear it from the organ. A normal clearance is dependent on good hepatic blood flow, functioning liver cells and lack of obstruction in the biliary tract. This is the most sensitive of the liver function tests. It is the first test to become abnormal and the last to return to normal. False readings may be due to CHF, bleeding, previous contract dye injection, extravasation of dye at time of injection and the patient not being in a fasting state (postprandial increased hepatic blood flow produces increased excretion).

Gastrointestinal ammonia is decreased by the elimination of protein from the diet; by the administration of strong cathartics to cleanse the bowel, and by the use of nonabsorbable antibiotics (such as neomycin) to sterilize the bowel.

Ammonia is also a by-product of the kidneys as they break down amino acids. Ammonia from the kidneys is increased following the administration of diuretics; following the restriction of dietary sodium; and in patients with potassium depletion. Blood ammonia is also increased during exercise, as it is liberated from the contracting muscle cell.

Loss or impairment of liver cell function results in multiple body disturbances. In addition to ammonia intoxication, there are defects in carbohydrate, fat and protein metabolism; in blood coagulation, resulting in bleeding tendencies; in fluid and electrolyte balance; in the detoxification mechanism; and in renal function (the reason for renal malfunction is unknown).

Liver cells can regenerate if the disease process is not too toxic to the cells. The end result of severe parenchymal disease is a firm (cirrhotic), normal to small sized liver, which may be smooth or irregular (due to scar tissue); portal hypertension due to intrahepatic obstruction is also present.

When the flow of bile into the intestine is not normal, it is dammed back into the liver and reabsorbed into the bloodstream. This results in yellow staining of the skin and sclera (jaundice). The pigments of bile in the blood cause the skin to become very dry and to itch. The bile is excreted in the urine, making it a deep orange color and foamy. Because of the decreased amount of bile in the intestinal tract, the stools become white or clay colored. Dyspepsia and an intolerance to fatty foods occur due to the impairment of fat digestion. Prolonged obstructive disease of the biliary tract may cause biliary cirrhosis of the liver.

management

The ill hepatic failure patient requires careful attention and nursing care that is based on sound judgment. This patient usually arrives in the intensive care unit in some state of unconsciousness. Some type of seizure activity may be present. The skin and sclera will be jaundiced. Coagulation times are prolonged and bleeding is apt to occur from any mucous membrane, an injection and/or infusion site, the gastrointestinal tract, and/or the genitourinary tract. Mouth sores, if not present, may develop due to the debilitated state of the patient.

In order for the liver to restore itself, the demands of the body on it must be limited. Therefore, the whole body is put at rest. With the whole individual resting, the blood supply to the liver will be increased (as the muscles and the gastrointestinal tract will not require as much blood) and it may heal itself. During this period of liver cell regeneration, the treatment of the patient will consist of (1) maintaining those bodily functions (such as respiratory function) not impaired by the disease, (2) intervening when assistance is required to maintain specific functions (such as fluid balance), and (3) taking over the function of those systems where failure may be complete (such as maintaining albumin levels).

Because of the patient's inability to maintain fluid and electrolyte balance and the everpresent possibility of impaired renal function, an accurate intake and output record must be kept. Weighing the patient daily will assess fluid retention.

Patients with hepatic failure require a large stable intravenous conduit because of the need for large quantities of blood, plasma, albumin and fluids necessary to maintain bodily functions until the diseased liver cells are regenerated. Maintenance of electrolyte balance is achieved by the intravenous route. These patients tend toward potassium depletion due to (1) the diarrhea induced from the enemas, laxatives and antibiotics administered to evacuate and/or sterilize the bowel, (2) the use of diuretics to reduce water retention, (3) frequent paracentesis to relieve the symptoms of ascites, and (4) the liver failure itself.

Because of his generalized deteriorating health state, the patient is very susceptible to infection. Disturbances of the respiratory system, such as pneumonia; of the circulatory system, such as thrombophlebitis; and of the skin, such as decubitus ulcers, need to be avoided. All the invasive equipment and procedures used, including the intravenous line, the bladder catheter, the gastrointestinal tubes, and paracentesis, must be treated as the source of infection they are. An alert and conscientious nurse can prevent this type of complication with continuous application of her nursing skills.

The use of medications poses a particular danger due to the inability of the diseased liver to detoxify certain drugs. The nurse must be particularly attentive to the amount of the medications administered. Most sedatives, analgesics and narcotics are detoxified in the liver; therefore, the level of responsiveness before and after the administration of these drugs is important.

Skin care must be meticulous in the hepatic patient. Subcutaneous edema, immobility, and poor nutrition are all present and are all prime factors in the development of decubitus ulcers.

Due to the incapacity of the patient, a complete and applicable knowledge of respiratory care is essential. (Please refer to Chapters 11 to 14 on respiratory care in this book.)

The complications of liver disease are numerous and varied. Their advent is ominous and their treatment is notoriously difficult. Among the most difficult to manage are gastrointestinal hemorrhages, excessive water retention with ascites and edema, impairment of the central and peripheral nervous systems, abnormal bleeding tendencies, and hepatic coma (ammonia intoxication).

Recovery is neither rapid nor easy. There are frequent setbacks and an apparent lack of improvement. The survival of the patient is greatly dependent on optimal medical and nursing management.

BIBLIOGRAPHY

Brunner, L. S., and D. S. Suddarth, *Textbook of Medical-Surgical Nursing,* ed. 3 (Philadelphia: J. B. Lippincott, 1975).

Holvey, D. N. (ed.), *Merck Manual of Diagnosis and Therapy,* ed. 12 (Rahway, N. J.: Merck & Company, 1972).

Meltzer, L. E., et al., *Concepts and Practices of Intensive Care for Nurse Specialists,* ed. 2 (Bowie, Md.: Charles Press Publishers, 1976).

HELEN C. BUSBY, R.N.

26

management of acute gastric-intestinal bleeding

The appearance of the patient presenting with upper gastrointestinal tract bleeding varies considerably, depending upon the amount and rapidity of blood loss. The patient who is vomiting blood is usually bleeding from a source above the ligament of Treitz (at the duodenojejunal junction). Reverse peristalsis is seldom sufficient to cause hematemesis if the bleeding point is below this area. The vomitus may be bright red or coffee-ground in appearance, depending on the amount of gastric contents at the time of the bleeding and the length of time the blood has been in contact with gastric secretions. Bright red blood results from profuse bleeding and little contact with gastric juices. Gastric acid converts bright red hemoglobin to brown hematin, accounting for the coffee-ground appearance of the drainage. Massive hemorrhage from the upper gastrointestinal tract, along with increased intestinal motility, may result in stools containing bright red blood. A tarry stool may be passed if as little as 60 ml. of blood has entered the intestinal tract; tarry stools occur more frequently with duodenal ulcers than with gastric ulcers. The picture of shock will usually appear following a blood loss of 1 to 2 pints.

Care of the patient includes assessing the severity of blood loss, replacing a sufficient amount of blood to counteract shock, and planning a definite type of treatment. The decision for surgical intervention is based on many factors of the medical history and physical examination (gastric ulcer, duodenal ulcer, esophageal varices, etc.). Repetitive bleeding will likely require surgery as soon as possible.

The patient admitted with gastrointestinal bleeding needs an immediate intravenous infusion route by means of a large caliber intracatheter or cannula. Blood is typed and cross-matched and transfusion treatment is based on the presence of shock as well as on the blood count and blood volume levels. Vital signs are checked frequently until stable. Apprehension accompanied by thirst may indicate additional bleeding. Urinary output is monitored to confirm the presence of shock. The blood pressure is usually adequate to prevent cerebral or cardiac damage if the kidneys are able to produce 20 to 30 ml. of urine per hour. The moderate elevation of the BUN is due to absorption of decomposed blood from the intestine as well as diminished blood flow through the kidneys, secondary to shock.

A Levin tube is inserted to keep the stomach empty, to remove irritating gastric secretions and to lavage with iced normal saline (decreasing bleeding tendencies). If the patient is presenting with hematemesis, the stomach is irrigated with iced saline until the returned solution is clear. It is important to keep accurate records of the amount of fluid used for irrigation so that this fluid can be subtracted from the total amount of aspiration to ascertain the true amount of bleeding.

If continuous irrigation with iced saline does not decrease the amount of bleeding, the instillation of topical thrombin into the stomach may be ordered. Thrombin clots blood at the site of bleeding by acting directly with fibrinogen. Because of this action, topical thrombin is used only on the surface of bleeding tissue and is never injected into blood vessels where extensive intravascular clotting would result. The speed with which thrombin clots blood is dependent upon its concentration; i.e., 5,000 units of topical thrombin in 5 ml. of saline is capable of clotting 5 ml. of blood in 1 second. Remember, to clot the site of bleeding in the stomach, the topical thrombin must come in contact with the capillary that is bleeding. This may not be possible; therefore, topical thrombin will not be beneficial in every case of upper gastrointestinal tract bleeding.

The procedure for instillation of topical thrombin is more time consuming than difficult.

1. Aspirate stomach contents and measure.
2. Instill per nasogastric tube 2 ounces of a buffer solution and clamp the tube. Dilute acid is detrimental to thrombin activity; therefore, stomach acids must be neutralized prior to administration of thrombin. Milk may be used until the pharmacy can prepare a buffer solution. This phosphate buffer solution is stable only for 48 hours, so solutions cannot be stored for future use.
3. After 5 minutes, instill 2 more ounces of the buffer solution, containing 10,000 units of topical thrombin. Clamp tube.
4. After 30 minutes, aspirate stomach. If no fresh bleeding is evident, instill 2 ounces of the buffer and clamp the tube.
5. Repeat instillation of 2 ounces of the buffer solution every 1 to 2 hours for 24 to 48 hours.

6. If bleeding is not controlled after the 30 minutes, or if bleeding begins again, repeat steps 1 through 4. Repeat this procedure until bleeding is stopped.
7. Remember to total the aspiration and mark as output. Since the buffer solution is absorbed, mark this amount as intake.

Another method that may be used to control gastric bleeding is a continuous irrigation of the stomach with iced saline containing levarterenol (Levophed). The usual dilution is two ampuls of levarterenol per 1,000 ml. of normal saline. The principle action of this agent is vasoconstriction. Following absorption in the stomach, levarterenol is immediately sent to the liver via the portal system where metabolism of the drug takes place; therefore, a systemic reaction is prevented.

If the patient is not vomiting, or after the bleeding is controlled, a feeding program is instituted. Milk is given every 1 to 2 hours, day and night. Often Maalox or a similar antacid is also given every 1 to 2 hours. The milk and antacid should be given at alternating times. This means the patient is getting a neutralizing agent every 30 minutes if on an hourly alternation, or every hour if on a 2-hour alternation. Milk is absorbed; therefore, it is measured and added to the intake tally. Non-absorbable alkali antacids are not considered part of the intake volume.

Diagnostic studies are done as soon as possible for the purpose of establishing a definite diagnosis. A prothrombin time is performed to rule out (1) the presence of long-term anticoagulant therapy (which may not immediately be made known in the excitement of admitting a patient during an episode of gastrointestinal bleeding) and (2) liver disease. A prolonged prothrombin time may be indicative of liver disease. A normal Bromsulphalein test (BSP) is generally considered to be adequate in ruling out esophageal varices as a source of bleeding.

As soon as the patient's clinical condition stabilizes, an upper gastrointestinal series and/or gastroscopy may be performed (Fig. 26-1). Both are of immense value to the physician in deciding definitive treatment.

Esophageal varices should be suspected in the patient who has been addicted to alcohol and who presents with upper gastrointestinal bleeding. To control the hemorrhage from the varices, pressure is exerted on the cardia of the stomach and against the bleeding varices by a double balloon tamponade (the Sengstaken-Blakemore tube) (Fig. 26-2).

Once the tube is in the stomach, the stomach balloon is inflated with the amount of air necessary, predetermined by measuring the amount of air necessary to inflate the balloon prior to insertion. After inflation, the tube is slowly withdrawn until the gastric balloon fits snugly against the cardia of the stomach. Traction is then placed on the tube where it enters the patient. Traction is achieved by means of a piece of sponge rubber, as shown in Fig. 26-2. This procedure may be sufficient to control the bleeding if the varices are in the cardia of the stomach.

If bleeding continues, the esophageal balloon is inflated to a pressure of 25

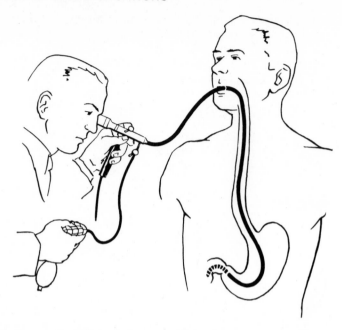

Fig. 26-1. Patient undergoing gastroscopy. Note the extreme flexibility of the tube with the patient in the sitting position. (Adapted from G. McNeer and G. T. Pack, *Neoplasms of the Stomach*, Philadelphia, J. B. Lippincott, 1967)

to 40 mm. Hg and maintained at this pressure for 24 hours. Pressure for longer than 24 hours could cause edema, ulceration or perforation of the esophagus.

If bleeding still persists, traction is applied to the end of the balloon. This may consist of suspending a weight from the end of the tube or putting a football helmet on the patient and securing the tube, under traction, to the face bar.

The potential dangers of this treatment require constant observation and intelligent care. It is essential that the three tube openings be identified, correctly labeled and checked for patency prior to insertion. The pressures in the balloons must be maintained and the balloons must be kept in their proper position. If the gastric balloon ruptures, the entire tube may rise into the nasopharynx and completely obstruct the airway. In the event this happens, deflate the esophageal balloon and withdraw the entire apparatus. It is wise to

Fig. 26-2. Diagram showing esophageal varices and their treatment by a compressing balloon tube (Sengstaken-Blakemore). (A) Dilated veins of the lower esophagus. (B) The tube is in place in the stomach and the lower esophagus but is not inflated. (C) Inflation of the tube and the compression of the veins which can be obtained by inflation of the balloon. (From L. S. Brunner and D. S. Suddarth, *Textbook of Medical-Surgical Nursing*, ed. 3, Philadelphia, J. B. Lippincott, 1975, p. 609)

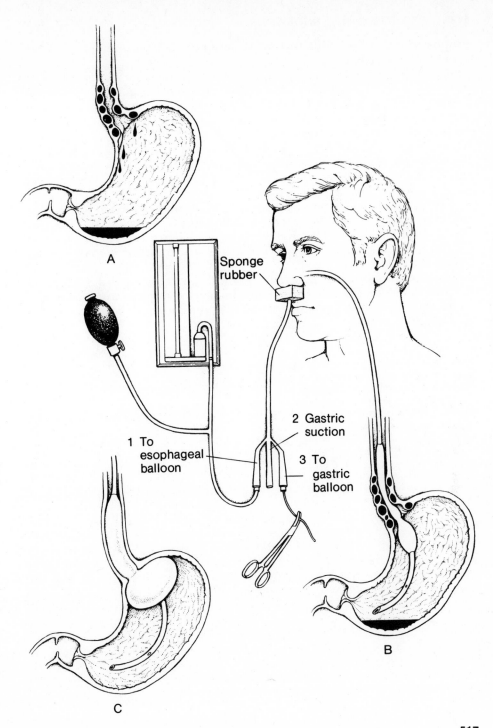

A

Sponge rubber

2 Gastric suction

3 To gastric balloon

1 To esophageal balloon

B

C

prophylactically restrain the patient's arms if he is agitated and restless to prevent him from dislodging the tube.

The patient is kept at complete rest since exertion, such as coughing or straining, tends to increase intra-abdominal pressure that predisposes to further bleeding. The head of the bed is kept elevated to reduce the flow of blood into the portal system. Since the patient is unable to swallow, saliva must be suctioned frequently from the upper esophagus. The nasopharynx also needs frequent suctioning due to the increased secretions resulting from irritation by the tube. The nostrils are checked frequently, cleansed and lubricated, for the tube causes pressure. The nasogastric tube should be irrigated every 2 hours to assure that it is patent, and the stomach must be kept empty.

Patients with liver damage tolerate the breakdown products of blood in the intestinal tract very poorly. Bacterial action on the blood in the intestinal tract produces ammonia which is absorbed into the bloodstream. The ability of the liver to convert ammonia to urea is impaired, and ammonia intoxication ensues (see Chapter 25).

The nurse will probably experience many frustrations while caring for such patients; however, constant observation and expert nursing care are essential to stabilizing them. Surgery for a portal systemic shunt may be indicated after this crisis is reversed.

BIBLIOGRAPHY

— Brunner, L. S., and D. S. Suddarth, *Textbook of Medical-Surgical Nursing*, ed. 3 (Philadelphia: J. B. Lippincott, 1975).

Holvey, D. N. (ed.), *Merck Manual of Diagnosis and Therapy*, ed. 12 (Rahway, N. J.: Merck & Company, 1972).

Meltzer, L. E., et al., *Concepts and Practices of Intensive Care for Nurse Specialists*, ed. 2 (Bowie, Md.: Charles Press Publishers, 1976).

Watson, J. E., *Medical-Surgical Nursing and Related Physiology* (Philadelphia: W. B. Saunders, 1972).

HELEN C. BUSBY, R.N.

hyperalimentation: total parenteral nutrition

One of the breakthroughs in the medical management of patients who have lost the ability to eat and/or absorb nutrients is *parenteral hyperalimentation*. Enough calories and nitrogen to sustain life can be supplied to the body through this process. Burns, gastrointestinal disorders, and liver disorders are but a few of the indications for this sophisticated therapy (Table 27-1).

The solution for parenteral hyperalimentation begins as a base solution of 1,000 calories (20 percent glucose) and nitrogen (5 percent amino acids) per

table 27-1
indications for total parenteral nutrition

Malnutrition	Diverticulitis
Malabsorption	Alimentary tract fistula
Chronic diarrhea	Alimentary tract anomalies
Chronic vomiting	Reversible liver failure
Failure to thrive	Acute and chronic renal failure
Gastrointestinal obstruction	Burns
Ulcer disease	Hypermetabolic states
Granulomatous enterocolitis	Complicated trauma or surgery
Ulcerative colitis	Short bowel syndrome
Pancreatitis	Protein-losing gastroenteropathy
Severe anorexia nervosa	Nonterminal coma
Indolent wounds and decubitus ulcers	Malignant disease (adjunctive therapy)

S. J. Dudrick, "Total Intravenous Feeding: When Nutrition Seems Impossible," *Drug Therapy*, Hospital Edition, Vol. 1, No. 2 (February 1976), p. 92.

1,000 cc. To preserve the nitrogen balance of the body, hypertonic glucose is given for caloric requirements, thus allowing the amino acids to be used for protein synthesis rather than being burned up for energy. Daily additions to the base solution of potassium, sodium and chloride are necessary. The daily requirements of these are greatly increased because of the increased volume of water intake and output. With the increased intake of glucose and amino acids, hypokalemia will soon result if additional potassium is not administered in sufficient quantities to maintain normal serum potassium levels. Potassium is also necessary for the transport of glucose and amino acids across the cell membrane. Magnesium, calcium, phosphorus and other trace elements are added as deficiencies occur. Since cations are poorly absorbed in the intestinal tract, the intravenous requirements of these elements are less than one would suspect. A multiple vitamin preparation is usually mixed in 1 liter of base solution per day. A unit of albumin may also be included daily to supplement protein intake.

Decisions concerning the amount of additives necessary to keep the patient in electrolyte balance are determined from serial blood tests. Positive nitrogen balance is monitored by serial BUN and creatinine levels. A hyperalimentation panel as shown in Table 27-2 is done twice daily initially, and then daily until

table 27-2
tests that may be on a hyperalimentation panel

CHEMISTRY	NORMAL RANGES	RESULTS
pH	7.35–7.45	
Sodium	135–149 mEq./L.	
Potassium	3.5–5.3 mEq./L.	
Chlorides	100–109 mEq./L.	
Calcium	4.5–5.7 mEq./L.	
Phosphorus	1.45–2.76 mEq./L.	
Magnesium	1.5–2.4 mEq./L.	
Glucose	70–115 mg./dL.	
BUN	8–22 mg./dL.	
Creatine	0.8–1.6 mg./dL.	
Bicarbonate	22–26 mEq./L.	
Total protein	5.5–8.0 gm./dL.	

the electrolytes are stabilized. Once stabilization is achieved, the serum levels may be checked every other day.

Glucose intolerance may occur at the onset of treatment if the pancreas does not respond to the increased glucose load. Fractional urines must be done every 4 hours on every patient receiving hyperalimentation therapy. Parenteral insulin should be administered when necessary to maintain the quantitative urine glucose at the 2 percent level. Insulin may be added to the base solution (5 to 25 units crystalline insulin per 1,000 calories) to enhance the utilization of glucose and protein in patients with borderline glucose tolerance or pancreatic disorders, in critically ill patients and in cases of severe malnutrition. Insulin has the peculiarity of settling to the bottom of the solution; therefore, intravenous solutions with insulin added must be agitated every hour to prevent too large an insulin infusion in too short a time.

The rate of infusion of the hypertonic solution must be constant over a 24-hour period to achieve maximum assimilation of the nutrients and to prevent hyper- or hypoglycemia. The flow rate cannot be increased to compensate for interruptions or slowing of the infusion, as glycosuria with osmotic diuresis (diuresis from body compartments and cells leading to dehydration) can occur. Headache, nausea and lassitude are early symptoms of too rapid an infusion. Too slow an infusion results in the administration of fewer nutrients, and hypoglycemia with a rebound of insulin may occur. The aim of treatment is a continuous infusion that meets the caloric requirements of the patient by allowing maximum utilization of the carbohydrate and protein substrates with minimal renal excretion. The flow rate must be checked faithfully every 30 to 60 minutes. If a slowing does happen to occur (as from an obstruction in the infusion line from a kink in the tubing), an increase of flow not to exceed 10 percent of the original rate may be instituted to bring the caloric intake back to the desired level. An infusion pump will help insure continuous accurate infusion. However, such pumps are mechanical devices subject to malfunctions, and the nurse must still keep a close watch on the flow rate.

Volume is given according to established water metabolism levels (2,500 cc. per 24 hours in adults and 100 cc. per kg. per 24 hours in infants), and carbohydrate metabolism (0.5 gm. per kg. hour). One thousand to 2,000 cc. in 24 hours is the initial intake with a gradual increase according to the patient's tolerance, established by careful clinical and chemical monitoring. Three liters is generally the maximum daily volume. However, patients undergoing massive catabolism, such as that occurring in severe or extensive burns or severe traumatic injuries, often require 4 to 5 liters per day. If there is a problem with the integrity of the liver and/or kidneys, fluid volume must be carefully calculated to prevent cardiopulmonary overload. One can readily see that the nurse must be very familiar with determining flow rate in drops per minute calculated on the size of the drop in order that the correct volume of the infusion is delivered. If the patient is receiving adequate nutrition, his weight gain should be $\frac{1}{4}$ to $\frac{1}{2}$ pound per day. If he is gaining much more, it is probably water retention and not tissue gain, and the volume infused will be adjusted downward.

Knowing the nature of this solution, one can easily understand why the usual normal intravenous routes are not utilized. This hypertonic solution would rapidly cause thrombosis at the tip of the intravenous catheter. Since this high caloric/nitrogen solution must be rapidly diluted and dispersed within the blood vessels, the superior vena cava is an excellent site. Figure 27-1 indicates the different routes which can be utilized. Passing the intravenous catheter into the superior vena cava via the subclavian vein is the route of choice, for it allows the patient the greatest freedom of movement without disturbing the injection site and the incidence of infection at this level of the body is lower. Jugular veins may be used but are not as comfortable for the patient. Basilic vein routes are too prone to irritation and infection for long-term therapy. The femoral vein as a route to the inferior vena cava is rarely selected, for it is highly susceptible to contamination from body pathogens, i.e., abdominal wound drainage, urine and stool.

Two key factors are involved in the success of hyperalimentation therapy. (1) the long-term presence of the indwelling catheter directly in the superior vena cava and (2) the hypertonic solution. Both are prime sites for the source of infection. The puncture site is a potential portal of entry of organisms, and the solution is an excellent culture medium for many species of bacteria and fungi. Meticulous asepsis in the care of the line and in the preparation of the solution cannot be overstressed.

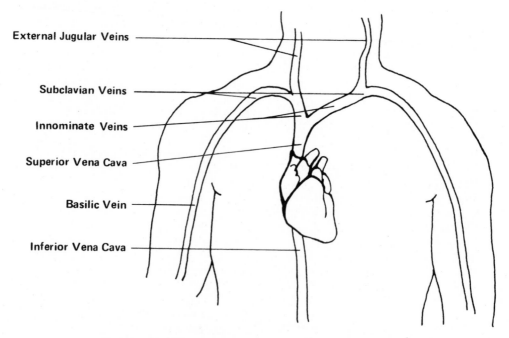

Fig. 27-1. Venous anatomy for hyperalimentation routes.

Asepsis starts with the insertion of the subclavian catheter. This is performed under strict sterile technique, and a sterile dressing is applied to the site. This dressing should be changed every 24 to 72 hours. At the time of the dressing change, the site should be examined for signs of leakage, edema and/or inflammation and the catheter should be checked for any kinking of the tube. The skin should be cleansed with a solvent such as acetone to remove surface skin fat that harbors pathogenic organisms and adhesive tape which, if allowed to accumulate, will cause irritation and skin breakdown. A large area surrounding the catheter is cleansed with an antibacterial solution (e.g., an iodine preparation) and a broad-spectrum antibiotic ointment is applied to the puncture site. An occlusive dressing is applied over the area. Open and/or draining wounds around the area or a tracheostomy in place, require extra precautions to insure sterility of the site. A transparent plastic waterproof surgical drape over the entire dressing will help prevent contamination from fluid or exudates. With sound infection control procedures, the sterility of the insertion site can be maintained for the length of the treatment, even if the treatment lasts for months.

Maintaining sterility of the solution is mandatory. As stated, it is an excellent culture medium for pathogens. The solution is usually prepared in the pharmacy with aseptic techniques. Preferably, additives are added under a laminar air-flow hood to assure a particle-free environment. If the nurse must add electrolytes and other elements to the base solution, she must be aware of any contamination that may occur from syringes, needles, flasks, etc. Each new flask is hung with particular attention to avoid contamination of the solution and the recipient set. A new bottle hung every 8 hours (with disposal of any solution left in the flask after 8 hours) may be employed. Solutions are inspected for clouding and/or particular matter when the flow rate is checked every 30 to 60 minutes.

All of the intravenous tubing should be changed once a day at the time a new flask is hung. If dressings are changed daily, the new tubing, the new bottle and the dressing change should be correlated to take place at the same time. If dressings are changed every 48 to 72 hours, the indwelling catheter and tubing connection sites should be situated so the change of tubing does not interfere with the integrity of the dressing. The tubing change is made with the patient in a low Fowler's position or flat in bed to prevent an air embolism from occurring with a deep inspiration.

No intravenous push or piggyback medications should be given in the same line as the hyperalimentation solution. No steroids, pressor drugs, antibiotics or other parenteral drugs are ever added to the base solution as they may interact with the fibrin hydrolysate or with each other, forming a precipitate that would not be visible to the naked eye. In addition, the mixing of drugs (other than the electrolytes) in the solution could necessitate adjusting the flow rate according to their requirements rather than those of the nutritional hypertonic solution. If any intravenous medication or blood transfusions are necessary, an alternate route should be started for their administration. Only the hyperalimentation solution with its electrolyte additives added under aseptic conditions should be administered through the subclavian line. The subclavian catheter should not be used to draw blood samples, either. Any break in the system is an entrance for infection; maintaining the sterility of the system is of the utmost importance.

Nursing care is based on individual patient requirements. The degree of illness may vary from that of the severely burned, critically ill patient to that of the postoperative gastrectomy patient who is up and about, progressing satisfactorily. Daily weights are recorded; the patient should be weighed with the same scale at the same time each day. Accurate intake and output records give a picture of the patient's fluid balance. Vital signs are recorded depending on the problems of the patient. Any elevation of body temperature must be reported immediately. The intravenous tubing and solution flask are changed and cultures taken from the discarded tubing and solution. If the fever persists, the treatment may be discontinued and the subclavian catheter removed. A culture is taken immediately from the tip of the catheter. An elevated temperature may be due to an allergic reaction to the nutrients, an infection around the catheter, contamination of the fluid and/or infusion tubing with resulting septicemia, or the patient's own disease process.

Patients must be observed closely for signs of solution infiltration. Any pain or swelling in the shoulder, arm, neck or face must be reported. Activity and ambulation are encouraged whenever possible to decrease the risks of phlebitis, cardiopulmonary problems and muscle wasting. Lack of exercise and muscle inactivity also lead to a catabolic state with protein breakdown and excretion.

Many patients receiving hyperalimentation therapy are afraid, worried and anxious. Their reactions to their illness vary greatly, and the nurse must help them with their psychological needs as well as their physical and physiological needs.

An expert team is essential for this therapy—the physician, the pharmacist and the nurse—and the nurse needs to be the expert in the administration of hyperalimentation.

BIBLIOGRAPHY

Coppage, C., "Describe Qualifications, Training, Functions of Nurse Epidemiologist," *Hospital Topics* (June 1972), p. 90.

Dudrick, S. J., "Total Intravenous Feeding: When Nutrition Seems Impossible," *Drug Therapy*, Hospital Edition, Vol. 1, No. 2 (February 1976), p. 92.

Grant, J. A., "Preventing Infection, Maintaining Flow Called Primarily Nurses' Responsibility," *Hospital Topics* (June 1972).

———, E. Moir, and M. Fago, "Parenteral Hyperalimentation," *American Journal of Nursing*, Vol. 69, No. 11 (November 1969), pp. 2392–2395.

professional practice in the critical care unit

NAOMI D. MEDEARIS, B.S., M.A., M.B.A.

28

planning for the training and development of the critical care nursing staff

a case in point

As the charge nurse of the critical care unit replaced the telephone in its cradle, she silently prayed enough people would respond to the Cor Zero page. She had been having these feelings of panic more frequently of late. She could not accurately anticipate the number of people who would respond. Sometimes there would be too many, sometimes there would be too few.

Without hesitation she moved into action and began dealing with the crisis. Fortunately enough people began to appear. The right things began to happen. The patient began to move out of crisis. Things began to ease off a bit.

It was then that she really began to have the shakes. "What if enough people had not shown up? What if they had not accurately assessed the situation? What if people had hesitated to do the things that needed to be done?"

That night while nursing her exhaustion and recalling the events of the day, she thought of the crisis and the panic it caused. "Why," she said to herself, "should I push the panic button every time there is a crisis on the unit? Is such wear and tear on the nervous system implicit in the job? Isn't there something I can do to reduce the tension and anxiety? Maybe I should give more leadership. Maybe I should do more staff training."

She began thinking back over the critical care course she attended some months ago. She recalled a training session focused on the teaching role of the nurse in the critical care unit. The instructor spoke of the growing trend to decentralize inservice training programs. She had said, "The rapid change

527

in medical and nursing knowledge and the new techniques and procedures which evolve from these changes have created the need to decentralize training and share on-the-job inservice responsibility with professional nurses working in clinical areas. Ask your inservice educator to assist you in developing this new facet of your role as a nurse. She can help you acquire the knowledge and skill you need for teaching and developing your staff."

What the instructor said didn't seem to fit at the time. The hospital had an inservice program which seemed to be getting the job done. When she went home she talked it over with the inservice education director and they had set up a course on critical care nursing for the entire hospital. They set up lectures by clinical specialists in nursing service, physicians, and school of nursing faculty; demonstrations of equipment by salesmen and distributors; practice sessions in reading monitor strips; and reading materials.

Things went better after the training, too. Cor Zero situations were pretty well handled. The right number of people usually showed up and did their part with few questions and with little or no hesitation. She had been pleased with the results of the training and had felt that the problem was solved.

What had happened since then? Things were certainly different now. As the charge nurse reflected on her situation, she began to suspect that several things had happened: For one thing, the inservice training program had been a "one shot" event—there was no follow-up. For another, there had been a number of staff changes in the nine months since the event. She couldn't prove this was a factor since she had never known for sure who had taken the training. Still another thing that seemed to have happened was that she had too easily assumed that everyone who had attended the inservice training would magically appear when they heard Cor Zero. And obviously this was not the case.

Even though she had been charge nurse for almost three years now she had never taken time to give such matters much thought. Nursing administration obviously had assumed she had the qualities needed for the charge nurse job; she had accepted the promotion with the same assumption. Since they hadn't talked to her about her need for supervisory training, she hadn't given it much thought.

She began to feel angry about her dilemma and her feeling of incompetence to train and develop her staff. She asked, "How can I change this situation?"

Perhaps you empathize with this charge nurse. Everyone has been there at one time or another—either in reality or in her imagination.

an overview

Alvin Toffler in his book *Future Shock* described what happens to people when they are overwhelmed by change. The acceleration of change produces a fantastic stress. Handling such stress demands special coping mechanisms. The case in point symbolizes such a situation.

To cope with job stress, the charge nurse decided to use education as a strategy for managing change. This decision became significant for three reasons. First, it challenged inservice education and the way it was organized to serve nursing personnel. Second, it expanded the role of the charge nurse and the way she developed nursing resources. Third, it changed the dynamics of staff involvement by offering each staff member different ways to respond to learning needs related to the job.

For your guidance, the first part of this chapter describes the changing focus of inservice education and its decentralization; the second part outlines the process of training and developing staff. The approach to content is presented as a guide for charge nurses in critical care units.

In describing the implications that decentralization of inservice education has for clinical areas, certain assumptions have been made regarding the charge nurse. She is competent in her nursing knowledge and skills. She is comfortable supervising the work of other people. She is aware of the acceleration of change in her unit. She is curious about potential alternatives to cope with needed changes. And she is willing to explore the possibility of decentralized inservice education and to experiment with the role of teacher-learner (or co-learner).

the changing focus of inservice education

What needs to take place in the modern hospital organization to improve inservice education of personnel working in acute settings?

Some background data on the development of inservice education will clarify its current status and support the premise that inservice for the critical care units should be decentralized to clinical areas.

current administrative structure of inservice education

In a few hospitals you will find that staff development departments are emerging which incorporate inservice functions. These departments have expanded services to facilitate the development of both the professional nursing staff and the paraprofessional staff. However, you will discover that the usual inservice department today is locked into a system which limits its effectiveness. Inservice education has struggled to establish a viable program within nursing service, and it has struggled against unbelievable odds. However, a new role for the inservice educator is gradually evolving.

Over the years, many of the time-consuming reports and surveys and disciplinary actions requiring counseling have been assigned to the inservice director, along with functions that range from conducting fire drills and updating procedural manuals to presenting films, lectures and nurse aide training programs.

Another handicap has been the budget. As a rule, the budget has been limited to the salary of the inservice director, and perhaps a part-time clerk. Operating expenses for the inservice program were "taken out of" the nursing service budget.

Physical facilities were limited to office space and an occasional classroom. Frequently the cafeteria or administrative conference rooms were utilized for training sessions.

Another deterrent to effective inservice education was the fact that the inservice educator lacked not only a realistic job description and adequate support but also the relevant educational preparation.

As you can see, it has often been an impossible job. When you combine a potpourri-type job with minimum financial support, inadequate facilities, and an underprepared inservice director, the need to reorganize administration of inservice programming is evident.

program characteristics of inservice education

If you take a moment to review the characteristics of most inservice education programs, you will discover another reason why clinical inservice should be decentralized to the unit level.

Some of the unique characteristics of inservice programs have evolved from mass education and the medical education model.

From mass education, designed to meet the needs of "anybody and everybody," classic inservice has drawn its form and methodology. It has characteristically assumed that all participants have the same abilities and interests in the subject being offered. Posters, public-address announcements, and pressure on head nurses to "send anyone who can be spared from the floor" provided criteria for selection of learners. The successful inservice program was measured by the number who attended. As in the typical academic classroom, the basic purpose of education was simply to transmit information and assume that the content was assimilated by the learner.

In following the medical model, inservice programming often got trapped into equating role status with credibility of information. Thus it often relied on lectures, slide presentations, papers, and the like, usually presented in the language of medicine. The programs were presented to an audience of nonmedical listeners, namely nurses and paraprofessional nursing personnel who were scheduled for inservice. The intent of such programming was to teach by presenting information in an authoritative manner by an authoritative status figure. And the expectation was that everyone who attended would learn.

When you look for coordinated inservice programming in most hospitals, the evidence is at best minimal. Some of the reasons for this lack include the absence of long-range, collaborative programming with staff and prospective participants; the lack of relating each inservice activity to specific learning objectives for the participants; and the sporadic attendance of personnel who seem powerless to alter their working schedule to attend a planned sequence of inservice programs. As a rule, only persons on the day shift attend. It is still a rare inservice program that is offered "live" to personnel on all three shifts. Such fragmented learning significantly weakens the chances of the learner to acquire either knowledge or skill.

Confronted with these realities, it is impossible for the inservice coordinator to follow up on inservice sessions to see whether or not the knowledge has been effectively utilized throughout nursing service. Therefore the relevance and applicability of clinical inservice offered on a mass scale to nursing personnel is at best fragmented, superficial, and transitory. Combine these facts with the explosion of new techniques, procedures, medications, equipment, and material in a multiplicity of clinical settings within the hospital and you find that the need to restructure inservice is inescapable.

Consequently, you, as a charge nurse in the critical care unit, may want to pursue the prospect of developing a training and staff development program of your own. Such a program would be tailored to meet the needs of *your* unit, *your* staff, and *your* patients. We hope that the description of decentralization of inservice to clinical areas will offer data upon which you can base a decision to undertake such a task.

a look at decentralized inservice education

ASSESSING FEASIBILITY OF DECENTRALIZATION

To answer the question of feasibility you will need to gather data upon which to base your decision to add inservice and staff development to your job responsibilities. You will need to assess your current functions. To accomplish this assessment, the following suggestions are offered:

1. List the responsibilities for which you hold yourself accountable. By writing out a detailed list of these functions you will develop a concrete picture of what you do.
2. Next, rank-order these functions according to your own priorities. Perhaps this will be difficult to do, for you can easily convince yourself that everything you do is equally important. However, by numbering 1, 2, etc., you lay the foundation for the next important step in your job assessment.
3. Critically evaluate each of these functions. Consider: should you delegate, discontinue, reschedule or reorganize the function — or should you retain the function as it is? The outcome of this evaluation will provide data for reallocating your time and redesigning some aspects of your job, so that you can assume the new training functions.
4. Now, going back to your priority listing of responsibilities, insert inservice and staff development functions in a realistic position. By doing this, you crystallize your intent to engage in creating new job functions and your willingness to allocate time and effort to do so.
5. Evaluate the personal resources you bring to this new function of training and developing your staff. Again, write down the teaching you are already doing. Find answers to questions like, What help do I give new employees and floats? How do I introduce new ideas, procedures, equipment, supplies? After attending a meeting, conference, or intensive course, how do I share the information? When a critical incident occurs, how do I deal with it? When I am working side by side with my staff in a crisis situation, what is my staff learning from me? When the census is low, how do I use the time? Do personnel on the other shifts understand and follow nursing care plans that I write?

How is "report" given and received? What plans do I make prior to calling a staff meeting, and how does my staff respond? What do employees learn in the periodic performance appraisals?

Add questions which occur to you to this list and analyze more completely the teaching and learning going on in your unit at the present time. The process of disciplining yourself to write down what you do will help you (1) determine the training currently done, (2) recognize and build on the teaching you are already doing, and (3) clarify those areas that you may want to change to maximize learning potential.

The next data you will need to assemble come from other people whose functions relate to your own. These people include the Director of Nursing Service and the Director of Inservice Education. Following the pattern used in assessing your own resources, list the administrative resources available to you that will provide the needed support for launching your inservice program. Consider specifically the interest, style, and leadership, as well as the contribution the Director of Nursing Service could offer you in your undertaking. Your observations, based on such questions as these, will help you list available resources: What is the attitude of nursing service toward experimenting with new ideas, new functions, new programs? What position does nursing administration take when plans do not work out as predicted? What kind of financial support would administration give if either additional coverage, compensatory time, or overtime pay were indicated in my staff development plan? Would money be available for outside consultation should such consultation resources be needed? Would administration underwrite costs for continuing education (tuition, fees, travel, lodging, and the like) outside our hospital to prepare me and members of my staff to increase our clinical competence as such opportunities arise? What kind of space do we have to hold staff conferences and how available is this space to us?

Next, assess the resources that the inservice education department offers. What support will the Director of Inservice Education give a decentralized inservice program? What materials are available to me, such as film and tape catalogues and programmed instruction materials on clinical aspects of nursing related to my specialty service? What unique resources, such as persons within the hospital, related health agencies and associations, colleges and universities, and health consumers, are available to me?

As a result of this assessment of resources available from nursing administration, the inservice education department, and your own personal resources, you will have a basis of deciding whether or not it is feasible to continue your exploration of decentralization. If it shows promise, you are ready to pursue the study of the characteristics of a decentralized inservice program that is tailored to meet the needs of the adult learners in your unit.

CHARACTERISTICS OF DECENTRALIZED CLINICAL INSERVICE EDUCATION

The most unique characteristics of a reality-based inservice program in a clinical unit are its flexibility, spontaneity, timing, relevance, conscious exploitation of daily situations for learning, the active involvement of everyone present, and the supportive nonjudgmental climate. A brief descriptive statement of each of these characteristics may help you get a feeling for the dynamic nature of a small, interdependent staff, meaningfully involved in meeting their own learning goals and the general goals of their unit.

A flexible program implies that even though there are thoughtfully developed training plans to meet long-term goals within a predetermined time block, changes can be made in the light of unexpected developments which offer viable learning opportunities, but *now. Flexibility* is the freedom to change the master training plan, to improvise on ongoing training, or to alter priorities based on new data or needs. If the charge nurse and members of her staff develop an awareness of freedom to deviate from the training prescription in the light of pertinent facts, and then exercise this freedom, flexibility to move to meet the needs becomes evident. Appropriate action will then follow.

Spontaneity might be described as generating learning from daily on-the-spot incidents, or when the inspiration occurs. No plan exists. Out of a situation grows the opportunity to acquire insights, identify new knowledge, or recognize new skills. Sensitivity to the learning inherent in what is happening all the time can be developed in your staff. This quality spawns spontaneity and unexpected or surprise opportunities to learn. It makes learning fun!

A *sense of timing* is essential to planning inservice and designing individualized staff development. Respect for careful and thorough long-range programming is a vital part of sequencing learning activities. On the other hand, a quick, perceptive response to a current situation has a profound effect on timing. If you can develop a feeling for the pulse of what is happening in the unit and if you can feed in either programmed or spontaneous learning experiences, you utilize time effectively and your staff responds positively.

Every potential training event should be assessed very specifically to see how directly it relates to the patient, the staff, and the unit. To validate *relevance* of potential learning, identify such basic issues as (1) how this information will be used, (2) why it should be offered, (3) what changes it will require, (4) what changes will individuals need to make, and (5) what results are expected. Taking time to articulate these relationships of learning will pinpoint their relevance to patient service, to the situation, to staff capacity, and to the goals of the unit.

In looking at the *exploitation of the daily situation for learning purposes*, you select those situations that occur infrequently or offer unique content and experience. Another criterion for selecting a situation is the opportunity for all those involved to see the same occurrence and share their different perceptions of it and how they experienced it. From this it is possible to create new procedures, anticipate similar problems, and check out the understanding of what might be expected the next time a comparable event occurs. It affords an opportunity to demonstrate role and task relationships. The art of managing time, staff, and the situation creates meaningful involvement and learning for each person present.

Active involvement of everyone present has been alluded to in the aforementioned characteristics. However, active involvement of the total person in the teaching-learning process deserves to be lifted out for special emphasis. Research on the learning process shows people remember

10% of what they read
20% of what they hear
30% of what they see
50% of what they see and hear
80% of what they say
90% of what they say as they do a thing*

A *nonjudgmental climate* supports a creative inservice program in the clinical unit. Such a climate allows moderate risk-taking on the part of staff who want to grow personally and professionally while working, and who want to accept responsibility for their experimentation and are willing to be held accountable for the results. This climate permits more self-direction, once the level of competency has been identified cooperatively by the worker and members of the staff and the charge nurse. It creates a support system of interdependence when each member clearly sees the situation and the role and level of competency of her co-workers, and understands and accepts her relationship, level of competency, and responsibility in the unit. A nonjudgmental attitude supports the staff as they learn to move toward higher levels of competency. The emphasis is not on what is right or wrong, but rather, what is the most effective way to accomplish the task. Perhaps this attitude is the most significant one to develop when a new training program which is based on involvement of the staff is undertaken.

Even though these descriptions of characteristics have been given separately, they are in fact blended, balanced, and counterbalanced in a well-conceived inservice program. To the degree that you develop your skill in integrating these components in your inservice and staff development programming, you can measure the degree of artistry and effectiveness you have in handling this responsibility.

expanded role = charge nurse in critical care unit + learning specialist

Probably the most exciting part of your new role in assuming responsibility for training and developing your staff is the fact that there is little precedent for it. Part of the reason for this is the recent major shift in emphasis from "teaching" to "learning." Becoming a learning specialist in the critical care unit offers a unique opportunity to pioneer—develop the role as you live it.

In writing about this change in education the eminent psychologist Carl Rogers points out that as a teacher he discovered he couldn't teach anyone anything. He believes the student learns what *he* wants and needs to learn. This fact imposes a significant change in the role of the teacher. Rogers believes his role as teacher is to help the student learn. To provide the kind of

---

*Special survey/research project conducted by the Industrial Audiovisual Association.

help the student needs in order to learn, the teacher will need to assume the new role of co-learner. As a co-learner, the teacher is free to learn many things about the learner, from the learner, and with the learner.

In the process of learning these things, the teacher will assume her part of the responsibility in the teaching-learning process—that is, planning and organizing learning activities and materials which have as their goal the satisfaction of learner needs. The teacher's responsibilities center around having "the right resources and materials, at the right time and in the right place" so that the learner can learn when she is ready.

Transferring this concept to the teaching and learning activities in the critical care unit, your role as teacher does not carry full responsibility for training and developing your staff. In fact, you and members of your staff will enter into a co-learner relationship in the teaching-learning process. You will need to learn together. Their role as learners will change from passively listening to you, as teacher, to actively assuming responsibility for what they want and need to learn, and when they need to learn it.

Employees are more than workers, they are adults who want to learn. Powell and Aker point this out (bracketed material added):

> Adults do not need, nor do they wish, to be overly directed or controlled in their learning experiences. They are self-directed, autonomous human beings, and desire a strong sense of dignity and individual worth. Nothing will offend this sense of dignity more than to have an individual throw bits of information at them, like raw chunks of meat, and demand that they accept them.
>
> The adult is a learner; as such, the responsibility for learning should be placed upon him. He will choose, if allowed, what he learns and how he learns it, and will also decide the rate and speed at which he learns best. He will need helpful advice and suggestions, however, as to how he should best continue his self-directed learning . . . and this is where the teacher [charge nurse] comes in, as a helpful aide who is prepared, not to answer the student's [employee's] every question, or to solve his problem, but to help him develop the skills to solve his own problems. *The teacher* [charge nurse] *should not attempt to play God.* Her adult students [employees] are as mature as she, and in certain ways probably more so. With a deep interest in the student [employee] the teacher [charge nurse] can help him find his own way, but find his own way he must.[1]

If you embrace this concept of the role of teacher, you will probably have to unlearn many of your preconceived ideas about how you train and develop your staff. If, however, you can engage in this newer concept of the teaching role, the excitement of sharing responsibility for learning activities with your staff will bring its own rewards.

Characteristics of effective learning specialists include the following: (1) they spend considerable time planning; (2) they individualize instruction and make it practical in terms of the interests, needs and wants of their employees; (3) they are highly flexible; and (4) they use a wide variety of methods and techniques.

Planning is needed in order to develop unit goals, staff goals and individual goals; planning is needed in order to determine which method or technique or material will facilitate the achievement of objectives, and planning helps develop criteria for evaluating progress and change. Much of the planning, however, can be shared with staff members, as can the instructional responsibilities. The good teacher carefully plans the learning experience on the one hand but is extremely flexible on the other—by being able to use various techniques and resources to achieve the overall objectives as opportunities arise. A sensitive teacher constantly adjusts and changes the plan for the learning experience as new opportunities for doing so are presented and as "feedback" is obtained from the staff.

Many techniques and methods are available to you. Your choice of technique will be governed by the learning need and the situation. A brief summary follows:

1. *Presentation techniques:* lecture, television, videotape, dialogue, interview, group interview, demonstration, slides, dramatization, recordings, exhibits, trips, and reading.
2. *Discussion techniques:* guided discussion, article or book-based discussion, problem-solving discussion, group-centered discussion.
3. *Simulation techniques:* role playing, critical-incident process, case method, games, participative cases.
4. T-Group (sensitivity training).
5. Nonverbal exercises.
6. Skill-practice exercises, drill, coaching.

The best way to develop a repertoire of techniques is to experiment and evaluate effectiveness. Keep in mind the objective, and match the technique with it. Certain techniques are more effective in bringing about behavioral change than others. Another point to remember is the principle of participation. If you have a choice between techniques, choose the one that involves your staff in active participation.

To increase your knowledge and skill in the teaching-learning process and your knowledge of adults and how they learn, read the current professional journals. An increasing number of journals present innovative ideas, and writers share their experiences in using action learning approaches.

dynamics of staff involvement

As you become increasingly aware of the teaching-learning process as it applies to the responsibility you and the staff of your unit share, it becomes obvious that the staff will actively participate in the training and development enterprise. If you can release the need for achievement, reduce the fear of failure, enhance the curiosity drive, develop new interests and stimulate the desire for learning and self-fulfillment, you will have effectively performed your tasks and fulfilled your role as charge nurse-learning specialist. To accomplish these tasks, several principles may make your job easier. These principles, taken from Powell and Aker, support the concept of active participation and staff development programming. If you bear these principles in mind, they will provide a viable guideline for securing participation that is meaningful to staff and productive in good achievement.

PRINCIPLES OF ADULT LEARNING

1. *Adults learn better when they are actively involved in the learning process.* The more they participate through discussion groups and in other group techniques, the more responsibility they are given for what happens in a learning situation, the more effectively they will progress.

2. *Adults can learn materials which apply to their daily work more quickly than they can learn irrelevant materials.* Adults will be receptive to new information only if they are sure it is useful to them immediately.

3. *Adults will accept new ideas more quickly if these ideas support previous beliefs.* Adults come to learning situations with a well-fixed set of values and beliefs, regardless of whether or not they verbalize them. They tend to reject information which attacks or destroys their beliefs.

4. *Adults' needs and backgrounds must be understood and integrated into their learning experiences as much as possible. Out of feelings of inadequacy, many adults believe they cannot learn.* This belief will be evident in their attitude toward learning situations and toward themselves. Before they are placed in a learning situation, adults should first feel encouraged enough to attempt to learn; otherwise they are likely to fail before they begin.

5. *To the extent possible, adults should be allowed to pursue their own areas of interest at their own rate, and to find answers to questions on their own.* Regardless of how they may react to an authoritarian learning atmosphere, adults are not likely to grasp knowledge that is forced upon them. A teacher should act as a resource person, available to guide or discuss a problem with the learner. The teacher should *not* have all the answers, or even pretend to have them.

6. *Adults, because of possible unhappy past experiences, should be prepared for learning so it will be a pleasant, rather than an unpleasant, experience.* Drill and repetition of material will not help them to learn. It will only make them dislike the learning experience even more than they did before.

7. *Adult learners should be rewarded immediately for success, and should never feel as if they are being punished for making a mistake.* When rewarded, they will want to continue the experience. If punished, they are apt to reject the entire situation either by leaving it physically or by refusing to become involved.

8. *Adults learn in a series of "plateaus";* that is, they do well for a while, then level off in performance, but they will move on again if they have not become discouraged. This is a natural process, and adults should understand that it is, so that they will not give up.

9. *Adults should always know why they are learning and toward what goal they are aiming.* They should understand what steps are necessary to reach a particular learning goal, and in what order they should come. If

adults become confused about where they are going, or why they are going there, they will lose interest in going any place.[2]

In summary, the decentralization of inservice education and staff development to the critical care unit offers the charge nurse an opportunity to experiment with innovative ways of meeting the learning needs of her staff and to achieve a higher level of nursing service for her patients. The characteristics of a decentralized training program, built on sound adult education principles and supported concretely by nursing administration, provide a framework upon which the charge nurse can begin to create a new role for herself—co-learner and learning specialist. The risks in undertaking this task should be moderate and the rewards should be great . . . for staff and charge nurse alike.

Moving on to the second part of this chapter, the process of training and staff development is outlined for the purpose of providing a practical and systematic approach which may prove useful to the charge nurse in a critical care unit.

the process of training and staff development

Training has as its primary purpose the discovery, development, and change of employee behavior and attitudes in such a way that job performance will be improved. Staff development includes this purpose of training as a component, but adds another vital purpose—staff development is predicated on meeting some of the employee's need for self-worth, growth and development, and satisfaction through her work.

If you, as charge nurse, undertake the responsibility for training and developing members of your staff in the critical care unit, you will need to give careful thought to these two components of staff development and their implications for your leadership style. It will mean integrating the needs and goals of the critical care unit with the personal growth needs and goals of members of your staff. For only by blending and balancing these diverse needs can you hope to achieve the ultimate goals of delivering appropriate and effective care to each patient and his family, as well as growth opportunities for you and your staff.

To provide some background for your orientation, consider the contribution of progressive industrial management.

For the past two decades many industries have experimented extensively with ways of dealing with both organizational needs and objectives, and employee needs and objectives. Researchers have attempted to discover and develop the key to releasing motivational energy of employees toward achievement of company objectives. The research findings showed that the concentrated effort on the part of management and the willingness to participate on the part of employees resulted in participative and collaborative planning in job and staff development. Over a period of time the results of these cooperative efforts in job and staff development have been measured in cold cash—lower operating costs, lower turnover, creative product development, new marketing techniques, new management techniques, and increased profits.

Shifting from industry to health care systems, and to hospitals in particular, the problem of tapping the full potential of the people-resources is of genuine concern. With the increased pressure to deliver more effective health care to the community, control costs to patients, and more fully utilize the unique capabilities of employees, hospitals must look for alternatives to the narrowly conceived assembly-line way of delivering health service to patients.

There was a tendency (and still is in some cases) for hospital administration and nursing service to buy into the assembly-line, minute-division-of-labor approach to organizing work which stems from Henry Ford's mass production concept, and was almost written in stone by Frederick W. Taylor in his scientific management theory.*

With the multiplication of the number of professional specialties and skilled technicians in the health sciences, the challenge to integrate into the health care system persons who come with special educational preparation and rich and varied work experiences is somewhat overwhelming. To this complex situation add the fact that all of these people come initially with a desire to make maximum use of their special expertise and the need to keep growing in their occupational life as well as their personal life. It appears that the key to genuine motivation rests within the employee and is released when the need to keep growing on the job is met. How to release this energy in the interests of providing effective health care to patients is the focus of practical and realistic training and staff development.

The need to respond to a different concept of management confronts not only hospital administrators but also directors of nursing administration, and specifically supervisors of direct patient care.

Experience in training and developing a small group of people into an organization acknowledges the reality of interdependence, the need for mutual work goals, and an awareness of the process needed to achieve both organization and individual goals. It utilizes the participative decision-making process in those areas of work that directly involve the resources of the employee.

The process model for training and staff development is offered as a means of facilitating the planning of specific, realistic, and needed training which can be made manageable and measurable (Fig. 28-1). By familiarizing yourself with the process model, you can begin to develop an overall program for your unit. In addition, you will find it equally applicable in designing your

---

* Taylor assumed that the majority of employees were undereducated and unskilled. Therefore a system which divided the task into routinized fragments which relatively unskilled workers could perform adequately under close supervision would maximize production. This theory also assumed a high need for control and centralized decision making. This theory may be useful in some industrial processes, but is not useful in the delivery of health care. In fact, it seriously inhibits and curtails the service to patients as well as stunts the growth and development of the professionals and paraprofessionals involved.

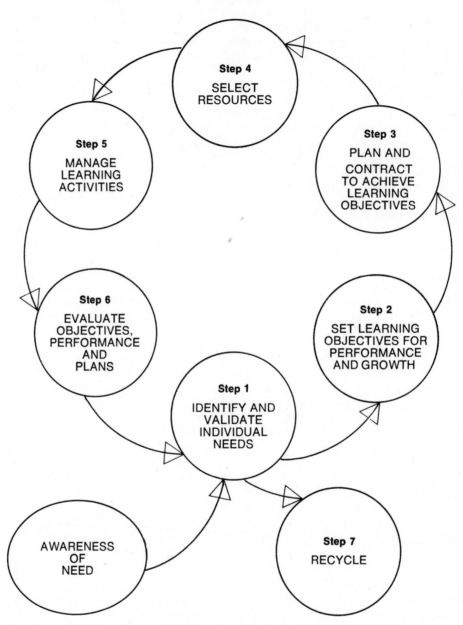

Fig. 28-1. Process model for training and staff development.

own personal and professional developmental plan, and it will serve you well as a guide for working and planning with each member of your staff. Moreover, it will provide a continuing framework for training and developing staff through its recycling design. The process model uses seven steps:

Step 1. Identify and validate individual needs.

Step 2. Set individual learning objectives for performance and growth.

Step 3. Plan and contract to achieve learning objectives.

Step 4. Select resources.

Step 5. Manage learning activities.

Step 6. Evaluate objectives, performance and learning plan.

Step 7. Recycle.

Perhaps right now, as a result of the assessment you made of your personal resources, you are very much aware of how good you feel about the training you are already doing in your unit; however, you are also becoming increasingly aware of the value of involving your staff more actively in planning training which will meet some of their own needs. From this new awareness, a healthy dissatisfaction with the present way you are functioning as a teacher may trigger your taking time to validate the need to change the way you handle training in terms of staff involvement. This initial awareness is shown in the model (Fig. 28-1) in a kind of free form. It represents the consciousness of a need, but this need lacks validation which is necessary to determine whether or not it is a viable learning need.

step 1 – identify and validate individual needs

How do you determine what the needs are?

How do you check them out to make sure they are real?

Are they educational needs that can be met through training or staff development?

In reply to the question, "How do you determine what the training needs are?" your best source of information will be the people with whom you work in delivering care to patients in the critical care unit. Different needs will come from each shift and from persons who "float" or "relieve" on the days the regular staff is off.

You can obtain data on needs in many ways; however, here are three with which you are familiar: interviewing, observation, periodic performance evaluations.

INTERVIEWING

If the individuals in the critical care unit are interviewed either formally or informally, on a one-to-one basis, or as a group, data based on "conscious needs" will be collected. Preparation on your part prior to interviewing will facilitate gathering specific data and guide the discussion; however, the use of some open-ended questions will permit some free-flowing input from employees and provide data that otherwise you would miss.

OBSERVATION

Gather data based on guided observations of the job performance of each member of the staff, on their interactions with patients and with each other. Observe staff contacts with persons who provide direct services to patients in the critical care unit, but who are not a part of the critical care staff. As a professional nurse in charge of nursing care delivered in the critical care unit, your observations are those of the expert. Your perceptions provide the criteria for determining the required level of competence for effective performance. Therefore, base your observations on a set of criteria which you prepare prior to making your observations. Your observations will reveal the "unconscious needs"—those needs that were not revealed in the interviews, but are evident from the point of view of an expert.

PERIODIC PERFORMANCE EVALUATIONS

Data on these reports provide an indication of the needs and resources both you and the employee are aware of and have dealt with in some way. In some cases, reports may cover several years and reflect changes in the performance level of an employee. In studying these data, consider the abilities and skills each employee demonstrates, as well as her attitude toward herself and her job.

Now, to refine the needs which the data produced, a suggestion from Malcolm Knowles will help pinpoint how the educational need is defined. He states that need is defined as the gap between present level of competency and a higher level required for effective performance as defined by the individual, the organization or society. His concept is illustrated in Figure 28-2.

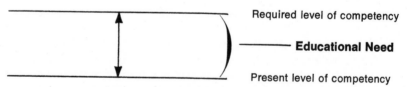

Fig. 28-2. Definition of an educational need.

In reply to the question, "How do you check it out to make sure it is real?" the issue becomes one of validating the need. Validation requires that you seek out sources of data that verify the reality and the extent of the need—it supports the fact that the gap, or educational need, exists and justifies further consideration. The best source for validation and the one most frequently overlooked is the person for whom the training is being planned—the learner. Sources such as the supervisors, administration, research studies, speakers, and consultants usually provide verification. In some instances their input is essential; however, the learner must not only be aware of the need to increase her competence, she must want to do it—for her own reasons. Therefore the learner provides one of the soundest answers to the question, "How do you check out the need to make sure it is real?"

Knowles phrases it like this:

> The more concretely an individual can identify his aspirations and assess his present level of competencies in relation to them—the more exactly he can define his educational needs—the more intensely will he be motivated to learn. And the more congruent the needs of the individual are with the aspirations of the organization . . . [and vice versa] the more likely will effective learning take place.[3]

Now for the last question: "Is it an educational need that can be met through training or development?"

Assuming that the need identified and validated is an educational need, the capabilities of the critical care unit and its staff must form the first criterion to determine whether or not the need can be met. The probability that training needs can best be met in the unit is a basic assumption. To increase the effective level of competency on the job, the reality situation offered by the unit provides the best learning laboratory. If the need is more long-range in nature, staff development may be the logical approach to meet the need. This may involve assistance outside the critical care unit.

One of the final considerations you will want to deal with is determining the priority of needs that result from your assessment. You would be wise to involve the staff in helping to establish priorities. This practice will begin to create the expectation that they share responsibility in the training and development program. Another thought to bear in mind in setting priorities is the desirability of a successful first experience. If the first need is "bite size" and chances of meeting it are very good, you probably have a winning combination to move to the next step in the process.

step 2—set individual learning objectives for performance and growth

The second step in the process model is concerned with setting goals and objectives so that the training efforts will have direction. For purposes of this model, goals will be identified as long-term and broad in scope. For instance, a goal for a training and staff development program might be stated:

> To involve each staff member in planning and implementing an inservice program for the critical care unit.

Another might be:

> To provide more effective nursing care to patients in the critical care unit by helping to increase the level of competency of each person who gives direct patient care.

Although these goals are rather explicitly stated, and in fact provide guidelines upon which to structure a training program, more specific objectives are needed to insure achievement of the goals.

These more specific learning objectives are usually stated in behavioral terms which describe outcomes or results.*

For example, these short-term objectives usually include these characteristics: they represent behaviors that are observable by others; they are specific, limited in scope, and include certain conditions, such as time and method; and they are measurable.

As an example, an objective for a learning experience designed for a new associate degree nursing graduate who has been employed as a staff nurse in a coronary care unit might be stated:

Given basic instruction on the use of monitoring equipment by the head nurse, within five days be able to prepare a patient and properly attach equipment.

As an approach to involving your staff in setting their own objectives, such questions as these may stimulate their active involvement: What would I be doing differently if I were accomplishing my goal? How might someone else know that I have changed? When will I be doing it? Where would I be doing it? What will I need to know and do to actually reach my goal? What can I do for myself? What help will I need from others? Who, specifically?

After each employee has identified her goal or goals, co-workers can review their goals with each other. With the help of feedback, each employee can clarify her goal, making it more specific, more realistic, and more observable.

In one training situation the author suggested that all the participants do a little dreaming about what they would want as a goal if they could utterly divorce themselves from reality. Each participant was encouraged to go off by herself, away from the distractions, and work on it. Most of the participants were able to do the assignment and found it a rather useful means of getting a goal initiated.

The next step suggested was that of refinement of the goal. Participants were encouraged to get together in pairs and share their goals with each other. In the process of sharing they could sharpen each other's goals by asking each other questions about them, and by trying to determine what kind of goal it was. Was it a "must" goal? Was it a "want" goal? Was it attainable? Was it an ideal goal that could never be attained, but one that set a direction for the maker? Was it a maintenance goal which merely keeps the performance on an even keel? Or was it a growth goal which partakes of the ideal and at the same time is close enough to reality to be attainable?

To get the goals broken down into workable units, or objectives, all participants were given the assignment of assembling the blocks that stood in the way of the attainment of the goal. They were also encouraged to assemble all of the assets they had going for them.

After having listed all the "blocks" and the "assets" to deal with these blocks, participants were asked to state an objective, or outcome, to deal with each block they had identified. They were asked to state the objective as simply as

---

* For a programmed instruction book on writing learning objectives, see Robert F. Mager, *Preparing Instructional Objectives* (Palo Alto, Calif.: Fearon Publishers, 1963).

possible, and in terms that could be measured when the time came to evaluate the outcomes.

While the learning experience proved to be a lot of hard work, each participant found it a useful discipline. Some considered it very difficult to develop a goal that could be broken down into objectives. But when it was finally possible to do this, the participants could see the practicality of the process. They could understand how functional objectives can be in generating action that is aimed directly at the target of the problem addressed.

The step of goal-and-objective formation is probably the most difficult of the steps, but is essential and should never be overlooked. As your staff becomes more comfortable working together in planning the initial steps which need to be taken to lay the groundwork for Step 3, goals and objectives may change. It should be remembered that this element of change is implicit when you work with the concept of process.

step 3 — plan and contract to achieve learning objectives

ACTION PLAN

In order to reach objectives, you will need to develop a strategy that will zero in on the restraining forces which slow down learning. There is a natural resistance to change, and the removal of this resistance is essential if the desired learning is to take place. Honestly acknowledging the existence of resistance to learning and accepting it as a normal phenomenon will remove some of the resistance. This strategy helps the learner identify the reasons for resisting, and this awareness makes it easier to move toward building on the assets, abilities, and strengths that will support learning. Encourage the learner to specifically identify the resources she can use or request that will help overcome the blocks to learning, and free her energy to accomplish her own goal. Help identify the driving forces — those things that tend to propel her into action and move her toward the learning goal. These forces provide the motivation. When she capitalizes on these and applies her personal resources to offset the resistance to learn, she is ready to develop a plan for determining responsibilities others share in supporting the goal achievement. Work with her in assigning specific responsibilities to yourself and to other resources. Help her clarify her self-assignment of responsibilities. In each instance, encourage her to identify the specific contribution each person is expected to make in her learning plan.

CONTRACT

One of the most helpful elements of collaborative plans for achieving learning goals is the concept of a contract or working agreement among those involved. The contract is not of a formal nature. It evolves as you, your staff, and individuals openly discuss expectations of each other in terms of what needs to be done to achieve learning. For instance, in discussing the assignment of responsibilities, the dialogue clarifies what is needed and why a particular resource seems most relevant. At this point, agreement to accept the responsibility is sought from the resource person. As a part of clarifying the assignment, the persons involved need to discuss reasonable checkpoints and set deadlines. This practice provides specific data for mutually shared expectations. As you can see, the agreement takes on the overtones of a contract to which you, the staff, and individuals are committed. This agreement provides the mechanism that anyone who is involved in the work of achieving learning can use to check the progress that is being made and the status of assignments, identify problems encountered, renegotiate the agreement, and deal with other matters that center around the achievement of learning objectives.

If you keep in mind the development of a strategy that will help adult learners understand and accept the tension between their desire to grow and their desire to remain the same, you will help them move through the process of unlearning, learning, and relearning.

Adults resist unlearning things which have worked for them in the past, or seemed to be adequate in most situations. In the process of really giving up familiar ways of responding to situations, adults accept the necessity of learning new ways that increase competence. However, learning is not enough; adults need to internalize the learning—make it a regular part of their behavior. Thus they need the opportunity and time to relearn or "refreeze" the new learning so that it becomes their typical response to a situation.

RISKS AND PAYOFFS

One of the basic factors in the learning process is the power and influence of risks learners take and the payoffs they receive. Since learning imposes change, you will want to make sure that the risk the learner takes is a moderate one. Moderate risks result in a fair degree of safety and a good chance for success. Knowing the degree of risk they are taking enables adult learners to accept responsibility for learning. Equally important to adult learners are the payoffs in store for them. Frequently these payoffs are taken for granted, but you will want to plan very carefully for genuine payoffs for learners. An open discussion of "both sides of the coin" of the learning experience—the risks and the payoffs—will make it much easier for learners to buy into a learning experience and for you and the co-workers to give support during the learning process. Learners will have a gauge by which they can anticipate the results of changed behavior as they strive for increased competency or self-fulfillment.

One further point: adults want immediate payoffs in return for learning. They want to be able to use the learning *now*, not at some future time. Being able to use the learning effectively and feeling competent in using it is probably the most valued payoff. Coupling this with your recognition of effective performance doubles the payoff.

step 4 — select resources

After the action plan has been developed, and even as it is taking shape, the identification of appropriate learning resources follows. You will want to look for situations, people, and materials that will enhance learning opportunities.

Situations offer unique resources. For example:

1. *Participative learning as a resource.* Unstructured learning groups provide rich resource material for learning about "people things." Task groups are useful for integrating theory inputs into operational objectives.

2. *The learner as a resource for planning and implementing programs.* The creative and practical forces generated by employees who accept the role of learner release resources that can only be obtained from such involvement.

3. *Daily living experiences as a resource for learning.* When employees accept role playing and role training as a way of improving their competency, daily happenings in the unit provide the content for the learning situations. These offer a rare potential for reality-checking attitudes, values, and habitual responses to situations and afford the opportunity to try on different behaviors. This enables employees to expand their behavioral repertoire of meeting common experiences. As resources, these are among the most stimulating and exciting.

4. *Spontaneity as a resource in learning.* When spontaneity is present, learning is precious, stimulating, and fun. The problem becomes one of how to develop spontaneity, how to make room for it, and how to capitalize on it. Spontaneity develops in a supportive, nonevaluative climate. The norms which govern behavior in the critical care unit hold the potential of inhibiting the development of spontaneity.

5. *Conflict as a resource for learning.* From genuine differences in values, expectations, techniques, roles, priorities, comes the grist for conflict. Working through these differences to resolve the conflict provides another viable resource for learning. Here again the issue is how to develop a climate in which people can learn from conflict; to create a norm where conflict is legitimatized or sanctioned; to set ground rules so that the conflict can be resolved. Probably one of the most effective resources for learning is found in the differentness that can openly be dealt with.

6. *Failure as a resource for learning.* If the staff within the unit can lower the sensitivity, or help desensitize, so that persons who believe they have failed can learn from the experience, failure can become a motivational force to learn new ways of handling situations or performing certain procedures. Role training is helpful in assisting learners to find new ways of approaching the problem. Using an approach of "how would you do it differently" may help learners develop spontaneous responses which they can capitalize on later.

RESOURCE PEOPLE

Selecting competent resource people requires careful planning. Criteria for this selection are threefold: (1) Consider the resource person's ability to adapt his professional knowledge and expertise to "layman-type listeners." This ability is essential if the resource person is to be understood and his expertise utilized. (2) Consider his ability to adapt his "expertise" to your objectives. Unless the resource person has been given a well-developed set of objectives for his appearance, he will need to fall back on his own experience and perception of what your staff needs to know. This may subvert the achieving of your learning objectives. (3) Consider his ability to listen to and respect the knowledge and experience your staff members bring to the session. The assessment of this quality places a special responsibility on you. If the resource person believes in the competence and effectiveness of your unit and communicates his respect for you and your staff, and builds on this, he will be an acceptable resource.

Organizing the inservice program will mean carefully preparing resource people and employees to work together in the learning activities. Resource people will need well-prepared answers to questions like these: Why me? How do I fit in with your overall inservice training? What do you want from me? What are the people like that you want me to work with? What will they want to know? What do you expect to happen when it's over?

These, or similar questions, need to be answered for staff members involved in the inservice and staff development program. They, too, provide a reservoir of resources that needs to be tapped. To tap such resources, however, your people will need to know honestly what is in it for them. In other words, what's the payoff? If they can see a payoff, they will be motivated to learn and to become involved and to accept the change that learning creates and demands.

MATERIALS

With the help of your inservice educator and learning laboratories in schools of nursing which may be in your vicinity, you can locate excellent materials to use in group sessions for your staff; materials for individuals to work through on their own, such as programmed instruction units; reading materials for personal reading or group discussions.

In summary, select the resource for achieving specific learning objectives, and keep in mind the work situation, the timing, and the learners. Accommodating all of these elements becomes an art, so allow yourself time to develop this particular ability.

step 5—manage learning activities

Once the potential resources have been selected, the next step in the process model is managing the learning activities in such a way that learning objectives and unit objectives are achieved. To gear learning to the work cycle in a practical and realistic manner demands sheer artistry in juggling the components that shape a satisfactory learning experience. These components include time, place, material, equipment, situations, and human resources. You may have to settle for something less than the ideal educational setting and schedule learning in conjunction with work in progress. As these functions become more complementary, you will use less time and energy in their integration.

READINESS OF THE LEARNER

To manage opportunities for individual learning, you will need to be thoroughly familiar with the level of performance of all members of your staff. In addition, you will need to be aware of the explicit learning objectives which will lead to their increased competency on the job. Their readiness to learn is important. Recognizing this, you will need to schedule training for a specific time, or rely on the possibility that training can be done in the process of the day's activities on an unscheduled basis. Here again you can manage through specific teaching assignments, and the use of a variety of techniques, if you choose. Your responsibility is really to see that training happens when the learner is prepared and ready to learn, and that appropriate techniques have been used.

You will need to provide periods of time for learning which are long enough to capitalize on the learning potential of the employees. Consider the fact that each time the learners experience a new behavior they are in effect relearning it in each new situation. Becoming aware of this fact will help you taper off any coaching or special attention when it becomes evident that the new behavior has been well integrated into performance.

SITUATION

When you tune in to the daily experiences within the critical care unit which offer content for learning, your readiness and spontaneity facilitate learning. Getting people together and orienting them to the situation and content to be presented require presence of mind and quick action. At first this practice will be awkward, but as your staff becomes comfortable with it, such cooperative effort can be directed or suggested by any person. Being sensitive to feedback (which comes in the employee's verbal and nonverbal response to the learning situation) allows you to adjust your teaching as the activity progresses. This flexibility in your style of managing the situation and yourself will increase the potential for learning.

CONTENT

Handling content can pose problems for the instructor. Several cautions in managing content may save time and effort. So often the tendency is to tell the learners what you want them to know and rarely to take time to find out what they already know—or even need to know. The usual response of the learners in this situation is mixed; they feel put down by the instructor, or are bored and tune out the instructor, so that the possibility of missing important information is real. A guideline might be to take time to find out "who knows what" and build from there.

When you need to provide a considerable amount of information or content, organize it into a sequence of segments that can be grasped by the learner. An overload of information with little or no breathing space between inputs discourages the adult learner. When extensive content in a particular sequence is indicated, look at the potential resources within your staff. If sharing responsibilities for training is expected on the part of the employees, they can prepare specific content in collaboration with you. In this way you can decrease your responsibility and increase the versatility of your unit's resources. This approach to managing content will give you more time to manage the overall critical care unit and direct the resources toward both unit goals and growth goals of individuals.

HUMAN RESOURCES

This subject is covered rather extensively in Step 4. However, a point that bears repeating is this: Take time to carefully prepare your resources—outside resources, hospital resources, staff resources, as well as yourself. Check out the guidelines suggested in Step 4.

A great deal of the success and effectiveness of the resource person depends on how you have managed the scheduling, the goals for the event, the information announcing the session, the rationale for the content and method of presentation, the plan to involve the learners, the preparation of the learners, and the setting in which the session is to be held.

Attention to these details creates a climate which supports the teaching-learning activities and those actively involved in them.

PLACE, MATERIAL, AND EQUIPMENT

One asset not to be overlooked is the dual function of the critical care unit. It serves as a treatment area and as a learning area. This fact simplifies your management problem of providing an educational facility. The standard equipment and materials used in the unit serve the needs of both patient and employee-learner. As you begin to blend the service of nursing care to patients with on-the-spot teaching, you will develop a keen appreciation of the versatility, efficiency and capacity of the critical care unit.

step 6—evaluate objectives, performance and learning plan

The next step is to evaluate the learning which in effect means measuring the degree of change in the performance of persons who have been involved in the training activities; it also means measuring the degree to which the learner's own objectives have been achieved. These changes may be observed in terms of overt behavior. Your guided observation over a period of time will result in the evaluation of the employee's ability to integrate the new learning into the performance of the job.

Another form of evaluating learning is open staff meetings. This allows the staff to give feedback on the significance of the learning opportunity and how they have been able to utilize what they learned. In this process, evaluation of the effectiveness of how the staff functions can be made. Successes, failures, conflicts, creative solutions—all these data are part of the evaluation process

and contribute information essential to developing objectives for the next sequence of training activities.

Another facet of evaluation is determining the adequacy of the objectives.
After evaluating the degree to which they were achieved, some objectives may
need to be modified, others have to be phased out because they have been
met, and new ones have to be developed. Still others must be discontinued because they were unrealistic or the situation had changed.

The action plan will need to be evaluated. How effectively the learning
forces were identified and handled will be the focus of this evaluation. The
resources used by the learner will be evaluated in terms of how effectively
they overcame the blocks to learning. The working agreement and deadlines
will be reviewed in terms of how they contributed to the accomplishment of
the learning objectives.

How well the learning activities were organized in terms of the working situation, the readiness of the learners, the preparation of the resource people
or materials, and the timing will be grist for the evaluation mill.

Perhaps the most difficult aspects to measure will be the results. If you can
gather data that will support such long-term results as lower turnover, effective patient care on a cost basis, a high level of staff competence based on specific learning activities, you will be a winner. To facilitate the gathering of
these data, use resources such as the hospital's personnel director, inservice
educator, and cost accountant. There may also be a researcher on the hospital
staff that could help you design such an evaluation tool. Local colleges and
universities will have resource people who could help design such an evaluation.

Use feedback from everyone involved in the learning activities. Data from
these sources of information will provide viable information to use in moving
into the recycling process, which is Step 7.

step 7—recycle

This last step requires us to start all over again. Based on the validation of
new needs or unmet needs which emerge from the evaluation process, and
from changes which have evolved during the intervening time, recycling inservice in the critical care unit begins.

All of these steps in the process model involve other people. In the final
analysis, the process model is also a participative model as you have discovered
by now.

conclusion

After reading this chapter, and reflecting on how adults learn to cope with
significant changes in their professional and personal lives,

GO!

GROW!

LIVE TO LEARN!

LEARN TO LIVE!

COLLECT THE PAYOFFS FOR LEARNING!

REFERENCES

1. Toni Powell and George F. Aker, "Teaching and Learning in Adult Basic Education," unpublished paper, Department of Adult Education, Florida State University, Tallahassee, Florida, 1971.
2. *Ibid.*
3. Malcolm Knowles, *The Modern Practice of Adult Education* (New York: Association Press, 1970).

BIBLIOGRAPHY

Argyris, C., and D. A. Schon, *Theory in Practice: Increasing Professional Effectiveness* (San Francisco: Jossey-Bass Publishers, 1975).

————, *Integrating the Individual and the Organization* (New York: John Wiley & Sons, 1964).

————, *Interpersonal Competence and Organizational Effectiveness* (Homewood, Ill.: Dorsey Press, 1962).

Blansfield, M. G., and R. Ayers, *The Professional Nurse Looks at Appraisal of Personnel* (Washington, D.C.: Leadership Resources, 1966).

Byrne, M. S., "The Clinical Specialist: Her Role in Staff Development," *Staff Development* (Wakefield, Mass.: Contemporary Publishing, 1975).

Herzberg, F., "One More Time: How Do You Motivate Employees?" *Harvard Business Review* (January-February 1968).

Kindall, A. F. and J. Gatza, "Positive Performance Evaluation," *Harvard Business Review* (November-December 1963).

Knowles, M., *The Modern Practice of Adult Education* (New York: Association Press, 1970).

————, *Self-Directed Learning: A Guide for Learners and Teachers* (New York: Association Press, 1975).

————, and R. Ayers, *The Professional Nurse Looks at the Learning Climate* (Washington, D.C.: Leadership Resources, 1966).

Levinson, H., "Management by Whose Objectives?" *Harvard Business Review* (July-August 1970).

Likert, R., *New Patterns of Management* (New York: McGraw-Hill Book Company, 1961).

Mager, R., *Preparing Instruction Objectives* (Palo Alto: Fearon Publishers, 1963).

McGregor, D., *The Human Side of Enterprise* (New York: McGraw-Hill Book Company, 1960).

Medearis, D. W., and N. D. Medearis, "The Uniqueness of the Adult Learner," *AORN Journal* (April 1975).

Medearis, N. D., "Training Your Staff Effectively," *Nursing '74* (March 1974).

————, and E. S. Popiel, "Gudelines for Organizing Inservice Education," *Journal of Nursing Administration* (July-August 1971).

Miles, M. B., *Learning to Work in Groups* (New York: Teachers College Press, 1959).

Morton, R. B., "Straight from the Shoulder—Leveling with Others on the Job," *Personnel Magazine* (November-December 1966).

Powell, T., and G. F. Aker, "Teaching and Learning in Adult Basic Education," unpublished paper, Department of Adult Education, Florida State University, Tallahassee, Florida, 1971.

Rogers, C. R., "Personal Thoughts on Teaching and Learning," *Improving College and University Teaching, National Journal* (Eugene, Ore.: Graduate School of Oregon State University, 1958).

Warr, P. (ed.), *Personal Goals and Work Design* (New York: John Wiley & Sons, 1976).

VIRGINIA S. PAULSON
EXECUTIVE DIRECTOR OF
COLORADO NURSES' ASSOCIATION

29 29

legal responsibilities of the nurse in a critical care unit

The legal responsibility of the registered nurse in the critical care unit does not differ from the legal responsibility of the registered nurse in any work setting. Five principles to which the registered nurse adheres for the protection of both patient and practitioner are:

1. A registered nurse performs only those functions for which she has been prepared by education and experience.
2. A registered nurse performs these functions competently.
3. A registered nurse delegates responsibility only to personnel whose competence has been evaluated and found acceptable.
4. A registered nurse takes appropriate measures as indicated by her observation of the patient.
5. A registered nurse is familiar with policies of the employing agency governing nursing functions, and practices within these policies.

Nurses need particularly to be reminded that they can be as liable when they fail to take necessary action as when they act in a negligent manner. There have been numerous cases in which a nurse has been held liable for inaction. This is especially true when a nurse fails to act appropriately based on her observation of the patient. A typical situation might involve a patient with recognizable signs of acute cardiac embarrassment which the nurse fails to call to the immediate attention of a physician.

Nurses can be found liable of *misfeasance, malfeasance,* and *nonfeasance.* These terms will be considered in relation to the administration of medications so that they may be more understandable.

Misfeasance is an act which is lawful in itself, but which results in injury to the patient. Thus a nurse may be legally administering sulfisoxazole under the written orders of a licensed physician, but may fail to recognize signs of toxic reaction. If she continues to give the drug until the patient sustains kidney damage, this would constitute misfeasance.

Malfeasance is the doing of an act which should not be done. For example, if a patient's chart indicates that this patient is allergic to penicillin, and a physican is informed over the telephone that the patient has symptoms of a postoperative infection, the physician may order a medication containing penicillin. If the nurse proceeds to give the medication, this action on the part of the nurse would constitute malfeasance.

Nonfeasance is the failure to do something which ought to be done. Thus if a medication vital to the patient's survival is not administered by the nurse, the nurse is liable for nonfeasance.

There are six ways in which functions once the exclusive prerogative of the medical profession become an accepted part of nursing practice. Frequently, procedures are absorbed by nursing when the physician finds them repetitive and time-consuming. When this occurs simultaneously throughout the community, it has become "standard practice in the community." Opinions of the state board of nursing or state board of medical examiners stating that there is no violation of either practice act can expand nursing responsibilities. Joint practice statements mutually arrived at by representatives of the medical society and nursing association, and ratified by their respective boards, become the standard unless challenged legally. A legal opinion of the attorney general on a specific practice can determine the legality of the act; and statements of the professional nursing association will resolve whether or not specific practices fall within the purview of nursing practice. Of the four ways mentioned thus far, all are subject to reversal in a court of law. The fifth method would be legislative action amending the medical practice act to permit other categories of practitioners to perform functions which only physicians are entitled by law to perform.

During the 1970s many state licensure laws regulating nursing have been revised. These new practice acts generally enhance the role of nursing by specifically defining such terms as "case finding," "diagnosing" and "nursing regimen."

The law covering extreme emergencies is broad in its protection of the nurse when there is no physician present to make judgmental decisions. If the nurse believes the situation critical enough to call for immediate action on her part, she should take the following steps: (1) evaluate the relative hazards of action and inaction, and (2) determine whether there is a reasonable chance of success.

If the hazard of inaction is greater than that of action, and if there appears to be a reasonable chance of success, the nurse should not hesitate to act for fear of possible legal implications.

All nurses should carry malpractice insurance. There seems to be a common misunderstanding that the employer, rather than the nurse, would be liable. It is true that a joint suit might be filed naming both the employer and the nurse as defendants; however, the fact remains that the nurse as a professional practitioner is responsible, at all times, for her acts in relation to other people. However, nursing malpractice insurance does not cover the nurse if she is performing functions which only a physician is licensed to perform.

The pitfall the nurse must assiduously avoid is to be pressured into performing functions for which she feels herself unqualified. The nurse must have the courage and integrity not to permit herself to be stampeded into unwise acts as a matter of expediency. The nurse's primary concern must always be the life of the patient.

index